Handbook
of
Sensory Physiology

Volume VII/6B

KV-177-772

Comparative Physiology and Evolution of Vision in Invertebrates

B:
Invertebrate Visual Centers and Behavior I

By

M.F. Land   S.B. Laughlin   D.R. Nässel
N.J. Strausfeld   T.H. Waterman

Edited by

H. Autrum

With 319 Figures

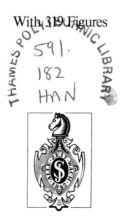

Springer-Verlag Berlin Heidelberg New York 1981

Hansjochem Autrum

Zoologisches Institut der Universität, Luisenstr. 14, D-8000 München

ISBN 3-540-08703-6 Springer-Verlag Berlin · Heidelberg · New York
ISBN 0-387-08703-6 Springer-Verlag New York · Heidelberg · Berlin

Library of Congress Cataloging in Publication Data
Main entry under title: Comparative physiology and evolution of vision in invertebrates.
(Handbook of sensory physiology; v. 7/6A-) Bibliography: p. Includes indexes.
Contents: A. Invertebrate photoreceptors. — B. Invertebrate visual centers and behavior I. 1. Vision. 2. Invertebrates — Physiology.
3. Physiology, Comparative. I. Autrum, Hansjochem. II. Series [DNLM: 1. Evolution. 2. Invertebrates — Physiology. 3. Vision —
Physiology. WL700 H236 v. 7 pt. 6].
QP351.H34 vol. 7/6A, etc. [QP475] 591.1'82₆ 78 21470 ISBN 0-387-08837-7 (v. A) [592'.01823]

Printed in Germany
Typesetting, printing and binding: Brühlsche Universitätsdruckerei Giessen
2122/3130-543210

Preface

Morphology and physiology are two fields which cannot be separated. This statement needs to be amplified: purely factual results of a morphological or physiological nature only have real value when they are gained in the context of certain guiding, embracing questions. By themselves they are mostly of little value, because only a guiding hypothesis or theory is of any importance. Equally, a physiological question will always raise questions as to the morphological substrate, and vice versa. Thus, Wiedemann's discovery, for instance, that the visual cells in each ommatidium of the dipterans have differing fields of vision has revived the question as to what the optical properties of individual visual cells, and the complete ommatidium, might be and how neighboring ommatidia interact. These questions in turn led to that of the morphological, neuronal wiring diagram of the visual cells in the optical ganglia. Within the realm of invertebrates, the morphological and physiological problems of visual perception have been resolved in very different ways on various levels, from the photo-receptor to higher centers; despite many investigations, however, there remain unsolved problems.

The first chapter of Vol. VII/6B deals with the neuroarchitecture in the visual system of two groups: crustaceans and insects. These systems are best known through recent investigations. The second chapter is devoted to the neural principles in the visual system of insects. It could not have been written without parallel research into morphology. The same is true for the third chapter: Polarized light sensitivity, discovered by Karl von Frisch in 1948, is more widespread in invertebrates and vertebrates than had until recently been supposed. It raises questions of anatomy, molecular biology, neuronal processing and behavior. While the first two chapters are confined to arthropods as the best-researched illustrative examples, the third and fourth chapters give a comprehensive overview over polarized light sensitivity and the optics of vision in all groups of invertebrates. In this last chapter particular emphasis is laid on the enormous diversity of the kinds of eyes which is a reflection partly of the different evolutionary history and partly of the different visual needs of the animals that bear them.

The following volume, VII/6C, will treat the general question of visual adaptation, followed by a discussion of that diverse group of molluscs in which a great variety of very different visual organs is to be encountered – from the most primitive to the most highly complex. Volume VII/6C will also treat in detail the morphology and physiology of the ocelli, which do indeed correspond in several basic principles to other arthropod eyes (see Chap. 2 of this volume), but which at the same time display a number of pecularities, both in their morphology and their physiology. Finally, the last chapter of Vol. VII/6C will treat the behavioral aspects of spatial vision in arthropods. In all of these chapters one is reminded of the various levels of sensual physiology:

1) The properties of the individual neuronal elements – their mode of functioning and their signals;
2) The individual mechanisms for the processing and summation of signals;
3) The gradual metamorphosis of signal patterns in the neuronal system; and
4) The result of these metamorphoses, i.e., behavior. Chapter 4 of Vol. VII/6C, "Pattern Recognition," is given over to this very topic.

Many problems have still to be solved. It is one of the aims of this book to point up those unsolved problems, encountered in innumerable individual papers and books, without the reader's having to work arduously through the original texts themselves. By gathering, sifting, and critically evaluating under one cover the details of research otherwise scattered over a wide literature, this book will prove itself a basis for new discoveries.

The editor would like to express his gratitude to Springer-Verlag for accepting "Vision of Invertebrates" in three volumes for publication in the handbook. That completeness of presentation cannot be achieved and, indeed, has not been sought is already stated in the preface to Vol. 1: "The purpose of this handbook is not encyclopedic completeness, nor the sort of brief summaries provided by periodic annual reviews."

Munich   H. AUTRUM

Contents

List of Contributors

LAND, M. F., Biology Building, School of Biological Sciences, University of Sussex, Brighton, Sussex BN1 9QG, Great Britain

LAUGHLIN, S. B., Department of Neurobiology, Research School of Biological Sciences, Australian National University, P. O. Box 475, Canberra, A.C.T. 2600, Australia

NÄSSEL, D. R., Europäisches Laboratorium für Molekularbiologie, Meyerhof-straße 1, D-6900 Heidelberg

STRAUSFELD, N. J., Europäisches Laboratorium für Molekularbiologie, Meyerhof-straße 1, D-6900 Heidelberg

WATERMAN, T. H., Kline Biology Tower, Department of Biology, Yale University, New Haven, Connecticut 06520, USA

Chapter 1

Neuroarchitectures Serving Compound Eyes
of Crustacea and Insects

N. J. STRAUSFELD and D. R. NÄSSEL, Heidelberg, Germany

With 70 Figures

Contents

A. Summary

The purpose of this account is to summarize the basic principles of nerve cell organization in crustacean and insect optic lobes. In recent years a number of publications have dealt with this subject, and the amount of information available is large. However, for the sake of simplicity we have emphasized mainly two species, the crayfish and the fly, to actually illustrate generalizations about structural organization.

The present chapter is divided into two parts, one dealing with Crustacea and the other with insects. The first describes the basic arrangements of single nerve cells in the three main synaptic regions (the lamina, medulla, and lobula complex) and illustrates how parallel channels from the lobes converge to relatively few neurons that descend from the brain to the ventral cord. In addition, the organization of lamina neurons is described for a number of Crustacea to illustrate species-specific differences of cell relationships on the one hand and, on the other, to illustrate that a limited number of neuron types are involved in specific geometries.

Most of our knowledge about the synaptology of optic lobes is derived from Golgi-electron microscopy studies of the crayfish lamina and the lamina of the house fly, *Musca domestica*. The second part (Sect. C) begins by describing all that is presently known about the fly lamina, in terms of structure, and serves as a useful comparison with that of the crayfish, representing Crustacea, and some other species of insects. The synaptology and cell arrangements of the fly lamina are discussed with reference to the most recent studies by other workers on the laminas of Hymenoptera, Odonata, and Hemiptera.

When seen in its entirety the structure of even a simple synaptic region appears to be highly complex, even though it comprises rather few cell types. This is clearly illustrated by the fly lamina where only 13 types of nerve cell contribute to each retinotopic channel. In deeper levels of the system 40 or more species of nerve cell may contribute elements to a single retinotopic column, and we may expect a corresponding increase in the number and combinations of functional connexions. The prospect of analysing these by combinations of stochastic impregnation (the Golgi method) and electron microscopy is daunting.

In order to start sorting out some basic patterns of connexions we need to perceive neural arrangements in a way that allows a step-for-step analysis. This can be achieved by means of cobalt impregnation methods that resolve entire populations of neurons. Seen in this way, the structure of the optic lobes begins to look far simpler than has been previously imagined. These features are described in the remaining parts of Sect. C and are drawn almost exclusively from cobalt studies of *Calliphora erythrocephala*. They outline how single nerve cell populations contribute to simple arrangements of parallel retinotopic pathways and how these are sorted out to specific regions of the lateral midbrain and thence to descending pathways. In addition, cobalt studies reveal features of organization that have been refractory to other methods. These include the resolution of local cell populations, or local gradients of structure that subserve characteristic regions of the retina, and forms of neurons that are typical of one or the other sex.

Most of the present account is derived from original observations. However, we would like to thank at its outset several colleagues who have contributed data, some of it published here for the first time. In particular, we acknowledge major contributions by J.A.CAMPOS-ORTEGA to studies of the lamina's synaptology; several of the illustrations are from joint studies by him and one of us (N.J.S.) and are hitherto unpublished. We would also like to thank H.SCHIFF-SERTORIO for cooperation on a joint project in 1973 studying the visual system of *Squilla mantis*. The present Golgi studies on *Squilla* are derived from this project , and the projection patterns of *Squilla* receptors are from her reduced-silver preparations.

Drs. W.RIBI, K.WOLBURG-BUCHHOLZ, and P.OHLY kindly provided material or gave permission to reproduce material from their studies as did Prof. H.F.ROWELL and Dr. J. BACON. Illustrations of procion yellow-stained nerve cells were derived from Dr. K.HAUSEN's investigations of motion-sensitive neurons in the optic lobes of *Calliphora*. We are grateful for his permission to use these and to adapt the summary diagram presented in his thesis account.

B. Neural Arrangements in Crustacean Visual System

I. Introduction

This review restricts discussion to those neuropils that subserve the lateral compound eyes and will ignore other photosensory systems such as, for example, the nauplius eye. All orders of Crustacea except Copepoda and Cirripedia possess compound eyes (though the cirriped *Cypris* larvae have simple compound eyes), but of these only a limited number have been studied with respect to the neural organization of the optic lobes. The following decapods deserve special mention: the lobster *Homarus* (Hámori and Horridge, 1966a, b); the shrimp *Pandalus* (Nässel, 1975, 1976a); the crayfishes *Procambarus* (Shivers, 1967; Hafner, 1973, 1974; Hafner and Tokarski, 1978), *Pacifastacus, Astacus*, and *Orconectes* (Nässel, 1976a, 1977a, b ; Nässel and Waterman, 1977; Nässel, in preparation); the crabs *Leptograpsus* and *Scylla* (Stowe, 1977; Stowe et al., 1977), *Ocypode* (Nässel, 1977b) and *Pachygrapsus* (Hanström, 1924); and the anomuran *Emerita* (Hanström, 1924).

Some non-decapod crustaceans have also been studied, three of which are malacostracans: the mysid shrimp *Neomysis* (Nässel, 1977b), the euphausiacean *Meganyctiphanes* (Nässel, 1977b) and the stomatopod *Squilla* (Schiff-Sertorio and Strausfeld, unpubl.). Hanström (1928) further studied malacostracans, representing the orders Isopoda and Amphipoda but, characteristically, these works are not detailed and, from current observations, appear to be unreliable. These are not treated in the present account.

Non-malacostracans studied include the anostracan, *Artemia* (Hanström, 1924; Nässel et al., 1978) and the cladoceran, *Daphnia* (Retzius, 1906; Leder, 1915; Wolff and Güldner, 1970; Macagno et al., 1973; Macagno and Levinthal, 1975; Macagno, 1978; Nässel et al., 1978).

In contrast, retinal morphology (that is, the structure of the ommatidia and the dioptric apparatuses) has been studied in numerous crustacean species representing most groups and revealing a vast variety of eye organization. The reader is referred to a few contributions containing bibliographies that probably cover the entire literature (Bullock and Horridge, 1965; Ball, 1977; Hallberg, 1977; Nilsson, 1978; Andersson et al., 1978; Meyer-Rochow, 1978a, b; Land et al., 1979 and this volume).

Of the crustaceans the crayfish will be described in most detail and serve as a paradigm with which other groups will be compared. We have adopted a simple and, we hope, logical format which is to start with the retina and work through the optic lobes as they are located. Very few physiological or behavioural experiments have been performed on crustaceans that can be related to the anatomical descriptions in this account, and only where there is anatomical relevance will there be reference to such work. It is to be hoped that in the future there will be further attempts to bridge the existing gap between anatomy on the one hand and physiological and visual behaviour studies on the other.

II. The Crayfish Visual System

1. Plan of the Crayfish Visual System and Terminology

The eyestalks of the crayfish contain three successive columnar neuropil regions underlying the compound retina and which are connected by crossed projections of retinotopic fibres, i.e., the first and second optic chiasmata (Figs. 1 and 2; cf. also Fig. 18). Central to these columnar neuropils lie lateral portions of the protocerebrum which are drawn out into the eyestalks. These are connected to cerebral centers by the so-called optic nerve.

In insects the three columnar neuropils are referred to as the lamina, medulla, and lobula complex. However, classically, the analogous structures were named "lamina ganglionaris," "medulla externa," and "medulla interna," respectively (HANSTRÖM, 1928). Recent studies of the crayfish visual system showed that the analogy between these neuropils in the crayfish and insects is so clear that it was felt a radical change in the terminology for the crayfish and other crustacea was justified (NÄSSEL, in preparation). Thus, the insect terminology is simply applied here to crustacea. It is hoped that this will be common usage in the future.

Furthermore, the term medulla terminalis will be avoided and replaced by lateral protocerebrum or by appropriate terms for neuropil regions or glomeruli in this lateral region of the brain. This is called for because the lateral protocerebrum comprises a conglomerate of delineated neuropil regions that serve not only vision but also several other modalities. Amongst the visual regions there are at least four fourth-order visual neuropils which by analogy with insects are termed optic foci. The term optic nerve will still be used even though it is not fully appropriate considering that it also refers to chemosensory, mechanosensory, motor and multimodal neurons (BULLOCK and HORRIDGE, 1965; WIERSMA and YAMAGUCHI, 1966). Its actual structure is a compound one, consisting of several fibre bundles that project from the lateral brain into its most central regions.

The three neuropils – lamina, medulla, and lobula – will be described in some detail in the following sections, with emphasis on the columnar and stratified arrangements of neurons. As in insects, photoreceptor axons are "implicator elements" of retinotopic columns in the lamina and in the medulla. Associated through-going columnar relay neurons connect the three neuropils and relay the retinotopic mosaic through the medulla into the lobula. Superimposed on the columnar mosaic are also relay neurons whose spacing is in proportion to the columns, but which do not occur in every column. Others, such as anaxonal (amacrine) or tangential relay neurons, contribute to planar networks across the columnar mosaic. The stratification of the neuropil is derived from relay neuron terminals, as well as from their collaterals and dendrites, and from amacrine and tangential cells. This general feature of structural organization in retinotopic neuropil applies also to the insects (see Sect. C).

Finally, the retinotopic mosaic is projected onto the dendrites in higher order neuropil of the optic foci (Fig. 1) where small groups (or unique) higher order interneurons (possibly analogous to the descending neurons of insects) derive a structurally summed input from a specific population of lobula relay neurons

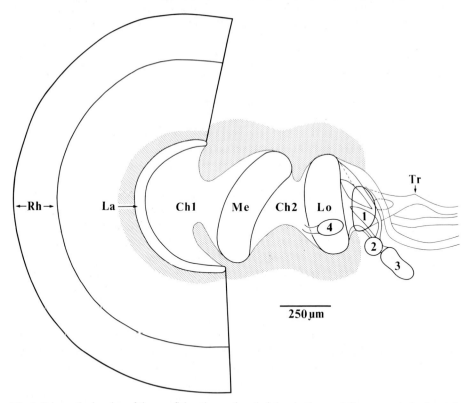

Fig. 1. Schematic drawing of the crayfish retina and optic lobes in the eyestalk, as seen in horizontal cross-section. The receptor layer of rhabdoms (*Rh*) is shown to the left. The dioptric elements of the ommatidia reside external to this layer. The eyestalk contains three columnar neuropils: the lamina *(La)*, the medulla *(Me)*, and the lobula *(Lo)*. Between these the axons form chiasmata which reverse and then re-reverse the anteroposterior order of the retinal mosaic (*Ch 1* and *Ch 2*). At least four neuropil regions are recognized *(1–4)* as receiving axons from the ipsilateral columnar neuropils. These are termed the *optic foci*. Tracts of axons derived from the lobula and these foci *(Tr)* project centrally. The cell body regions are shaded light grey

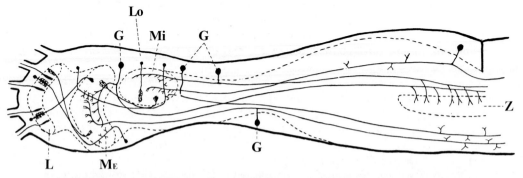

Fig. 2. Horizontal section through the protocerebrum of the isopod crustacean *Ligydia occidentalis* with some of its "main neuron tracts." *L*, lamina; *ME*, medulla; *Mi*, lobula. Large axons *(G)* project to protocerebrum and to contralateral optic lobes. *Z*, central body. After HANSTRÖM (1924) in HANSTRÖM (1928); the illustration shows a level of resolution typical of HANSTRÖM's neuroanatomical descriptions

prior to their entry into the optic nerve. The cerebral visual centres have not been adequately studied anatomically; nor have neurons that descend down the circum-oesophageal commissures to thoracic ganglia. These are omitted from the present account.

2. The Crayfish Retina

The compound retina of the crayfish consists of between 2,000 and 3,000 ommatidia (PARKER, 1897). Our present knowledge of the anatomy of the ommatidial and retinal arrangements is based on descriptions by PARKER (1897), EGUCHI (1965), KREBS (1972), and NÄSSEL (1976a).

Each ommatidium consists of a corneal lens, a crystalline cone, a crystalline tract and eight receptor cells forming a microvillar rhabdom. Two types of pigment cells screen each ommatidium, one type distally and another proximally. The latter type contains a reflecting pigment. In addition, seven of the receptor cells of the ommatidium contain screening pigment granula.

The positions of these pigments (BERNHARDS, 1916; PARKER, 1932; KLEINHOLZ, 1961), in light- and dark-adapted states, allow different acceptance angles for the individual receptors. In the light-adapted state the acceptance angle is $4° \pm 2°$ and in the dark-adapted, $24° \pm 8°$ (WALCOTT, 1974). Light entering several facets can reach one individual receptor in the light-adapted state (SHAW, 1969), and this is accentuated in the dark-adapted state (WALCOTT, 1974). Classically, the crayfish compound eye is referred to as a superposition type of eye (EXNER, 1891).

Two main classes of photoreceptors can be distinguished. The receptors R 1–R 7 constitute the first class and form the large proximal rhabdom which is spindle-shaped and has orthogonal layers of microvilli. The other class comprises the R 8 cells. Each of these forms a small separate rhabdomere with horizontal microvilli situated distally in the ommatidium (NÄSSEL, 1976a; see also WATERMAN, 1977; HAFNER and TOKARSKI, 1978).

Cobalt and Golgi studies of R 1–R 8 receptor axons show that axons from R 1–R 7 terminate in the lamina's plexiform layer, whereas R 8 axons terminate in the medulla, further suggesting that the two morphological types represent two functional classes of receptors. The R 1–R 7 cells can be divided into two subclasses on the basis of their microvillar orientations. Those of R 1, R 2, R 5, and R 6 are oriented vertically, while those of R 3, R 4, and R 7 form horizontally arranged microvilli (numbering according to PARKER, 1897).

RUTHERFORD and HORRIDGE (1965) suggested that the two microvilli directions found in the lobster rhabdom comprise a mechanism for two-channel e-vector analysis (see also EGUCHI and WATERMAN, 1966). A differential sensitivity of retinular cells to the e-vector of polarized light was demonstrated by SHAW (1966, 1969), WATERMAN and HORCH (1966), WATERMAN and FERNANDEZ (1970), and MULLER (1973). These authors found two classes of cells sensitive to horizontal and vertical e-vectors, respectively, and other studies resolved polarization sensitivity ratios of up to 1:9 and 1:12 (SHAW, 1966, 1969; WATERMAN and FERNANDEZ, 1970). The mechanisms for detection and analysis of polarized light are dealt with in detail by WATERMAN (1980). Evidence that information about the e-vector of polarized light is actually transferred to higher-order neurons is derived from recordings of neurons in the crab medulla externa and crayfish and stomatopod optic nerves (LEGGETT, 1976; YAMAGUCHI, 1967; YAMAGUCHI et al., 1976).

Two visual pigments have been demonstrated in the crayfish retina. These are both rhodopsins (WALD and HUBBARD, 1957; WALD, 1967) imparting to the receptors maximum sensitivities at 565–570 nm and 425–445 nm, respectively (KENNEDY and BRUNO, 1961; GOLDSMITH and FERNÁNDEZ, 1968; WALD, 1968).

Dichromatism has been suggested from intracellular recordings of photoreceptor cells. NOSAKI (1969) and WATERMAN and FERNÁNDEZ (1970) showed that two classes of colour receptors are present in each ommatidium, the majority of the cells were shown to be yellow-green sensitive, whereas only a small fraction (10%–19% of the total impalements) were violet sensitive.

Since the recorded cells were not intracellularily labelled, there is yet no correlation between morphological and physiological units that are violet or yellow-green sensitive, respectively. GOLDSMITH (1978), however, demonstrated with microspectrophotometry that a pigment with an λ_{max} in the shorter wavelengths is absent in the proximal (R 1–R 7) rhabdom. It is thus possible that R 1–R 7 are yellow-green sensitive and R 8 (which has not yet been analysed in this respect) is violet sensitive. Recordings from higher-order interneurons have so far shown convergent inputs from both the violet and yellow-green channels (TREVINO and LARIMER, 1970; WOODCOCK and GOLDSMITH, 1970).

3. Projection of the Retina into the Lamina

The pattern of retinal projections onto the lamina has recently been studied in the crayfish by means of cobalt uptake. By contrast, earlier attempts at tracing individual axon bundles by serial section analysis were hindered, inter alia, because of the vast distance between the retina and the lamina as well as the dense packing and heavy pigmentation of the receptor axons. STOWE (1977), however, showed conclusively that in the crab *Leptograpsus* the receptor mosaic is projected retinotopically into the lamina. Serial sections from the retina to the lamina revealed that the axons from one ommatidium innervate one underlying columnar module (optic cartridge) and retain their neighbourhood relationships amongst themselves between the retina and lamina. The sampling raster of receptors is probably mapped homotopically to deeper neuronal levels, as it is in insects.

Since so many other features of the crab visual system are similar or identical to those of the crayfish (see STOWE et al., 1977, and following sections) it could be assumed that the crayfish retina lamina projection has an identical retinotopic organization. The proposal by MEYER-ROCHOW (1975), NÄSSEL (1976a), and MEYER-ROCHOW and NÄSSEL (1977) that receptor axon penetrations through the retinal basement membrane permutate a map of the retina (below the retina) was based upon observations of short stretches of receptor axons. It was thought that initial crossover patterns were of a divergent and combinatorial nature. This is, however, quite erroneous. The cited studies were incomplete in so far as the axons were not traced through the total distance between the retina and the lamina. Apparently, as is the case in *Leptograpsus* (STOWE, 1977), groups of axons below the basement membrane, derived from three ommatidia, collect into single bundles. These then separate proximally above the lamina where retinotopic unpermutated, mappings of receptor axons are re-established.

Cobalt diffusion into the crayfish retina reveals sets of retinotopic axon bundles that project to the lamina, each accompanied by one long visual fibre axon from the R 8 photoreceptor of each commatidium. Together, R 8 axons project retinotopically through the lamina and then across the first optic chiasma to the medulla where they map an anteroposterior inversion of the retinal mosaic (NÄSSEL in preparation).

4. Neural Arrangements in the Lamina

The lamina is the best studied of the crustacean visual neuropils and will therefore be described in some detail.

Compared to the homologous region in Diptera, or, for example, Hymenoptera, the columnar and layered organization of the crayfish lamina is less precisely arranged but more orderly than, e.g., the lamina of a nocturnal superposition lepidopteran. The structural "noise", or imprecision, can be related to variations of shapes of receptor axons and the structural variations amongst a class of interneurons. However, despite this, all species of interneurons – anaxonal or relay monopolar cells – are relatively simple to classify as distinct types according to characteristic features of their profiles. It is also apparent from electron microscopy studies that the connectivity patterns of receptor axons and interneurons are precise and seem to be reiterated in each cartridge. Parallel channels maintain the retinotopic mosaic, and lateral interactions between discrete stets of elements provide substrates for inhibition, excitation, or adaptation pools, amongst large domains of nerve cells.

The neural components, and some of their synaptic relations within and across the lamina's columnar array, will be described below. Layering in crayfish neuropil is more pronounced in deeper optic neuropil. However, it is also present in the lamina and serves as a structural paradigm for layered laminae of other Crustacea and many species of insects, particularly those suspected to have trichromatic vision.

5. Types of Neurons

Centripetal input to the optic lobes is provided by R 1–R 8 photoreceptor axons. The short photoreceptor axons (R 1–R 7) end at two levels in the lamina, indicating two main lamina strata, whereas axons from the 8 th receptor cells project through the lamina, alongside the R 1–R 7 cells from the same ommatidium, and finally terminate superficially in the medulla. Ten species of neurons have so far been distinguished in the crayfish lamina (NÄSSEL, 1976 a, 1977 a, b; NÄSSEL, in preparation). These are as follows: five types of monopolar neurons, two types of tangential T-neurons, one type of small field T-neuron, one type of centrifugal cell, and one type of amacrine cell. All neurons, bar the anaxonal amacrine cells, connect the lamina with the medulla (Fig. 3), or vice versa, according to their structural-functional polarity.

Interneurons can be characterized with respect to their dendritic or terminal domains in the lamina (Fig. 3) and in the medulla, as well as with respect to their

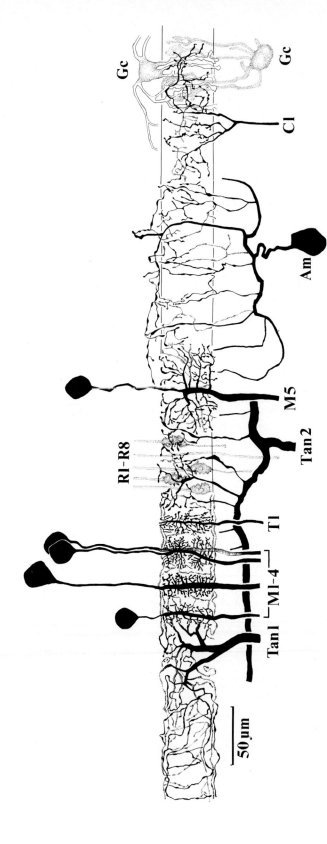

Fig. 3. Diagram of lamina cells in the crayfish. Columnar elements invade every cartridge. These are the monopolars *M 1–M 4* and the T-neuron *T 1* as well as receptor axons *R 1–R 8*. Two types of wide-field tangential neurons, *Tan 1* and *Tan 2*, form dense arbors comprising large lamina domains and overlap freely. Cells with intermediate fields of arborizations include the monopolar cell *M 5* and centrifugal neurons *C 1*, both of which are present as a proportion of the lamina columns. Large amacrine cells *(Am)* invade the lamina from below. Glial cells *(Gc)* form velate processes in the lamina plexiform layer

cell body locations. Dendrites of relay neurons are restricted to either of the two lamina strata or are distributed in both. Their fields have characteristic domains extending either to one single columnar unit (optic cartridge) or extending through a number of columns.

Monopolar neurons of the lamina are derived from cell bodies distal to the neuropil, whereas the amacrine cells and T-neurons are derived from cell bodies beneath the lamina or proximal to the crossover of fibres in the first optic chiasma, respectively.

6. Columnar and Layered Organization of Lamina Cells

Seven receptor axon terminals define each cartridge, four in the distal and three in the proximal lamina stratum (Fig. 4). As in the crab, retinotopic receptor projections bring the channels of one sampling unit (an ommatidium) to a single unit of organization in the neuropil.

Each cartridge comprises, then, a set of seven receptor terminals (plus the en passant R 8) and a set of relay neurons, the monopolar cells. By analogy with insects these are termed "columnar" neurons. Axons of columnar (relay) neurons project alongside axons of long visual fibres (R 8) and transfer the retinotopic mosaic of the lamina into the outer surface of the medulla. Cobalt studies show that each R 8 axon shares a coherent bundle with the relevant set of relay axons, and there is no evidence of any lateral permutation of neighbourhood relationships.

a) Monopolar Cells

Observations of cobalt-filled neuron populations (see STRAUSFELD and HAUSEN, 1977), together with Golgi preparations and electron microscopy, reveal that several types of monopolar cells are found reiterated in each cartridge (NÄS-SEL, 1977 a, b; NÄSSEL, in preparation). Among these are the monopolar neurons M 1–M 4, whereby there is a pair of M 1 cells in each cartridge (M 1 a, b). M 1–M 4 are all small-field elements, with their dendritic arbors restricted to the parent cartridge. Their division into four categories in the lamina is based upon their overall Gestalten and on the distribution of their dendrites in this region. M 1 and M 2 are non-stratified, having dendrites in both lamina strata, whereas M 3 and M 4 are stratified, M 3 with dendrites in the outer stratum and M 4 with dendrites exclusively in the inner stratum (Fig. 3).

b) T-Cells

Another columnar neuron, the small-field T-neuron (T 1), has small-field processes disposed in both lamina strata. Each T-cell is derived from a cell body situated above the medulla and each gives rise to a small distal arborization in each medullary column. In this respect, monopolar cells and small-field T-cells bear direct analogy with lamina relay cells (L 1, L 2, L 3, L 5) and medulla-to-lamina T-cells (T 1) of dipterous insects (STRAUSFELD, 1970, 1976 a). All species of relay neurons can be identified by electron microscopy, and each has a characteristic set of connexions in each cartridge. These are summarized in Sect. B.II.7.

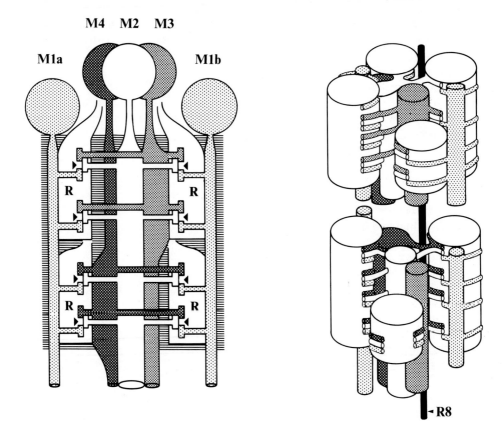

Fig. 4. Schematic representation of the synaptic connexions between photoreceptors (white profiles labelled *R*) and five columnar monopolar cells *M 1 a*, *M 1 b*, and *M 2–M 4* (*M 2*, white; the rest; stippled) in the crayfish. The arrowheads indicate the triad arrangements of synapses in the left hand figures. *M 3*, *M 2*, *M 1 a*, and *M 1 b* receive input in the distal lamina stratum (from four receptor terminals), whereas *M 4*, *M 2*, *M 1 a*, and *M 1 b* are postsynaptic to three terminals in the inner stratum. *M 1 a* and *M 1 b* divide the receptor output so that *M 1 a* receives input from two distal and two proximal receptor endings and *M 1 b* from the two other distal and the remaining single proximal terminal. The long visual fibre *R 8* projects centrally through the cartridge and appears devoid of synaptic relationships in the lamina. The right-hand figure shows a dissected view of these elements

c) Resolution of Cell Assemblies

The remaining types of neurons (tangential cells, centrifugal cells, and amacrines) are regularly distributed, one to several cartridges, according to cobalt uptake experiments (Nässel, in preparation). However, their processes appear to participate in the mosaic organization of the entire neuropil and, most probably, each cell type has a precise and reiterated relationship within each column. Cobalt studies have shown that each optic cartridge contains specializations from all types of lamina elements, as is the case in the lamina of many species of insect. The following observation serves as an example of this. Injection of Co^{++} directly into crayfish neuropil has resolved populations of amacrines and, in other preparations, wide-field centrifugals or tangential elements. Within the range of the cobalt pool (see STRAUSFELD and HAUSEN, 1977; BACON and STRAUSFELD, 1980), what is presumed to be the entire local population of any given cell is resolved. Observations of these "cell assemblies" (STRAUSFELD and HAUSEN, 1977) reveal that even though single amacrine cells vary in their lateral domain, all amacrine cells together contribute to a homogeneous network or "isomorphic neural assembly" whereby each cartridge receives the same complement of neural elements, irrespective of size variations of large-field nerve cells (see Sect. C). The same kind of distributions have been resolved for other wide-field elements. One example is the supraperiodic monopolar neuron, M 5. These are wide-field neurons that spread through several columnar units and which together comprise a regular palisade of neurons, one to every six or eight cartridges, with dendritic assemblies that invade every cartridge of the lamina. Similar spatial arrangements have been documented from cobalt studies of the dipterous lobula (Sect. C).

Another class of neurons that comprise the mosaic, but are numerically fewer than the number of cartridges, are the wide-field tangential neurons (Fig. 3). These elements have processes that extend over large portions of the projected retinotopic mosaic. Two types of such neurons have been distinguished; both contribute to regular and isomorphic networks of fibres.

d) Tan 1

This species of tangential neuron cell (Tan 1) has long processes whose arborizations invade both the lamina strata in a bistratified rather than a diffuse pattern. The arrangement of these cells across the lamina make up a distal hexagonal network of processes which, deeper in the neuropil, is compressed to a rectilinear lattice. Adjacent Tan 1 cells overlap each other extensively. Their thick axons connect the lamina with the medulla where they also give rise to extensive arborizations.

e) Tan 2

The second type of tangential neuron (Tan 2) has large vertically arranged branches beneath the lamina from which processes ascend distally into the lamina's plexiform layer. This neuron is connected to the medulla by a thick axon that gives rise to a large dendritic arborization.

f) Centrifugal Cells

One type of centrifugal neuron has a regularly distribution amongst optic cartridges. By morphological definition (CAJAL and SÁNCHEZ, 1915) this cell type in insects is classed as a centrifugal neuron (Fig. 3) derived from a unipolar cell body proximal to the medulla. Its ascending axon gives rise to a characteristic, layered pattern of collaterals or dendrites at several levels in the medulla, and thereafter its axon projects distally, across the first chiasma, to arborize diffusely over several cartridges in the lamina.

g) Amacrine Cells

One type of anaxonal or amacrine element has been found in the lamina and is derived from cell bodies that are located below the lamina's inner surface (Fig. 3).

Cell body fibres give rise to tangential branches from which numerous processes project through the plexiform layer, finally giving rise to lateral branchlets at the distal surface of the lamina. There is considerable overlap between adjacent amacrine neurons. Cobalt uptake by amacrines show this cell type to be spaced one to several cartridges.

7. Synaptic Arrangements in Cartridges and Stratification of the Lamina

a) Synaptology

The lamina columns (optic cartridges) of the crayfish are less regular and less extensively separated by glial elements than is the case in several studied insects (Fig. 5). It is, however, clear that seven photoreceptor endings at two strata define each columnar unit, with a synaptic output onto five monopolar neurons. This pattern is most likely identical throughout the complete set of cartridges in the lamina. Each cartridge also contains several other components derived from columnar and non-columnar neurons, as described above.

The shapes and arborization patterns of crayfish visual neurons are too imprecise to allow identification of dendrites by conventional electron microscopy alone. However, combined Golgi and EM techniques (Fig. 5) prove a valuable tool for routine analysis (Nässel and Waterman, 1977). With this technique each cell is first identified by light microscopy and is then resectioned for electron microscopical observation. It was found that the five monopolar neurons (M 1 a, M 1 b, M 2–M 4) of each cartridge are characteristically wired up to specific receptor terminal combinations and thus comprise five distinct parallel channels (Fig. 4) that project to medulla relay cells of each central column.

Channel 1. M 2 has numerous postsynaptic sites to all seven receptors of the cartridge. This neuron is thus capable of relaying from both levels of R 1–R 7 receptors and would be likely to mix discrete channels that carry information about the *e*-vector of polarized light.

Channels 2, 3. M 3 is postsynaptic to the four shallow receptor terminals and M 4 to the three deep ones (Fig. 4).

Channels 4, 5. The two M 1 neurons share the receptor terminations in that one receives input from two shallow and two deep terminals, whereas the other derives an input from two shallow and one deep receptor terminal (Fig. 4). Possible separation of the receptor input might provide two *e*-vector channels; however, the significance of five parallel pathways, all of which derive a first-order input, is not clear. The evidence is that the R 1–R 7 receptors have identical spectral sensitivities (Goldsmith, 1978), and colour-coded channels appear to be unlikely amongst these elements.

In spite of some variations in the morphology of the individual lamina neurons, at least at the light microscopical level, precise synaptic arrangements are manifested by the receptor-monopolar junctions. Characteristically, the receptor terminals form membrane evaginations (with a presynaptic dense bar and clear vesicles)

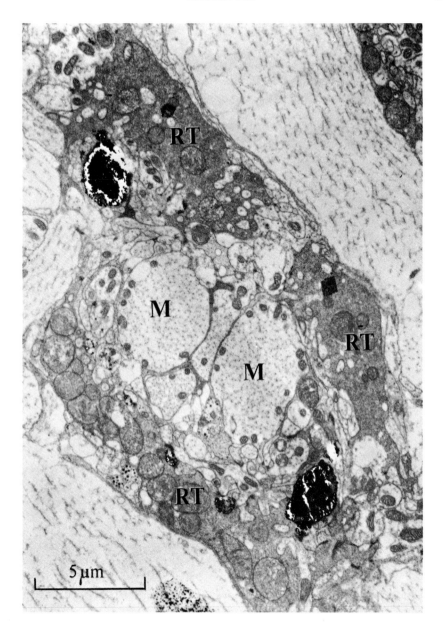

Fig. 5. Electron micrograph of a Golgi preparation (Golgi-EM) showing a fortuitous resolution of two *M 1* neurons (*M 1 a* and *M 1 b*) which have been impregnated with silver chromate in the same cartridge of the crayfish lamina (black profiles). The micrograph originates from the lower part of the lamina where three photoreceptor terminals *(RT)* have their expanded endings. In the center of the cartridge (lined by two tangential profiles) the axis fibres of other monopolars can be seen, two of which are labelled *M*. (These are probably *M 2* and *M 3*, whereas *M 4* in this region is represented by diffuse arborizations rather than a single large profile.)

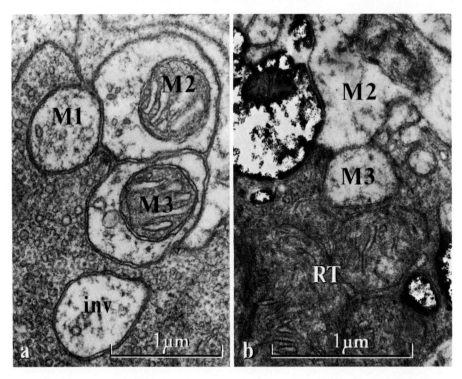

Fig. 6. a Electron micrograph of a photoreceptor-triad synapse from the distal lamina stratum in the crayfish where the postsynaptic profiles are *M 1*, *M 2*, and *M 3*. A small arrow-shaped presynaptic structure resides in the evaginated membrane area of the receptor terminal. A profile *(inv)* is also shown invaginating into the receptor from the *M 3* dendrite. **b** A Golgi-EM micrograph of a receptor terminal *(RT)* and a postsynaptic triad where the black profile, with its invaginating spines, belongs to an M 1 monopolar

adjacent to triads of postsynaptic profiles (Fig. 6 a, b). The central profile in these postsynaptic triads is always a spine from M 2, irrespective of its level.

In the distal lamina stratum, one of the lateral profiles is derived from M 3 and the other from one of the M 1 neurons. In the proximal stratum the one lateral profile is derived from M 4 and from the M 1 s, respectively. The M 1 neurons establish their contacts with receptors in the specific pattern described above. Triadic and diadic arrangements have also been resolved in the lamina of Diptera (R 1–R 6 to L 1, L 2, L 3 monopolar cells) and in Odonata (see Sect. C of this chapter, and Boschek, 1971; Campos-Ortega and Strausfeld, 1973; Strausfeld and Campos-Ortega, 1977; Armett-Kibel et al., 1977).

The lateral postsynaptic profiles of M 1, M 3, and M 4 neurons form small knob-like invaginations into the receptor terminals (Fig. 6 a, b). No specialized membranes, synaptic bars or vesicles have been found in or adjacent to these invaginations that could be suggestive of chemical synapses. The significance of these structures is unknown.

Wide-field, T-cell and other lamina neurons have not yet been studied by electron microscopy in detail. It seems, however, from combined Golgi and electron microscopical observations that neither M 5 nor Tan 1 neurons are directly post-synaptic to receptor elements, and they most probably interact with sets of relay neurons in the lamina, as do L 4 monopolar cells, tangential cells and amacrines in insects. It would not be surprising if some of the circuitry described from the fly, purportedly candidates for lateral inhibition and neural adaptation (STRAUSFELD and CAMPOS-ORTEGA, 1977), are also present in the crayfish; however, there is at present no physiological evidence for corresponding electrophysiological phenomena at the level of the lamina in Crustacea. If such circuits are present, neurons such as Tan 1, C 1 and amacrine cells would also bear good comparison with wide-field centrifugal neurons, C 2, C 3, centrifugal cells and α-processes in the lamina of the fly (Sect. C).

b) Stratification

In addition to the two main lamina layers, defined by the receptor terminals and M 3–M 4 dendrites, there are additional strata which reflect the layers of synaptic specializations of other cell types.

Neurons such as Tan 1 and the amacrine cells have processes distal and proximal to the lamina plexiform layer. They thus form strata outside the main synaptic region of photoreceptor-monopolar neuron synapses and possibly comprise special levels of synaptic connectivities amongst themselves, distal and proximal to their functional relationships with relay neurons.

Electron microscopical observations of these two levels have detected numerous neural profiles containing dense-cored vesicles. The profiles are of two types, one containing large (100–160 nm) and the other small (60–80 nm) vesicles (ELOFSSON et al., 1977). In addition, both contain clear vesicles (20–40 nm) characteristically associated with chemical synapses. Profiles containing dense-cored vesicles are, by contrast, seldom detected in the main plexiform layer.

8. Aminergic Neurons in the Lamina

Formaldehyde-induced fluorescence (FALCK et al., 1962) reveals a specific pattern of catecholaminergic fluorescence in the optic lobes of the crayfish (see also Fig. 9 a, b) (ELOFSSON et al., 1966; ELOFSSON and KLEMM, 1972; ELOFSSON et al., 1977). The lamina normally displays a weak fluorescence or a complete absence of fluorescence with the standard method. However, if optic lobes are incubated in α-methyl noradrenalin or dopamine, after reserpine treatment, a clear fluorescent pattern arises in the lamina (ELOFSSON et al., 1977). This pattern most likely represents two superimposed neuron types, by analogy with the patterns of fibres revealed after Golgi impregnation or cobalt injection. The most prominent pattern (which is occasionally revealed without inducement) appears to be derived from a small-field lamina T-neuron, linked to shallow arborizations in the medulla. The cell bodies of this neuron reside in the chiasmatic region between the two neuropils. The entire structure of each cell much resembles the T 1 neurons that link the lamina to the medulla and which have been observed as single stochastically impregnated elements by the Golgi technique and as assemblies of cells after cobalt uptake.

The second fluorescent cell type is characterized by the presence of large cell bodies below the lamina from which axis fibres invade the lamina to give rise to tangentially oriented processes, distal and proximal to the main lamina plexiform layer. The only neurons resolved in Golgi and cobalt preparations that match this pattern are the lamina amacrine neurons.

Profiles detected by electron microscopy, containing large dense-cored vesicles, partly coincide with these fluorescent patterns (ELOFSSON et al., 1977). Their tangentially arranged components reside distal and proximal to the plexiform layer. However, since the uptake of exogenous catecholamines is cytoplasmic, it is possible that neurons resolved by conventional electron microscopy, characterized by their contents of dense-cored vesicles, do not fully match the fluorescence pattern, and it may be that some lamina neurons are still refractory to either Golgi methods or to cobalt – silver analysis.

9. Physiology of Lamina Neurons

Surprisingly few electrophysiological studies performed on crustacean optic lobes shed any light on the functional significance of a lamina neuron. The only recordings from neurons of this level are from the crab *Leptograpsus* (ERBER and SANDEMAN, 1976). These authors demonstrated that the crab lamina cells (unspecified and unmarked) exhibit the same kind of hyperpolarizing potentials as found in some insects, where modulations of light intensity cause a modulation of the amplitude of the interneuron membrane potential, rather than eliciting spikes.

10. Organization of the Medulla

The medulla is divided into an outer and inner neuropil by a layer of thick tangential axons that separate the outer three-quarters of its depth from the inner eighth (Fig. 7). These axons, which comprise the serpentine layer, are destined for regions in the midbrain and contralateral optic lobes (see also BETHE, 1897a, b; HANSTRÖM, 1924, 1926, 1928).

The distal three-quarters of the medulla [termed ME(o)] contain the terminals of M 2–M 4 lamina monopolar cells, the paired M 2 terminals, the shallow endings of the long visual fibres (R 8) and the arborization of lamina tangentials, Tan 1 and Tan 2 (Fig. 7). In addition, the majority of the dendrites of medulla columnar neurons (transmedullary neurons), as well as amacrine arbors, are observed to reside within the outer layers of the region (Fig. 7).

The inner eighth of the medulla [ME(i)], beneath the serpentine layer, contains axon collaterals of some transmedullary neurons as well as dendrites from some cell types, such as T-neurons, that project to the lobula from exclusively this layer. Thus, the basic principle organization is most reminiscent of the medulla in insects, particularly the diurnal Lepidoptera, Hymenoptera, and Diptera.

The retinotopic mosaic is carried through the medulla by small-field transmedullary neurons which are arranged periodically (1: 1) with respect to the columnar arrangements of long visual fibres and their accompanying sets of five monopolar cell endings and T 1 cell terminals. In Fig. 7 examples of types of transmedul-

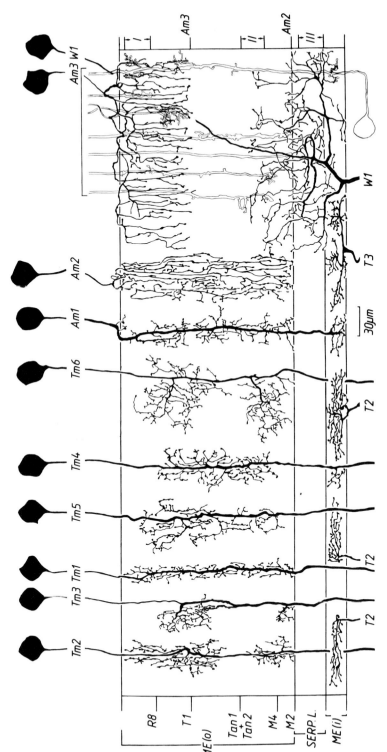

Fig. 7. The medulla of the crayfish. On the left-hand side are indicated levels of terminations of some lamina elements as well as the main layers; *ME(o)*, serpentine layer (*SERP.L*) and *ME(i)*. The amacrine *Am 2* and *Am 3* layers, as well as three main tangential layers (*I–III*), are indicated to th e right. In this simplified diagram only examples of medulla relay cells are shown. *Tm 1–Tm 6* are six characteristic types of transmedullary neurons classified according to their arborization patterns. *Am 1–AM 3* are T-neurons restricted to the *ME(i)* layer. *W 1* is a type of wide-field non-columnar superperiodic transmedullary cell. *T 2–T 3* are T-neurons restricted to the *ME(i)* layer. Lastly, the input from the lamina is indicated by open profiles (inside bracket). Fro̅m left to right these are *M 3, M 4, M 1, M 2, T 1, R 8,* and *C 1,* some of which are partly obscured in this illustration

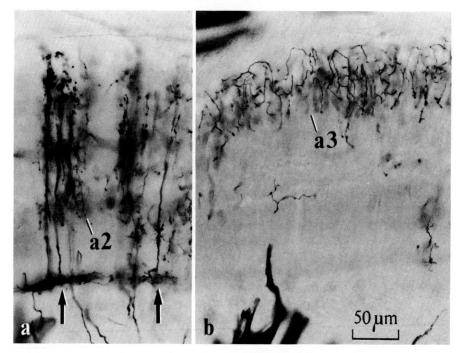

Fig. 8 a, b. Three types of amacrines in the crayfish medulla seen in Golgi preparations: **a** Amacrines *Am 1* and *Am 2* from Fig. 7. *Am 1* connects *ME(o)* and *ME(i)* (arrowed) where processes from some T-neurons are also seen. *Am 2* extends through about two-thirds of the medulla depth. **b** The third kind of amacrine *(Am 3)* which has a large-field arborization in the distal portion of the medulla

lary neurons are illustrated, as observed in Golgi preparations. These neurons are characterized by a perpendicular axis fibre, one or several sets of dendritic arborizations in the ME(o), some types also having collaterals in ME(i), and axons projecting to the lobula via the second optic chiasma. The dendritic arbors of transmedullary neurons are disposed at several levels which bring them into apposition with arborization domains of other species of neurons and/or with one or more terminal specializations derived from the lamina. Despite their diffuse appearance these cells impart precision to layered structures of the neuropil as is shown by mass staining with cobalt. Another class of neurons that most clearly contributes to the stratification of the medulla is the amacrine cell. Three such examples are illustrated in Figs. 7, 8 a, b.

Characteristically, amacrines are either restricted to a single column or a specific domain of medulla columns and project to different depths of the neuropil. Whether these merely provide local circuitry within a stratum is not clear.

The remaining cell types resolved in the medulla have extensive arborizations throughout large portions of the projected retinotopic mosaic. These can be divided into three main classes: (1) large cells that connect the medulla with the lobula; (2) cells that connect the medulla with the lobula and optic foci; and (3) cells that project directly to protocerebral centers or contralateral optic lobes (see also Fig. 2).

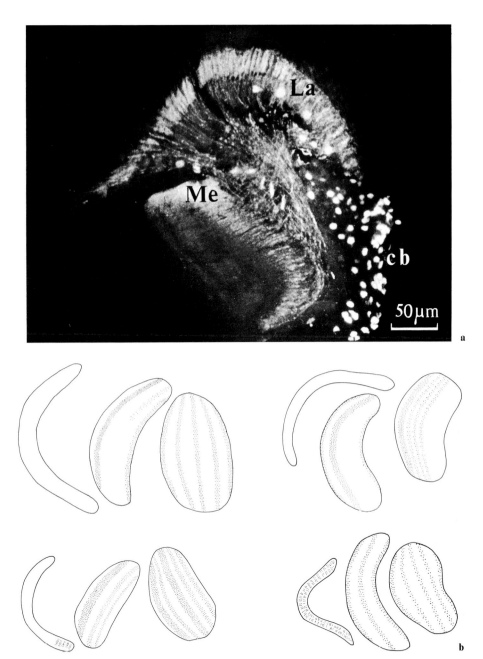

Fig. 9. a Horizontal section through the crayfish lamina *(La)* and medulla *(Me)* displaying catecholamine fluorescence after reserpine treatment followed by dopamine incubation. The neurons resolved are small-field columnar T-neurons connecting the lamina with the medulla. The cell bodies *(cb)* are situated outside the chiasma between the two neuropils. The two proximal bands of fluorescence are too weak to be seen in this micrograph. (ELOFSSON, NÄSSEL, and MYHRBERG, 1977). **b** Schematic drawings of catecholamine fluorescence patterns in the optic lobes of four Crustacea. The neuropils are, from left to right: lamina, medulla, and lobula. Upper left, *Pandalus borealis* (decapod shrimp); upper right, *Neomysis integer* (mysid shrimp); lower left, *Astacus astacus* (crayfish); lower right, *Portunus depurator* (crab). (The different animals are not to scale.) After ELOFSSON and KLEMM (1972) with permission of R. Elofsson and Springer-Verlag

Cell types that constitute these classes either have diffuse arborizations or form precise planar layers. Large cells of group 3 invade the serpentine layer and also have branches in two more distal strata as indicated in Fig. 7. The thickest axons within these three tangential layers have perpendicularly oriented secondary branches invading specific strata in the ME(o), suggesting functional relationships with columnar efferents from the lamina.

As in the larvae of *Aeschna* (Insecta: Odonata) one type of neuron, resembling class 3 elements, forms three extensive strata of thin varicose processes in the medulla. These cells are peculiar in both crayfish and dragonfly in that they are resolved in sulphide-treated, silver-intensified brains which have not been exposed to cobalt ions. Possibly these neurons contain endogenous metal cations, such as zinc or cadmium which, in the form of the corresponding sulphide, catalyses silver reduction.

Catecholamine fluorescence is demonstrated in three layers of the medulla, a broad band distally and two thinner bands proximally, just above the serpentine layer (Fig. 9) (ELOFSSON et al., 1966; ELOFSSON and KLEMM, 1972; ELOFSSON et al., 1977). Only in the case of the distal band can the fluorophore be correlated with any single type of neuron, the lamina medulla small-field T-neuron (ELOFSSON et al., 1977), as mentioned previously.

11. The Lobula

Inputs from the medulla to the lobula comprise bundles of retinotopic columnar relay neurons and columnar T-neurons from ME(i). Postsynaptic columnar relay cells in the lobula seem, however, to be arranged as a subperiod of this lattice, thus coarsening the retinotopic mosaic as is the case in insects (see Sect. C). Accordingly, all cell types in the lobula which are arranged as columnar palisades have dendritic tree domains which correspond to specific groups of input columns projected from the medulla. Figures 10 and 11 illustrate the dendritic arbors of some columnar cells, in either one of two main distal strata. These layers correspond to two main levels of input from the medulla. Two other levels of medulla terminals are distinguished more proximally in the lobula (Fig. 10) at levels of columnar neurons whose dendrites span large portions of the projected mosaic. Interspersed between the distal and proximal strata are diffusely arranged dendritic or terminal expansions of other cell types whose topological relationships seem to be concomitant with axons of lobula relay neurons rather than with primary input of medulla-derived efferents. Lobula stratification is also apparent in the distribution of catecholamine fluorescence in five layers of the neuropil (ELOFSSON and KLEMM, 1972), three of which appear to correspond to three of the lobula input layers (Fig. 9).

Amacrine cells have not been seen in the crayfish lobula, though one type of large intrinsic T-neuron has been resolved which appears to join the outer layer of the lobula with its innermost layers, reminiscent of T-cells in undivided insect lobulae, such as, for example, in the bee (CAJAL and SÁNCHEZ, 1915; STRAUSFELD, 1970, 1976b). This region is also invaded by large-field tangential neurons comprising diffusely arborizing elements that connect the lobula with one of the optic

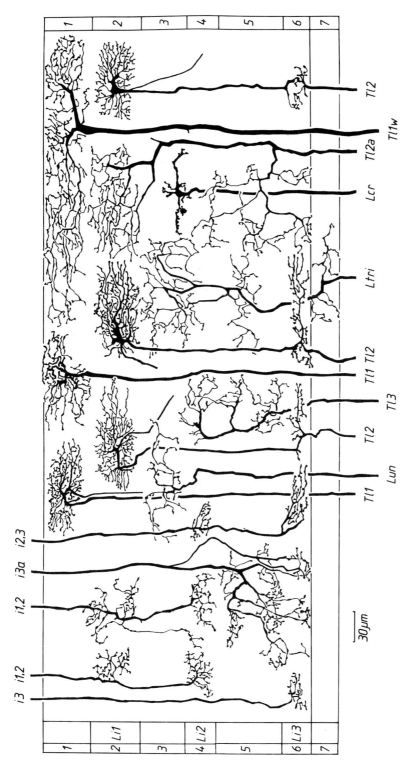

Fig. 10. Diagram of elements in the crayfish lobula. The lobula has seven main strata (1–7), three of which receive input from the medulla (Li1–Li3). Input elements from the medulla are shown to the left (i3: i1,2; i3a; i2,3), most of which are derived from transmedullary neurons. Columnar elements have processes in either of two distal strata: Tl1 elements at the distalmost and Tl2 at the second level. Tl2 also has processes in stratum 6. A third kind of columnar element, Tl3, has processes in the lower half of the lobula. Lun, Ltri, and Lcr are neurons that appear to be non-columnar in structure

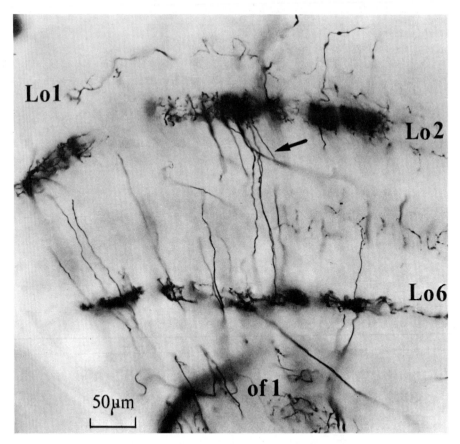

Fig. 11. A set of columnar *(Tl2)* neurons in the crayfish lobula with arborizations in two strata *(Lo 2, Lo 6)* as seen in a Golgi preparation. Note the obliquely emerging cell body fibres (indicated by the arrow). All the columnar neurons of the lobula are T-neurons with the characteristic T-shaped origin of the cell body attached below the dendritic arbors. A wide-field lobula element is stained distally in the outermost stratum *(Lo 1)*. Proximal to the lobula part of the first optic focus can be seen *(of 1)*

foci and large axonal neurons that project to ipsi- and contralateral protocerebral centres.

The lobula is the most proximal neuropil in the lobes to show a clear-cut columnar and stratified organization. The retinotopic mosaic is thereafter transposed onto prominent higher-order neurons in optic foci where, it seems, spatial segregation amongst single columnar elements is maintained by virtue of their presynaptic pattern on the recipient dendritic tree.

Several types of output structures from the lobula have been observed: (1) topical projection of neurons onto four different optic foci (see next section); (2) large axonal neurons that project to ipsi- or contralateral protocerebral centers from the lobula, directly, rather than via an intermediate station; (3) large-axon neurons that project to cerebral centers and have collaterals to one of the optic foci and/or to other parts of the lateral protocerebrum in the eyestalk.

12. Projection of Columnar Neuropils onto Higher-Order Centres

Axons leaving the lobula comprise a number of discrete tracts. These project to single higher-order neurons, many of which most likely project to neuropils of the body ganglia, as they do in the insect central nervous system. In crayfish four lobula-derived tracts end in ordered neuropil of the lateral eyestalk protocerebrum (Fig. 12). These visual neuropils are here termed "optic foci" by analogy with their insect counterpart (STRAUSFELD, 1976a). Other tracts enter the optic nerve directly or after donating collaterals to different foci in the eyestalk's lateral protocerebrum.

In crayfish the optic foci are delineated regions of neuropil, each with a characteristic fibroarchitecture and location within the eyestalk. Within most of these regions the spatial arrangement of axon terminals, derived from palisades of lobula columnar cells, seems to be quite orderly. The evidence is that a coherent bundle of axons of one cell type establishes a characteristic pattern of terminations on the dendrites of each single optic focus relay cell. Spatial segregation of efferents is demonstrated by four foci in particular. In one, which resides just beneath the lobula, spatial segregation of efferents is in fact columnar, giving this fourth-order neuropil a retinotopic structure *(of 1)*. This focus also receives retinotopic inputs both from collaterals and terminals of, respectively, large- and small-diameter axons derived from the lobula. Many of these elements also project further centrally. Two other fibre types that terminate in the focus *of 1* are shown in Fig. 12: one is a diffuse wide-field neuron from the lobula; the other is peculiar in that it is derived from a large-field neuron of the medulla. This cell also gives rise to collaterals that extend from distal layers in the lobula, traverse this region and finally terminate in *of 1*. All types of columnar neurons ending in *of 1* appear to impinge upon large and extensively ramifying neurons (see Fig. 13) that lead to cerebral centers. These are accompanied by thinner, diffusely branching nerve cells (Fig. 14). In several aspects the presence of a fourth retinotopic region of neuropil as an addendum to the lobula is reminiscent of the lobula plate structure of some insects (Coleoptera, Lepidoptera, and Diptera) or lobula plate-like areas associated with the lobula neuropil in Ephemeroptera and Odonata (STRAUSFELD, 1976b).

The second optic focus to be described here, *of 2*, (Figs. 12 and 15c, d) is innervated by one type of lobula columnar cell (Tl2 in Fig. 10). The projection to the focus is retinotopic, and the terminals in the focus are flattened, rosette-like structures (arbors) packed as discs in the dorsoventral axis; the focus itself is cylindrical. Concomitant with its long axis, large centrally projecting relay neurons, with orderly patterned dendrites, receive the orderly rosette input from the lobula cell terminals. This finding demonstrates that although there is an abrupt convergence of several hundred columnar elements to a single (or very few) protocerebral relay cells, projections onto them by columnar neurons is precise. Order is maintained and the retinotopic map is translated into a different, but characteristic, distribution of terminals that maps onto a single dendritic tree.

Observations of cobalt- or Golgi-impregnated material show that the third focus, *of 3*, is more diffusely organized in comparison to *of 1* or *of 2* (Figs. 12 and 15a, b). Large axons from large-field lobula neurons comprise glomerular endings in an amphora-shaped neuropil. Higher-order relay neurons that project from this

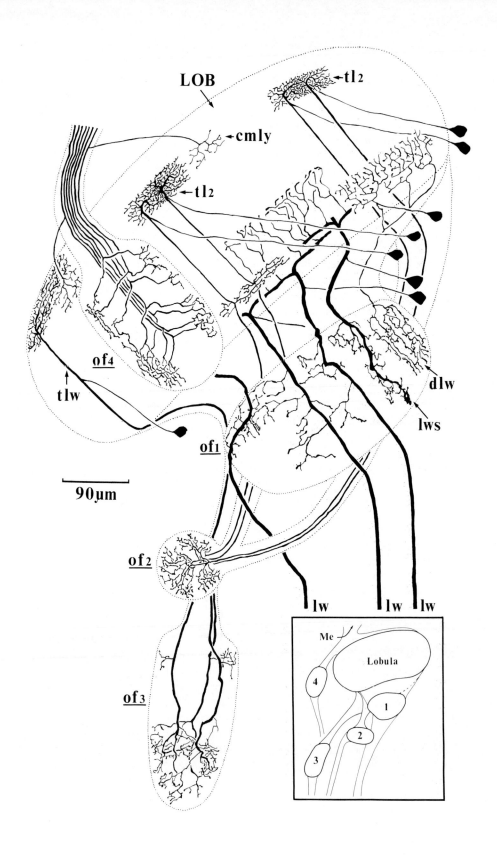

LOB

cmly

tl₂

tl₂

of₄

tlw

of₁

dlw

lws

90μm

of₂

of₃

lw   lw   lw

Me

Lobula

4

1

2

3

focus have diffuse dendrites that form a plexus over the neuropil and amongst the presynaptic glomerular terminals within it. It seems that in this case geometrical precision is *not* preserved between the optic focus and lobula neuropil.

The fourth example of an optic focus *(of 4)* is peculiar in that it receives collateral input from neurons that connect the medulla and the lobula (Fig. 12). Although the complete morphology of these in the medulla is not yet clear, observations of the lobula show them to have processes in the second main stratum, regularly distributed amongst the dendritic trees of one type of columnar lobula cell and the terminal specializations of several kinds of transmedullary cells (Fig. 12). In the optic focus itself terminals are arranged as a set of layers. The output neurons from *of 4* have dense, orderly arranged, dendritic trees whose layered branching pattern matches the spatial arrangement of the lobula-derived terminals (Fig. 16).

The axons of higher-order neurons (Fig. 16) leading from optic foci are collected into four tracts that project centrally (see inset of Fig. 12). Unfortunately, the destinations of these large and important relay cells are not yet clear since tracing of axons across the optic nerve to cerebral or thoracic centres has proved difficult with present techniques.

Finally, a few words should be said about the remaining neuropil masses in the eyestalk. Classically, these have been referred to as the "medulla terminalis" or "terminal medulla" but are here termed the lateral protocerebrum, for reasons mentioned previously. The majority of electrophysiological studies of the crustacean visual system have been recordings from within this region, or they have been from neurons that lead from it into the optic nerve. However, the lateral protocerebrum is, even today, the least understood and least studied part of the optic lobes with respect to its structural organization. Apart from numerous axon tracts, the lateral protocerebrum comprises several distinct glomeruli or neuropil areas and, excepting the optic foci, only a few structures have been identified as serving a particular sensory modality. Some are predominantly visual (see below), while another is known to be mechanosensory or chemosensory: this area consists of an anteriorly situated "hemiellipsoid glomerulus" that is classically referred to as the "corpora pedunculata," innervated by relay neurons that originate in the antennal glomeruli (HANSTRÖM, 1928) and, as such, is analogous to the mushroom bodies of insects.

Central regions of the lateral protocerebrum are less well-defined in terms of their fibro-architecture. However, some have been recognized as deriving collateral projections from visual interneurons that are primarily derived from the lobula. There is also evidence that other areas in the lateral protocerebrum are possibly

----

◄ **Fig. 12.** Reconstruction of four optic foci from serial horizontal Golgi-impregnated sections *(of 1–of 4)* in the crayfish optic lobes. These illustrate examples of the terminals from lobula relay neurons or, in the case of *of 4*, from interneurons shared by the medulla and lobula. The latter donate collateral branches *(cmly)* to the second stratum of the lobula *(LOB)*. Some types of lobula interneurons, ending in *of 1 (lws, dlw)* or sending en passant collaterals *(lw)* to *of 1*, are shown. In contrast, the terminals in *of 2* are derived exclusively from columnar (Tl2) neurons of the lobula. The inset shows the optic foci *1–4*, as they are seen in a vertical section, and illustrates the distribution of tracts of descending or higher-order neurons leading from the foci towards the midbrain proper

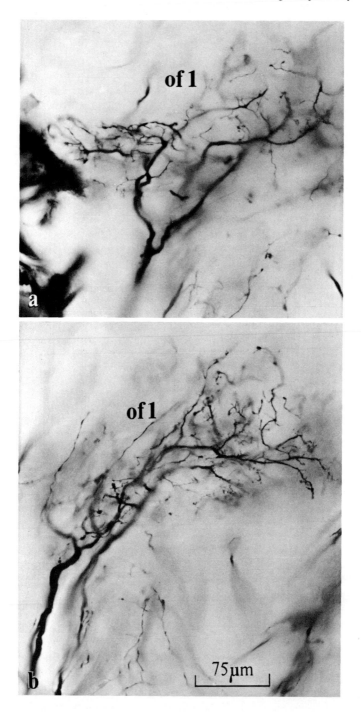

Fig. 13. a Large-field descending neuron with dendrites in the first optic focus *(of 1);* Golgi preparation.
b Two large-field descending neurons from the same focus (crayfish)

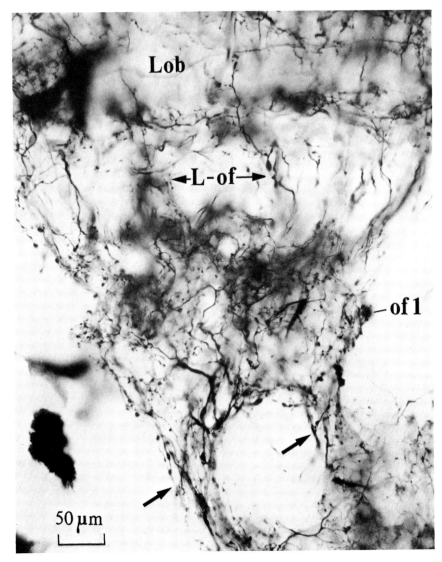

Fig. 14. The lower part of the lobula (*Lob*) and the first optic focus *of 1* of the crayfish. Two tracts are illustrated, which emerge from the proximal part of *of 1* (arrowed); these are destined for deeper centres. The retinotopic projection between the lobula and the optic focus is seen in the region labelled *L-of*. The whole focus is penetrated by diffusely branching wide-field output neurons whose axons enter the tracts (arrowed)

second- or third-order mechanosensory regions. Observations of Golgi and cobalt preparations have resolved exceedingly large unique neurons that connect several of these neuropil masses and project to centres of the midbrain proper.

In addition to axons derived from the antennal lobes the "optic nerves" also contain axons of mechanosensory neurons, motor neurons destined for eye withdrawal muscles (which should not be confused with oculomotor neurons; MELLON,

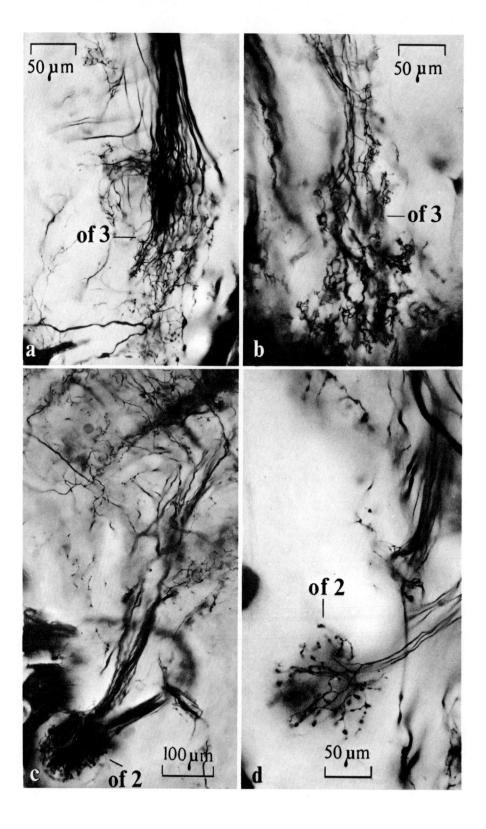

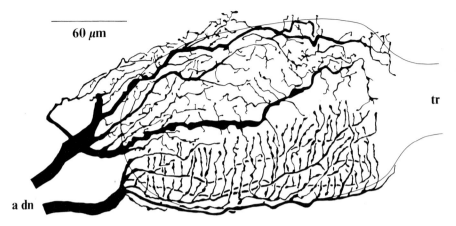

Fig. 16. The output neurons of the optic focus *(of 4)* in the crayfish have orderly arranged dendrites which coincide with the pattern of terminations from invading medulla-lobula neurons (cf. Fig. 12). *a dn*, axons of the two output neurons; *tr*, tract from the lobula and medulla

1977), and visual or "multimodal" neurons (WIERSMA, 1967; WIERSMA and YA-MAGUCHI, 1966; SANDEMAN, 1977). These electrophysiological findings emphasize the multimodal nature of lateral protocerebral neuropil.

Physiological studies cited previously have demonstrated that visual inter-neurons in the optic nerve display highly integrated properties. However, these can shed little light on any interpretation of structural findings of more distal regions, described earlier in this account, all of which are situated peripheral to sites of previous electrode recordings.

Three main classes of visual interneurons have been distinguished from extracellular recordings in the optic nerve. These are, "sustaining fibres" (tonic on-fibres), "dimming fibres" (tonic off-fibres), and "movement fibres" (phasic off-fibres) (WATERMAN et al., 1964; WIERSMA and YAMAGUCHI, 1966; YORK and WIERSMA, 1975; FRASER, 1977; GLANZ, 1977). All have large visual fields and can be divided into subclasses depending on response characteristics, such as space-constant sustaining fibres, multimodal sustaining fibres, direction-sensitive movement fibres, and cells responding to erratic movement of objects ("jittery movement fibres"). Responses also depend on the size and location of the presumed visual fields. The complexity of these units is further demonstrated in their responses to different wavelengths (TREVINO and LARIMER, 1970; WOODCOCK and GOLDSMITH, 1970) and polarized light patterns (YAMAGUCHI, 1967; YAMAGUCHI et al., 1976) and the "memory" of temporal patterns in movement fibres (SHIMOZAWA et al., 1977). Although valuable and interesting in their own right, these data are hardly useful

◀ **Fig. 15. a** Terminals of lobula neurons in the third optic focus *of 3* of the crayfish as seen in a Golgi preparation. **b** The same terminals in *of 3*, seen after cobalt backfilling from the lobula. Cobalt diffusion through all the invading axons shows up the glomerular structure of this neuropil quite clearly. **c** The lower part of the lobula *(lob)* and the second optic focus *of 2* in a Golgi preparation. Two main tracts from the lobula of this focus can be resolved. **d** An enlargement of *of 2*, showing details of its structure for correlative structural studies. The shapes and dispositions of recorded cells have not been resolved, either because historically no such techniques were available or because of the technical difficulties involved. Yet the crayfish optic lobes are possibly as amenable to structural and functional studies as are their insect counterparts – in particularly those of Diptera. The significance of the various kinds of spatial arrangements and mappings of the retinotopic mosaic onto single relay cells is not known. The organization of optic foci is possibly most amenable to experimental analysis. Structures are generally larger than in optic foci of studied insects (e.g., Diptera and Hymenoptera), and they could provide general information about integration of this level of the system.

III. Other Decapod Crustaceans

Amongst the species of decapods hitherto studied, *Pandalus* shows the most orderly arranged lamina (Nässel, 1975, 1976b). The optic cartridges are distinctly delineated and comprise elements with relatively constant shapes and locations. In *Pandalus*, cartridges are arranged in horizontal rows separated by plexuses of tangential neurons. This is in contrast to other decapods studied where the optic cartridges are hexagonally packed, but are less regular, and show a relatively high level of structural variation with respect to the arrangements of neurons in them.

The shapes and projections of neurons resolved are more or less identical in all decapod species. Variations between species relate to the finer details of dendritic branching pattern and the distribution of synaptic specializations. The shapes and arrangements of the receptor terminals and the monopolar neurons M 1–M 4, as studied in Golgi preparations and by electron microscopy, show identical patterns of connectivity between the crayfish (Nässel and Waterman, 1977; Nässel, 1977b), the lobster (Hámori and Horridge, 1966a, b), and the prawn *Pandalus* (Nässel, 1976b).

In contrast, the M 5 monopolar neuron of the crayfish and the M 6 monopolar of *Squilla* (p. 49) are two examples of cells that are not resolved in all the studied decapods and may indeed be absent in some. However, their absence can only be shown by electron microscopy, and it is possible that these cell types are merely refractory to Golgi techniques in some species.

Some variation is found in the anatomy of the tangential T-neurons between the different decapods. All decapods have basically the same forms of two classes of tangential fibres in the lamina (Tan 1 and Tan 2), but their lateral extents and the elaboration of their lamina arborizations vary from species to species. Recent observations of tangential neurons, such as those described from *Pandalus* (Nässel, 1975), have been resolved in detail by improved Golgi techniques. In comparison with the crayfish these cells are more elaborately branched though their general morphology clearly resembles Tan 1 and Tan 2 in the former species. A third type of tangential neuron has been resolved in the crabs *Leptograpsus* and *Scylla* (Stowe et al., 1977) and *Ocypode* (Nässel, 1977b). This neuron has a slender axis-fibre from which arise small-diameter processes arranged at right angles to the main tangential branches beneath the lamina plexiform layer and projecting in parallel with optic cartridges. The neuron might possibly be analogous to the centrifugal (C 1) neuron of crayfish or it may represent a novel cell type.

In addition to tangential neurons described above, the crab *Ocypode* also has two plexuses of thin tangential processes above and beneath the lamina's plexiform layer (NÄSSEL, 1977 b). Thin fibres penetrate the lamina and connect the two plexuses. However, no axon has been resolved connecting these plexuses with a component in the medulla, and it is possible that these fibres are, in fact, intrinsic to the lamina, derived from amacrine cells, as observed in the crayfish.

Descriptions of crab (STOWE et al., 1977) and *Pandalus* (Fig. 14 in NÄSSEL, 1975) laminae include forms of neurons classified as centrifugal on the grounds of their structural polarity, from proximal medulla to distal lamina and by analogy with similar elements in the insects. The morphologies of centrifugals differ little between the species.

One striking feature of the lamina's organization amongst decapod crustaceans is the general identicality between different species. It seems, therefore, that neural organization between species with superposition eye (*Pandalus*, *Homarus*, *Nephrops*, and the crayfishes) and those with appositional eyes (the crabs *Scylla*, *Leptograpsus*, and *Ocypode*) is surprisingly consistent and is not reminiscent of gross differences described for lamina organization between some insects such as *Notonecta*, on the one hand, and the beetle *Phausis*, on the other. However, there should be one word of caution: differences of lamina neuroarchitecture may possibly be more pronounced between diurnal and nocturnal insects, both with superposition eyes, than between apposition and superposition retinae of diurnal species (cf. *P. brassicae* and *Apis mellifica:* RIBI, 1975 a).

IV. Mysid and Euphausiacean Crustaceans

The two species of the two orders described here, *Neomysis integer* and *Meganyctiphanes norwegica*, have clear-zone superposition eyes, and their rhabdoms are fused and banded as in decapod crustacea (HALLBERG, 1977; KAMPA, 1965; MEYER-ROCHOW, 1978 b).

Neomysis integer, a shallow-water mysid, was studied from selective-silver and reduced-silver techniques (NÄSSEL, 1977 b) by light microscopy. Each ommatidium of *Neomysis* is said to consist of only seven photoreceptors, and it is claimed that an eighth distal receptor is absent in this species but is present in some related mysids (HALLBERG, 1977). The apparent absence of long visual fibres (R 8 axons) to the medulla of *N. integer* (NÄSSEL, 1977 b) lends some support to the above observation. The lamina is clearly bistratified with R 1–R 7 photoreceptors ending at two levels, corresponding to the dendritic arbors of the stratified monopolars M 3 and M 4 (Fig. 17). The lamina neuropil is also columnar, and M 2 type monopolars lie centrally to the axis of each cartridge. The cell bodies of the M 2, M 3, and M 4 monopolars do not reside over their respective cartridges, but are displaced to the lateral margins of the lamina. M 1 monopolars have not yet been identified from selective impregnation, but their presence is strongly suggested from observations of reduced-silver preparations. The putative M 1 neurons have their cell bodies lo-

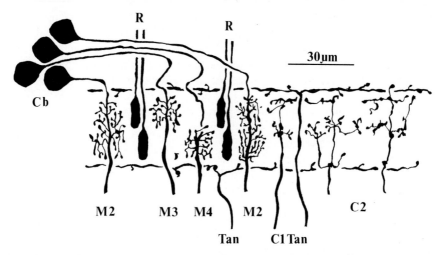

Fig. 17. Lamina of *Neomysis integer*. The monopolars of M 2–M 4 have their cell bodies *(Cb)* disposed laterally with respect to the neuropil. The receptors *(R)* terminate at two levels. Tangential neurons *(Tan)* are found distally and proximally in the lamina. Centrifugal (or possibly T-neurons) *(C 1, C 2)* have arborizations in one or several cartridges. No long visual fibres have been resolved

cated as a single layer abutting the distal surface of the lamina's plexiform layer, as in decapods (Nässel, 1975).

Observations of Golgi-impregnated material have shown that tangential fibres, distal and proximal to the plexiform layer, are derived from medulla-to-lamina tangential neurons, and that the two synaptic regions are also linked by small-field T-neurons whose arborizations spread through between one and three cartridges.

Meganyctiphanes norwegica (Fig. 18), a deep-sea euphausiacean, has been superficially studied with respect to neuron arrangements in the lamina (Nässel, 1977 b). As in previous examples, its lamina is bistratified with two levels of short receptor terminals and two levels of monopolars whose forms correspond to the M 2–M 4 types. No M 1 neurons have been detected by selective silver impregnation, and there is no evidence from reduced-silver studies that they are present. Accordingly, in this species all the monopolar cell bodies are located at the lateral margins of the lamina (see also Hanström, 1928). Two layers of tangential neurons can be seen in reduced-silver preparations, one distally the other proximally, in the lamina plexiform layer as in *Neomysis*.

V. Branchiopod Crustaceans

These non-malacostracan crustaceans have much-simplified visual systems. The retinae of the compound eyes of the two animals described here are of the appositional type and comprise only a few ommatidia: 22 in the water flea *Daphnia* and about 300 in the brine shrimp *Artemia*. No special pigment cells are present in the retina and the rhabdoms are fused and non-banded (Röhlich and Törö,

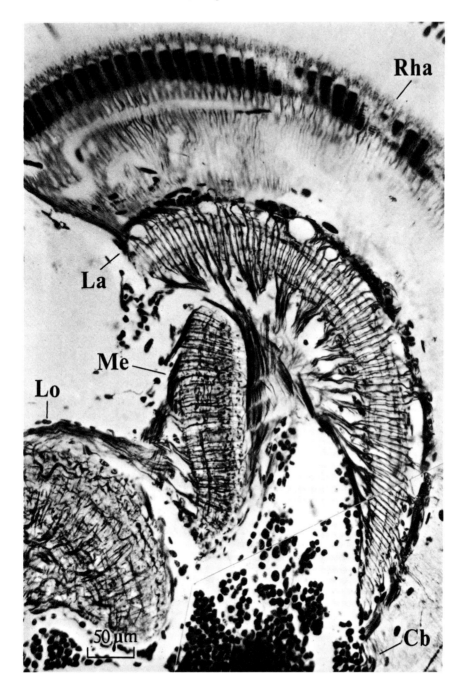

Fig. 18. Bodianreduced-silver preparations of retina and optic lobes of the euphausiacean *Meganycti-phanes norwegica*. The lamina *(La)*, medulla *(Me)*, and lobula *(Lo)* are each separated by chiasmata, seen in this horizontal section. The rhabdoms of the receptor cells are shown darkly stained *(Rha)*. Note the characteristically displaced perikarya *(Cb)* of lamina monopolar cells. Their cell body fibres run from this cluster parallel to the surface of the lamina to enter their respective cartridges

1965; Waterman, 1966; Güldner and Wolff, 1970; Elofsson and Odselius, 1975).

The optic lobes are small and reduced in number. Only a lamina and a medulla neuropil are present in the *Artemia* eyestalk (Hanström, 1924; Elofsson and Dahl, 1970), and the same is true in *Daphnia* except that the two eyestalks are fused to form a cyclopean eye. This means that in *Daphnia* the two retinae are fused, as are the two laminae. However, the medulla is partly divided (Retzius, 1906; Elofsson and Dahl, 1970), and there is no chiasma formed by the fibres connecting it with the lamina, as is the case in previously discussed malacostracans (Elofsson and Dahl, 1970). However, as in all the other species described, the projection of photoreceptor axons onto the lamina is strictly retinotopic (Retzius, 1906; Macagno et al., 1973; Nässel et al., 1978).

1. Artemia

The lamina of *Artemia* is bistratified and shows in its distal portion a clear subdivision of structural units (cartridges). Deeper, in the lamina's synaptic neuropil, this orderliness cannot be so easily detected (see below). The ommatidia of *Artemia* consist of six photoreceptor cells, one of which forms a small distal rhabdomere (Debaisieux, 1944; Elofsson and Odselius, 1975). Axons of five receptors terminate at two levels in the lamina, and the sixth axon comprises a long visual fibre that terminates shallowly in the medulla (Nässel et al., 1978). The lamina terminals of the photoreceptors give rise to slender lateral processes which overlap each other extensively. This rather unusual feature means that photoreceptors in different optic cartridges could interact directly with each other via lateral extensions rather than through interneurons.

Monopolar cells that appear analogous to M 3 and M 4 can be distinguished in Golgi preparations; they contribute to the lamina stratification (Fig. 19). Also, M 2-type neurons are resolved with dendrites disposed at both lamina strata. It is, however, not clear if any M 1-type monopolars are present although some neurons similar in appearance have been shown up by selective silver impregnation.

Large T-neurons *(Tan)* give rise to tangentially arranged processes in both lamina strata. Their axons connect the lamina directly with protocerebral centres (Fig. 20) without collaterals to the medulla. Centrifugal neurons arise from cell bodies in the proximal medulla cell body layer. Their axons arborize in the medulla and in both lamina strata (Fig. 20).

The columnar organization of the lamina is best seen in its distal layers. Pseudocartridges with six photoreceptor axons and between four and five other axons are identifiable above the plexiform layer. The axons enlarge and are heavily invested with branches upon entering the synaptic region. No distinct cartridges can be discerned, though the elements of the pseudocartridges maintain coherence, imparting a distinct periodic appearance of subunit organization to the lamina's distal cross-section. Two receptor axons terminate in the distal stratum of the lamina, three in the proximal stratum.

Synapses between photoreceptors and second order neurons are of the dyad type. An evaginating membrane area of the receptor terminal contains a presynap-

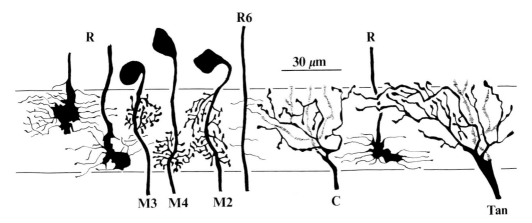

Fig. 19. Lamina cells of *Artemia salina* contain three types of monopolars *(M 2–M 4)*, stratified receptor cell terminals *(R)*, and long visual fibres *R6*. Together these comprise the columnar sub-unit organization. Tangential cells link the lamina directly to the protocerebrum *(Tan)*. Medulla-to-lamina centrifugal neurons (C) are found in proportion to columnar units (one to every six to eight columns). After
NÄSSEL et al. (1978)

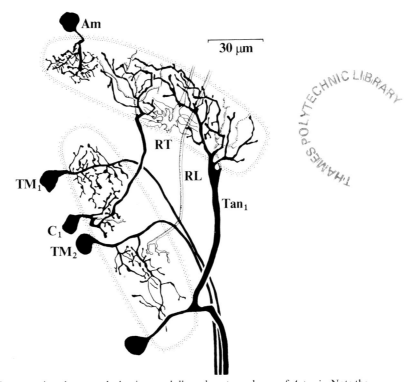

Fig. 20. Some of the connexions between the lamina, medulla and protocerebrum of *Artemia*. Note the
direct non-chiasmal retinotopic projection between the lamina and the medulla. *Am*, amacrine neuron;
RT, receptor terminal; *RL*, *R6* long visual fibre; *Tan 1*, tangential T-neuron connecting the lamina directly with protocerebrum; *TM₁* and *TM₂*, transmedullary neurons; *C₁*, centrifugal neuron. NÄSSEL et
al. (1978)

tic bar, and clear vesicles face the two postsynaptic profiles. The receptors are also reciprocally postsynaptic to second-order neurons by means of similar synapses where the photoreceptor is one of the two postsynaptic profiles, with another element of unknown origin.

ARAMANT and ELOFSSON (1976) have demonstrated catecholaminergic neurons in the *Artemia* lamina. These could possibly be related to neural profiles with small dense-cored vesicles which form a tangential network in the lamina as they do in the crayfish (NÄSSEL et al., 1978). No fibres with large dense-cored vesicles were resolved, in contrast to decapods (SHIVERS, 1967; NÄSSEL, 1975, 1976a; ELOFSSON et al., 1977) and *Daphnia* (WOLFF and GÜLDNER, 1970; NÄSSEL et al., 1978).

The medulla of *Artemia* is relatively simple compared to that of decapods. Relatively few distinct types of transmedullary neurons can be recognized and these connect the medulla directly with the protocerebrum. Together with a few forms of amacrine cells, medulla relay neurons form a simple stratified neuropil. Wide-field, large axon neurons serve to interact with large areas of the projected mosaic and project these from the medulla to deeper centres.

2. Daphnia

Although tiny, the compound eyes of *Daphnia* are as precisely arranged as the large eyes of decapods which consist of several thousand ommatidia. The eyes of *Daphnia* have a fixed number of ommatidia (22 units) and exactly the same number of underlying cartridges. There are eight photoreceptors per ommatidium and five second-order neurons per cartridge. Thus, 176 plus 110 elements comprise the periodic structure of the lamina neuropil (MACAGNO et al., 1973; MACAGNO and LEVINTHAL, 1975). Because of its numerical constancy and because *Daphnia* can give rise to parthenogenetic (isogenic) offspring, this organism has been extensively used for the study of variations in neural connectivities of the visual system, as well as for the analysis of its development (MACAGNO et al., 1973; MACAGNO, 1978, 1979).

The photoreceptor axons end at three levels (Fig. 21) and are characterized by enlarged terminations that have long and slender lateral processes which extend radially for a distance of about 20 μm, suggesting an extensive overlap amongst receptors (NÄSSEL et al., 1978). One form of receptor endings has elongated terminations in the middle stratum of the lamina. Two forms of receptor terminations appear flattened and reside either distally or proximally in the lamina. Possibly, however, some of the proximal flattened terminations are actually situated superficially in the medulla, as suggested by MACAGNO and LEVINTHAL (1975), and not in the lamina. This statement may appear surprising to the reader; however, *Daphnia* is extremely small, and it is difficult to resolve the precise levels of Golgi-impregnated elements without additional landmarks. The medulla lies almost immediately below the lamina, and the slightest tilting of the plane of section will confuse the resolution of stratifications. The lamina is thus bi- or tristratified, depending on the exact location of these terminals. If, however, the last-mentioned elements truly reside in the medulla, this would mean that *Daphnia* is the only species of Crustacea yet investigated to possess a paired arrangement of long visual fibres. Two morphological types of monopolar cells have been resolved in Golgi preparations

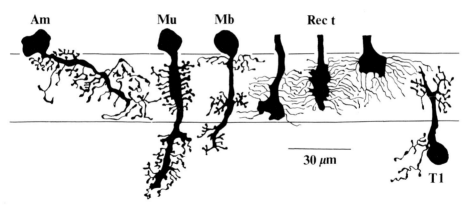

Fig. 21. Lamina elements of *Daphnia*. Three kinds of receptors are resolved *(Rec t)* which terminate at three levels (note the long lateral processes). Two types of monopolars have been resolved, one unistratified *(Mu)* and the other bistratified *(Mb)*. One kind of large-field amacrine cell *(Am)* (cf. Retzius, 1906, and Fig. 21) and a small-field medulla-lamina T-neuron *(T1)* have also been shown up by Golgi impregnations. Nässel et al. (1978)

(NÄSSEL et al., 1978) (Fig. 21). One of these is unistratified, the other bistratified. RETZIUS (1906), LEDER (1915), and NÄSSEL et al. (1978) showed two types of connexions between the lamina and the protocerebrum (Figs. 22 and 23). One type of tangential T-neuron connects the lamina directly with the protocerebrum; the other connects both the lamina and the medulla with the protocerebrum. One type of small-field T-neuron (NÄSSEL et al., 1978), as well as large-field amacrine cells (RETZIUS, 1906; NÄSSEL et al., 1978), also invade the lamina (Fig. 21).

It is difficult to resolve a columnar pattern of elements except in the most distal part of the lamina. "Pseudocartridges" with eight photoreceptor axons and five other profiles are readily resolved by electron microscopy. However, more proximally, the columnar organization seems to be concealed by the extensive branching of receptors and second-order neurons. Using computer-aided reconstructions from serial sections for electron microscopy, MACAGNO et al. (1973) did identify a periodic subunit organization of photoreceptor endings accompanied by second-order neurons that established characteristic synaptic connexions (MACAGNO et al., 1973). All the synapses hitherto described appear to have rather simple monadic relationships namely, one pre- and one postsynaptic profile (WOLFF and GÜLDNER, 1970; MACAGNO et al., 1973; NÄSSEL et al., 1978).

The *Daphnia* lamina contains fibres with small and large dense-cored vesicles (WOLFF and GÜLDNER, 1970; NÄSSEL et al., 1978) and, again, the Falck-Hillarp histochemical method demonstrated catecholaminergic neurons both in the lamina and the medulla (ARAMANT and ELOFSSON, 1976), indicating that this species shares many properties of optic lobe organization typical of the more elaborate Crustacea.

Monopolar neurons terminate in the distal layer of the medulla, and projections are carried through this region by a few types of relay cells originating from cell bodies in the proximity of the second synaptic region. These include neurons that link the lamina and the medulla with the protocerebrum as well as one cell type that connects the medulla alone with protocerebral neuropil.

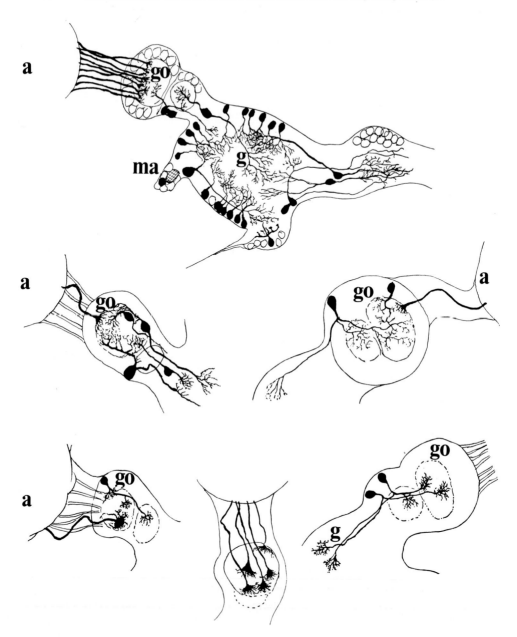

Fig. 22. The optic lobes of *Daphnia*, as drawn by RETZIUS (1906). The top illustration shows a sagittal view of the brain and the optic lobes. Different neuron types and the photoreceptors are illustrated. *go*, lamina, below which is situated the medulla; *g*, midbrain; *a*, retina of the cyclopean compound eye. Note the retinotopic projection between the retina and the lamina

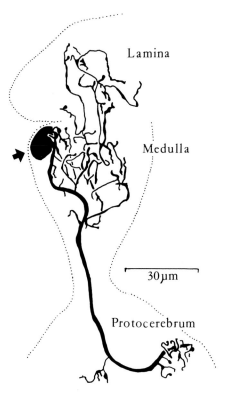

Fig. 23. One type of T-neuron which connects the lamina and the medulla directly to the protocerebrum in *Daphnia*. Nässel et al. (1978)

VI. Insect-Like Lamina in a Crustacean, *Squilla mantis*

1. Introduction

This species of stomatopod crustacean is described last in the section because its lamina shares many features typical of complex two- or three-tiered insect lamina. For example, the number and arrangement of cell types identified allows comparison with the lamina of another fast-moving aquatic predator, the hemipterous insect *Notonecta glauca* (see Sect. B), as well as with the simpler lamina of the crayfish. *Squilla* manifests at least six separately identifiable monopolar cells including a true midget neuron, similar in form to the L 5 cell of Diptera. Widefield monopolar neurons are also present and their axon collaterals project to adjacent cartridges in a way that is reminiscent of the dipterous L 4 monopolar and its homologues in Hymenoptera.

The eye of *Squilla* is hugely elongated along the vertical axis, and its hemi-cylindrical profile is deeply indented at the equator to give it the appearance of a double eye whose "two" retinae are dorsoventrally mirror symmetric. The lamina neuropil is likewise divided into two discrete areas, each subserving the dorsal and ventral eye half, respectively. The two sheets of lamina neuropil are linked by tangential plexuses whose processes are derived from amacrine cells and three types of medulla-derived terminals of wide-field centrifugal neurons. In this aspect the neuropil is not strictly divided into two separate and discrete areas. The two halves share possible substrates for wide-field adaptation circuits about the equator. The division of dorsal and ventral neuropil is no longer discernible in the medulla, which, in the present species, comprises a kidney-shaped region of neuropil whose construction is isomorphic across its dorsoventral extent.

2. The Retina and Its Projection to the Lamina

The structure of the retinal subunits has been extensively described from scanning and transmission electron microscopy by Schönenberger (1977). This author describes the retina's lattice as consisting of between 3,600 and 3,700 ommatidia, where each subunit has the following composition.

A lamellated corneal lens surmounts an eucone-type crystalline cone. A pair of distal pigment cells entirely enwrap the cone, and the photoreceptor elements of each ommatidium are sheathed by between 12 and 16 pigment cells which extend from the crystalline cone down to the basement membrane. Schönenberger describes seven large, and an eighth (basal), retinal cells. Although not explicitly stated in his account, the eighth retinal cell is illustrated as giving rise to a rhabdomere that extends distally. The remaining seven retinal cells contribute to a long, fused rhabdom that extends from the base of the crystalline cone to just above the basement membrane. The seven retinal cells, presumably, share the same optical alignment.

Light microscopical studies by Schiff-Sertorio and Strausfeld (unpublished observations) distinguished eight photoreceptor axons from each ommatidium that penetrated the basement membrane. These eight elements contribute to a coherent bundle which passes proximally to the lamina's plexiform layer. However, adjacent bundles sometimes converge and mix up their positions within an extensive fenestration layer (Fig. 24), giving the wholly erroneous impression that there is a lateral permutation of the peripheral retinotopic mosaic. This is, however, not so: although each bundle may shift its location by up to as much as 50 μm laterally (within a trajectory of between 400 and 600 μm), each bundle separates from its companion to become relocated at its proper (homotopic) retinotopic position at the level of the cell body layer. Axon bundles project further into the lamina's plexiform layer where they give rise to three levels of terminals (Figs. 24 and 25).

Terminals of receptor cells in the lamina (here presumed to be those seven elements that contribute to the fused rhabdom) give rise to a pair of outer endings stacked above two pairs of inner endings that overlap in depth (Fig. 25). A seventh unaccompanied terminal ends somewhat deeper (Figs. 25 and 26), and occasionally these give rise to slender processes that extend between 10 and 30 μm into the first optic chiasma (Fig. 26). These observations detect an unambiguous projection of two receptor fibres to a depth that exceeds the proximal limit of the external plexiform layer (Fig. 26). However, only one axon from each ommatidium has been unequivocally followed to the medulla. These long visual cells impart a map of the retinal mosaic directly into second-order neuropil. A simple anteroposterior inversion of the retina is mediated via the first optic chiasma.

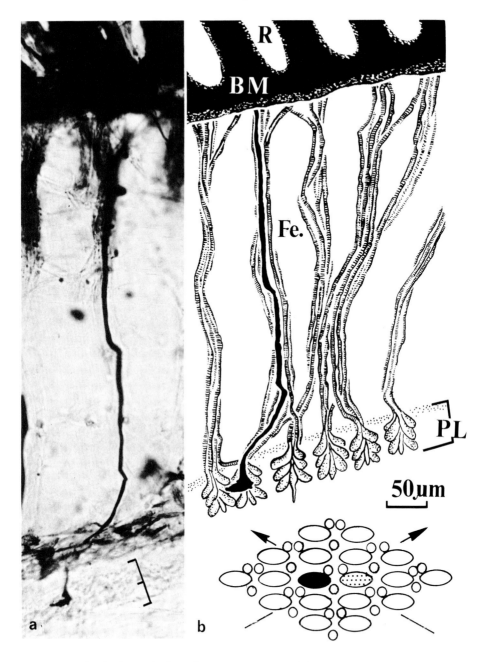

Fig. 24 a, b. Retina-lamina projections of *Squilla mantis*. To the left is shown a singly impregnated receptor axon with a terminal in the outer stratum of the plexiform layer *(PL)*. The drawing to the right illustrates the homotopic trajectories of axon bundles from five ommatidia to five adjacent optic cartridges. One Golgi-impregnated cell is shown amongst the characteristic triple-layered endings (stippled). The deepest terminal is shown as a clear profile. Beneath is illustrated the compressed orthogonal tessellation of optic cartridges (vertical axis is from left to right of the picture). *BM.*, basement membrane; *R*, retina; *Fe*, fenestration layer

3. Structure of the Lamina

The lamina neuropil can be subdivided into three strata on the basis of the different levels of receptor terminals. This tripartite organization is reflected in the structure of many types of lamina interneuron.

Although the *Squilla* nervous system is difficult to stain with Golgi methods, there is some information about the shapes of cells, their structural variations, and their topological relationships within and between optic cartridges.

4. Monopolar Cells

The seven endings from each ommatidium impart a strict orthogonal lattice to the lamina whose two axes are aligned between 30° and 60° from the horizontal (Fig. 24). Velate glial cells are interposed between each of the terminal cartouches. Their nuclei reside beneath and above the plexiform layer and between each cartridge (Fig. 25).

Two large-diameter monopolar cells reside on the axis of each cartridge (M 1 a, M 1 b; Fig. 26). M 1 a gives rise to dendrites at the level of the outer and second tier of receptor endings, whereas M 1 b processes are disposed at the level of the second and third tier of endings. Both cell types give rise to a single process that extends ventrally or dorsally towards the equatorial midline, depending on which side of it they are located. Their lateral processes extend across the equatorial midline to the first row of ventral or, conversely, dorsal cartridges.

A second neuron, M 2, has a narrow field of dendrites disposed at the level of all seven short receptor endings and so arranged as to establish contact with their surfaces most central to the axis of their parent cartridge. In contrast, each M 3 cell is characterized by two stout lateral "arms" whose tips are festooned with short protuberances. Golgi observations reveal these as clasping the outermost receptor-axon terminals of their respective cartridge.

Two wide-field neurons have been resolved by Golgi impregnations. One, here labelled M 4, consists of a set of long, but sparse, axon collaterals. These reside at the level of the second tier of axon terminals, and extend dorsally and ventrally as far as the two most adjacent cartridges. By comparison, the wide-field neuron, M 5, possibly subtends only two cartridges. However, it is rarely impregnated, and at present its precise topological relationships remain unresolved.

5. Amacrine Cells and Large-Field Centrifugals

Amacrines must now be considered a standard component of both insect and crustacean laminae. In *Squilla* one form of amacrine has been resolved whose processes are derived from perikarya beneath the proximal margin of the external plexiform layer. Possibly other forms exist, hitherto unresolved, and it should be borne in mind that the recent discovery of a second species of amacrine in the most extensively researched of any arthropod neuropil (the lamina of *Calliphora* and *Musca;* NÄSSEL and SEYAN, in preparation) means that the likelihood of achieving

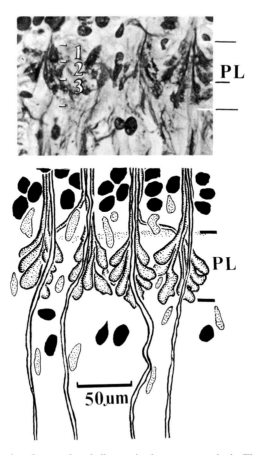

Fig. 25. The upper illustration shows reduced-silver stained receptor terminals. The lower illustration is a tracing from a reduced-silver preparation which shows the triple-tiered arrangement of short visual fibre endings in the plexiform layer *(PL)*. This can be approximately divided into two main strata as shown above. A single long visual fibre passes alongside the axis of each cartridge and penetrates the inner face of the lamina, en route to the medulla. Nuclei of neurons are shown as black profiles. Nuclei of glial cells are stippled. (Reduced-silver preparation by courtesy of H. SCHIFF-SERTORIO)

a complete inventory of cell types requires the use of many variations of the Golgi method, each of which is selective in its own right.

Amacrines of *Squilla* extend through the lower tiers of terminals and may just reach the outermost endings of receptor axons. Their processes are characterized by rosette-like specializations which are mainly concomitant with arborizations of lamina-to-medulla T-cells. This topographical relationship is analogous to α-β-relationship in the lamina of the fly (CAMPOS-ORTEGA and STRAUSFELD, 1973).

Three large-field centrifugal afferents have been resolved in the *Squilla* lamina. One contributes to a dense tangle of processes at the outer margin of the plexiform layer, whereas another contributes to a rather precise orthogonal network of processes at its inner layer (see Fig. 27 B). Both cell types arborize extensively in the lamina and are linked to multistratified or diffuse wide-field domains of processes

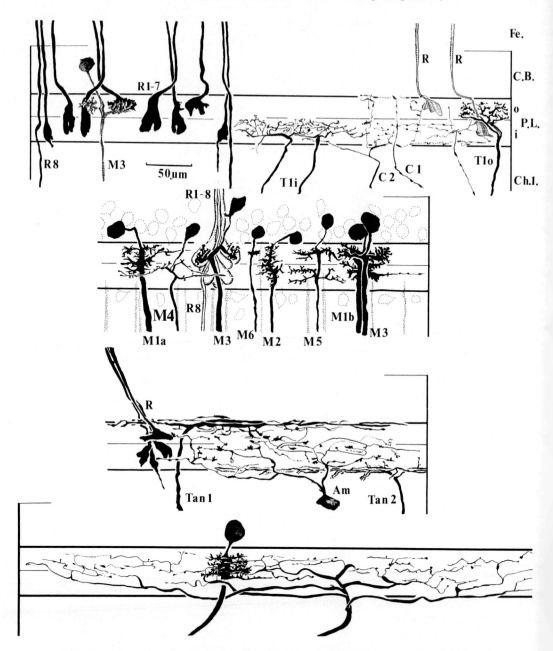

Fig. 26. Neurons in the lamina of *Squilla mantis*. The upper diagram illustrates the forms of receptor terminals *(R1–R7)* and the passage of long visual fibres *(R8)*. Note that each level of endings is characterized by a particular receptor profile. Deepest endings sometimes give rise to a prolongation into the outer 10–30 μm of the first optic chiasma. The *M 3* monopolar cell is shown clasping one distal receptor ending. To the right are shown the two forms of lamina-medulla T-cells *(T1o* and *T1i)* disposed at two distinct levels of the plexiform layer. *C 1* and *C 2* centrifugals are classified according to their lateral spread in the lamina and the relative depth of penetration into the centre stratum and distal stratum of the plexiform layer. *Fe.*, fenestration layer; *C.B.*, monopolar cell body layer; *P.L.*, outer *(o)*

in the medulla. Their cell bodies reside above the distal surface of the second synaptic region. A third form of tangential cell has diffuse processes through all the lamina layers (Fig. 26).

6. Small-Field Lamina-to-Medulla T-Cells and Medulla-to-Lamina Centrifugal Neurons

One type of small-field T-cell, derived from cell bodies above the medulla, links the medulla to the lamina. Its processes arborize within the two inner strata of the external plexiform layer and extend through a vertical domain of between two and four cartridges. Their fields in the medulla have identical lateral extents. Two forms of small-field centrifugals have been resolved, both of which are derived from perikarya beneath the medulla's inner face. These cells have characteristic arborizations in the lamina, one extending through all its layers, the other restricted predominantly to the level of the second and third tier of receptor endings. Both centrifugal elements invade between two and four cartridges, and their fields are elongated vertically. Both cell types are also characterized by slender blebbed processes, in contrast to the spiny and varicose branches of the lamina-to-medulla T-cells.

7. Tangential Organization

As in other Crustacea the wide-field tangential centrifugal cells contribute to dense plexuses of lateral processes above and beneath the plexiform layer. Amacrines arborize freely within this layer. However, the M 1 a and M 1 b monopolar cells also contribute to the lamina's lateral organization, as does the M 4 neuron. Figure 27 A shows an oblique section across the plexiform layer in which the Tan 1 arbor is resolved with intercartridge plexuses derived from M 1 a and M 1 b cells with contributions from the type C 1 centrifugal.

Figure 27 C illustrates the cross-section of a single M 3 monopolar cell, showing its bilaterally arranged arms which are, in fact, restricted to a single optic cartridge. In contrast, Fig. 27 D shows an M 1 a monopolar cell with a lateral process that extends to at least the nearest neighbour cartridge, if not beyond.

◄ and inner *(i)* layers of the plexiform layer. *Ch. 1.*, the distalmost part of the first optic chiasma. The centre illustration shows the types of monopolar cells hitherto found in *Squilla. M 1 a* and *M 1 b* are analogized with *M 1* elements of decapod crustacea, as is *M 2*. Note the unilateral fibres extending away from the axis of both *M 1* types. These project to adjacent cartridges. The *M 3* monopolar neuron is characterized by a bilateral arrangement of two stout dendrites (arms) whose specializations appear to clasp the two outermost receptor endings of a cartridge. The *M 4* neuron is more reminiscent of the *L 4* monopolar in flies than its nominal counterpart in decapods. The *M 6* (midget monopolar) has been resolved on many occasions and must be classified as a separate cell type on the basis of its cell body position and the paucity of distal dendrites at the level of the outer tangential plexus. The third illustration shows the dispositions of two types of wide-field medulla-to-lamina centrifugal cell, *Tan 1* and *Tan 2*. Their terminal processes are disposed at the upper and lower surfaces of the lamina, above and below dendrites of monopolar cells. In contrast, the arborizations of the amacrine cell *(Am)* branch freely within the lamina's plexiform layer. The bottom illustration is of a third type of tangential ending of an axon from the medulla

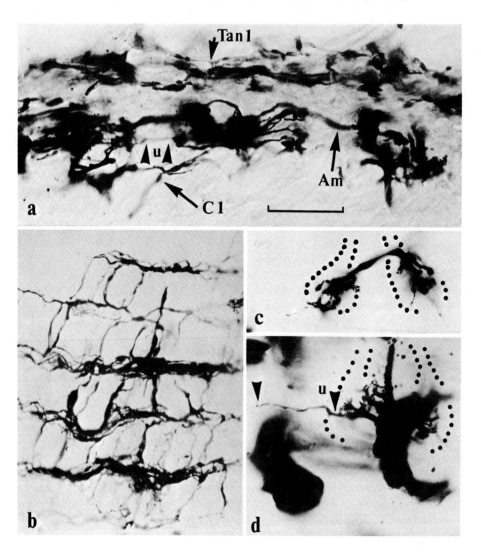

Fig. 27a–d. Lateral projections in *Squilla* lamina. **a** Processes of *Tan 1* reside above dendrites of mono-polar cells and project over many optic cartridges. However, centrifugal elements and tangentially di-rected fibres also provide a structural substrate linking several optic cartridges, as do serial arrange-ments of unilateral processes of *M 1* neurons (arrowed). **b** *Tan 2* contributes to a regular orthogonal network of fibres beneath the lamina's inner face. Monopolar cell and long visual fibre axons pass as coherent bundles through the meshes of this network. **c** At first sight the bilateral branches of *M 3* ap-pear to be disposed in such a way as to link neighbouring cartridges. However, this is not so, as illus-trated in Fig. 26. The lateral spread of the *M 3* neuron is equal to the distance between the outer edges of a pair of shallow receptor terminals *(R)*. **d** In contrast, the unilateral process of *M 1* monopolars ([*u*] resolved in the lower half of the lamina, beneath the equator) extend for a distance equivalent to at least two optic cartridges, adjacent along the vertical axis

In summary, the lamina of *Squilla* is rigidly compartmentalized into discrete optic cartridges. However, the great majority of associated centrifugal and relay neurons do not respect the constraints of a single retinotopic pathway, but contribute to systems of extensive overlap between pathways, as they do in other insects and Crustacea. The M 1, M 4 and M 5 cells contribute to lateral pathways between adjacent cartridges, as is the case in many insect laminas.

8. The Midget Monopolar Cell M 6

This element is characterized by a set of short distal dendrites at the level of the Tan 1 arborization. In this respect it is analogous to the L 5 neuron of Diptera (STRAUSFELD, 1970) which is now known to be postsynaptic to the Tan 1 neuron of *Musca* and, possibly, one of six short receptor endings. The M 6 cell of *Squilla*, like its counterpart in *Musca*, is also characterized by a perikaryon which is closest to the outer surface of the external plexiform layer.

C. The Optic Lobes of Insects

I. Introduction

Retinotopically organized neuropils are arranged beneath the insect compound eye much in the same way as already demonstrated from the crayfish and some other Crustacea. Axons of photoreceptors penetrate the basement membrane of the retina and project into the lamina neuropil, sometimes traversing long distances in the fenestration layer. The majority of photoreceptor axons terminate in the first optic neuropil, usually at two distinct levels. However, in most insects a special pair of photoreceptor axons penetrate through the lamina and eventually terminate within the outer medulla. In some Hymenoptera three axons from an ommatidium reach the medulla. This is in contrast to all the unambiguous descriptions of Crustacea where only a single "long visual" fibre has been recognized as passing from an ommatidium into a medullary column.

As in the crayfish, three major neuropils contribute to the optic lobes. These are: the lamina, medulla, and lobula. However, in three orders (Coleoptera, Lepidoptera, and Diptera) the lobula is clearly divided into an anterior and a posterior neuropil, each connected to the medulla by retinotopic projections. T-shaped fibres also link the medulla to both parts of the divided neuropil, and there are separate homotopic-retinotopic projections between its two divisions. The posterior component of the "lobula complex" has been termed the "lobula plate" by BULLOCK and HORRIDGE (1965), the word "plate" adequately describing its shape which is a thin tectum of neuropil posterior to, and facing, the distal (input) surface of the lobula. In some other orders of insects such as the Orthoptera, the undivided lobula is accompanied by a satellite region of neuropil, much like the *of 1* optic focus of the crayfish, that receives a point-for-point projection from the lobula and the medulla. This arrangement has been observed in *Locusta* and *Schistocerca*. Similarly, there is a plate-like sheet of retinotopic neuropil situated dorsally, satellite to the lobula, in species of Odonata and Ephemeroptera (Strausfeld, 1976b).

In the "undivided" lobulae of Hymenoptera the neuropil is bipartite, characterized by a longitudinal division of the tissue. The lobula neuropil comprises a thin outer leyer that includes more or less one-quarter of its depth, separated from a thicker inner layer by bundles of tangential cell axons that sweep out into the optic pedunculus. This tangential layer is here termed the "lobula serpentine layer." Inner and outer layers are linked by retinotopic, small-field, short-axoned relay neurons whose shapes are most reminiscent of short-axoned T-neurons connecting the lobula and lobula plate (in Lepidoptera, Diptera, and Coleoptera). In general, the insect lobula should be considered as a divided neuropil, whether or not the two divisions are contiguous.

Likewise, the second optic neuropil (the medulla) is bipartite, and its division is a general feature of all insects hitherto studied. Characteristically, its outer levels are composed of neuronal arrangements which show rigid precision of their retinotopic arrangements. Palisades of neurons maintain their geometrical spacing proximally as far as a pronounced layer of tangential axons comprising the medulla's serpentine layer or "cuccati bundle." A similar layer has been resolved in Crustacean optic lobes. As in Crustacea, the serpentine layer divides the medulla into two distinct levels of neuro-architecture where strata proximal to the serpentine layer contain the dendrites of T-shaped or Y-shaped neurons that project to the lobula and/or to the lobula plate or the equivalent levels in "undivided" lobulae. At the inner medullary level, retinotopic channels are again multiplied, and the arrangement of axons and dendrites contribute to a complex lattice in which structural imprecision is inherent.

In the following sections the medulla is treated as two separate subregions of neuropil: an outer and an inner layer. Evidence from developmental studies (see review by Meinertzhagen, 1973) indicates that the inner region is derived from the same embryonic origin as the lobula complex, whereas the outer layer of the medulla and the lamina are derived from a separate anlage.

It is apparent that there are obvious structural affinities of cell arrangements in the outer medulla and in the lamina on the one hand, and between the inner medulla and the lobula complex on the other. Possibly these reflect two general classes of functional connexions that are characteristic to one or the other level. In summary, the insect optic lobe, and by analogy, that of Crustacea, is apparently composed of five discrete neuropils: (1) the lamina (the external plexiform layer); (2) the outer medulla (the internal plexiform layer); (3) the inner medulla; (4) the lobula; and (5) the lobula plate, or an equivalent neuropil beneath the lobula's serpentine layer (e.g., in Hymenoptera).

II. The Resolution of Neurons
and Their Basic Arrangements in Optic Lobes

Single nerve cells can be resolved either by selective impregnation by the Golgi method or by mass uptake of cobalt cations or by uptake and dye coupling of STEWART's (1979) Lucifer yellow (STRAUSFELD and BACON; in preparation). In all cases the entire spread of the neuron is resolved as has been demonstrated by combined Golgi and electron microscopy methods (CAMPOS-ORTEGA and STRAUSFELD, 1973; STRAUSFELD and CAMPOS-ORTEGA, 1973a) or by combined cobalt-silver staining and electronmicroscopy (ALTMAN et al., 1979, 1980; HAUSEN and WOL-BURG-BUCHHOLZ, 1980). However, whereas the Golgi method mainly provides a compendium of nerve cell shapes, cobalt impregnation resolves novel structures in neuropil. These are assemblies of nerve cell populations. Recently horse-radish peroxidase and cytochrome c have been used to resolve entire neurons, and combined with electronmicroscopy, reveal synaptic connections in both labelled and unlabelled neurons (NÄSSEL et al., 1980).

A rough impression of the analytical power of Golgi methods, in terms of resolving features of neural architecture, can be seen in Fig. 28, a composite drawing of single nerve cells in the medulla, lobula, and lobula plate of the fly lobe. It demonstrates the complexity of form of each individual cell and the apparent heterogeneity of structure which, in the light of recent cobalt studies, is, in fact, misleading. This impression is due to the stochastic nature of the Golgi method, for it is impossible to demonstrate spatial relationships amongst a specific nerve cell population. The Golgi method does, though, allow statements about layer relationships as well as the forms and destinations of single neurons.

Cobalt impregnation best demonstrates cell assemblies (p.97), and the passage of axons leading off from the lobes, and reveals their typical patterns of terminals onto descending neuron's dendrites. As described from the crayfish (Sect. B), relay neurons which are retinotopically spaced in the lobula lose this geometry during their passage to the lateral midbrain. Their axons bundle together and usually terminate predominantly in non-columnar neuropil of the "optic foci." Each focus receives an input from one or several classes of lobula cells, and the patterns of their terminations onto the dendrites of descending neurons are characteristic for that class of relay elements. These patterns may possibly represent transformations of their maps in the lobula mosaic to those which are appropriate to the message they carry. For example, nerve cells that subserve the anterior retina and which may terminate nearest to the base of the dendritic tree of the final output neuron from the brain may act differently than those subserving posterior retina and terminating at the tips of the tree and therefore confer positional information onto the postsynaptic cell.

Figure 29 summarizes the kinds of structural organization in the insect lobes as seen from observations of the three light microscopy methods: reduced silver, Golgi and cobalt impregnation.

Channels from the retina diverge twice, once in the lamina onto sets of monopolar cells and centripetal T-neurons and a second time to columnar relay neurons in the medulla. Endings from long visual fibres and lamina relay cells diverge to

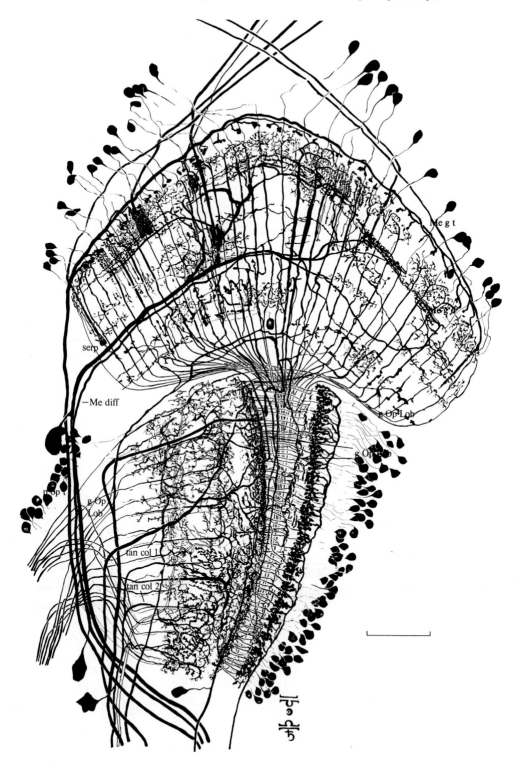

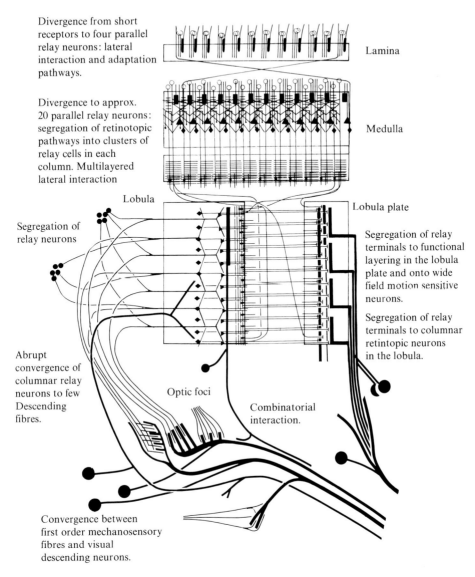

Divergence from short
receptors to four parallel
relay neurons: lateral
interaction and adaptation
pathways.

Lamina

Divergence to approx.
20 parallel relay neurons:
segregation of retinotopic
pathways into clusters of
relay cells in each
column. Multilayered
lateral interaction

Medulla

Lobula

Lobula plate

Segregation of
relay neurons

Segregation of relay
terminals to functional
layering in the lobula
plate and onto wide
field motion sensitive
neurons.

Segregation of relay
terminals to columnar
retintopic neurons
in the lobula.

Abrupt
convergence of
columnar relay
neurons to few
Descending
fibres.

Optic foci

Combinatorial
interaction.

Convergence between
first order mechanosensory
fibres and visual
descending neurons.

Fig. 29. Summary diagram of the principle organization of the optic lobes (lamina, medulla, lobula, and lobula plate) and projections from the lobula complex to optic foci of the lateral protocerebrum

◀ **Fig. 28.** Drawings of Golgi-impregnated neurons in the medulla, lobula, and lobula plate of *Musca domestica*. Nerve cells are arranged as columnar palisades (relay neurons) or tangentially (wide-field relay neurons leading off to the midbrain), or anaxonal amacrine cells. Some terminals are shown derived from the lamina, projecting to levels of columnar relay-cell dendrites. Medullary columnar cells project across the second chiasma to the lobula plate or to the lobula. Together, Golgi-impregnated cells demonstrate layer relationships of forms of neurons and their destinations in other regions. The scale bar equals 50 μm. (Adapted from STRAUSFELD, 1976)

as many as 20 types of transmedullary neurons which project to the lobula complex. Layers of amacrine cells provide systems of local circuitries: lateral interaction, feedback loops, and so forth. These presumably provide the relevant connectivities for various filters which compute edge detection, motion, centre-surround fields, colour features, and the like. Recent electrophysiological studies on the medulla have shown that cells exist there with quite complicated response properties, and some of these small field neurons have been identified by dye-marking (see p. 115).

Medulla relay neurons can be separately classified according to their profiles, the levels at which they end in the lobula or the lobula plate. These levels are also distinguished by the dendritic assemblies of columnar or wide-field relay neurons leading off to the midbrain. Pathways from the medulla converge at the level of lobula (third-order) neuropil in such a way that a single lobula relay neuron has a space relationship of one to several identical retinotopic inputs (usually a ratio of 1:9). Possibly there is at least one morphological type of lobula relay cell postsynaptic to each functional pathway of the medulla, though this has yet to be demonstrated. Some evidence is provided by wide-field cells of the lobula plate that structurally summate the entire projected retinotopic field. Two examples are the horizontal or vertical motion-sensitive neurons that reside in the distal and proximal layers, respectively (HAUSEN, 1976a, b, 1977). Small-field input neurons presumably relay information about horizontal motion computed in the medulla and terminate superficially in the lobula plate. These seem to be distinct from a parallel system of neurons that relay information about vertical motion and which end deeply in the lobula plate. Other wide-field relay neurons at these layers link the left- and right-hand neuropils or project to optic foci of the ipsi- and contralateral protocerebrum that receive the terminals of exclusively ipsilateral neurons. A schema of connectivities for the horizontal motion-sensitive system is summarized at the end of this account and is derived from procion yellow staining of recorded neurons (HAUSEN, 1976a, b).

In the strict sense, output from the optic lobes is carried by very few neurons indeed. Recent electrophysiology and structural identification suggests that output neurons are multimodal, carrying visual and mechanosensory information (see section C VIII). Neurons that are postsynaptic to lobula cells pass from optic foci to other brain regions or, more commonly, project from the foci to the neuropils of the body ganglia. This means that a population of one type of lobula relay neuron comprising 300 cells may terminate on a single descending relay neuron. This is an abrupt reduction of the numbers of parallel pathways: namely, a reduction ratio of between 300:1 and 30:1, depending on whether the lobula relay neurons are distributed throughout the retinotopic mosaic or are restricted to a special zone of it (see Sect. C.III.3). In terms of columnar pathways that lead from the medulla the final reduction of the number of channels is at least 3,000:1.

Exact structural analysis of these cellular relationships is important for electrophysiology. Recording from a single descending neuron can exploit its relationships with all converging pathways, the neuron itself serving as a multi-electrode probe of cellular activity and integration. However, proper interpretation of the electrophysiological record can be made only after cell-cell connexions are known.

Information about the synaptology of the optic lobes is mainly confined to the first optic neuropil of the dipteran lamina. Although some combined Golgi and electron microscopy has been performed on Hemiptera (WOLBURG-BUCHHOLZ, 1979) and Hymenoptera (MEYER, 1979) and conventional electron microscopy on species of Odonata (ARMETT-KIBEL et al., 1977), it is the fly that has received most attention and provided most of the data about complex synaptology. In this species *(Musca domestica)* principal connexions have been resolved between receptors and centripetal neurons that lead off from the lamina and between small- and wide-field centrifugal cells that project distally from the medulla. Also, it is only in *Musca* that connexions between amacrine cells and other neurons are known.

The following sections describe the fly lamina in some detail and compare its structure with the same region in *Notonecta* (Hemiptera), *Phausis* (Coleoptera), *Apis* and *Cataglyphis* (Hymenoptera), and *Sympetrum* (Odonata). The remainder of the account outlines the way in which the retina is mapped through the neuropil as a set of retinotopic projections and illustrates how neurons are arranged within this framework. Most of the descriptions are derived from reduced-silver studies and cobalt impregnations and describe the arrangements of cells that subserve the whole or parts of the retina. These include sex-specific neurons and binocular projections between the two lobulae. Descriptions of single cell anatomy have been kept to an absolute minimum because a recent account has dealt with this at length (STRAUSFELD, 1976 b). And, in any case, single-cell descriptions are largely irrelevant to the main theme of the account which is concerned with the organization of groups of cells. This being the case, orders of insects other than Diptera figure less predominantly simply because they have not yet been studied in sufficient detail.

III. The Lamina

1. Projections of Receptor Axons to Relay Neurons

Open rhabdomere retinae are found amongst dipterous insects (DIETRICH, 1909; KIRSCHFELD, 1967; BRAMMER, 1970; ZEIL, 1979), Hemiptera (LANGER and SCHNEIDER, 1970) and some species of Coleoptera (WACHMANN, 1977) and Orthoptera (ECKERT, 1968). However, correlations between the pattern of projections of receptor fibres and the open rhabdomere optics of the compound eye are known only from Diptera (see studies by KIRSCHFELD, 1967, 1973; KIRSCHFELD and FRANCESCHINI, 1968; SCHOLES, 1969; ZEIL, 1979). KIRSCHFELD (1967) showed that seven rhabdomeres of each ommatidium have divergent optical axes. However, six wide-diameter receptors, distributed amongst a trapezoid configuration of six ommatidia, but sharing the same optical axis, project to a common locus in the lamina neuropil. This is the optic cartridge (see KIRSCHFELD 1967; TRUJILLO-CENÓZ, 1965; BRAITENBERG, 1967). The central rhabdomere of each ommatidium is composed of two receptors (R 7, R 8) that are arranged in tandem (TRUJILLO-CENÓZ and MELAMED, 1966) and share a common optical alignment which is identical (or nearly identical) to the optical axis of the lens above it (KIRSCHFELD and FRANCESCHINI, 1968). Axons of R 7 and R 8 receptors project down alongside the optic cartridge beneath their ommatidium of origin, and containing the R 1–R 6 endings of like optical alignment, bypassing all other elements of the cartridge and apparently devoid of synaptic connexions. The R 7 and R 8 axons comprise pairs of long visual

Re   La

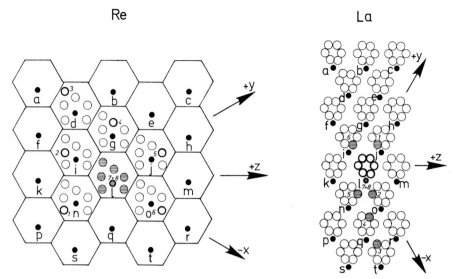

Fig. 30. Arrangements of R 1–R 6 and R 7+R 8 receptors in retina (*Re*) and lamina (*La*) of *Musca, Calliphora* etc. Each lens surmounts the rhabdomeres of six short visual elements (R 1–R 6) and a pair of long visual fibres (R 7 and R 8). This diagram illustrates R 1–R 6 elements beneath seven lenses and R 7+R 8 fibres beneath 20 lenses. The six short retinal cells and pair of long visual fibres beneath each lens have seven different optical alignments. R 1–R 6 (cross hatched in ommatidium *l*) project to six different lamina cartridges (*i,j,n,o,q,t*) in the way described by BRAITENBERG (1967). Six retinal cells that share the same optical alignment are arranged in six different ommatidia (heavy circles numbered 1–6 in ommatidia *n,i,d,g,j,* and *o*). These project to the same optic cartridge (*l*) in the lamina (KIRSCHFELD, 1967; BRAITENBERG, 1967). The long visual fibre pair which shares the same alignment as the set of R 1–R 6 (KIRSCHFELD and FRANCESCHINI, 1968) resides in a seventh ommatidium (*l*) and projects more or less straight down into the lamina alongside optic cartridge *l*. Other R 7+R 8 receptors (black in ommatidia *a–k* and *m–t*) likewise project homotopically beside the corresponding optic cartridges beneath them. (CAMPOS-ORTEGA and STRAUSFELD, 1972; permission by Springer-Verlag)

fibres that map the receptor mosaic into the medulla (Fig. 30). Degeneration studies (CAMPOS-ORTEGA and STRAUSFELD, 1972a, b) and cobalt or horse-radish peroxidase injections into the retina (NÄSSEL, 1980) have shown that the neighbourhood relationships between adjacent pairs of long visual fibres are maintained between the retina and medulla despite the anteroposterior reversal of their linear order by the first optic chiasma (STRAUSFELD, 1971 b). Long visual fibre projections of Diptera are non-permutating and homotopic, as are the projections of R 1–R 8 (and R 9) described from apposition eyes of the bee (Fig. 31). Species of Lepidoptera (STRAUSFELD and BEST, 1970) and the beetle *Phausis splendidula* also are characterized by non-permutating projections of R 7 and R 8 axons (OHLY, 1975).

Fig. 31 a–d. Different levels of the retina and lamina in the bee (left, micrographs; right, tracings). ▶ These reduced-silver sections show **a** cross-sections of retinulae just under the nuclei of R 1–R 6 visual cells; **b** sections across the proximal retina above the level of their penetration through the basement membrane; **c** sections across the cell body layer of the lamina; and **d** across the external plexiform layer. In **d** the short endings of receptor cells are absent. Projections of axon bundles of each ommatidium keep their lateral relationships with bundles of neighbouring ommatidia. (Reproduced by permission of W.RIBI and Springer-Verlag)

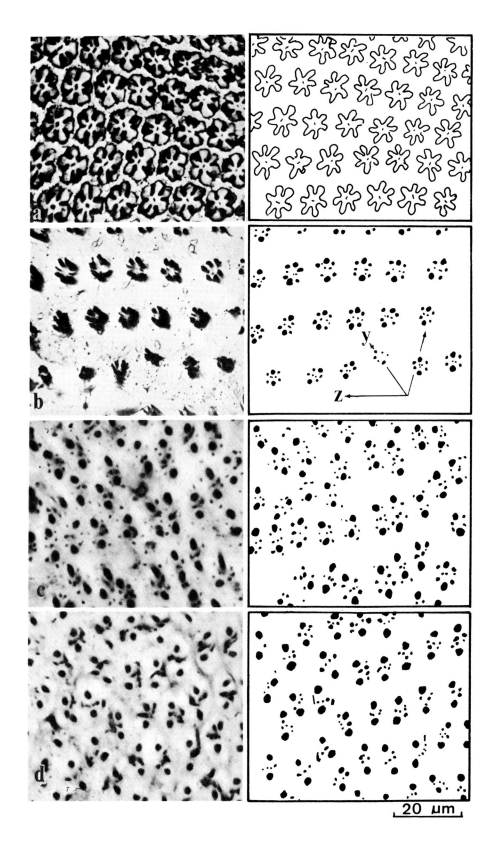

20 μm

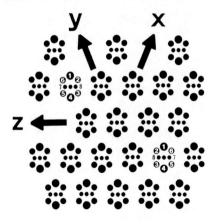

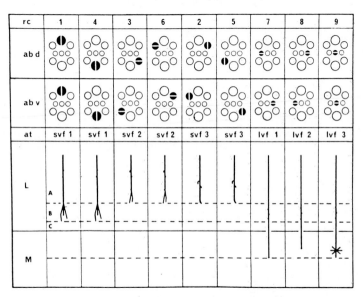

Fig. 32. Cyclic arrangement of short receptor axons around triplets of long visual fibre axons in the bee lamina optic cartridges (upper diagram). The lower diagram classifies the numbered *(rc)* receptor cell types *(at)* according to the level of penetration into the lamina and the shape of their profiles (see also RIBI, 1979). Golgi thin-section studies relate each type of receptor cell to the relevant profile of an optic cartridge in the dorsal *(ab d)* and ventral *(ab v)* lamina, either side of the eye's horizontal equator. Note the mirror symmetry of cyclic order with respect to cells *svf 2*, *svf 3*, *lvf 1*, and *lvf 2*. Note also that three types of long visual fibres pass to deep layers of the outer medulla *(M)*. The major strata of the lamina *(L)* are indicated A,B,C. (Reproduced by permission of W.RIBI and Springer-Verlag)

MEINERTZHAGEN'S (1976) study of insects with fused rhabdomeres has shown that the groups of short visual fibres to the lamina project coherently to the nearest cartridge beneath their ommatidium of origin. Thus, in apposition eyes each optic cartridge receives a set of terminals that shares the same optical alignment. RIBI's (1979) studies of the bee substantiate this. Serial sections from the level of ommatidia down to the lamina show that bundles do not mix and do not permutate the receptor mosaic. The axons from one ommatidium retain their neighbourhood

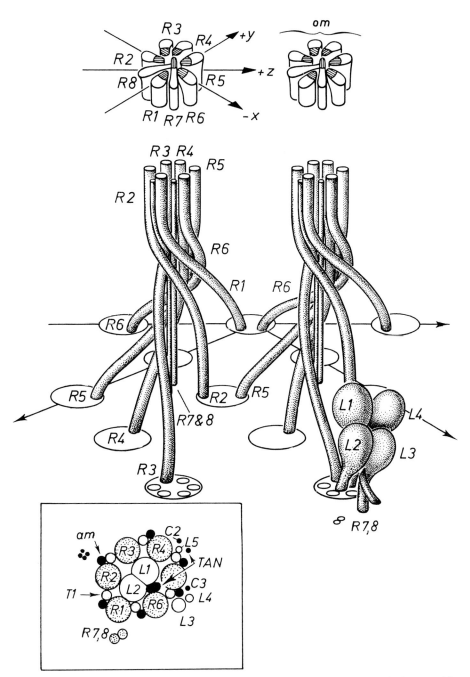

Fig. 33. Updated diagram of the projections of six short receptor cells *(R1–R6)* from single ommatidia into six optic cartridges. The cyclic arrangement of rhabdomeres in ommatidia of the fly retina *(om)* is shown with the orientations of microvilli in the distal segments. Receptor axons *R1–R6* have divergent optical axes in an ommatidium and their trajectories accordingly diverge to appropriate cartridges in the lamina. *R2* of the left-hand ommatidium shares the same optical alignment as *R5* of the right-hand ommatidium, and both fibres project to the same target in the lamina. The inset illustrates the cyclic order of receptor terminals in the upper lamina of the right-hand eye and shows the typical cross-sectional locations of lamina neurons. Monopolar and T1 relay cells are open profiles; centrifugal *(C2, C3, Tan 1, Tan 2)* and amacrine elements *(am)* are black profiles. (Adapted from STRAUSFELD, 1971 a)

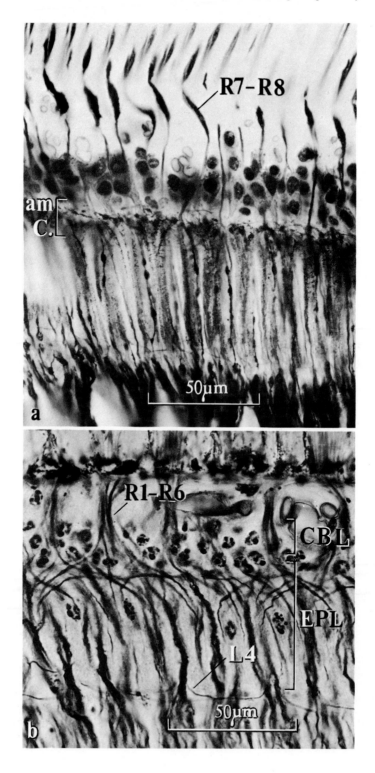

relationships in the bundle from the level of the basement membrane into the lamina. As in the fly, specific types of receptors reside at specific locations about the axis of the rhabdomere. This cyclic order is maintained amongst the set of terminals of the cartridge (Fig. 32). In bees, as in Diptera, the cyclic arrangement of the receptors is mirror symmetric between the upper and lower eye halves. This also applies to geometrical relationships between receptors and axis fibres of relay neurons (monopolar cells). TRUJILLO-CENÓZ (1965) and, later, BRAITENBERG (1967) showed that in Diptera, sets of six short-axoned receptors follow a complex, divergent pathway to six destinations in the lamina (Figs. 33 and 34). The cyclic arrangement of six terminals in a single cartridge (derived from six ommatidia) is the same as that of six receptors distributed amongst a trapezoid arrangement of six ommatidia in the retina but rotated through 180° (BRAITENBERG, 1967) (see Fig. 30). As predicted by VIGIER (1907a, b, 1909) and demonstrated by KIRSCHFELD (1967) the parallel optical axes of six rhabdomeres amongst six ommatidia and the subsequent convergence of their (R 1–R 6) axons to a common locus in the lamina serve to channel information from identically aligned receptors to a common set of relay neurons, the monopolar cells (Fig. 33).

In contrast to the dipterous "neural superposition" eye, and apposition eyes, axon projections from superposition retinae (EXNER, 1891; KUNZE, 1969, 1972) are less precisely organized. In the nocturnal moth *Sphinx ligustri* axons from a set of fused rhabdomeres penetrate roughly the same point of the lamina and then spread laterally in a somewhat messy fashion amongst the dendrites of wide-field monopolar neurons. Dendrites of these relay cells overlap extensively and could, in principle, derive an input from as many as 20 bundles of afferents (cf. CAJAL and SÁNCHEZ, 1915; STRAUSFELD and BLEST, 1970). By comparison, in the apposition eye of the diurnal butterfly, *Pieris brassicae*, the lamina appears to be organized in columns and the lateral spread of axon terminals is less pronounced. The largest dendritic domain of a monopolar cell extends through a maximum of only nine receptor axon bundles. In the superposition eye of the nocturnal beetle, *Phausis splendidula* (OHLY, 1975), the lamina is not strictly compartmentalized into cartridges. Receptor cells are seen to diverge laterally and possibly there is some mixing of their lateral relationships even though their retinotopic distribution is approximately maintained. A greater precision of axon projections has been observed in the diurnal beetle *Hoplia farinosa* (STRAUSFELD, 1976b) and, in this species, some receptors were observed with axon collaterals. In these Coleoptera there are two forms of wide-field monopolar cells at the level of receptor terminals which possibly derive their input from several sets of projections. One other form of wide-field element gives rise to processes beneath the level of axon terminals, as is the case for some

---

◄ **Fig. 34a, b.** Two views of the lamina of *Musca* showing non-permutating projections of R 7/R 8 fibres from each ommatidium selectively backfilled from the medulla by cobalt chloride injection. The lower figure illustrates divergence of R 1–R 6 fibres from ommatidia and convergence at optic cartridges revealed by reduced-silver. **a** Also shows mass impregnation of backfilled T 1 baskets, C 2 centrifugals and monopolar cells. *c* and *am* layer indicates the distal level of centrifugal connexions and tangential pathways of amacrine cells. *CBL* is the cell body layer (shown in **b**). *EPL* is the external plexiform layer which is bordered proximally by the network of L 4 axon collaterals

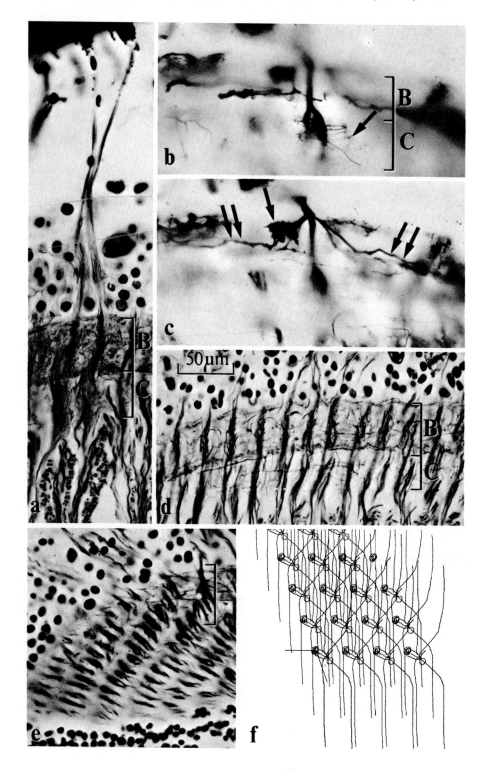

species of monopolar cells in the bee and in the fly. These may constitute substrates for lateral interactions (e.g., the L 4 monopolar cell; see p. 81).

In hemipterous insects, receptor projections are superficially even more complex than in Diptera. The open rhabdomere eye of Hemiptera (LANGER and SCHNEIDER, 1970) consists of four large-diameter rhabdoms that are distributed asymmetrically around the margin of an ommatidium and partly surround a pair of long-axoned R 7 and R 8 receptors. R 7 and R 8 are flanked by two small-diameter, short-axoned receptor elements. As in the neural superposition retina of Diptera, or the apposition eyes of Odonata and Hymenoptera, hemipterous R 7 and R 8 axons project as a pair directly to the medulla (STRAUSFELD, 1976). As in Hymenoptera and damsel flies (Odonata), R 7 and R 8 also give rise to lateral processes in the lamina. These may reflect some distal synaptic connexions between long visual fibres and interneurons (STRAUSFELD, 1976; RIBI, 1975 a, b, 1979; WOLBURG-BUCHHOLZ, 1979).

In Hemiptera, only two small-diameter, short-axon receptors project to the outer and inner layers of the lamina, penetrating the optic cartridge that resides beneath their ommatidium of origin. The remaining four large-diameter receptors of an ommatidium give rise to rather slender axons that pass to the outer layer of the lamina and then abruptly diverge to give rise to tangentially directed endings (Fig. 35 e, f).

Reduced-silver studies of *Notonecta* show that all the receptor axons from an ommatidium project as a single bundle to the lamina surface, even though the distance between the lamina and basement membrane of the retina is quite extensive (between 40 and 200 μm) (Fig. 35 a). Observations of serial 2-μm araldite sections, stained with toluidine blue, show the arrangements amongst the photoreceptor axon cross-sections of each bundle to be consistent across the fenestration layer. In *Notonecta* axons from the four wide-diameter receptors project between 10 and 20 μm into the outer stratum of the external plexiform layer and then bend through 90° to run tangentially through the distal neuropil for a distance equivalent to about six adjacent optic cartridges (see WOLBURG-BUCHHOLZ, 1979; STRAUSFELD, 1976 b). Observations of reduced-silver and Golgi impregnations show that the orientation of tangentially directed receptor axons is vertical, two above and two beneath their point of entry into the lamina (Fig. 35 e, f). Thus, they invade two

---

◄ **Fig. 35 a–f.** The lamina of *Notonecta glauca*. **a** Homotopic projection of two adjacent bundles of receptor axons from the retina across a 200-μm distance in the fenestration layer. The lamina of this species and other Hemiptera is bistratified at the level of the plexiform layer (levels B and C after WOLBURG-BUCHHOLZ's terminology). **b, c** Terminals from the retina end as tangentially directed processes in layer B (double arrows in Fig. 34 c) or as displaced terminals in layer B (single arrow in Fig. 34 c). A single ending from each receptor bundle ends in layer C (Fig. 34 b) and gives rise to vertically directed processes (arrowed). **d** The arrangements of processes from relay cells and other interneuron types are roughly arranged according to the two main levels of receptor endings. However, it can be seen that several other strata are disposed in layers B and C that are not directly correlated with the structure of receptor terminals. **e** This oblique section through the lamina shows the regular arrangement of cartridges and vertically oriented receptor tangential ending (from left to right, bracketed) in layer B. **f** A computer reconstruction of the pattern of projections from ommatidia (open circles) to optic cartridges in the lamina (filled profiles) to illustrate the tangential network of four short receptor endings from each ommatidium. In **f** the vertical axis is oriented from top to bottom, in **b** and **c** it is left to right

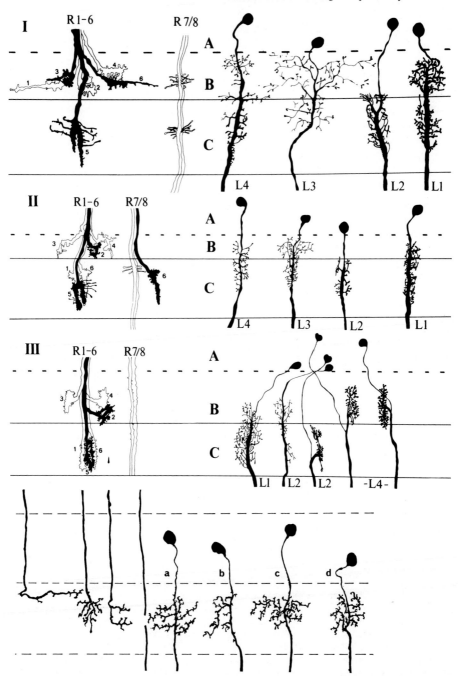

Fig. 36. Comparisons between monopolar cells and levels of receptor terminals in three species of Hemiptera, *N.glauca (I)*, *C.punctata (II)*, and *G.lacustris (III)*, showing species-specific differences of receptor terminal morphology and corresponding differences in the branching patterns and levels of relay cells (see text). The lower figure illustrates forms of branched receptor endings and a tangentially directed receptor ending in the lamina of the cockroach, *Periplaneta americana*. (*I–III* by permission of K.WOLBURG-BUCHHOLZ; lower diagram by permission of W.RIBI)

parallel rows of cartridges, extending from a centre locus; this is the cartridge containing the paired axons of the long visual fibres from the same ommatidium and the two short terminals from its small-diameter receptors. One short terminal is displaced laterally, away from the cartridge's long axis, and ends shallowly in the lamina's outer stratum (Fig. 35 b, c). The other short terminal projects deep into the second layer of the plexiform layer where it gives rise to a bilateral arrangement of slender processes which project dorsally and ventrally towards the nearest neighbour cartridges (see STRAUSFELD, 1976 b; WOLBURG-BUCHHOLZ, 1979, and Fig. 35 b, c).

The receptor projection pattern of hemipterous photoreceptor axons appears to depart radically from that of any other species and, by analogy with Diptera, is suggestive of a neural superposition eye. However, the optical alignments of the receptors of a single ommatidium are not yet known, and it may be that the permutation of the receptor map by tangentially directed axon terminals is trivial. This distribution may only reflect a pattern of connexion between one class of receptor and one type of wide-field lamina monopolar cell (L 3; WOLBURG-BUCHHOLZ, 1979) whose dendrites are vertically aligned and extend over a considerable distance of the superficial strata of this region. Illustrations in a comparative study by WOLBURG-BUCHHOLZ are suggestive of this (Fig. 36). In *Notonecta* wide-field monopolar cells (arbitrarily named L 3) have distal dendritic spreads that are equal to the spread of tangential receptor endings. In *Notonecta* both dendritic fields of L 3 and the receptor passage are extensive. However, in *Corixa punctata* and in *Gerris lacustris*, both hardly pass to the next cartridge. In *Gerris* the lateral spread of the receptor axons is, in fact, so insignificant that there is no monopolar cell worth labelling "L 3."

Similar matching between receptor terminal alignments and the disposition of monopolar dendrites has been shown in the cockroach lamina (see RIBI, 1977, and Fig. 36). At least one type of receptor axon projects tangentially even though it is derived from a fused rhabdomere which presumably shares a common optical alignment with seven other elements. Correspondingly, the dendritic tree of one form of monopolar cell (type c, lower diagram of Fig. 36) is widespread at the level of the tangentially directed receptor terminal. It is therefore important to consider the significance of lateral projections of receptors with respect to the shapes of monopolar cells: lateral projections of photoreceptor axons do not automatically imply neural superposition or mixing between retinotopic channels. In laminae whose receptor endings are strictly arranged as columns, monopolars usually have narrow fields. Only in laminae of superposition eyes is it feasible that many sets of receptors converge onto a single wide-field monopolar cell, and in *Sphinx*, for example, it is possible that overlapping monopolar cells are mutually pre- and post-synaptic (see also Fig. 39; *Phausis splendidula*).

2. Cell Types

Golgi studies of the insect lamina have distinguished four major cell classes. [Lepidoptera (STRAUSFELD and BLEST, 1970), Hymenoptera (RIBI, 1975, 1976, 1979; MEYER, 1979). Coleoptera (OHLY, 1975; STRAUSFELD, 1976), Odonata (STRAUSFELD, 1976; ARMETT-KIBEL et al., 1977), Hemiptera (PFLUGFELDER, 1937;

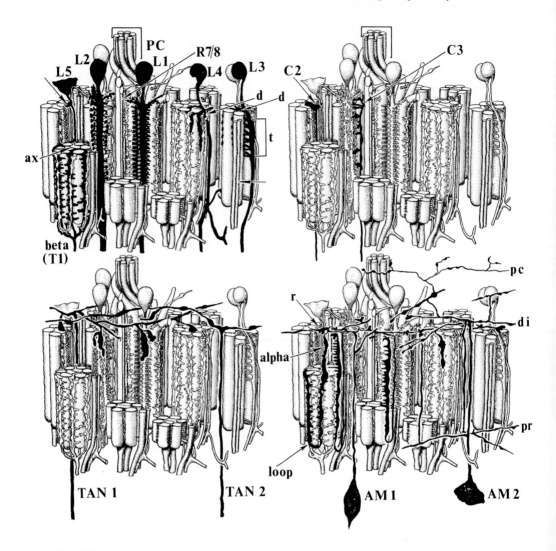

Fig. 37. Neuronal element in the lamina of *Musca domestica*, shown against a background of ten "dissected" optic cartridges. *L1*, *L2*, and *L3* are the three monopolar cells which derive input from a set of six receptor endings. *T1* (beta) is the basket of dendrites of a fourth direct centripetal relay to the medulla. *C2* and *C3* are narrow-field centrifugal endings associated with *L1–L3* and receptors, and *L1/L2*, respectively. Two forms of tangential centrifugals are shown, lower left. The two species of amacrine cells are shown lower right. *Am 2* has special relationships with bundles of receptor axons above the level of their decussation to optic cartridges. *Am 1* is characterized by looped processes that give rise to alpha fibres and by tangential processes that give rise to rosette *(r)* and blebbed specializations. *ax*, pairs of axial fibres of L 1 and L 2; *pc*, pseudocartridge (bundles of R-axons before their decussation) *d*, dendrites of L 3 and L 4 in the outer one-third of the lamina; *t*, level of triad dendritic configurations between receptors and *L1*, *L2*, and *L3* monopolars. (Adapted from Strausfeld, 1971)

STRAUSFELD, 1976; WOLBURG-BUCHHOLZ, 1979), and Diptera (STRAUSFELD, 1970, 1971 a, b, 1976 b; CAMPOS-ORTEGA and STRAUSFELD, 1972, 1973; STRAUS-FELD and CAMPOS-ORTEGA, 1973, 1977).] The classes are (1) terminals of short receptor axons and the en passant segments of long visual fibres; (2) columnar relay neurons (monopolar cells and T-cells); (3) centrifugal neurons: and (4) amacrine cells. Columnar relay neuron dendrites at receptor endings are commonly restricted to one optic cartridge in laminae that subserve apposition or neural superposition retinae. In laminae that subserve superposition retinae, monopolar dendrites may extend through several sets of axon projections from the retina. In all laminae there are two forms of relay neurons: monopolar cells, derived from cell bodies situated distal to the lamina, and small-field T-cells whose cell bodies are situated above the surface of the medulla. The forms of lamina elements in the fly are shown in Fig. 37, drawn against a background of "dissected" optic cartridges.

The lamina has neuronal arrangements that are typical of all deeper levels of the system. These include tangential cells such as the wide-field endings of medulla-to-lamina centrifugal neurons and complex systems of amacrine cell interconnexions. As in the medulla, the amacrine cell provides a two-fold system of functional pathways: local circuits within single retinotopic columns and connexions that extend over quite long distances between columns. These probably serve as lateral interaction pathways between retinotopic channels. As in the medulla and lobula, relay neurons are not invariably postsynaptic to a centripetal input, but instead can be connected to the afferent input via intermediate amacrine synapses. Examples of these are serially arranged amacrine-amacrine circuits or amacrines arranged in series with centrifugal terminals. Some types of relay neurons are characterized by axon collaterals that link neighbouring retinotopic channels. These also probably serve as substrates for lateral inhibition or excitation. Possible functional-structural correlates between synaptology and electrophysiology are discussed in a recent account with reference to the fly lamina and recordings from fly and dragonfly relay neurons (see STRAUSFELD and CAMPOS-ORTEGA, 1977).

3. Lamina-Medulla Connexions and Forms of Medulla Terminals

Bundles of fibres can be traced the whole distance from the base of the lamina to the medulla. Reduced-silver preparations of *Musca* show that output bundles derived from horizontal rows of cartridges comprise sheets of fibres that link these two neuropils. Each sheet is folded over on itself in such a way that the sequence of cartridges is mapped in the reverse order at the medulla's surface (STRAUSFELD, 1971 b; BRAITENBERG and STRAUSFELD, 1973). This simple crossover is called the first optic chiasma and is found in every species of insect hitherto studied. Reduced silver preparations unambiguously resolve the axons of the R 7 long visual fibre and the L 1, L 2, and L 3 monopolar cells. Small-diameter fibres cannot be discerned by this method. Nevertheless, Golgi preparations indicate that small-field centrifugal elements, R 8 receptor axons and axons of T 1, L 4, and L 5 neurons maintain their lateral relationships between the two regions. Recently, cobalt injections have proven without doubt that all relay cells preserve the retinotopic mosaic between the two visual neuropils contrary to an isolated observation from *Pieris*

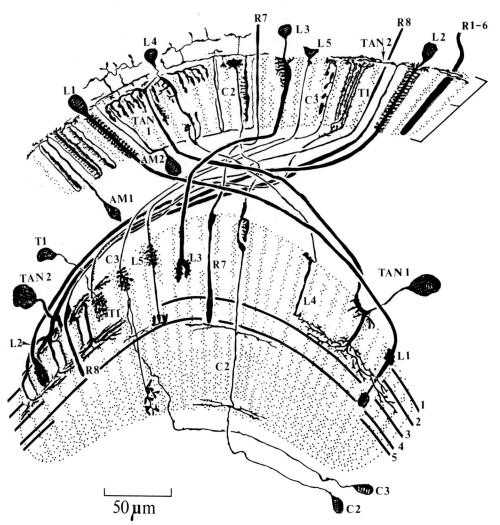

Fig. 38. Summary diagram of types of neurons in the lamina and between the lamina and medulla (see text). *1–5* are the levels of medulla neuropil characterized by neurons to or from the lamina (*Musca*)

brassicae (STRAUSFELD and BLEST, 1970). Injection of cobalt cations into the medulla backfill entire populations of medulla-to-lamina neurons (C2 and C3) as well as the L4, L5, and T1 elements. Cobalt pools generated in the retina allow all pairs of long visual fibres to be followed to the second synaptic region (see Fig. 34a).

Golgi impregnations reveal that each cell type recognized at the level of the lamina has a characteristic profile in the medulla. Figure 38 summarizes the known cell types connecting these regions in the fly and illustrates the clear differences of morphology between the L1 and L2 monopolar neurons with respect to their levels of endings. As in the crayfish (see Sect. B) centrifugal cells arborize at several levels in the medulla and presumably derive their input from sub-serpentine layers as well as levels of monopolar and long visual fibre endings. In contrast, wide-field centri-

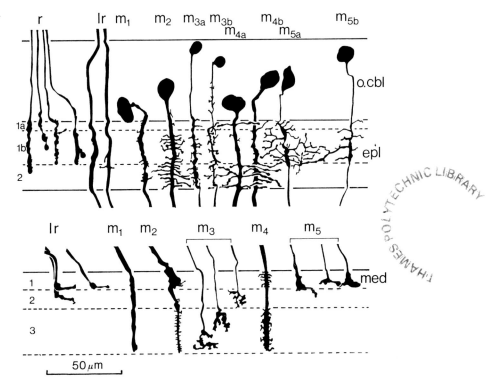

Fig. 39. Forms of receptor terminals and monopolar cells in the lamina, and terminals in the medulla, of the beetle *Phausis splendidula* (for explanation, see text). (OHLY, 1975, with permission of Springer-Verlag)

fugal cells (Tan 1 and Tan 2) arborize exclusively at the level of endings from the lamina and the retina. Golgi-electron microscopy has shown that some terminals have quite complex interrelationships. L 5 monopolar cells, for example, end closely apposed to the L 1 from the same cartridge (CAMPOS-ORTEGA and STRAUS-FELD, unpublished observations). Electron microscopy observations have shown that L 1 either establishes direct synaptic contact with medulla-to-lobula relay neurons or is presynaptic via serial synapses mediated by the L 1/L 5 complex.

The forms of long visual fibre terminals in the medulla are known for the bee (RIBI, 1975a), the ant *Cataglyphis bicolor* (MEYER, 1979), the butterfly *Pieris brassicae* (STRAUSFELD and BLEST, 1970), the fly, *Musca domestica* (CAMPOS-ORTEGA and STRAUSFELD, 1971), and the beetle *Phausis splendidula*. A study of *Phausis* (OHLY, 1975) has shown that long visual fibres end shallowly in the medulla, in contrast to the bee and the fly, at the same level as the terminals of wide-field monopolar cells, M 5a and M 5b (Fig. 39). OHLY's studies describe eight forms of monopolar cells in the lamina, which could be grouped together as five separate types, M_1–M_5. There are, correspondingly, five distinct forms of endings in the medulla. Some variation is shown by the depths of penetration of one cell type (M_3), but apart from this there is less variation of shapes between the endings of monopolar cells than between their distal components (Fig. 39).

In the ant, *Cataglyphis bicolor*, five monopolar cells have been distinguished from Golgi preparations (MEYER, 1979) of which two (L 1 a and L 1 b) are distinguishable only by their medullary endings. This is also the case for the dipteran L 1 and L 2 monopolar cells (Fig. 38). In the ant, long visual fibres terminate deep in the medulla's outer strata.

In both the ant and the bee at least three forms of neurons link the medulla centrifugally to the lamina. However, it is not known whether these elements are centrifugal in terms of their synaptic relationships or whether they are centripetal in nature, as is the T 1 cell of dipterous insects (see Sect. IV.4).

RIBI's studies on the bee optic lobes (1975, 1976) also indicate that the projections between the lamina and medulla are unpermutated except for a simple anteroposterior crossover. His studies describe six forms of monopolar cells in the lamina, each characterized by a typical branching pattern in the medulla. However, later accounts generalize four monopolar cell types. In the bee there are three forms of long visual fibres which end deeply in the medulla.

IV. Complex Cell Relationships: The Organization of the Fly Lamina

1. Receptor Terminals

The fly lamina contains only one morphological type of receptor terminal. Physiologically, all R 1–R 6 elements seem to share the same spectral sensitivities (STARK et al., 1976) and absolute sensitivity properties (JÄRVILEHTO and MORING, 1976; KIRSCHFELD and FRANCESCHINI, 1969). This is in contrast to the bee, and possibly the cockroach, where different levels of photoreceptor terminals may possibly be correlated with different spectral sensitivity properties of the respective receptor components in the retina (see discussion in RIBI, 1979).

In Diptera *(e.g. Musca, Calliphora, Drosophila, Lucilia, Tabanus, Sarcophaga)* short receptor endings terminate at the same level in the cartridge and comprise a hollow crown of tube-like structures closed at their proximal end. Occasional Golgi impregnations show that receptor endings sometimes have spines that project towards the centre of the crown. However, this is unusual and may be correlated with the occasional paucity of dendritic spines from the axial monopolar cells. Instead of contact between a receptor terminal and monopolar by dendritic expansions, connexions may possibly be established by outgrowths from a receptor ending to the axis fibre of the relay cell.

The cyclic order of receptor terminals in the crown is precise and is reiterated between optic cartridges. The arrangement of cross-sectional profiles can be described according to geometrical axes that are inherent to the neuropil mosaic (two oblique and one horizontal axis [BRAITENBERG, 1967]). Similarly, cross-sectional profiles of interneurons can be exactly described with reference to receptor terminal positions (see Fig. 33).

2. Monopolar Cells

A pair of axis fibres resides within each receptor crown. These are the "axial" monopolars, termed L 1 and L 2 by BRAITENBERG (1967) or "giant monopolars" of CAJAL and SÁNCHEZ (1915) and TRUJILLO-CENÓZ (1965). A second pair of monopolar cells is situated outside the crown, adjacent to the endings of R 5 and R 6. These neurons have been labelled L 3 and L 4 and correspond to the brush monopolar cell and tripartite monopolar cells, respectively (BRAITENBERG, 1967; STRAUSFELD, 1970, 1971 a; STRAUSFELD and BRAITENBERG, 1970). A fifth monopolar resides outside the cartridge beside the terminals of R 4 and R 5. Because of the paucity of lateral processes this element has been termed the "midget" monopolar cell, abbreviated to L 5 (STRAUSFELD 1971 a). L 1–L 5 have been resolved in all the abovementioned species of Diptera and in the hoverflies *Eristalis tenax* and *Syrphus nitidicollis*. Their dispositions are shown in Fig. 33 with respect to the cartridge cross-section, and their forms are illustrated in Fig. 37 against a dissection of ten optic cartridges whose structure has been derived from comparative studies of Golgi and reduced-silver impregnations.

Golgi studies show that the pair of axial monopolar cells is almost indistinguishable in the lamina. In cross-section their fibres are aligned along the "Y-axis" linking the cross-sections of receptor terminals R 4 and R 1. The profile labelled L 1 is arbitrarily assigned to the cross-section nearest the pole of the lamina neuropil beside the receptor endings R 3, R 4, and R 5. Both L 1 and L 2 are characterized by spines down their length in the plexiform layer. At any level these spines radiate to all six receptor endings.

The monopolar cell L 3 gives rise to dendritic branches only within the outer one-third of the plexiform layer. These extend into the lumen of the cartridge, wrap around the axis fibres of L 1 and L 2, and insert between adjacent receptor endings (CAMPOS-ORTEGA and STRAUSFELD, 1971). In contrast, L 4 and L 5 dendrites are not apposed to receptor terminals. Dendrites of L 4 are profuse in the anterior medial lamina, especially beneath the male fovea (see p. 103) where they number between six and eight processes. These extend through the outer one-third of a cartridge's length. Further posteriorly and at the poles of the lamina, L 4 dendrites are small and fewer in number. In contrast, all L 5 monopolar cells give rise to between one and two short processes that reside at the surface of the plexiform layer. Entire populations of L 5 neurons have been resolved by cobalt backfills from the medulla (STRAUSFELD and HAUSEN, 1977) and show that their dimensions and shape are uniform across the lamina's extent.

3. Synaptology of L 1, L 2, and L 3 and Receptors

Each of the six receptors establishes presynaptic connexions with the dendrites of L 1 and L 2 monopolars. Pairs of L 1/L 2 specializations are arranged as dyads opposite a single presynaptic T-shaped ribbon at the receptor membrane or with L 3 dendrites as triads opposite a single ribbon or with a glial profile, or a profile

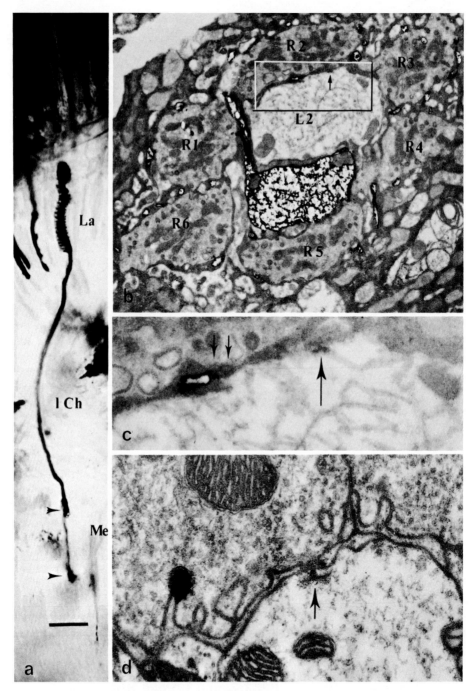

Fig. 40. a Golgi-electron microscopy analysis of lamina connexions *(Calliphora)*. This figure illustrates an impregnated *L1* monopolar cell which was later sectioned for electron microscopy. **b** Its silver-chromate-impregnated profile is shown lying adjacent to the impregnated cross-section of *L2*, and both elements are seen encircled by cross-sections of *R1–R6* receptor endings. x 10,000. **c** Dyad arrangement between a T-shaped presynaptic site (double arrows) and the profile of *L2* (clear) with a silver chromate-filled profile from *L1*. The single arrow shows the monadic relationship of a reciprocal synapse from *L2* to the receptor. x 30,000. **d** Conventional electron micrograph showing the *L2*-to-*R* relationship. x 38,000

of some other neuron, as tetrads (BURKHARDT and BRAITENBERG, 1976). Typically, each L 1 and L 2 neuron gives rise to six rows of dendrites. Each row consists of between 12 and 18 outgrowths from the axis fibre. Each dendrite ends as a rosette-like specialization. A petal of the rosette represents one postsynaptic site. L 1/L 2 pairs receive an identical input in terms of the numbers of receptor synapses onto their dendrites. These vary between 300 and 400. However, as is the case in the dragonfly *Sympetrum* (ARMETT-KIBEL et al., 1977) only one of the two large monopolar cells of each cartridge (their M 1–M 2 being analogous to the fly L 1–L 2) is postsynaptic to receptor membranes that are immediately adjacent to the monopolar main axis. In flies this is shown by monadic connexions between receptors and L 2, and in *Sympetrum*, between receptors and M 2. In the fly such synapses are resolved only in the lower synaptic stratum of the lamina, at the level of reciprocal pathways between L 2 monopolars and receptors, and where L 2 is presynaptic to its partner, the L 1 monopolar (Figs. 40, 41).

Dendrites of L 3 extend to all six receptors, dividing into branchlets and rosettes. These contribute to triads or tetrads of postsynaptic configurations, being flanked by a dendritic spine of L 1 and L 2. There are approximately two-thirds fewer presynaptic sites from receptors onto L 3 than onto either L 1 or L 2 (STRAUSFELD and CAMPOS-ORTEGA, 1972).

4. The Fourth Centripetal Pathway (T 1): The β-Fibres

Conventional electron microscopy reveals two sets of climbing fibres (α and β) that enwrap each set of receptor endings (TRUJILLO-CENÓZ and MELAMED, 1970). These are distinguishable on the basis of specific electron microscopical criteria such as their relative electron opacity and the presence of peculiar electron-dense indentations into only one (the α-fibre) of each pair (the so-called gnarls; BRAITENBERG and STRAUSFELD, 1973). It was found that both the α- and its mimetic β-components were postsynaptic to receptors and that the two fibres were pre- and postsynaptic to each other (CAMPOS-ORTEGA and STRAUSFELD, 1973). This finding was in contrast to previous descriptions by TRUJILLO-CENÓZ and MELAMED (1970) and by BOSCHEK (1971). No evidence was found that the two fibres twisted about each other (cf. BOSCHEK, 1971), and only the α-fibre could be identified as presynaptic to receptor endings. These findings appose earlier claims that α and β elements represented a system of presynaptic centrifugal fibres (cf. TRUJILLO-CENÓZ and MELAMED, 1970; BOSCHEK, 1971). However, Golgi-electron microscopy substantiated TRUJILLO-CENÓZ and MELAMED's findings that the β-fibres are in fact derived from a T-shaped neuron that connects the lamina and medulla. Each cell gives rise to a basket of six climbing fibres from the axon (STRAUSFELD, 1970, 1971a) and these contain the six terminals of short receptor axons at an optic cartridge. Comparative studies of *Lucilia* and *Musca* (CAMPOS-ORTEGA and STRAUSFELD, 1973) showed that the basket elements of the lamina are predominantly postsynaptic to receptors. This being so, each set of receptors must be considered as contributing directly to four parallel centripetal channels, L 1, L 2, L 3, and T 1. T 1 (β) terminates in the outer stratum of the medulla at the same level of L 2 monopolar cell endings (see Fig. 42).

5. Centrifugal Cells C 2, C 3, Tan 1, and Tan 2

Cross-sections of optic cartridges reveal many small profiles whose diameters range from 0.05 μm to 3.0 μm and whose positions are more or less constant with respect to the geometry of the receptor and monopolar cell cross-sections (Fig. 33). Golgi studies (Strausfeld, 1971 a) and combined Golgi-electron microscopy (Campos-Ortega and Strausfeld, 1972, 1973; Strausfeld and Campos-Ortega, 1973 a, b, 1977) reveal the largest of these as belonging to four types of centrifugal cells (two narrow-field and two wide-field) and to amacrine cells. As outlined on p.68, narrow-field centrifugals are derived from cell bodies beneath the medulla. The C 2 element is characterized by a swollen terminal that inserts into the distal opening of the receptor crown. The terminal is derived from a thin fibre that ascends through the lamina alongside R 4, outside the receptor crown. The second type of centrifugal fibre (C 3) resides alongside the axis fibre of the L 4 monopolar cell and gives rise to a set of unilateral tuberous outgrowths that enter into the centre of the cartridge. These terminate between the L 1 and L 2 monopolar cells and are dispersed down the entire length of the cartridge (see Figs. 37 and 38).

Wide-field centrifugal endings (Tan 1 and Tan 2) are derived from cell bodies above the medulla. Their bi- or tristratified dendritic fields are connected to wide-field telodendria distally in the external plexiform layer (Fig. 38). Tan 1 endings give rise to varicose collaterals that "hang" into the distal openings of receptor crowns. In contrast, the Tan 2 endings consist of thin tangential fibres that give rise to swellings distributed periodically along their length. The swellings are usually situated at either side of each L 5 monopolar spine. The fields of Tan 2 are large and overlap 2 extensively. Mass impregnation by Golgi methods, or resolution by reduced silver, has shown that although the two types of tangential cells are arranged one to every several cartridges, the total populations of tangentials give rise to uniform networks of fibres covering the whole of the lamina's extent. Each Tan 2 field spreads horizontally through between four and eight cartridges; its vertical extent is through between 20 and 36 cartridges. The horizontal extent of Tan 1 is identical, but its vertical extent reaches between 8 and 20 cartridges.

a) Synaptology of Centrifugal Inputs C 2 and C 3

C 2 establishes contact with the necks of the L 1, L 2, and L 3 monopolar cells. The L 2 monopolar neuron gives rise to a collar of between six and eight stubby dendrites that partially wrap around the C 2 terminals. C 2 is presynaptic to all three monopolars and, as far as is known, the distribution of synapses is shared equally amongst them. However, unlike synaptic relationships between receptors and triads of relay neurons (L 1–L 3), the terminals of centrifugals invariably establish monadic contacts: an isolated profile of a monopolar faces a presynaptic site in the centrifugal ending.

Unilateral terminals of C 3 are presynaptic to the axis fibre of L 1 and L 2. There is a clear distinction between synaptological relationships of the two narrow-field centrifugals and the levels at which they insert into the cartridge (Fig. 41). In the case of C 3, dyad arrangements of L 1 and L 2 sometimes faces a single presynaptic site in the centrifugal ending.

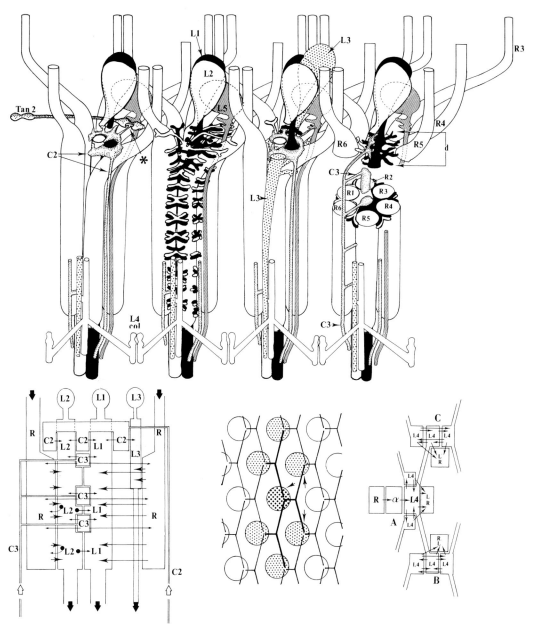

Fig. 41. Summary diagram of synaptic relationships between receptors, *L1–L3* monopolars and *L4* with receptors and *L1,L2*. The upper figure illustrates a cut-away view of a vertical row of cartridges in *Musca* showing distal relationships between the *C2* centrifugal terminal and *L1/L2*. *L1* and *L2* have a special group of neck-dendrites at this leved (*d* in right-hand cartridge) and that the *C2* ending has a small branch onto *Tan 2* which, in turn, contacts the spine of *L5* (see Fig. 42 for the relationships *Tan 2* to *L5*). *C3* inserts between the axis fibres of *L1/L2*. *L4* collaterals abut each other. The lower left diagram schematizes synaptic contacts between *C2* and *L1*, *L3*, *L2*, and *R/C3* and *L1/L2* and *L2* to *R* and *L1*. Note the stratified arrangements of these levels of connexions. *C3* is occasionally presynaptic to *R* fibres at the level of reciprocal *L2* to *L1* and *R* pathways. The middle lower diagram illustrates connexions to a single cartridge by three converging *L4* collaterals which link the centre *L1/L2* pair (cartridge is coarsely stippled) with a vertically oriented surround of six neighbouring cartridges and, hence, six neighbouring sets of *R*-to-amacrine-to-*L4* contacts. The right lower diagram summarizes receptor pathways over α-processes and *L4* to axial monopolar cells and receptors (labelled *L/R*). (After STRAUSFELD and CAMPOS-ORTEGA, 1973 and unpublished data by CAMPOS-ORTEGA and STRAUSFELD)

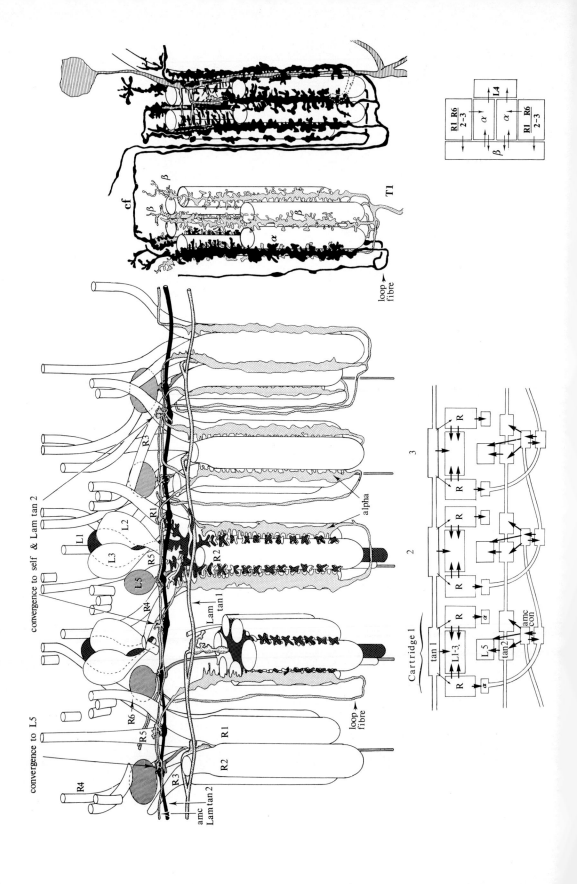

b) Type-1 Wide-Field Centrifugal (Tan 1)

Each cartridge is invaded by varicose terminal specializations of at least three Tan 1 neurons whose fields overlap extensively (STRAUSFELD and CAMPOS-ORTEGA; unpublished observation). Golgi-electron microscopy has located Tan 1 varicosities in a cartridge, and conventional electron microscopy shows these to be presynaptic to L 1, L 2, L 3, and the R 1–R 6 endings distally, within the outer third of the plexiform layer (Fig. 42).

c) L 5 Monopolar Cell and Type-2 Wide-Field Centrifugal (Tan 2)

Combined Golgi-electron microscopy studies and degenerative ablation of tangential fibres (CAMPOS-ORTEGA and STRAUSFELD, unpublished) reveal that the spines of L 5 are postsynaptic to a pair of tangentially oriented fibres; one degenerate, the other not. The non-degenerated fibre is a rosette specialization from the type-1 amacrine (see p. 66); the degenerated fibre was shown to be derived from a type-2 wide-field centrifugal (Tan 2). L 5 monopolars therefore receive inputs from two types of wide-field elements and there is no evidence to date that they are postsynaptic to receptors. They presumably monitor information from a large-field array of cartridges to a single retinotopic column in the medulla. Despite its size, the midget monopolar must be considered as a relay neuron that collects from a wide-field. L 5's terminal is tightly apposed to the ending of L 1 in the medulla. Pathways involving receptors – to L 1 to L 5 – to medulla relay neurons are complex and presumably carry information about wide-field interactions at several levels of the system (Fig. 42).

6. Amacrine Cells (Anaxonal Neurons)

a) The Type 1 Amacrine (Am 1)

Electron microscopy studies by CAMPOS-ORTEGA and STRAUSFELD (1973) identified the second set of climbing fibres around each crown of receptors (α-fibres) as belonging to a species of anaxonal neuron (the type-1 lamina amacrine: Am 1; Fig. 43 a, b). Light and electron microscopy studies demonstrated that each amac-

---

◀ **Fig. 42.** Summary diagram of synaptic relationships between receptors, type-1 amacrines, type-2 wide-field centrifugals *(Lam tan 2)* and amacrine-basket complexes in *Musca*. The upper diagram shows a vertical row of cartridges with L 5 monopolars. The fibres of *tan 2* endings converge with amacrine tangential processes to spines of *L 5* cells. Amacrines *(amc)* contact their own tangential processes and processes from other amacrines distally in the plexiform layer. α-Processes invaginate between receptors by spines whose density is about one-third that of *L 1/L 2* dendrites. Type-1 tangentials give rise to varicose components that project into the open (distal) ends of cartridges and contact receptors, *L 1*, *L 2*, and *L 3*. α-Processes from several amacrines comprise the amacrine donation of climbing fibres to each cartridge (upper right) mimetic to basket dendrites of medulla-lamina T-cells *(β-fibres)*. α-Processes are invested by the dendrites of *L 4* monopolars onto which they are presynaptic. Note specializations at the distal tips of some α-fibres; these are in synaptic contiguity with blebbed and rosette components from amacrine tangential fibres. The lower left diagram summarizes connexions from *Tan 1*, to *R, L 1–L 3* and from *Tan 2* to *L 5*. Amacrines are postsynaptic to receptors, reciprocally pre- and postsynaptic to other amacrines, postsynaptic to *Tan 2* and presynaptic to *L 5*. The lower right diagram summarizes receptor-to-amacrine-to-L 4 connexions, connexions from receptors to beta, and reciprocal connexions between beta and alpha at a single cartridge. (Adapted from STRAUSFELD and CAMPOS-ORTEGA, 1973, and from unpublished findings by these authors)

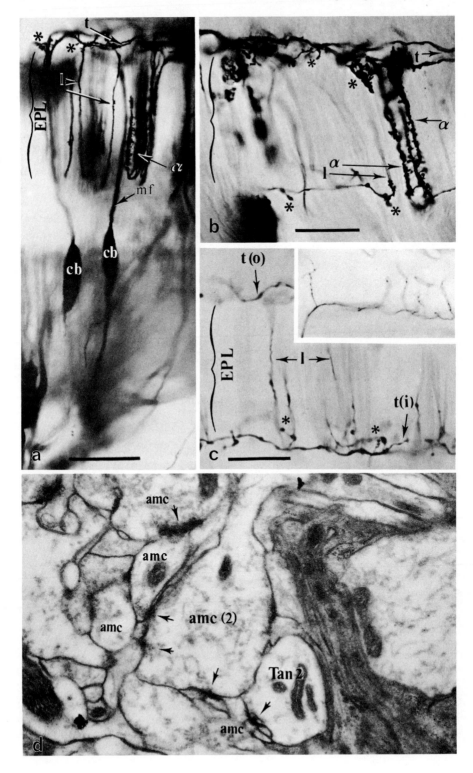

rine cell contributes between one and three α-processes to any cartridge and that many cartridges can receive an α-fibre contribution from a single amacrine cell. Between two and six amacrines are required to contribute six α-fibres to any single cartridge. Consequently, there is extensive overlap between these elements. Mass impregnation of amacrines by the Golgi-Cox method shows that many superficial tangential processes are derived from these cells. They give rise to a regular network of superficial interconnexions between cartridges, oriented along the two oblique axes of the neuropil and along the vertical and horizontal axes. Tangential processes of type-1 amacrines radiate dorsoventrally away from a structural "center" of α-elements. Tangential processes of Am 1 are characterized by rosette-like specializations and varicosities which have special distributions along their length (Fig. 43 b, c). Rosettes are closely apposed to branches that arise from the distal tips of each α-process. These connexions represent one type of amacrine-to-amacrine pathway. A second pathway involves serial synapse between Am 1 varicosities distributed along amacrine tangential fibres (Fig. 43 d).

In the front part of the male eye (beneath the fovea), type-1 amacrines typically show dense packing of centre α-fields from which radiate small "surrounds" of tangential processes. Further posteriorly centre fields are more diffuse, and the structural surround of tangential fibres is large.

b) The Type 2 Amacrine (Am 2)

As recently as 1977, it was claimed that all elements in the lamina had probably been identified (STRAUSFELD and CAMPOS-ORTEGA, 1977). Justification for this statement was that there seemed to be no space available for further cell types, because all profiles within an optic cartridge had been accounted for by Golgi-electron microscopy. However, this is incorrect. Recent improvements of the Golgi method, using borate-boracic acid buffers, have shown up a novel amacrine cell in *Calliphora* and *Musca* (NÄSSEL and SEYAN, in prep.). Its essential features are shown in Figs. 37 and 43. Basically, the shape of this cell (the type-2 amacrine, Am 2) is similar to bistratified tangential neurons that have been described from *Eristalis tenax* and *Syrphus* and which were illustrated as tangentials in BOSCHEK's account (1971) (Fig. 23, loc. cit.). Characteristically, Am 2 cells consist of a slender ascending fibre from the cell body that branches beneath and above the external

◄ Fig. 43 a–d. Amacrine cells of the lamina. a Two type-1 amacrines revealed by the Golgi-Cox method, illustrating the α-components derived from looped fibres *(l)* which branch off from amacrine tangential processes *(t) (Musca)*. Asterisks indicate specializations at the distal lateral margins of an optic cartridge. b Colonnier impregnations of the typically complex form of an amacrine cell, showing rosette specializations (asterisks), looped fibres with knotted protuberances at the proximal level of the lamina (asterisks) and α-processes *(Lucilia)*. c Elements of the type-2 amacrine *(Musca)* sharing two levels of tangentially directed processes at the distal and proximal margins of the plexiform layer which give rise to pre- and postsynaptic specializations (asterisks). The inset illustrates a type-2 amacrine of *Calliphora* showing a distal tangential process from which arise fibres that pass to pseudocartridges, just beneath the basement membrane of the retina. (Scale bar A, B, C = 25 μm.) d Amacrine-to-amacrine synapses in the distal lamina *(Musca)* and their characteristic flattened presynaptic specializations. These are unlike the T-formed synaptic ribbons found further proximally in the external plexiform layer or in tangential fibres at this level. x 20,000

plexiform layer. Both levels are characterized by extremely long "knotted" processes which cross as many as 20 cartridges along the vertical axis of the neuropil. Occasionally these processes contribute to part of the α-donation. However, their insertion into the α-set is from the distal surface of the lamina, and reaches downwards one-quarter of the depth of the plexiform layer. A similar structure has been described from a second type of amacrine in white-eyed mutant *Calliphora* (Strausfeld, 1976b, loc. cit. plate 7.10). In contrast, type-1 amacrines donate α-processes via looped fibres from the proximal lamina surface and α-components extend completely through the external plexiform layer (Figs. 42 and 43a, b). One rather astonishing feature of the type-2 amacrine is the presence of collaterals that ascend to the level of the so-called pseudocartridges. These are the bundles of receptor axons immediately beneath the retina's basement membrane at a level above their decussation to the physiologically and optically appropriate cartridge.

7. Type-1 Amacrine Synaptology

a) With Receptors L4 and Tan 2

A-processes are mimetic to climbing fibres of the T 1 basket (Campos-Ortega and Strausfeld, 1973). *A*-processes are postsynaptic to all six receptors and are pre- and postsynaptic to β-fibres (Fig. 42). In the outer one-third of the lamina, alphas (and other amacrine specializations) are presynaptic to the dendrites of L4 monopolar cells (Fig. 41) (Strausfeld and Campos-Ortega, 1973). The most numerous inputs to L4 neurons are where amacrines have small centre fields in the upper frontal lamina, beneath lenses with large-diameter facets of the type *La* lattice (Beersma et al., 1975; Strausfeld, 1979b). For example, there are more amacrine-to-L4 connexions at cartridges beneath the male fovea than elsewhere in that sex or in the female. Conventional electron microscopy reveals amacrine-tangential processes as pre- and postsynaptic to processes of other amacrines (possibly type-2 as well as type-1 cells) (Figs. 42 and 43d) and pre- and postsynaptic to the tangentially directed fibres of the type-2 centrifugal terminal (Tan 2).

b) With Basket Fibres (Beta or T1)

Basket dendrites of T-cells have been identified as the β-fibre components of an optic cartridge (see Golgi-electron microscopy studies by Campos-Ortega and Strausfeld, 1973; cf. Boschek, 1971; Trujillo-Cenóz and Melamed, 1970). Climbing fibres of the basket are apposed to two adjacent receptor terminals and partly invaginate between them. R 1–R 6 endings are presynaptic to dyadic configurations of β- and α-processes. Each β- and α- (type-1 amacrines) process shares an equal number of presynaptic sites from each receptor ending. Estimations from *Musca* indicate that a basket cell has between 100 and 150 postsynaptic sites to receptors, that is, one-third of the connexions between receptors and the axial monopolars (L 1, L 2) but equal to the number of connexions between receptors and L 3. Conventional electron microscopy shows β- and α-processes to be reciprocally pre- and postsynaptic. It can be assumed that since β-processes of one cartridge are postsynaptic to amacrines which invest several cartridges, T 1 cells are subject to some lateral modulation, possibly excitatory or inhibitory in nature (see also STRAUSFELD and CAMPOS-ORTEGA, 1977).

8. L 4 Monopolar Cell Relationships with R 1–R 6, L 1, L 2, and L 4

L 4 neurons are postsynaptic to α-processes of amacrines, and their axon collaterals are disposed beneath the inner surface of the external plexiform layer. Collaterals project to the parent cartridge and to the dorsoposterior and ventroposterior neighbouring cartridges (STRAUSFELD and BRAITENBERG, 1970; STRAUSFELD and CAMPOS-ORTEGA, 1973 a; BRAITENBERG and DEBAGGE, 1974). L 4 collaterals are presynaptic to axons of L 1 and L 2 and also establish pre- and postsynaptic relationships with converging collateral terminals from other L 4 neurons. Together, the entire population of L 4 neurons contributes a regular rectilinear network of intercartridge connexions at the most proximal level of the lamina. Each collateral establishes between four and six presynaptic sites onto receptor terminals. There are between three and five presynaptic sites onto L 1 and L 2, and about the same number with other L 4 collaterals. L 4 collaterals are reciprocally pre- and postsynaptic. These arrangements mean that an input to an L 4 cell from one or more cartridges via α-processes could theoretically be relayed across the entire extent of the lamina's inner surface. It is suggested that the receptor-to-amacrine-to-L 4–L 1/L 2 pathway mediates lateral inhibition between adjacent and subadjacent cartridges; the lateral spread of information from a single L 4 would possibly depend on the amplitude and duration of its initial input (see STRAUSFELD, 1976 b; STRAUSFELD and CAMPOS-ORTEGA, 1977).

V. Comparison Between Lamina Morphologies

Two comparative light microscopy accounts exist in the literature, the most important being the classic study by CAJAL and SÁNCHEZ (1915) which treats the three main visual neuropils of Diptera, Orthoptera, Hymenoptera, Lepidoptera, and Odonata.

CAJAL and SÁNCHEZ's studies are still valuable works of reference, although some discrepancies exist between their descriptions of the moth lamina (*Sphinx* sp.) and a later Golgi study on *Sphinx ligustri* (STRAUSFELD and BLEST, 1970). The Spanish authors describe several of the lamina's cell types in the following species: *Calliphora erythrocephala*, *Apis mellifica*, an (unidentified) orthopteran, *Sphinx* (possibly *S. ligustri*) and two odonate insects, *Libellula* sp. and *Agrion* sp. With the exception of *Sphinx*, modern Golgi studies of *Calliphora*, *Apis*, and the damsel fly *Coenagrion puella*, confirm CAJAL and SÁNCHEZ's major findings. The Spanish authors' descriptions of the dipteran amacrine neuron more resembles Am 2 than the type-1 amacrine cell, however.

Light microscopy comparisons (STRAUSFELD, 1976 b) between morphologies and dispositions of lamina elements were published recently with reference to the fly *Musca domestica*, the coleopteran, *Hoplia farinosa*, an odonate, *Coenagrion puella* and the hemipteran, *Notonecta glauca*. These four species represent four major types of lamina subserving four major types of retina. These are, respectively, the neural superposition eye (the N-type lamina of most Diptera [see also ZEIL, 1979]); the superposition eye (the S-type lamina of *Hoplia* and *Phausis* [OHLY, 1975]; see also studies by WOLBURG-BUCHHOLZ on the narrow-field neurons of the superposition eye of *Cloeon dipterum* [1977]); the apposition eye (the A-type lamina of *Coenagrion* and other species of Odonata [see ARMETT-KIBEL et al., 1977; CAJAL and SÁNCHEZ, 1915]; and the laminae of Hymenoptera [see CAJAL and SÁNCHEZ, 1915; RIBI, 1975, 1976; MEYER, 1979]). The open rhabdomere-appositional eye typical of Hemiptera has been termed the H-type lamina and is described from *Notonecta* (STRAUSFELD, 1976 b; WOLBURG-BUCHHOLZ, 1979), *Corixa punctata* and *Gerris lacustris* (WOLBURG-BUCHHOLZ, 1979), and *Benacus* and *Lethocerus* (MEINERTZHAGEN, 1971).

Three recent investigations are discussed here with reference to the fly lamina. These are WOLBURG-BUCHHOLZ's study of *Notonecta glauca*, RIBI's studies of the bee and MEYER's study (1979) of the ant *Cataglyphis bicolor*. The accounts are exemplary in that they identify the characteristic cross-sectional locations of receptor axons and monopolar cell axons within optic cartridges. Elucidation of these geometrical relationships is a prerequisite for synaptological studies where Golgi-impregnated elements must first be related to invariant patterns of profiles (see Fig. 40). Only then can profiles be properly related to each other by conventional electron microscopy.

Hemiptera and bee laminae are multistratified, with three levels of receptor terminals. In Hemiptera the receptor axons obviously cannot comprise a ring (or crown) of receptor terminals simply because only two of the short receptor endings penetrate down through levels of the external plexiform layer (see Figs. 35 and 36). Nevertheless, each type of receptor ending has a characteristic location with respect to the axes of the lamina's mosaic. Monopolar cell cross-sections are likewise organized according to characteristic loci amongst the constellation of receptor elements. This is typical of the medulla of the fly (CAMPOS-ORTEGA and STRAUSFELD, 1972) where the geometrical implicator elements of each column comprise two long visual fibre terminals that project alongside monopolar cell endings derived from the optically relevant optic cartridge. As in the hemipteran, constellations of axon cross-sections are more or less invariant across the medulla's extent, and their pattern can be described according to the major tangential axes of the mosaic.

In the ant and the bee, receptor terminals have cyclic arrangements at an optic cartridge. In both species the crown of short receptor endings encloses the profiles of three long visual fibres. Monopolar cells are arranged around the periphery of the crown, and their dendrites either insert into the receptor bundle or clasp it (Figs. 32 and 44).

MEYER's studies of the ant lamina describe two forms of spiny monopolar cell whose dendrites contact all six short receptor endings (monopolar cells L 1 a, L 1 c, and L 2). However, the L 1 c neuron appears to establish far fewer connexions with the receptor endings, and this aspect of it is reminiscent of the L 3 monopolar cell of Diptera. Golgi-electron microscopy studies of *Cataglyphis* illustrate long visual fibres contacted by the monopolar cell dendrites of L 1 a and L 2. This is in contrast

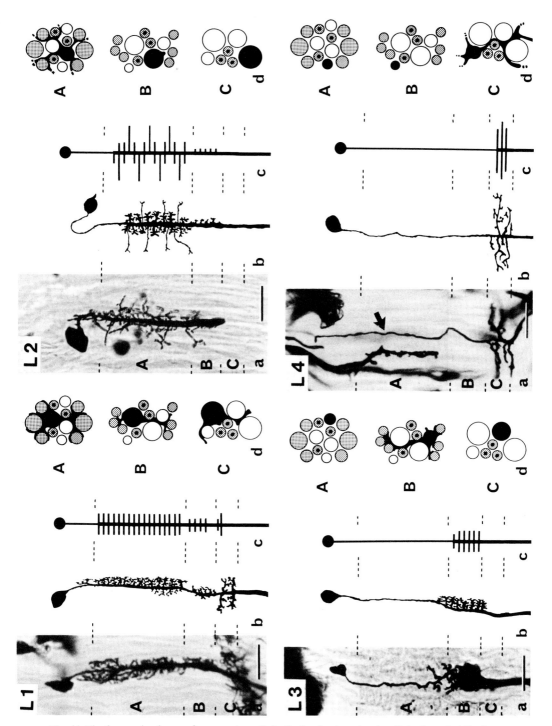

Fig. 44. The four major forms of monopolar cells in the bee lamina, showing their characteristic distribution of dendrites and collaterals and their locations in cartridge cross-sections (scale = 25 μm). Their levels should be compared with levels of receptor terminals shown in Fig. 32. Note the similarity between the form of the L 4 neuron and its counterpart in Diptera. (Reproduced by permission of W. Ribi and Springer-Verlag)

to Diptera where long visual fibres appear to have no connexions at all in the outer plexiform layer.

In both the bee and the ant, long visual fibres and some forms of spiny mono-polar cells (L 1/L 3) give rise to groups of collateral processes at the lower margin of the lamina, beneath the level of receptor terminals. These coincide with wide-field axon collaterals of the hymenopterous L 4 monopolar cell (Fig. 44) which is analogous to the tripartite L 4 monopolar cell of Diptera. Golgi-electron microsco-py studies of L 4 monopolars in the ant (MEYER, 1979) show that its collaterals pass to its parent cartridge and to three neighbouring cartridges. The domain of these processes is oriented roughly vertically, as it is in the bee. In *Musca*, L 4 collaterals project to the parent cartridge and two neighbours, one dorsoposterior and the other ventroposterior except beneath the male "La lattice" where L 4 collaterats extend to four cartridges (STRAUSFELD, unpublished observations). In flies, L 4 neurons provide a regular system of axon collateral connexions beneath the whole of the plexiform layer (STRAUSFELD and BRAITENBERG, 1970; STRAUSFELD and CAM-POS-ORTEGA, 1973) and, assuming that one L 4 cell exists in each cartridge of the bee and ant, a similar pattern should be present in these species. In Diptera, den-drites of L 4 neurons derive their input from amacrine processes at the outer one-third of the lamina. In bees and ants, L 4 neurons lack distal processes. However, as RIBI has shown, there are amacrines within the most proximal layer of the la-mina which could provide the relevant input from receptors.

The bee lamina is complicated by its several levels of receptor cell endings. Re-cent studies by RIBI (1979) have shown that three pairs of receptors in each om-matidium give rise to three characteristic terminal morphologies at two levels in the lamina. In addition, three types of long visual fibre from each ommatidium project through the lamina to the medulla. Each type is characterized by its branching pat-tern in the lamina and by its depth (and shapes) in the medulla.

HERTEL (1980) has shown that there are regional differences in the spectral sen-sitivities of ommatidia in the bee's eye. Trichromatic outputs characterize median and frontal retina; green dominates lateral ommatidia whereas ultraviolet recep-tors are prominent dorsally. However, according to RIBI, there does not seem to be a clear morphological correlate to these regions in terms of the shapes of recep-tor endings.

Comparisons between the bee and ant show significant differences with respect to stratification of the external plexiform layer. In *Cataglyphis* there is only one form of short receptor terminal, for example. Accordingly, dendrites of spiny mono-polar cells are distributed through the whole depth of the receptor-terminal layer. In the bee, dendrites of spiny monopolar cells are disposed at four distinct levels. L 1 invades all the receptor layers, as well as the L 4 collateral layer, where it gives rise to a separate and distinctive group of dendrites at the L 4 layer (layer C). L 2 invades exclusively the outer plexiform layer (layer A), and L 3 invades layer B at the level of the deepest receptor endings. Two other forms of monopolar cells (La and Lb) have dendrites disposed within the inner half of layer A. Their arrange-ments mimic the two forms of short receptor terminals (see R 181, 1974).

Golgi-electron microscopy studies of *Notonecta* show similar correlations be-tween the depth of receptor terminals and the branching patterns of monopolar cells. In this species there is a characteristic segregation of the receptor input to at

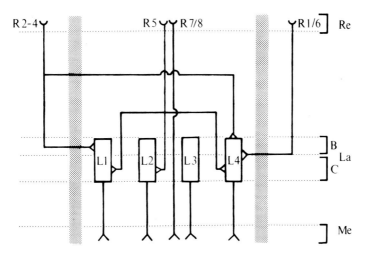

Fig. 45. Schema of convergence and segregation from receptor types onto monopolar cells in the lamina of *Notonecta glauca*. (See also Fig. 36) (Reproduced by permission of K. WOLBURG-BUCHHOLZ and Springer-Verlag)

least three parallel monopolar cell channels at each cartridge. In this species the divergence of parallel channels at the level of the lamina is combinatorial (Fig. 45). Specific combinations of receptors are presynaptic to specific monopolars. The neurons labelled L 1 by WOLBURG-BUCHHOLZ are postsynaptic to receptor channels R 2, 3, 4, and 5 whereas the neuron labelled L 4 is postsynaptic to all the short receptor endings (R 1–R 6). In contrast, the L 2 monopolar cell is exclusively postsynaptic to R 5. Segregation and combination of receptor-monopolar cell connexions has been described by NÄSSEL (1977 b) from the crayfish and by ARMETT-KIBEL et al. (1977) from the odonate *Sympetrum rubicundulum*. Typically in both crayfish and insect, monopolar cells that derive identical inputs from a receptor share the same presynaptic site. They thus constitute a dyadic, triadic or tetradic arrangement of postsynaptic spines opposite a single presynaptic ribbon in the receptor ending (ARMETT-KIBEL et al., 1977; NÄSSEL, 1977 b). In the ant *Cataglyphis*, tetradic relationships have been seen between receptor terminals and second-order elements, three of which are possibly relay neurons to the medulla and a fourth which has been suggested to belong to medulla-lamina neurons (T-cells) (MEYER, 1979). In the ephemerid lamina *(Cloeon dipterum)* cyclic arrangements of R 1–R 7 are presynaptic to dyads of relay neuron dendrites (WOLBURG-BUCHHOLZ, 1977).

Some generalities of lamina organization are beginning to emerge from the cited studies. Clearly not all monopolar cell types are necessarily postsynaptic to receptors as illustrated by the fly L 4 and L 5 cells. Similarly, MEYER was unable to detect apposition between the L 4 monopolar cell and receptor terminals. In *Sympetrum* (ARMETT-KIBEL et al., 1977) one small monopolar cell, MIII, was not observed to be postsynaptic to a receptor. In layered laminae (*Notonecta* and *Sympetrum*), between one and two monopolar cells are postsynaptic to all the short receptor terminals, and in both species each cell type is involved in specific connexions which distinguish it from any other. This has also been determined in the crayfish (Nässel and Waterman, 1977; Nässel, 1977b) and in dipterous insects (for summaries see Strausfeld, 1976b; Strausfeld and Campos-Ortega, 1977). Armett-Kibel et al. showed that differences of connectivity between monopolar cells and other elements are not trivially correlated with the layered relationships between monopolars and layered receptor endings. Differences of connectivity are encountered between elements that are in juxtaposition throughout the lamina's entire depth. For example, Armett-Kibel et al. describe feedback synapses from one form of large monopolar cell (M 1) to the receptors R 5 and R 8, specifically, in the proximal lamina. They also suggest that in the proximal lamina, relationships between R 1 and R 4 terminals and the triad arrangement of two large monopolar cells (MI and MII) with a small lateral monopolar cell (MIV) are characteristic of this layer; MI rather than MII is the median element of the triad, flanked by MII and MIV. Distally, MII appears to occupy the median position. In this respect, different levels of receptor endings seem to be irrelevant, and Armett-Kibel et al. suggest there must be more fundamental reasons for proximo-distal differences of synaptology. Layered arrangement of synaptic interactions is best shown in dipterous lamina where all R 1–R 6 receptors end at the same level. In *Musca*, synaptic interconnexions are precisely stratified according to at least six different levels (see Figs. 40, 41, and 42). The most distal of these is occupied by the interconnexions between amacrines and those relay neurons that do not receive direct input from receptors. The second level is occupied by centrifugal terminals onto monopolar cells or receptors. Third and fourth levels of connexions are between receptors and the three forms of monopolar cells (L 1–L 3) and the T 1 centripetal cells in conjunction with α-processes of amacrines. And a fifth level of connectivity is manifested by reciprocal synapses between each L 2 monopolar cell and its adjacent element (L 1), as well as between L 2 and receptors. The sixth and deepest level comprises presynaptic relationships between L 4 axon collaterals and outgoing axons of L 1 and L 2 monopolars. Considering this kind of diversity amongst identical receptor endings, it might be expected that very complicate synaptic relationships coexist amongst stratified receptor endings whose levels may segregate according to their spectral properties (see Ribi, 1979). One system of functional layering could simply comprise divergent and combinational channels between receptors and monopolar cells such as described by Wolburg-Buchholz from *Notonecta*. Other systems of synaptic stratification are likely to be as complex as that described from the fly and, possibly, a synaptic stratum may even reiterate and overlap, one for each receptor type.

VI. Retinotopic Organization and Neuroarchitecture

The previous chapters described the subunit organization of cells within the lamina, the smallest and simplest of the three optic lobe neuropils. The structure of this region is extraordinarily precise in Diptera, both in terms of its geometrical organization within each cartridge and the synaptic relationships between its constituent elements. Deeper regions of the optic lobes contain a multitude of neuronal forms, many of which spread through several columns, in contrast to the fly lamina.

Despite this apparent complexity, and despite the huge variation of cell shapes (see STRAUSFELD, 1976 b, loc. cit. Plates 7.11 and 7.12), reduced-silver studies reveal some general and significant features of columnar organization that distinguish medulla neuropil from other regions.

Figure 46 illustrates a series of sections taken tangentially across the columnar mosaic of the medulla of *Calliphora*. The first photograph (a) illustrates bundles of axons arriving at the medulla's distal surface, derived from optic cartridges of the lamina. Each pair of L 1 and L 2 fibres is resolved, accompanied by two small profiles belonging to R 7 and L 3. About 15 μm deeper in the neuropil (b), input elements clearly segregate into separate groups that form double rows mapped onto a rectilinear lattice. At the level of "line amacrines" (STRAUSFELD, 1970a), approximately 20 μm beneath the medulla surface, each input group is seen accompanied by the cross-sections of several medulla relay neurons. Here the mosaic is clearly composed of two superimposed rectilinear lattices, one comprising large diameter fibres displaced laterally from a set of small elements. This illustrates the principle of divergence from lamina input onto many parallel pathways destined for the lobula complex. Retinotopic maps are precisely maintained within the outer layers of the medulla. However, at the serpentine layer, axon bundles become displaced due to their passage amongst large meandering tangential axons (Fig. 46 e). Despite this, their lateral relationships are generally maintained. Just beneath this layer, columnar axons again adopt a precise pattern. In several aspects this shows geometries that are not seen further distally. Although axons of through-going relay cells maintain their neighbourhood relationships they do this only approximately, compared with the absolute precision above the serpentine layer (STRAUSFELD, 1979). This level shows some structural "noise" i.e., variation between the structures of single columns. Moreover, hexagonal patterns of fibre cross-sections are not resoluble. Instead, fibres are mapped according to two oblique coordinates of a rectilinear system, and this transformation has to be taken into account when dendritic fields at this or deeper levels are correlated with physiological maps of receptive fields.

The passage of relay fibres from the medulla to the lobula and the lobula plate is basically simple. It should be recalled that the outer surface of the lobula is oriented approximately at right angles to the inner surface of the medulla. Anterior cells project to that part of the lobula surface which is most distant from the inner medulla. Posterior medulla neurons project into the lobula closest to the region (see STRAUSFELD and BLEST, 1970). This crossover comprises the second optic chiasma and serves to re-invert the front-back reversal of the lamina mosaic onto the medulla which was carried by the first chiasma. Projections from the medulla to the lobula plate are uncrossed. The explanation for this is simple: the outer (distal) surface of the lobula lies opposite the distal surface of the lobula plate. For point-to-point correspondence between them, uncrossed projections have to link medulla and lobula plate. Equivalent points of the lobula and lobula plate are also connected by uncrossed fibres (STRAUSFELD, 1970).

Three rows of medullary columns contribute to each sheet of fibres of the second optic chiasma (Fig. 46 i). The lateral relationships between adjacent relay

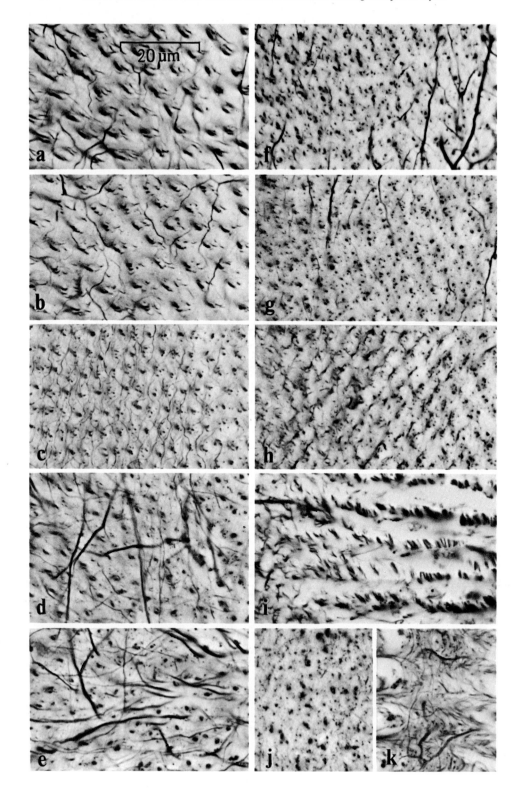

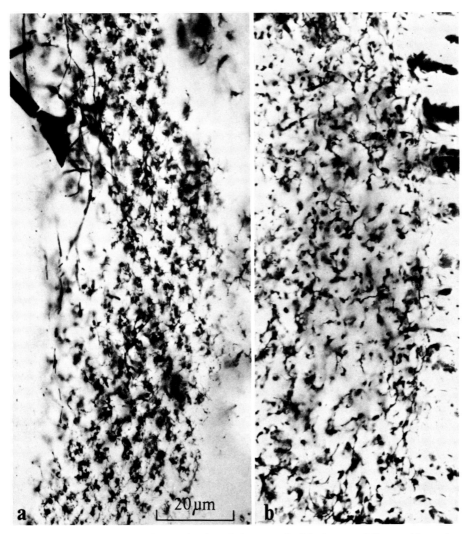

Fig. 47 a, b. Precision of dendritic mapping in orderly neuropil of the inner medulla **a** and imprecise arrangements of dendrites in the lobula plate **b**. Further explanation in the text *(Calliphora)*

neurons are approximately maintained. However, at the level of the lobula (and more so in the lobula plate), axon terminals are even less precisely arranged than in the lower levels of the medulla. This is well demonstrated by the shapes of large-field neurons whose dendrites are associated with "precise" or "noisy" retinotopic projections. Figure 47 a shows part of a giant dendritic field that invades the most

◄ **Fig. 46 a–k.** Patterns of retinotopic fibre bundles through the medulla of *Calliphora* and to the lobula **j** and lobula plate **k**. Above the level of the serpentine layer (**a–c** above **d, e**), bundles of axons are precisely aligned and oriented according to mosaic coordinates. Beneath the serpentine layer (**f, g, h**) bundles show variation in their alignment, are less orderly arranged, and appear to comprise a rectilinear lattice. Each row of chiasmal fibres **i** comprises three horizontal rows of medulla column projections. Their endings in the lobula and lobula plate are imprecise, and the two regions express a high level of structural "noise." Scale bar = 20 μm

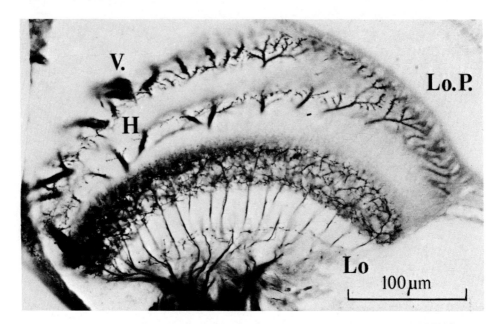

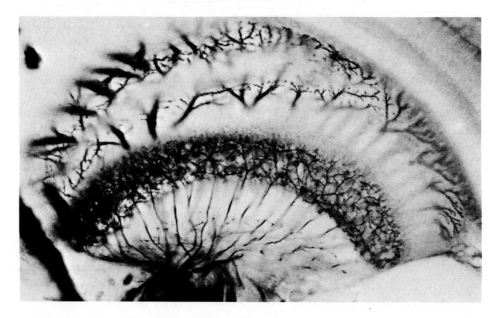

Fig. 48. The lobula (Lo) and lobula plate (Lo P) of two *Musca*, with assemblies of neurons filled with cobalt chloride and intensified with silver. Although there are more vertical (V) neurons in one lobula plate (lower micrograph), together they constitute the same distribution of summed dendrites over the region. Similarly, horizontal cells (H) and lobula columnar neurons constitute two nearly identical multicellular structures in the two animals

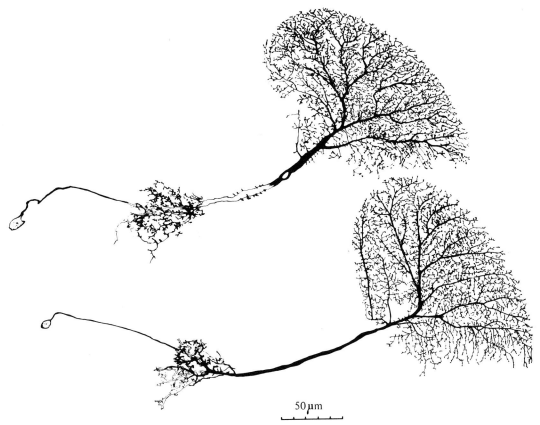

Fig. 49. Two horizontal motion-sensitive centrifugal cells (CH cells; HAUSEN, 1976a) drawn from procion yellow-injected lobula plates. Further explanation in text. (By kind permission of K. HAUSEN)

proximal medulla stratum at the level of Fig. 46h. Arrangements of dendritic rosettes reflect the precision of retinotopic mapping at this level. In contrast, a giant dendritic tree on the lobula plate (Fig. 47b), at a level equivalent to that shown in Fig. 46k, reflects the amount of structural imprecision between columnar inputs.

Despite the variabilities of structure at the inner medulla, lobula, and lobula plate cell arrangements between individuals of the same species are generally similar. Figure 48 compares three neural assemblies in the lobula complex of two (female) houseflies. The lobula is shown with an assembly of type-A columnar cells (HAUSEN and STRAUSFELD, 1980; STRAUSFELD, 1980) whose spacing and layer relationships are more or less identical between the two animals. The lobula plate is shown with two layers of wide-field dendritic trees, one derived from three horizontal motion-sensitive neurons (HAUSEN, 1976a, b; HAUSEN et al., 1980). The deeper set comprises the dendritic patterns of vertical motion-sensitive elements (HAUSEN, 1976a, b): These vary in number from individual to individual (between 8 and 12 neurons) and sometimes between the left- and right-hand lobes. However, their summed dendritic arborizations comprise nearly identical structures in both animals.

Identicalness between coverage in neuropils is also demonstrated by the shapes of large cells. Despite differences between the shapes of their main trunks, the final pattern of their branchlets comprises an isomorphic structure that invades a characteristic portion of the retinotopic mosaic. An example of this is shown in Fig. 49 derived from procion yellow fillings of two horizontal motion-sensitive (CH) centrifugal neurons (HAUSEN, 1976a,b) whose telodendria invade a superficial level of the lobula plate. In all animals a pair of these neurons cover the plate, one dorsal (see p. 117) accompanied by a smaller ventral element. The dorsal and ventral fields each occupy characteristic portions of the neuropil, and there is no significant disparity between their geometrical relations in different animals of the same sex.

VII. Simple Cell Relationships: Neuronal Assemblies

1. Introduction

Reiterated structures in insect neuropil were first described from reduced-silver stains of the dipterous lamina (BRAITENBERG, 1967; STRAUSFELD, 1971a) which resolved periodic arrangements of argyrophilic cross-sections of receptor terminals and relay neurons. Golgi impregnations combined with electron microscopy (STRAUSFELD and CAMPOS-ORTEGA, 1973b, 1977) correlated reduced-silver Gestalten and identified nerve cells. These studies demonstrated that each form of lamina nerve cell is reiterated in each cartridge. The entire population of any one type of nerve cell comprises a characteristic multicellular structure termed the "neuronal assembly" (STRAUSFELD and HAUSEN, 1977). When neurons are restricted to single retinotopic columns their summed structure is of little interest except to confirm that either cell shapes are generally consistent across the neuropil (e.g. L5) or they are arranged as special gradients (e.g. L4). However, the subunits of complex neuropil – such as the medulla columns – are composed of many neurons and also receive contributions from many kinds of wide-field elements (CAMPOS-ORTEGA and STRAUSFELD, 1972a, b) such as tangential relay cells or amacrines. Normally, the resolution of lateral arrangements between medullary columns is fraught with the simple problem of visualization. Stochastic impregnation by Golgi methods provides information about layer relationships and about projections of the single nerve cell; reduced-silver stains may occasionally resolve the Gestalt of one kind of neuron and show up its distribution within a region. But this kind of identification can be rarely achieved. Unless all the processes of all neurons are resolved, it is impossible to know if each column receives an identical contribution of processes. An earlier account speculated that this probably occurred (CAMPOS-ORTEGA and STRAUSFELD, 1972b), but proof of this was lacking. Resolution of organization across the neuropil by classic techniques is even more difficult in neuropils where retinotopic projections are rather imprecise and messy.

Recently it was found that in certain conditions cobalt ions can be incorporated in all the neurons of a single cell population. Resolution of such "neuronal assemblies" could also be achieved by backfilling neurons that descended from the brain into the ventral nerve cord (STRAUSFELD and OBERMAYER, 1976; STRAUSFELD

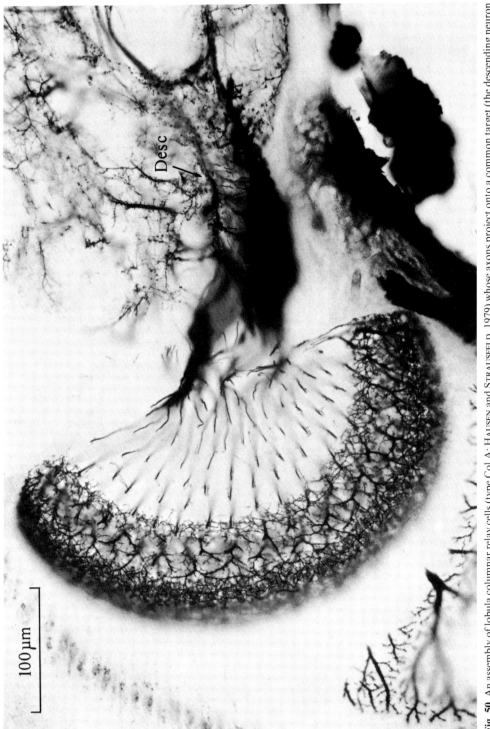

Fig. 50. An assembly of lobula columnar relay cells (type Col A; HAUSEN and STRAUSFELD, 1979) whose axons project onto a common target (the descending neuron *Desc*) in the lateral protocerebrum (*Calliphora*)

and Hausen, 1977). Cobalt ions migrate retrograde from the source of influx at a cut axon through the entire neuron. After a period of some hours cobalt passes from dendrites into populations of presynaptic relay neurons. Longer diffusion periods eventually filled the entire structure of the presynaptic assembly (Fig. 50). Similar patterns have recently been shown by dye coupling of Stewart's (1979), Lucifer yellow (Strausfeld and Bacon, in preparation) and horse-radish peroxidase also passes between contiguous neurons in the fly (Nässel, 1980).

These methods prove immensely powerful for structural analysis and provide the investigator with information about the arrangements amongst a selected population of nerve cells. They illustrate that axons of any one population of lobula-relay neurons converge together beneath the lobula and end at a common region of the lateral protocerebrum. The assembly of any species of nerve cell, whose dendrites and collaterals overlap and whose axons converge to a common focus, comprises a unique structure of the nervous system. In contrast to randomly impregnated neurons (or single cells filled with procion dye), such structures illustrate features of organization that were previously not visible. They include complex features of gradients, local variations of neuronal forms amongst a single population, restricted cell populations that subserve specific regions of the eye, and sexual dimorphisms, to mention just a few examples. Most recently, cobalt studies have revealed regions of lobula neuropil that are linked by retinotopic projections between the two optic lobes (Strausfeld, 1979). Examples of these are considered below.

2. Structure and Characteristics of a Neuron Assembly

Some predictions about how a population of cells should appear can be derived from single elements. Golgi-impregnated cells are traced, and their shape is simply spread according to some arbitrary period, as shown in Fig. 51. This is a computer's view of a neuronal assembly and assumes complete identically between neighbouring cells. More sophisticated synthetic structures can be derived, taking into account known distortions of packing density and curvature of the neuropil.

After cobalt uptake and silver intensification, structures can be resolved that are surprisingly similar to the synthetic one described above (Fig. 51 D). However, shapes of individual cells vary considerably in some assemblies of lobula columnar neurons. For example, the Col A layer appears to be composed of identical elements (Fig. 50). Indeed, the network of dendrites and the palisades of axons constitute an isomorphic structure and all cells converge to the same target. However, closer examination of single cells reveals an amazing variation of their shape. A selection of Col A cell is shown in Fig. 52, all sections of which are reproduced at the same magnification. Some have wide dendritic fields, others are narrow, extending only through a surround of nine projected retinotopic columns from the medulla. If these were seen as single Golgi-impregnated elements, at last three species of nerve cell might be classified. An earlier account of columnar cells at this level probably claimed more cell types than are actually present in terms of their summed structure (Strausfeld, 1970).

The functional significance of such variations is not yet known. Some differences of form would be expected amongst a single population on the basis of cur-

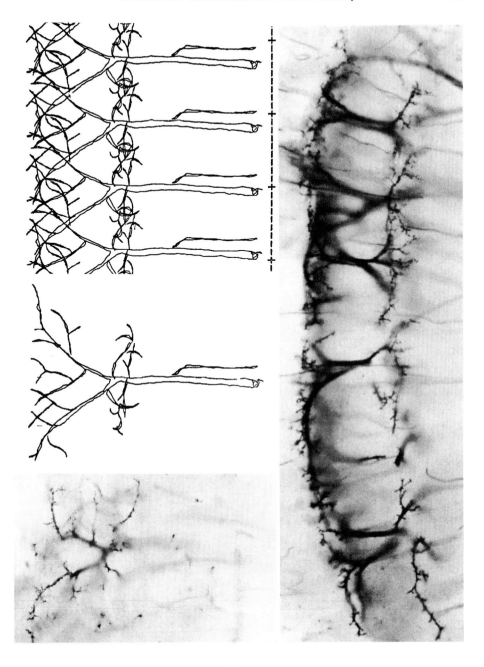

Fig. 51. Synthetic neuronal assemblies derived from a single Golgi-impregnated neuron (upper left) and a neuronal assembly resolved after uptake of cobalt by identical cells of a single neural population (see text)

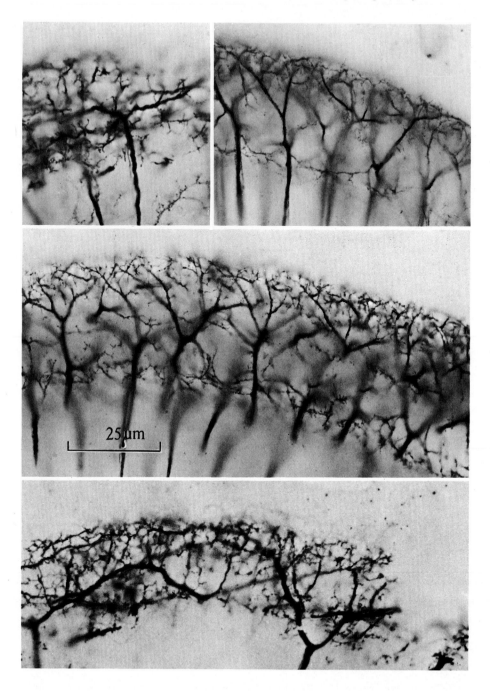

Fig. 52. Variations of individual dendritic shapes of cells comprising a neuronal assembly of Col A cells in *Calliphora* see text)

vature of the region and due to consequent variations of packing between retinotopic inputs at various locations across the neuropil. This feature is not trivial; in male eyes the neuropil that subserves the fovea of the retina (FRANCESCHINI et al., 1979) is composed of more neurons per retinotopic column than elsewhere in the optic lobes (STRAUSFELD, 1979). It is likely that differences of dendritic spread amongst an isomorphic assembly accommodate this kind of local input variation. Alternatively, dendritic field variations that are independent of the input pattern may imply that the form of the dendritic field is not necessarily related to its receptive field. It will be most interesting to see if the receptive field properties of any one Col A neuron is found to be equivalent to any other.

3. Local Isomorphic Assemblies, Unique Neurons and Sex Dimorphism

Some types of neurons are invariably restricted to specific zones of the neuropil. For example, in both male and female flies one population of small-field relay cell is located within a patch of posteroventral lobula accompanied by a single, unique, tangential cell. In both sexes one assembly of diffuse, multistratified, small-field neurons is specifically located within the ventral third of the lobula, whereas another invades only its dorsal two-thirds. Figure 53 shows the lobula of a female *Calliphora* that fortuitously took up cobalt into both these local assemblies from a single pool in the lateral protocerebrum. Accompanying them is the dendritic tree of a unique, female-specific, tangential cell that invades only the dorsalmost retinotopic columns. This neuron has been resolved on several occasions, and its domain is invariant.

Male flies, however, show the most pronounced local cell arrangements (STRAUSFELD, 1979, 1980; HAUSEN and STRAUSFELD, 1980). Male *Calliphora, Sarcophaga*, and *Musca* exhibit a special region of lobula neuropil in which the spacings of retinotopic input groups are expanded. Likewise, the type-A columnar relay cells (Col A) are spaced widest apart in these zones, although their periodic arrangement of one to every three retinotopic columns, every three horizontal rows, is maintained across the whole region (Fig. 54). This expansion is, in part, associated with projections from a region of the retina that is involved in binocular overlap. In the dorsal part of the male retina there is a special region of large facets (type *La lattice*, BEERSMA et al., 1977) which comprises a fovea of densely arrayed visual units (sets of identically aligned photoreceptor groups, R 1–R 7; FRANCESCHINI et al., 1979). Reduced-silver preparations (STRAUSFELD, 1979) reveal that the foveal region of the retina is represented by widely spaced columns in both the lamina and the medulla (Figs. 55 and 60). The number of retinotopic pathways into the lobula from the medulla is greatly increased from the medulla (Fig. 56c). Associated with these foveal projections is a foveal expansion of the lobula mosaic (Fig. 54) in which are located special local assemblies of columnar relay neurons. One type of neuron serves to superimpose the foveal expansion of the ipsilateral lobula onto its opposite counterpart (Fig. 56a, b) via axon projections that undergo a chiasma-like twist in the midbrain. Possibly the twist reverses the map of one foveal expansion anteroposteriorly onto the other. If this is so, then columns in both regions would be in binocular register.

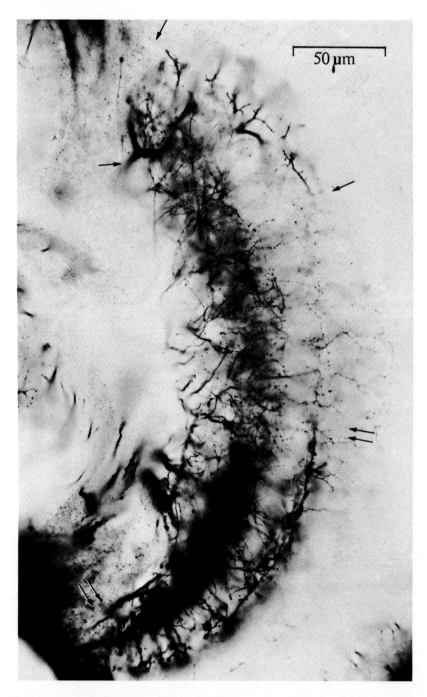

Fig. 53. Local isomorphic assemblies in a lobula of female *Calliphora*, showing also a dorsal unique sex-specific tangential neuron (arrowed). A ventral "local" assembly of neuron terminals is situated between the pairs of double arrows

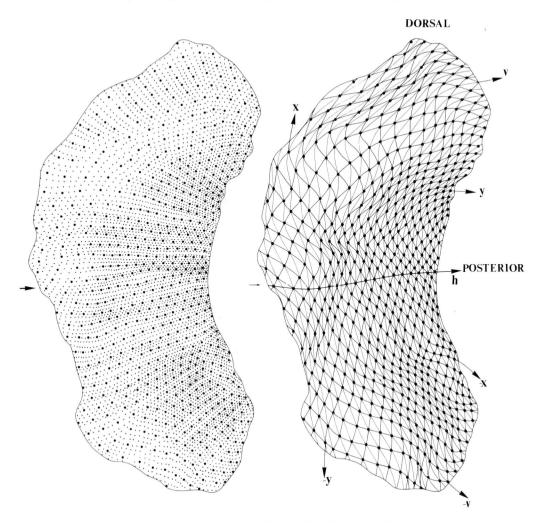

Fig. 54. Two maps of the lobula surface in male *Calliphora*. The left-hand map illustrates the retinotopic pattern of input channels from the medulla (small dots) on which is superimposed the supraperiodic distribution of one type of lobula relay cell axon (Col A cells: large dots). These are distributed one to every three columns, every third row. Note the expansion of column spacing frontally and dorsally. This is better shown to the right where axes of the mosaic are drawn between single Col A elements. The dorsoventral extent of the lobula surface equals about 450–500 µm

The foveal expansion comprises an area that is, in fact, much larger than the area of neuropil that presumably serves retina with binocular overlap (the binocular domain) and is exaggerated in the male fly. In male *Calliphora* there are three types of giant, unique, tangential neurons associated with this zone, and there is also a male-specific set of dorsal columnar relay neurons (STRAUSFELD, 1980; HAUSEN and STRAUSFELD, 1980). Typically, palisades of Col A cells are more or less identical between the two sexes. This is also true of a special frontal strip of large columnar cells (Col B neurons) which subserve the frontal region of binocular

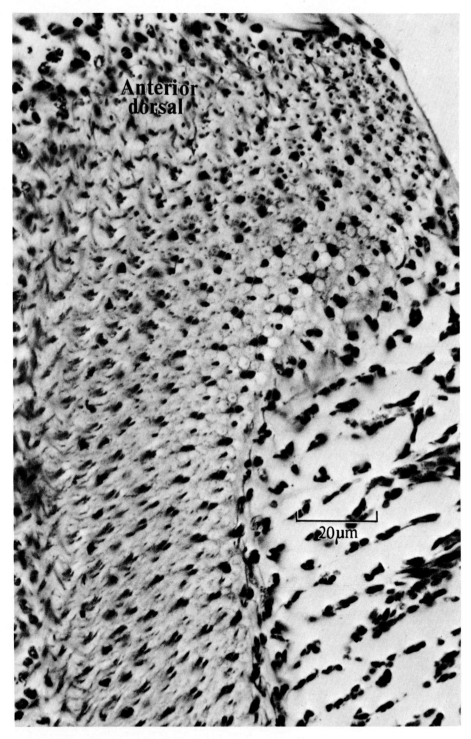

Fig. 55. Micrograph of a reduced-silver stained lamina of a male *Calliphora* showing the special region of wide diameter and widely spaced optic cartridges beneath the corresponding foveal region of the male retina (upper half of figure)

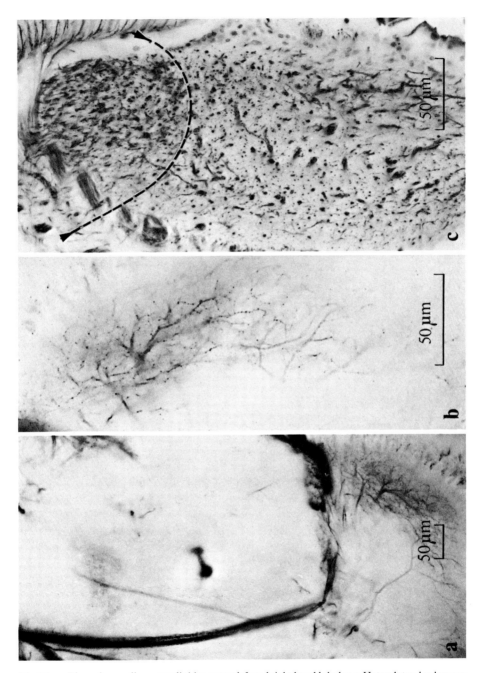

Fig. 56 a–c. Binocular small neurons linking upper left and right hand lobulas. **a** Heterolateral columnar relay neurons that project the lobula's binocular domain (arrowed in C) to the equivalent contralateral region. **b** Detail of lobula-lobula columnar relay cell dendrites. **c** The special dorsal region of lobula neuropil showing the specially dense distribution of axons of relay neurons and medulla inputs (see text). **a, b** are from *Calliphora;* **c** is from *Musca*

Col B, Col C assemblies   **MLG neurons**

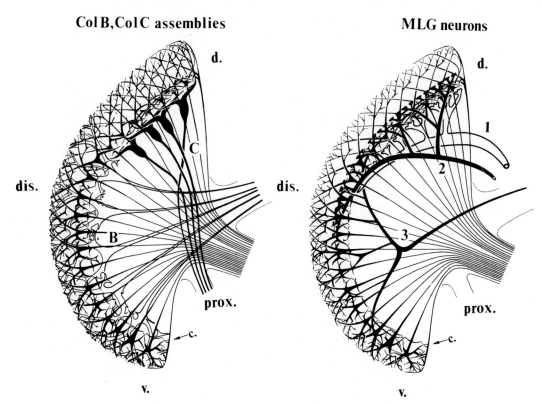

Fig. 57. Summary diagram of local and sex-specific neurons in the lobula of *Calliphora* (Col *B*, Col *C*; MLG *1,2,3*) shown against a palisade of columnar relay cells that are common to both sexes (see text)

overlap in both sexes and are termed sexually monomorphic elements. Figure 57 is a schematic drawing of the sex-monomorphic Col A background-superimposed upon sex monomorphs of the Col B local assembly, the male-specific dorsal columnar cells (Col C) and the three forms of giant neurons (MLG 1–3). The present data is derived from *Calliphora*. Homologous elements have been resolved in male *Musca* (HAUSEN and STRAUSFELD, 1980), *Sarcophaga*, *Syrphus*, and *Pollenia rudis*. Figure 58 is a dark-field photograph of cobalt-filled neurons in male and female *Calliphora* lobula which demonstrates that unique local neurons are also present in both sexes of this species (STRAUSFELD, 1980). In the male and female a small tangential fibre is shown against the Col A palisade.

4. Gradients and Local Specializations

It is to be expected that local curvature in neuropil contributes to variations of cell shape. This is demonstrated in the vertebrate cerebellum where Purkinje cell shapes vary in accordance with local curvature of the folium. However, in Diptera,

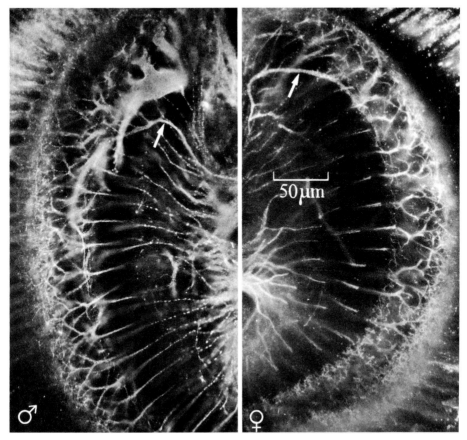

Fig. 58. Isomorphic assemblies of columnar relay neurons in male and female lobulae showing a small dorsal unique tangential cell (arrowed) that is common to both sexes and the dorsal lobula giant cell (type 1) of the male *Calliphora*

both reduced-silver studies and cobalt impregnations resolve arrangements amongst neurons which are also independent of local variations of neuropil volume and curvature.

Early examples of such gradients came from studies of the lamina. Dendrites of L 4 monopolar cells were found to be densest in the upper frontal part of the region where numerous dendrites pass to all six α-processes of an optic cartridge. Elsewhere, L 4 dendrites were found to be sparse (see p. 71). Two explanations for this were offered (STRAUSFELD and CAMPOS-ORTEGA, 1973 a). One speculated that the packing density of cartridges was such that many dendrites could be accommodated at some loci and fewer at others. The other proposed that the number and donation of L 4 dendrites was independent of cartridge packing and independent of lamina curvature. This is, in fact, the case. The L 4 cell is now known to exhibit a true structural variation that differentiates the upper frontal region of the lamina from other parts. In male flies this is specially noticeable beneath lenses of the *La lattice* (BEERSMA et al., 1977) that subserve the fovea.

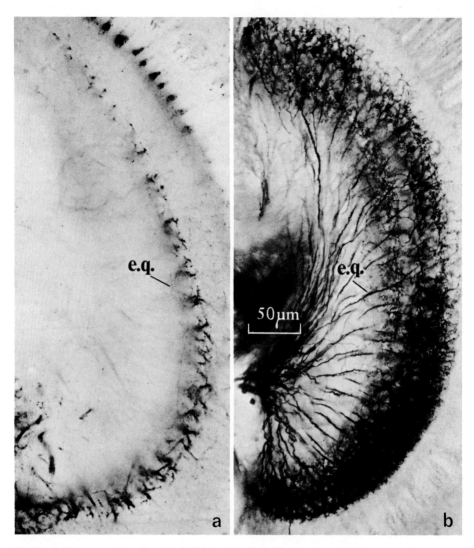

Fig. 59 a,b. Two types of gradients in the lobula. One (left) showing a gradual increase of fibre density from the upper to the lower poles of the lobula, the other showing an abrupt increase at the equator (eq.). Note the shadow of the male lobula giant in upper part of B *(Sarcophaga)*

A second gradient was described from the medulla, with reference to a set of vertically oriented, parallel fibres disposed in its third stratum ("line amacrines") which increase in density (and diameter) from posterior, dorsal and ventral columns towards anterodorsal columns (Braitenberg and Hauser-Holschuh, 1972). Again it was speculated that this gradient was independent of differences of packing density and curvature.

Electron microscopy studies of the lamina (Braitenberg and Hauser-Holschuh, 1972) resolved local variations of ratios between axon diameters of the L 1, L 2, and L 3 monopolar cells. These could not be related in a simple manner to the diameter of an optic cartridge, nor could they be related to local variations of curvature. In this study, BRAITENBERG and HAUSER-HOLSCHUH concluded that there are variations of axon diameters in the lamina, characteristic of one or the other sex, and they attempted to relate these variations to models of motion perception.

Application of cobalt ions unambiguously substantiates the existence of structural gradients within the neuropil, some running countercurrent, others independent of each other. Figure 59 illustrates two examples after cobalt fills to the *Sarcophaga* lobula: on the left is shown a graded dendritic density from dorsal to ventral in one type of giant lobula wide-field neuron, and to the right is shown a palisade of one species of relay neuron. The latter shows an abrupt increase of packing density beneath the lobula's equator. The example is derived from a male animal in which the dorsal, unique, giant neuron (MLG 1) is resolved as an empty profile. It is known that the packing density of columns is expanded in the frontal region of the male lobula (see Fig. 54). However, this would mainly affect packing along the horizontal axis, and less dorsoventrally than shown here. This assembly, therefore, demonstrates a special local variation of structure between upper and lower-front retinotopic projections. This is qualitatively different from the gradual change in packing density seen to the left which is derived from an equivalent strip of frontal neuropil.

Reduced-silver preparations of the medulla also show complex superimpositions of gradients as well as local differences of morphology. Figure 60 is a vertical section through the frontal medulla of the male *Calliphora*. Only the dorsalmost 48 columns are shown (the top of the right-hand picture continues from the bottom left). It can be seen that in the upper medulla (top left), columns are between two and three times further apart than elsewhere. The change in the packing density is abrupt and corresponds to the margin of the retina's *La lattice* (STRAUSFELD, 1979). A gradient of parallel fibres ("line amacrines") can also be seen. There is a gradual decrease of packing density, from top to bottom of the "foveal expansion", and then a sudden reduction in the number of fibres where columns are tightly packed. The gradient is then continued further posteriorly. Local morphological variations can be seen in the lower strata of the medulla, and closer inspection shows its cyto-architecture to vary between the representation of the retina's *La lattice* and elsewhere.

VIII. Output Pathways from the Optic Lobes

With the exception of the corpora pedunculata, olfactory lobes and central body, the greater part of the mid-brain is associated with neurons from the optic lobes. In particular, much of the mid-brain volume is taken up by an extensive system of tracts containing axons of relay cells from the medulla and lobula complex (Fig. 61). Some of these, such as the posterior optic tract, link the left- and right-hand medullas or the lobula plates. Others contain axons that pass centrally to optic foci on the same or opposite side of the brain.

Optic foci are discrete regions of neuropil characterized by the endings of axons from the lobula complex impinging upon parts of the dendritic trees of relay

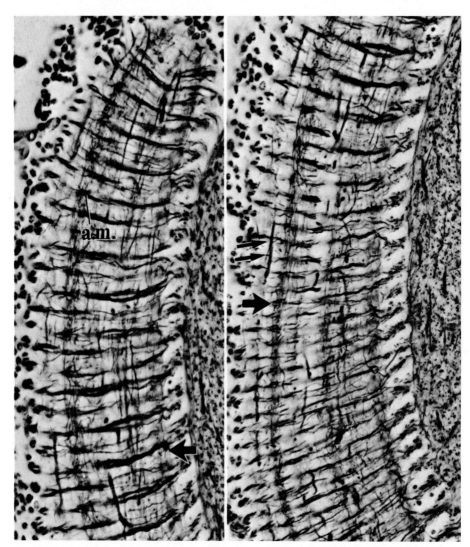

Fig. 60. Regional differences and superimposed gradients in the medulla of *Calliphora* (male). Columnar spacing is widest in the upper frontal medulla (left-hand micrograph, top, to right-hand micrograph
at double arrows) and represents the foveal region of the retina. Amacrine fibres in the third stratum
(am) abruptly decrease in density and number at the edge of the foveal expansion (single arrow, right).
Beneath the serpentine layer the structure of the neuropil shows graded and local differences of morphology (single arrow, left). Distance between upper columns is equal to 20–25 μm, between lower columns is equal to between 8 and 15 μm

neurons that leave the brain. Their axons project to thoracic and/or abdominal
ganglia and this cell class is therefore generally known as the "descending neurons"
(DN).

As a rule, small-field columnar relay neurons that are shared by the lobula and
lobula plate (or their analogues in undivided lobulas) project to optic foci in the
posterior supra-oesophageal ganglia. This part of the brain also receives the end-

ings of wide-field lobula plate neurons and some of the wide-field tangentials of the medulla. Previously, optic foci were described as being part of the protocerebrum. However, they lie at the same level as the posterior deuterocerebrum and would appear to be dorsal regions of neuropil according to the deuterocerebral neuraxis. Descending neurons that interact with optic foci also generally project down the dorsal part of the ventral cord (see also HENGSTENBERG and HENGSTENBERG, 1980).

Small-field and wide-field lobula neurons usually terminate in optic foci of the anterior brain (STRAUSFELD, 1976a, b). The great majority of small-field neurons terminate in ipsilateral optic foci although one locally arranged group of columnar neurons in dipterous lobula projects across the brain into the contralateral lobula (STRAUSFELD, 1979; see also p. 97). Tangential neurons from the lobula, or lobula plate, project either ipsi- or contralaterally. Many contralateral axons give rise to two or more groups of branches that invade ipsi- and contralateral foci. It could be envisaged that such cells mediate complex binocular interactions at the level of descending neuron dendrites. Complex heterolateral connections by lobula plate neurons in *Calliphora* have in fact been elucidated by electrophysiology combined with intracellular dye injection (HAUSEN, 1976a, b; see also HENGSTENBERG and HENGSTENBERG, 1980).

The anterior (lobula) and posterior (lobula plate) segregation of outgoing fibres from the optic lobes can also be seen in the brains of the bee and locust, representing species with an undivided lobula. Fibres above the lobula serpentine layer project to anterior optic foci.

Figure 61 illustrates axon bundles traced from the optic lobes into the midbrain through selected serial sections. Each population of neurons (that is, an assembly of similarly shaped neurons invading a characteristic stratum of neuropil) segregates out to a characteristic target in the lateral brain. This situation is identical to that found in the crayfish (see Sect. B). Figure 50 illustrated a typical pattern of axons, derived from an isomorphic assembly of Col A neurons (HAUSEN et al., 1980; HAUSEN and STRAUSFELD, 1980) converging onto the dendrites of a descending relay neuron.

Each type of nerve cell from the lobula gives rise to a characteristic form of ending. The collected endings from all of one type of neuron comprise a characteristic pattern onto a descending neuron's dendrites (see Sect. B). These patterns are invariant between individuals of the same species and if the same cell type can be recognized in two different species (e.g., *Calliphora* and *Sarcophaga*), then the patterns of endings in both are also similar. Cobalt injection into the lobula demonstrates the terminal arborizations from the lobula from which can be mapped the distributions of optic foci. Figure 62 illustrates 9 of the 40 or so optic foci in the lateral brain of *Calliphora*.

Relay neurons that pass to thoracic ganglia are associated with specific groups of terminals from the lobula. Occasionally there is a one-to-one relationship between a population of lobula neurons and a single descending neuron (e.g., the LGMD-DCMD connexion of *Schistocerca* [O'SHEA and WILLIAMS, 1974], the vertical neurons of *Drosophila* lobula plate and the vertical descending neuron [VDN] [STRAUSFELD, unpublished]). However, the more usual situation is that a descending neuron receives one major group of terminals and shares, with other descend-

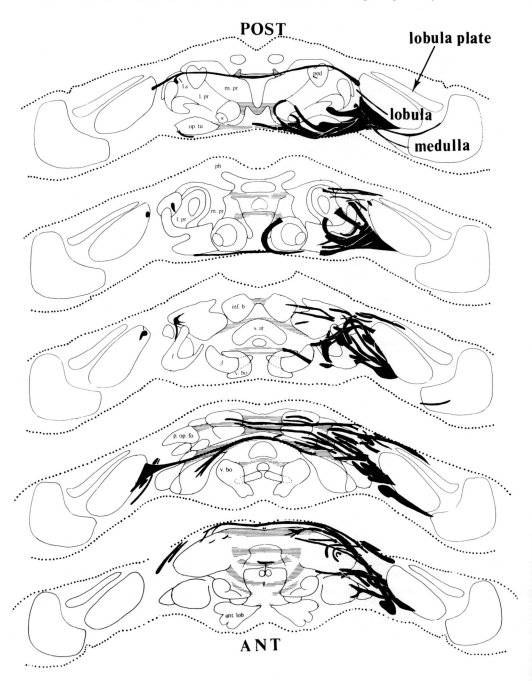

Fig. 61. Projections of axon bundles from the optic lobes into the midbrain of *Musca* showing segregation of anterior *(lobula)* and posterior *(lobula plate)* fibres. (Adapted from STRAUSFELD, 1976b)

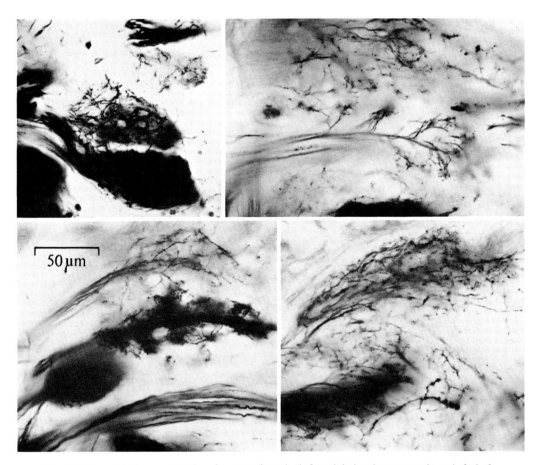

Fig. 62. Characteristic morphologies of groups of terminals from lobula relay neurons in optic foci of the deuterocerebrum (see text) *(Calliphora)*

ing neurons, terminals from other cell types from the lobula. This is apparently the case in male flies where the MLG 1 neuron arborizes extensively in the posterior slope (the most posterior region of optic foci) and interacts with dendrites of several descending neurons (STRAUSFELD and NÄSSEL, unpublished observations).

The *convergence* of many types of retinotopic neurons from the lobula complex onto relatively few descending neurons indicates that even at this deep level integration is being performed. Also, lobula terminals synapse onto more than one descending neuron, indicating that information from the lobula cells is also being *split* into parallel pathways. Studies of the LGMD-DN system have demonstrated this physiologically, showing that the LGMD converges onto an ipsilateral descending neuron which also receives input from other visual channels (O'SHEA and ROWELL, 1975), whereas the connexion to a contralateral descending neuron is through an electrical synapse modulated by chemical synapses derived from mechanoreceptor input. Complex pathways have been shown in Diptera by means of cobalt chloride diffusion. Two examples are shown in Fig. 63. In the upper

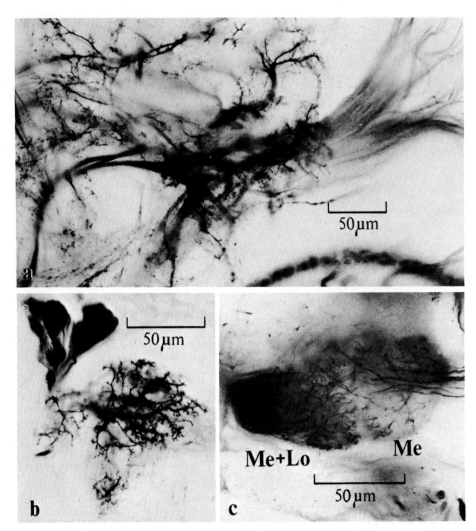

Fig. 63. a Convergence of one population of lobula relay neurons (Col A cells) onto the dendrites of a pair of descending neurons that project to the thoracic ganglia (see also Fig. 69). **b** Dendrites of four descending neurons that project from the optic tubercle and hence terminals derived from the lobula and medulla. **c** Typically bipartite structure of the optic tubercle showing its division into terminals from the medulla and lobula *(Me+Lo)* and from the medulla *(Me)*. a, b and c from *Calliphora*

micrograph, converging axons of lobula relay neurons are shown projecting onto the dendritic tree of a pair of descending relay neurons. The axon of one of them passes ipsilaterally down the ventral cord, and the other projects contralaterally down the cord, passing over the dorsal side of the oesophageal foramen (see also 68). When mechanosensory fibres are filled with cobalt from the antennae both these descending cells are resolved after migration of cobalt ions into them. Moreover, cobalt ions then pass in a retrograde fashion into the axons of lobula nerve cells. This pattern of cobalt migration illustrates that first-order receptor axons terminate on the main dendritic branches of descending visual neurons. The pattern is invariant (BACON and STRAUSFELD, 1980) and has been resolved in a number of different species of Diptera, including *Drosophila* (STRAUSFELD and SINGH, 1980: see also Fig. 68 a).

The structure of an optic focus is not just a simple convergence point. Indeed, some optic foci have very complex structures, particularly the most anterior region, the optic tubercle (STRAUSFELD and BLEST, 1970; STRAUSFELD, 1976a). This region receives input from the medulla and lobula and gives rise to at least four descending neurons (Fig. 63 b). The region is specially amenable to analysis because it is more or less isolated from the rest of the brain (COLLETT, 1972). Its structure is typical of a focus receiving heterogeneous input. The descending neuron dendrites are invested by lobula terminals, but only partly by axon terminals from the medulla. The remainder pass to the inner margin of the focus and wrap around the dendrites of neurons that connect the left- and right-hand optic tubercles. Heterolateral connexions between optic foci, carried by several axons, are typical of lobula-supplied foci in the anterior lateral brain.

The shapes of descending neurons are complex, both with respect to their dendritic trees and the patterns of terminals and collaterals in the ganglia of the body (for *Calliphora* see HENGSTENBERG and HENGSTENBERG, 1980). Again, the DCMD can be cited as the classic example (O'SHEA et al., 1974), and it is interesting to compare this cell with other descending neurons, such as the TCG (BACON and TYRER, 1979).

Characteristically, the dendritic trees of descending neurons are often subdivided into several distinct fields, some invading more than one group of lobula endings, others associated with terminals from other sensory regions, such as the corpora pedunculata (STRAUSFELD, 1976b; c.f. HENGSTENBERG and HENGSTENBERG 1980, loc. cit. Fig. 15–6). Each branch has a characteristic pattern of spines, or other specializations, and axon collaterals may also project into the posterior brain from a point just anterior to axon entry into the cervical connective.

Figure 64 illustrates some examples of descending neuron dendrites resolved by retrograde passage of cobalt or horse-radish peroxidase or by reduced silver staining. The latter shows quite well the general relationships between the cyto-architecture of the lateral deutero- and protocerebrum (which consists mainly of axon terminals and bundles from the lobula) and large argyrophilic dendritic trees. Retrograde diffusion with Lucifer yellow (STEWART, 1978) also reveals the general distribution of descending neuron dendrites and is particularly useful for mapping the positions of their cell bodies (STRAUSFELD and BACON, in preparation).

In conclusion, the final output pathway from the optic lobes is by descending neurons from the mid-brain. There is only one known exception. Horse-radish peroxidase or cobalt backfills consistently reveal a descending neuron in *Musca* whose dendrites ramify within the lobula itself. It has a second group of dendrites in the lateral deuterocerebrum. Interestingly, the neuron is postsynaptic to terminals in the lobula which are presumably derived from medulla interneurons (NÄSSEL and STRAUSFELD, 1980). As such it represents the most direct pathway to the ventral cord from the visual system. This cell has one further peculiarity. It is a typical descending neuron in that there is only one cell each side of the brain. However, whereas the pair of dendrites in the mid-brain is arranged symmetrically, left and

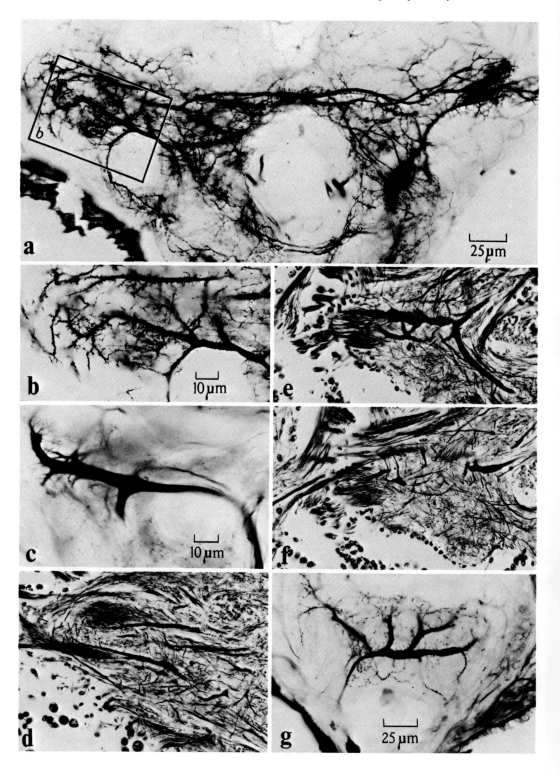

right, the dendrites in the right-hand lobula have always a much larger or much smaller field than the dendrites in the left-hand lobula. The cell imparts an asymmetry into the visual system's structure. Probably its dendrites interact with retinotopic projections, and it will be interesting to see whether the visual fields of these neurons are independent of the various forms of its dendritic fields.

IX. Functional Organization in Neuropils

a) Introduction

Previous sections outlined complex cell relationships (in terms of synaptic connexions) and general neuronal organization in terms of how cells are arranged in series, how they project between neuropils, and how cell populations contribute to special structures – neuronal assemblies.

Obvious conclusions about the visual system can be gained from the anatomy, the first being that the synaptology is already rather complicated in the lamina and is likely to be much more so in the medulla as the complexity of cell responses and the number of morphological cell types increases (see p. 115). However, although a receptor outputs to several divergent but parallel channels (p. 71), the number of neurons involved in each channel, though large, is not as defeating as it once seemed. Cobalt studies show that the shapes of cells vary considerably even though they contribute to a particular network whose structure is isomorphic (see Fig. 52).

The anatomical evidence is that parallel channels from the lamina structurally segregate in the medulla and carry through to specific cell assemblies in the lobula (STRAUSFELD, 1976 b). These then project to relatively few descending neurons that leave the back of the brain, via the ventral nerve cord, to body ganglia. There is abundant evidence that the two optic lobes communicate with each other, usually by neurons that have large dendritic fields and which possibly interact with large parts of the retinotopic mosaic (see COLLETT, 1970, 1971) or the whole of it (STRAUSFELD and BLEST, 1970; STRAUSFELD, 1976 a, b). Recently it has been shown that certain parts of the retina relay to special and local arrangements of neurons that are not found elsewhere (STRAUSFELD and HAUSEN, 1977; STRAUSFELD, 1979a, 1980; HAUSEN and STRAUSFELD, 1980).

Anatomy demonstrates much about the forms of cells, e.g., whether they are wide-field, multistratified and so on, or whether they are short axoned, long axoned or without an axon at all. Anatomy also shows the projections of cells and tells us how they might functionally connect with other cells in terms of synaptic

---

◀ **Fig. 64 a–g.** Examples of descending relay neurons from the protocerebrum. **a** Bilateral arrangements of dendrites either side of the oesophageal foramen. **b** Detail of dendrites showing local variations of dendritic spine morphologies and their distribution. **c** Horse-radish peroxidase filled giant visual descending neuron (GDN; see also Figs. 68, 69). **d–f** Reduced-silver preparations showing cyto-architecture of optic foci and the wide-diameter dendrites of descending neurons. **g** Bilateral descending neuron from sub-oesophageal ganglion and deuterocerebrum. **a, b, g** cobalt diffusion; **c** horse-radish peroxidase. Scale for figure also applies to **d–g**. All photographs from *Calliphora*

sites. But does the anatomy tell us anything about functional interaction in terms of what the animal sees?

Anatomists, by trade, would be unwilling to answer that question negatively. For example, CAJAL predicted a great deal about how neurons possibly function together, particularly in the spinal cord, and he was uncanny in the way he intuitively described the direction of axonal conductance in many systems, including the insect optic lobes (CAJAL and SÁNCHEZ, 1915). Nevertheless, predictions about functional properties of the visual system from how neurons are arranged can be no more than educated guesses. Without electrophysiological correlates and single cell dye injection, it is impossible to describe the functional circuit.

b) Structural-Functional Correlates

Neurons have been recorded and identified at every level of the system, amongst a variety of insects. The following is a brief and incomplete summary of the types of cells recognized.

1) SCHOLES (1969) first confirmed electrophysiologically that receptors sharing the same optical alignment converge to a single cartridge and to a single monopolar cell. The same was demonstrated in Odonata by LAUGHLIN (1973). Combined recordings and dye markings have shown that photoreceptor axons to lamina cartridges (and to the medulla) have depolarizing slow potentials, whereas the $L1/L2$ monopolars from the lamina have hyperpolarizing slow potentials (JÄRVILEHTO and ZETTLER, 1973). They convey information from receptors of an optic cartridge but are also influenced by signals to neighbouring cartridges, possibly via $L4$ neurons. ARNETT identified $L2$ monopolar cells with procion yellow, but the spiking cells he recorded (ARNETT, 1972) in the chiasma have not been identified by intracellular dye injection. Possibly they are wide-field centrifugals. In the fly, $L3$, $L5$, centrifugals and amacrine cells have not yet been resolved by dye injection. The $L4$ neuron and the $T1$ cell can be interpreted from dye marking experiments, and both appear to be involved in lateral inhibition (ZETTLER and JÄRVILEHTO, 1972; JÄRVILEHTO and ZETTLER, 1973; see also LAUGHLIN, 1973, 1974, 1975, on the dragonfly). The connectivities of $L4$ with amacrines, and then to $L1$, $L2$ neurons via their axon collaterals, leads us to expect that $L4$ neurons mediate lateral interactions. Also, the connexions of $T1$ with amacrines imply that this neuron receives input, excitatory or inhibitory, from a rather large field of receptors. In fact, the acceptance angle, or visual field, of $T1$ appears to be smaller than either $R1-R6$ receptors or $L1/L2$ monopolar cells (JÄRVILEHTO and ZETTLER, 1973). LAUGHLIN'S studies of dragonfly lamina neurons showed that neural adaptation circuits enable $L2$-type monopolar cells to detect changes in contrast at many ambient intensities and to standardize this information to higher-order neurons in the medulla. Two kinds of neural control mechanism have therefore been demonstrated in the lamina: one intracartridge which maintains constant contrast efficiency; the other, intercartridge, which mediates lateral inhibition and adaptation pools. In the light of LAUGHLIN'S studies on Odonata, and ZETTLER and JÄRVILEHTO'S studies on *Calliphora*, it is possible to make some sense of the logics of synaptic connexions and cell shapes in the lamina (see STRAUSFELD and CAMPOS-ORTEGA, 1977; LAUGHLIN and HARDIE, 1978).

2) Many insects are known to have two morphological classes of retinula cells, one which passes to the lamina, the other which passes to the medulla. In the fly, short retinula cell endings have the same shapes, whereas long visual fibres are of two kinds, one ending deep in the medulla (R 7) the other ending shallowly (R 8) (CAMPOS-ORTEGA and STRAUSFELD, 1971). In the bee there are three forms of long visual fibres and three main forms of short endings to the lamina (RIBI, 1979). Recordings and dye markings have shown that the shapes of these cells are peculiar to their physiology (spectral sensitivity and adaptation). In flies, R 1–R 6 are homogeneous. They show two S(λ) maxima at 470–490 nm and at 350 nm (ECKERT et al., 1976; HARDIE, 1979). R 7 has a single maximum at 344 nm (UV) or double maxima at 344 and 440 nm. R 8 has a single maximum at 440 nm (blue) and at 550 nm (blue-green) (see ECKERT et al., 1976; MEFFERT and SMOLA, 1976; STARK et al., 1977; SMOLA and MEFFERT, 1979; HARDIE, 1977, 1979; HARDIE et al., 1979). In the bee, UV receptors have long axons to the medulla, as they do in flies, whereas green receptors terminate either as deep branched axons in the proximal lamina or as thinner axons distally. Blue receptors have short stout axons (MENZEL and BLAKERS, 1975, 1976). Thus, the shape of a receptor axon (or a monopolar cell) has a functional correlate, and there is little or no ambiguity between different shapes with identical functional properties, or vice versa. However, the Gestalt of a nerve cell cannot give this information by itself. The L 4 neuron in the lamina, for example, was once proposed as a candidate for the primary motion detector (STRAUSFELD and BRAITENBERG, 1970) but, in fact, it most probably mediates lateral inhibition (STRAUSFELD and CAMPOS-ORTEGA, 1976; LAUGHLIN and HARDIE, 1978).

3) Recordings from the medulla of flies have electrophysiologically identified numerous types of activity, both small-field and large-field. Hyperpolarizing slow potentials have been recorded in the chiasma and outer medulla (monopolar axons), whereas medulla relay neurons are characterized by spikes (DEVOE and OCKLEFORD, 1976). These include directional and non-directionally sensitive neurons (BISHOP et al., 1968; MIMURA, 1971; DEVOE, 1980) and change-of-direction cells (DEVOE and OCKLEFORD, 1976). Cells recorded and dye marked include a directionally sensitive cell identified as a small-field T 2 cell that terminates in the deep strata of the lobula (DEVOE and OCKLEFORD, 1976). Another element stained represented a Y-neuron that projects to both the lobula and lobula plate. It was not tested for motion sensitivity, but was excited by light-on.

In the bee broad-band colour-sensitive neurons have been stained by procion yellow (KIEN and MENZEL, 1977). These were found to be wide-field "Y-neurons" which project into the outer and inner levels of the undivided lobula. Broad-band neurons of this kind had simply organized, sharply bordered fields. Neurons were also recorded with complex concentric fields dominated by UV, green or blue (KIEN and MENZEL, 1977). One such cell, dye-filled in the lobula, was shown to have a complex dendritic morphology where different dendritic specializations were arranged at two levels in the neuropil; each mapped differently into the retinotopic mosaic.

To date, the most extensive study of neuron shapes and response characteristics in the medulla has been made by HERTEL (1980), using intracellular injection of procion yellow, recording from the bee. Among the many classes of neurons found were broad-band colour-receptive neurons, narrow-band neurons with high sensitivity to a small part of the spectrum, and narrow-band neurons that reacted to a small intensity range and no others. These cells were sometimes antagonistic for different colours. Interestingly, the maximum sensitivity of many narrow-band neurons lay between the sensitivity maxima of different receptors. This suggests that receptor channels converge and interact more distally, supporting anatomical evidence that separate channels from the retina-lamina interact in the medulla. Possibly the abundance of amacrine cells at the level of monopolar endings and relay cell dendrites may mediate colour mixing.

HERTEL showed that the receptive fields of about 30% of recorded neurons in the medulla were smaller than 30°, whereas in the lobula they were always larger. This also supports the overall anatomy which shows that relay neurons in the medulla generally have a smaller dendritic field than they do in the lobula.

In general, neurons with complex shapes, such as asymmetric fields linked by tangential axons in the medulla, or multistratified neurons with several different sizes and levels of dendritic fields, showed the most complex responses. One asymmetric element, for example, showed different receptive fields for UV and orange light. When one field responded to UV, then orange evoked no reaction. When the other field was excited by orange, ultraviolet failed to elicit a response. Likewise, another neuron, shown to have two dendritic fields which converged to a common axon in the lobula, showed response patterns that varied in different areas of the visual field. Green was the excitatory stimulus posteriorly and inhibited anteriorly. Multistratified neurons are known to have various sizes of arborizations that radiate out from the main axis of the cell. One element recorded by HERTEL was shown to have a small receptive field and to be motion sensitive. The dimension of the field was closer in size to the cell's smaller arborization than to its deeper and wider radiations. Possibly the deeper levels represent mutually inhibiting axon collaterals rather than the receptive portion of the neuron. According to HERTEL, non-directional motion-sensitive neurons were generally found in the medulla. These had small receptive fields though their dendritic domains varied. Some extended through only a few columns, while others had wide fields. Direction-sensitive neurons were found in the lobula. However, their dendritic fields were not identical to their receptive fields and, in one case, the field of view was restricted to a horizontal strip above the equator. By comparison, the dendritic spread of this cell in the lobula was extensive.

4) The lobula and lobula plate of Diptera have attracted special attention since studies by BISHOP and KHEEN (1967) initiated electrophysiological investigations of directional motion-sensitive neurons. Studies by DVORAK et al. (1975), by HAUSEN (1976a, b), by ECKERT (1978, 1980), ECKERT and BISHOP (1978) and SOOHOO and BISHOP (1980) have demonstrated that "spiking" and "non-spiking" wide-field neurons (HENGSTENBERG, 1977) in the lobula plate are layered according to their functional properties. Neurons that are sensitive to horizontal motion reside superficially in the lobula plate, whereas neurons that are sensitive to vertical motion lie deep in the neuropil. Possibly, small-field elements, the primary motion detectors (yet unidentified), occupy two separate channels in each medulla column and segregate out to these two levels. Heterolateral neurons that connect left and right lobula plates, and which respond to horizontal motion, have terminals just beneath

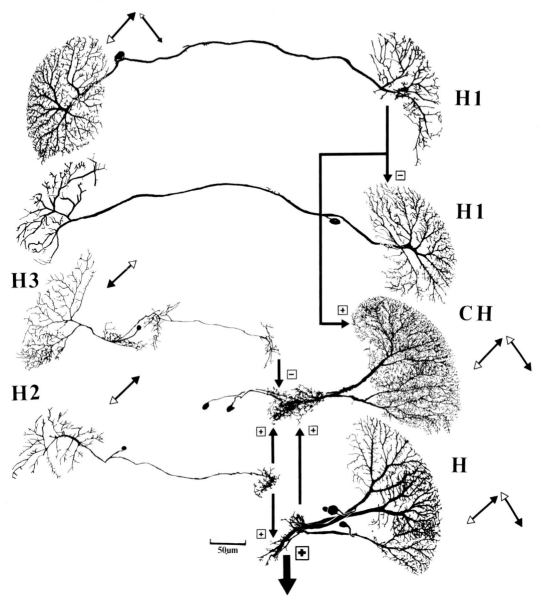

Fig. 65. Forms, and probable functional connexions, of horizontal motion-sensitive neurons of the lobula plate of *Calliphora*. A pair of heterolateral neurons *(H1)* link both plates. *H3* and *H2* link the contralateral lobula plate to ipsilateral optic foci of the rear of the mid-brain. These centers contain dendrites of two horizontal motion-sensitive centrifugal neurons *(CH)* that terminate as wide fields in the ipsilateral lobula plate. Preferred and null directions are indicated by closed and open arrows, respectively. Presumed inhibitory and excitatory relationships (from HAUSEN, 1976a) between cells are denoted by minus or plus. The three *H*-cells of the lobula plate are binocularly motion sensitive and terminate amongst the dendrites of *CH*. Presumably *H*-cells also derive inputs from small-field motion-sensitive neurons of the medulla as might the dendrites of *H1*. It is also possible that *CH* and *H1* terminals are functionally connected to *H*-cells. It is assumed that *H*-cell terminals are presynaptic to relay neurons that descend from the brain to thoracic ganglia motor neuropil. *(H1, CH* and *H* drawn from procion yellow preparations from K. HAUSEN; figures of *H3* and *H2* kindly provided by him. Other data is from HAUSEN [1976a, b] with kind permission of the author)

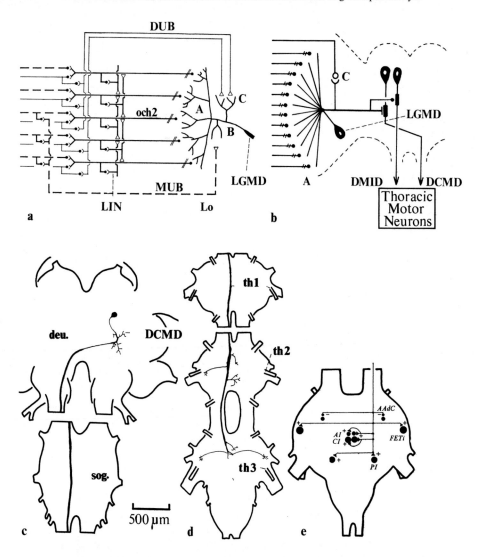

Fig. 66 a–e. Summary of connexions to the LGMD neuron and to the thoracic ganglia via the DCMD, derived from electrophysiological studies (see Rowell et al., 1977; O'Shea and Rowell, 1975, 1976; O'Shea et al., 1974; Burrows and Rowell, 1973). **a** Retinotopic ON and OFF units converge in the medulla to give phasic ON/OFF afferents that cross the second optic chiasma and end on the field *A* dendrites of the *LGMD*. These inputs are excitatory chemical synapses. However, they are labile and habituate readily. A lateral inhibitory network is envisaged to be in the medulla, between the ON/OFF pathways and to protect the system from habituation to whole-field stimuli. The inhibitory *DUB* pathway is envisaged to suppress the response of the *LGMD* to large-field stimuli (the OFF component) and the *MUB* presumably provides an inhibitory pathway for the ON component of large-field motion. Inhibition via *DUB* and, presumably, via *MUB* acts proximally to the site of input of small-field retinotopic ON/OFF units to field *A*. **b** A summary of the main elements of the *LGMD* system, showing the retinotopic inputs to *A*, the inhibitory wide-field input to *C* and the diverging input of *LGMD* to two descending neurons. One is via an electrical synapse onto the *DCMD*, the other is via an excitatory chemical synapse onto the *DIMD*. When cobalt is injected into the *LGMD*, only the *DCMD* is shown to be filled contiguously. **c** and **d** illustrate the dendritic form of the DCMD and its axonal passage into

the ipsilateral horizontal motion-sensitive cells and dendrites just superficial to them. This arrangement is invariant (see HAUSEN, 1976a, b; HENGSTENBERG, 1977; ECKERT, 1980).

The two major cell systems of the lobula plate were recognized by several anatomical methods: reduced silver (BRAITENBERG, 1970), reconstructions of semi-thin stained araldite sections (PIERANTONI, 1973, 1976) and by cobalt chloride backfilling and, fragmentarily, by the Golgi method (STRAUSFELD, 1976b). The cells are present in *Musca, Calliphora, Drosophila,* hoverflies *(Eristalis, Syrphus), Lucilia* and *Phaenicia,* to mention only a few Diptera. These cells are the first for whom a function was seriously proposed before physiological studies were performed (PIERANTONI, 1973, 1976). The vertically oriented cells were suggested to be detectors of vertical motion, the horizontal cells for horizontal motion.

The horizontal and vertical cell systems, with associated neurons, have been extensively investigated by HAUSEN (see also, ECKERT, 1980; HENGSTENBERG and HENGSTENBERG, 1980). This author has shown how the various forms of neurons (centripetal, centrifugal, and heterolateral) to and from the lobula plate respond and interact so as to give rise to binocular directional sensitivity to moving vertical or horizontal patterns. A summary of his findings for the H-system is shown in Fig. 65. The synaptic analysis of this system has been initiated using combined cobalt-electron microscopy techniques (HAUSEN et al., 1980) and preliminary results indicate that synaptology at this level might be simpler than in the lamina.

5) One pathway from the lobula to the thoracic ganglia has been extensively studied in the locust *Schistocerca.* In this species there are some bilaterally paired movement detectors which respond to vigorous and abrupt movement of small contrasting objects anywhere in the visual field. But although their dendrites cover the whole of the retinotopic mosaic, they do not respond to wide-field movement (HORN and ROWELL, 1968; PALKA, 1969; ROWELL, 1971). Combined structural and electro-physiological studies of the lobula giant movement detector (LGMD) have shown that (a) these neurons receive one retinotopic and two non-retinotopic inputs from the medulla onto three distinct dendritic areas, and (b) the LGMD is presynaptic onto a contralateral (DCMD) and an ipsilateral (DIMD) descending neuron (BURROWS and ROWELL, 1973; O'SHEA et al., 1974; O'SHEA and WILLIAMS, 1974; ROWELL et al., 1977). The retinotopic input onto the LGMD is excitatory. However, lateral inputs from the medulla onto special tufts of dendrites are inhibitory, non-retinotopic and near the site of spike initiation (Fig. 66). The retinotopic in-

---

◄ the sub-oesophageal and first through third thoracic ganglia. The main branches are in *th 2* and *th 3.* BURROWS and ROWELL (1973) deduced a pattern of connexions from the *DCMD* onto motor neurons from recordings of motor neurons. The filled circles are the sites of known motor neurons; the lines to them is the hypothetical terminal of the DCMD. PEARSON has also shown that the DCMD normally has a dorsal axon tuft to flight neuropil and that the DCMD synapses with interneurons that, in turn, provide inhibition to flexor motorneurons (PEARSON et. al., 1980; ROWELL, personal communication). **e** is at a larger magnification than **d**, and the outline of **e** is from a ventral view of *th 3* of *Schistocerca vaga. th 3* in **d** is a dorsal view, from *S. gregaria.* Despite the difference in species, physiological prediction and anatomical visualization are remarkably similar. *AAdC,* ant. coxal adductor motor neuron (MN); *FETi,* fast extensor tibiae MN; *AI* and *PI,* anterior and posterior inhibitory flexor tibiae MN; *CI,* common inhibitory MN (Figures by courtesy of C.H.F.ROWELL and M.O'SHEA)

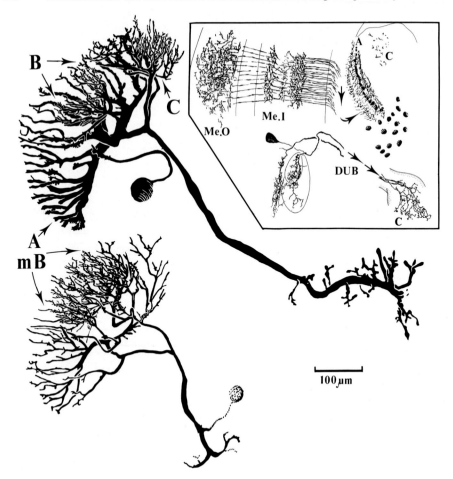

Fig. 67. The lobula giant movement detector (LGMD) and associated elements *(Schistocerca gregaria)*. Cobalt injection into the LGMD shows this cell to consist of a fan-shaped dendritic tree that maps into the lobula (the A field, *A*) and two smaller but denser trees, the B and C fields *(B, C)*. These invade lateral deuterocerebral outgrowths of the mid-brain neuropil that partly envelope the lobula dorsally (the C-field) and postero-medially (the B-field). The lower fan-shaped neuron is similar in shape to the LGMD and is sometimes shown up with the LGMD after cobalt-silver intensification. Typically this cell consists of an A-field and a B-field *(mB)* whose branches are blebbed and are possibly presynaptic onto the LGMD. This neuron would thus be a centrifugal cell and could possibly provide multimodal dishabituation input to the LGMD A and B-field. The cell-body of the second neuron lies centrally and is reminiscent of the centrifugal horizontal cell of the fly optic lobe (the CH-cell; see Fig. 65). At least three types of inputs are predicted onto the LGMD from physiology (see preceding figure). The first is a retinotopic projection of phasic ON/OFF units from the medulla, impinging onto sub-field A. It is predicted that an inhibitory network exists between neurons comprising this input, distal to its level of termination and probably in the medulla. The second input is supposed to collect from the phasic ON (and another from the phasic OFF) units in the medulla and provide inhibitory synapses onto the LGMD's central sub-fields (B and C). Golgi studies have shown that small-field tangential cells distributed across the whole of the inner medulla project axons to a dorsal uncrossed bundle that projects onto field C. Some of these cells are shown in the lower part of the inset. Silver intensified LGMDs also show accompanying small-field retinotopic elements, presumably filled transsynaptically and representing input cells. Some of these are shown in the upper part of the inset. The camera lucida drawing is from three consecutive sections and shows some T-cells that are arranged two per medulla column

puts habituate rapidly (O'SHEA and ROWELL, 1975, 1976). However, response to large-field motion is suppressed by the inhibitory input which derives its own input from spatial summation over the whole of the visual field. Anatomical correlates have been shown to exist for both pathways onto the LGMD. However, the site of an inhibitory network which protects this system from habituation to wide-field stimuli (which would otherwise render it blind to small-field stimuli after large-field movement) is predicted to reside peripheral to retinotopic convergence onto the DCMD. The structural correlate has yet to be found, but may reside even at the level of the lamina as suggested by LAUGHLIN and HARDIE, (1978).

The LGMD has been shown to be chemically presynaptic to the DIMD and electrically synaptic to the DCMD (O'SHEA and ROWELL, 1975). The former neuron receives input from other types of visual relay neurons. The DCMD, however, is modulated by other sensory modalities which may gate LGMD-DCMD transmission by means of chemical synapses. The DIMD and DCMD branch in all three thoracic ganglia where they synapse onto at least six motoneurons of the metathoracic (Fig. 66) involved in the escape jump reaction (BURROWS and ROWELL, 1973; PEARSON et. al., 1980). The system, from lobula to behaviour, is probably the most thoroughly studied of any visual pathway and demonstrates much about the shape of a neuron and the kind of multimodal output that can influence the messages carried by descending neurons from the brain. Anatomical correlates to the physiology (Fig. 66) are summarized in Fig. 67.

Other multimodal descending neurons have been identified. The giant descending neuron of *Drosophila* responds to both visual and mechanosensory stimuli (LEVINE, 1974; LEVINE and TRACY, 1973; see also KING, 1979; KING and WYMAN, 1980), and its relationships with antennal and visual fibres in wild-type and mutant *(bar-eyed) Drosophila* (Fig. 68) have been described by light microscopy (STRAUS-FELD and SINGH, 1980). Descending neurons that take up cobalt from primarily filled antennal axons and donate cobalt to Col A cells of the lobula (Fig. 50) have been recorded and filled with Lucifer yellow. These are also directionally sensitive to motion and respond to air flow (BACON and STRAUSFELD, 1980). In *Schistocerca* some small-diameter descending neurons respond exclusively to wide-field motion and have been singly marked with cobalt nitrate (KIEN, 1976). Others, such as the tritocerebral commissure giant (TCG), respond to light-on and light-off and to wind flow over the head (BACON and TYRER, 1978). Their relationship with projections from mechanosensory fibres is also known (TYRER et al., 1979), as is the branching pattern of the TCG in the thoracic ganglia (Fig. 70). In general, giant neurons

---

◄ and which project to the A-field of LGMD. Note that there are two forms of T-cell, one of which extends to the outer face of the medulla and another which resides beneath the serpentine layer. A pair of axons leaves each column and passes to the lobula. Some slender axons projecting to sub-field B were also found in preparations in which the LGMD had been filled with cobalt. These are not drawn here. However, they were traced into the medulla amongst the plexus of lateral connexions between the T-cells. Possibly axons onto sub-field B are collaterals from one type of these small-field medulla neurons. In any event, axons to B comprise a median uncrossed bundle which maps non-retinotopically onto B. [Preparations of silver intensified LGMD neurons (also found to contain fan cells an medulla-to-lobula T-cells) were provided by C.H.F.ROWELL. The drawing of the DUB neurons was provided by J.L.D.WILLIAMS.]

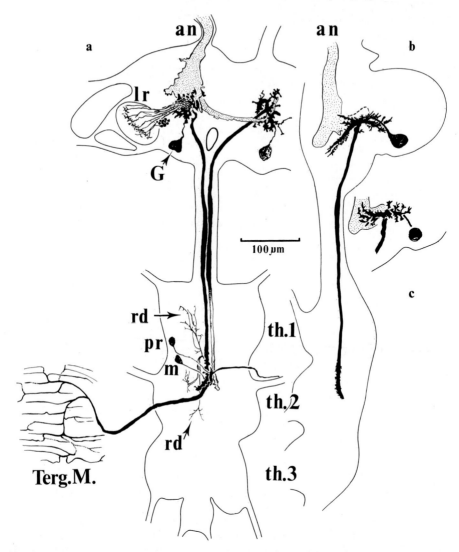

Fig. 68a–c. The giant descending neuron (GDN) of *Drosophila*. **a** The giant neuron with associated elements after cobalt diffusion from the antenno-mechanosensory nerve *(an)*. Cobalt migrates to some dendrites of the GDN ipsilaterally. A contralateral branch of *an* donates cobalt to the contralateral GDN. Silver intensification shows that most cobalt has entered the ipsilateral GDN and has spread across to Col A cells of the lobula (lobula relay neurons, *lr*). Cobalt also passes from the terminal of the giant *(G)* into a motor neuron (m) that terminates on the tergotrochantal muscle *(Terg.M)* and to a premotor relay neuron *(pr)* that leaves the second (meso-) thoracic ganglion *(th 2)* contralaterally. This neuron also has dendrites *(rd)* that extend into the dorsal medial tract, amongst sensory projections from the tergum and wings (see KING and WYMAN, 1980). **b** The form of a GDN from the side and **c** the dendritic tree of a GDN in a bar-eyed mutant in which ommatidia, lamina, medulla, and lobula complex are reduced to only a few columns. Mutations that affect the thoracic cuticle, such as bithorax, do not seem to give rise to an alteration of GDN's terminal

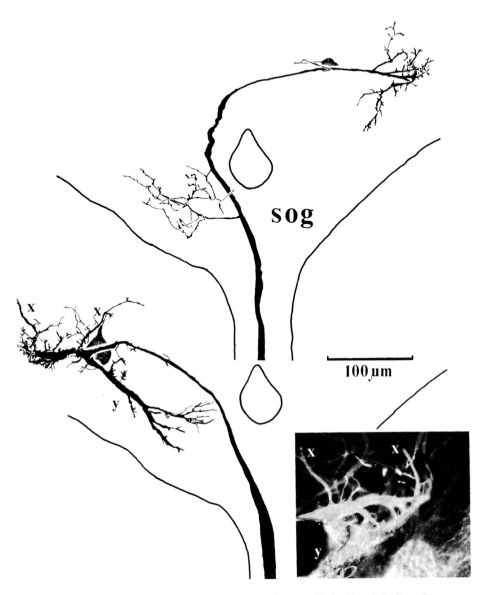

Fig. 69. A pair of descending neurons from the brain of *Musca* filled with cobalt-silver. The upper neuron projects contralaterally and gives off branches in the sub-oesophageal ganglion *(sog)*, whereas the lower neuron (the giant descending neuron, GDN) gives rise to a recurrent branch medially in the *sog*. The inset shows a GDN of the opposite side of the brain, but from *Calliphora*. The photograph is by dark-field illumination and shows first-order antennal sensory axons (bright, small diameter profiles) ending on the y-branch (see also BACON and STRAUSFELD, 1980a). The two cells, one in *Musca*, the other in *Calliphora*, are almost identical. *x* and *y* indicate similar and prominent branches. The contralaterally projecting cell was multimodal, directionally sensitive to regressive and up-to-downward movement of gratings and to wind flow. (See also Fig. 63a for convergence of visual cell axons onto these neurons)

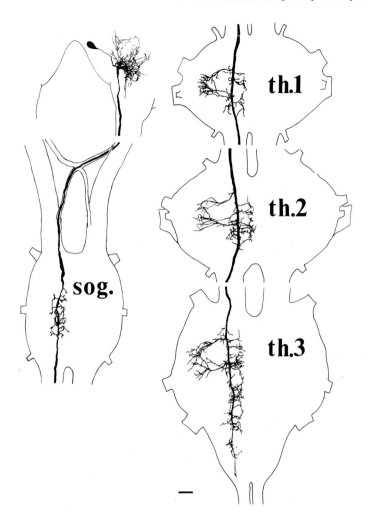

Fig. 70. The tritocerebral giant (TCG) of *Schistocerca gregaria*, so-called because its axon is the largest in the tritocerebral commissure (BACON and TYRER, 1978). The cell responds to air flow over the head. It receives an input frontally from the head hairs and is also excited by light-on and light-off. The axon gives rise to branches ipsilaterally in the sub-oesophageal ganglion *(sog)* and in the thoracic ganglia *(th. 1–3)*. Medially directed branches extend to the median tract which contains many of the wing sensory projections. Lateral branches extend into the lateral dorsal tract which contains the branched dendrites of flight motor neurons (see TYRER and ALTMANN, 1974)

of the lobula (or lobula plate) and descending neurons from the brain to the ventral cord are the most amenable for analysis. Both levels of the system predict functional connexions further peripherally and lead to precise questions about the anatomy. Also, both levels of the system are close to the final motor output. The last few years' research demonstrates that the insect visual system is wide open to analysis, from the retina to motor neurons, from the visual world to behaviour.

Acknowledgement. We would specially like to thank Malu Obermayer and Harjit Seyan for their enormous contribution to our research. The great majority of original light microscopy preparations of dipterous insects were made by them. Contributors of scientific material are acknowledged in the Summary (p. 3).

Note added in proof (see page 493).

References

Altman, J.S., Shaw, M.K., Tyrer, N.M.: Visualization of synapses of physiologically identified cobalt-filled neurones in the locust. J. Physiol. (Lond.) **296**, 2–3 P (1979)

Altman, J.S., Shaw, M.K., Tyrer, N.M.: Input synapses on to a locust sensory neurone revealed by cobalt-electron microscopy. Brain Res. **189**, 245–250 (1980)

Andersson, A., Hallberg, E., Johnsson, S. B.: The fine structure of the compound eye of *Tanais cavolini* Milne-Edwards (Crustacea: Tanaidacea). Acta Zool. (Stockh.) **59**, 49–55 (1978)

Aramant, R., Elofsson, R.: Distribution of monoaminergic neurons in the nervous system of non-malacostracan crustaceans. Cell Tissue Res. **166**, 1–24 (1976)

Armett-Kibel, C., Meinertzhagen, I. A., Dowling, J. E.: Cellular and synaptic organization in the lamina of the dragon-fly *Sympetrum rubicundulum*. Proc. R. Soc. Lond. [Biol.] **196**, 385–413 (1977)

Arnett, D. W.: Spatial and temporal integration properties of units in the first optic ganglion of Dipterans. J. Neurophysiol. **35**, 429–444 (1972)

Bacon, J., Strausfeld, N.J.: Nonrandom resolution of neuron arrangements. In: Experimental Entomology: Neuroanatomical Techniques (eds. T.A. Miller, N.J. Strausfeld) pp 357–372. New York–Heidelberg–Berlin: Springer 1980a

Bacon, J.P., Strausfeld, N.J.: Descending multimodal neurons from fly brains: 1. Functional organization by cobalt and lucifer yellow analysis (in preparation, 1980b)

Bacon, J.P., Tyrer, N.M.: The tritocerebral commissure giant (TCG): a bimodal interneurone in the locust. J. Comp. Physiol. **126**, 317–325 (1978)

Ball, E. E.: Fine structure of the compound eyes of the midwater amphipod *Phronima* in relation to behaviour and habitat. Tissue Cell **9**, 521–536 (1977)

Beersma, D.G.M., Stavenga, D.G., Kuiper, J.W.: Organization of visual axes in the compound eye of the fly *Musca domestica* L. and the behavioural consequences. J. Comp. Physiol. **102**, 305–320 (1975)

Beersma, D. G. M., Stavenga, D. G., Kuiper, J. W.: Retinal lattice, visual field and binocularities in flies. J. Comp. Physiol. **119**, 207–220 (1977)

Bernhards, H.: Der Bau des Komplexauges von *Astacus fluviatilis (Potamobius astacus)*. Z. Wiss. Zool. **116**, 649–707 (1916)

Bethe, A.: Das Centralnervensystem von *Carcinus maenas*. Ein anatomisch-physiologischer Versuch. I. Theil, II. Mittheil. Arch. Mikr. Anat. **50**, 589–639 (1897b)

Bethe, A.: Das Nervensystem von *Carcinus maenas*, ein anatomisch-physiologischer Versuch. I. Theil, I. Mittheil. Arch. Mikr. Anat. **50**, 460–546 (1897a)

Bishop, L. G., Kheen, D. G.: Two types of motion sensitive neurons in the optic lobes of the fly. Nature **212**, 1374–1376 (1966)

Boschek, C. B.: On the fine structure of the peripheral retina and the lamina of the fly, *Musca domestica*. Z. Zellforsch. **110**, 336–349 (1971)

Braitenberg, V.: Patterns of projection in the visual system of the fly. I. Retina-lamina projections. Exp. Brain Res. **3**, 271–298 (1967)

Braitenberg, V.: Ordnung und Orientierung der Elemente im Sehsystem der Fliege. Kybernetik **7**, 235–242 (1970)

Braitenberg, V., Debbage, P.: A regular net of reciprocal synapses in the visual system of the fly, *Musca domestica*. J. Comp. Physiol. **90**, 25–31 (1974)

Braitenberg, V., Hauser-Holschuh, H.: Patterns of projection in the visual system of the fly. II. Quantitative aspects of second order neurons in relation to models of movement perception. Exp. Brain Res. **16**, 184–209 (1972)

Braitenberg, V., Strausfeld, N.J.: Principles of the mosaic organization in the visual system's neuropil of *Musca domestica* L. In: Handbook of sensory physiology, Vol. VII/3 A: Central processing of visual information (ed. R.Jung). Berlin-Heidelberg-New York: Springer 1973

Brammer, J.D.: The ultrastructure of the compound eye of a mosquito, *Aedes aegypti* L. J. Exp. Zool. **175**, 181–196 (1970)

Bullock, T. H., Horridge, G. A.: Structure and function in the nervous system of invertebrates, Vol. II. San Francisco: W. H. Freeman and Co. 1965

Burkhardt, W., Braitenberg, V.: Some peculiar synaptic complexes in the first visual ganglion of the fly, *Musca domestica*. Cell Tiss. Res. **173**, 287–308 (1976).

Burrows, M., Rowell, C. H. F.: Connections between visual interneurons and metathoracic motor-neurons in the locust. J. Comp. Physiol. **85**, 221–234 (1973)

Cajal, S. R., Sánchez y Sánchez, D.: Contribución al conocimiento de los centros nerviosos de los insectos. Parte I. Rétina y centros opticos. Trab. Lab. Invest. Biol. Univ. Madrid **13**, 1–168 (1915)

Campos-Ortega, J. A., Strausfeld, N. J.: The columnar organization of the second synaptic region of the visual system of *Musca domestica* L. I. Receptor terminals in the medulla. Z. Zellforsch. **124**, 561–585 (1972a)

Campos-Ortega, J. A., Strausfeld, N. J.: Columns and layers in the second synaptic region of the fly's visual system: The case for two superimposed neuronal architectures. In: Information processing in the visual system of Arthropods (ed. R. Wehner). Berlin-Heidelberg-New York: Springer 1972b

Campos-Ortega, J. A., Strausfeld, N. J.: Synaptic connections of intrinsic cells and basket arborisations in the external plexiform layer of the fly's eye. Brain Res. **59**, 119–136 (1973)

Collett, T.: Centripetal and centrifugal visual cells in medulla of the insect optic lobe. J. Neurophysiol. **33**, 239–256 (1970)

Collett, T.: Visual neurones for tracking moving targets. Nature (Lond.) **232**, 127–130 (1971)

Collett, T.: Visual neurones in the anterior optic tract of the privet hawk moth. J. Comp. Physiol. **78**, 396–433 (1972)

Debaisieux, P.: Les yeux des Crustacés, structure, dévelopement, réactions à l'éclairement. Cellule **50**, 9–122 (1944)

DeVoe, R.D.: Movement sensitivities of cells in the fly's medulla. J. Comp. Physiol. **138**, 93–119 (1980)

DeVoe, R. D., Ockleford, E. M.: Intracellular responses from cells of the medulla of the fly, *Calliphora erythrocephala*. Biol. Cybern. **23**, 13–24 (1976)

Dietrich, W.: Die Facettenaugen der Dipteren. Z. Wiss. Zool. **92**, 465–539 (1909)

Dvorak, D. R., Bishop, L. G., Eckert, H. E.: On the identification of movement detectors in the fly optic lobe. J. Comp. Physiol. **100**, 5–23 (1975)

Eckert, H., Bishop, L. G.: Anatomical and physiological properties of the vertical cells in the third optic ganglion of *Phaenicia sericata* (Diptera, Calliphoridae). J. Comp. Physiol. **126**, 57–86 (1978)

Eckert, H., Bishop, L. G., Dvorak, D. R.: Spectral sensitivities of identified receptor cells in the blowfly *Calliphora*. Naturwissenschaften **63**, 47–48 (1976)

Eckert, H. E.: Response properties of dipteran giant visual interneurons involved in control of optomotor behaviour. Nature **271**, 358–360 (1978)

Eckert, H.: Functional properties of the H 1-neurone in the third optic ganglion of the blow fly, *Phaenicia*. J. Comp. Physiol. **135**, 29–39 (1980)

Eckert, M.: Hell-Dunkel-Adaptation in aconen Appositionsaugen der Insekten. Zool. Jb. Physiol. **74**, 102–120 (1968)

Eguchi, E.: Rhabdom structure and receptor potentials in single crayfish retinular cells. J. Cell. Comp. Physiol. **66**, 411–430 (1965)

Eguchi, E., Waterman, T. H.: Fine structure patterns in crustacean rhabdoms. In: The Functional Organization of the Compound Eye (ed. C. G. Bernhard), pp. 105–124. Oxford: Pergamon Press 1966

Elofsson, R., Dahl, E.: The optic neuropils and chiasmata of Crustacea. Z. Zellforsch. **107**, 343–360 (1970)

Elofsson, R., Kauri, T., Nielsen, S.-O., Strömberg, J.-O.: Localization of monoaminergic neurons in the central nervous system of *Astacus astacus* (Crustacea). Z. Zellforsch. **74**, 464–473 (1966)

Elofsson, R., Klemm, N.: Monoamine-containing neurons in the optic ganglia of crustaceans and insects. Z. Zellforsch. **133**, 475–499 (1972)

Elofsson, A., Nässel, D., Myhrberg, H.: A catecholaminergic neuron connecting the first two optic neuropiles (lamina ganglionaris and medulla externa) of the crayfish *Pacifastacus leniusculus*. Cell Tissue Res. **182**, 287–297 (1977)

Elofsson, R., Odselius, R.: The anostracan rhabdom and the basement membrane. An ultrastructural study of the *Artemia* compound eye (Crustacea). Acta Zool. (Stockh.) **56**, 141–153 (1975)

Erber, J., Sandeman, D.C.: The detection of real and apparent motion by the crab *Leptograpsus variegatus*. II. Electrophysiology. J. Comp. Physiol. **112**, 189–197 (1976)

Exner, S.: Die Physiologie der facettierten Augen von Krebsen und Insecten. Leipzig-Wien: Franz Deuticke 1891

Falck, B., Hillarp, N.-A., Thieme, G., Torp, A.: Fluorescence of catecholamines and related compounds condensed with formaldehyde. J. Histochem. Cytochem. **10**, 348–354 (1962)

Franceschini, N., Münster, A., Heurkens, G.: Äquatoriales und binokulares Sehen bei der Fliege *Calliphora erythrocephala* (abstract). Verh. Deutsch. Zool. Ges., **72**, 209 (1979)

Fraser, P. J.: Directionality of a one way movement detector in the crayfish *Cherax destructor*. J. Comp. Physiol. **118**, 187–193 (1977)

Glanz, R. M.: Visual input and motor output of command interneurons of the defense reflex pathway in the crayfish. In: Identified neurons and behaviour of arthropods (ed. G. Hoyle). New York: Plenum 1977

Goldsmith, T. H., Fernández, H. R.: Comparative studies of Crustacean spectral sensitivity. Z. Vergl. Physiol. **60**, 156–175 (1968)

Goldsmith, T. H.: The spectral absorption of crayfish rhabdoms: pigment, photoproduct and pH sensitivity. Vision Res. **18**, 463–473 (1978)

Güldner, F.-H., Wolff, J. R.: Über die Ultrastruktur des Komplexauges von *Daphnia pulex*. Z. Zellforsch. **104**, 259–274 (1970)

Hafner, G. S.: The neural organization of the lamina ganglionaris in the crayfish: A Golgi and EM study. J. Comp. Neurol. **152**, 255–280 (1973)

Hafner, G. S.: The ultrastructure of retinula cell endings in the compound eye of the crayfish. J. Neurocytol. **3**, 295–311 (1974)

Hafner, G. S., Tokarski, T. R.: Evidence for putative photoreceptor axon terminals in the medulla externa of the crayfish. Cell Tiss. Res. **195**, 331–340 (1978)

Hallberg, E.: The fine structure of the compound eyes of mysids (Crustacea: Mysidacea). Cell Tiss. Res. **184**, 45–65 (1977)

Hámori, J., Horridge, G. A.: The lobster optic lamina. I. General organization. J. Cell Sci. **1**, 249–256 (1966a)

Hámori, J., Horridge, G. A.: The lobster optic lamina. II. Types of synapse. J. Cell Sci. **1**, 257–270 (1966b)

Hanström, B.: Eine genetische Studie über die Augen und Sehzentrum von Turbellarien, Anneliden und Arthropoden. K. Svenska Vetensk. Akad. Handl. **66**, 1–176 (1926)

Hanström, B.: Untersuchungen über das Gehirn, insbesondere die Sehganglien der Crustaceen. Arkiv. Zool. **16**, 1–119 (1924)

Hanström, B.: Vergleichende Anatomie des Nervensystems der wirbellosen Tiere. Berlin: Springer 1928

Hardie, R. C.: Electrophysiological analysis of the fly retina. 1. Comparative properties of R 1–6 and R 7 and 8. J. Comp. Physiol. **129**, 19–33 (1979)

Hardie, R. C., Franceschini, N., McIntyre, P. D.: Electrophysiological analysis of fly retina. II. Spectral and polarisation sensitivity in R 7 and R 8. J. Comp. Physiol. **133**, 23–39 (1979)

Hausen, K.: Struktur, Funktion und Konnektivität bewegungsempfindlicher Interneuronen im dritten optischen Neuropil der Schmeißfliege *Calliphora erythrocephala*. Doctoral Dissertation. University of Tübingen (1976a)

Hausen, K.: Functional characterization and anatomical identification of motion sensitive neurons in the lobula plate of the blowfly *Calliphora erythrocephala*. Z. Naturforsch. **31**c, 629–633 (1976b)

Hausen, K.: Signal processing in the insect eye. In: Function and formation of neural systems (ed. G. S. Stent), pp. 81–110. Berlin: Dahlem Konferenzen 1977

Hausen, K., Strausfeld, N. J.: Sexually dimorphic interneuron arrangements in the fly visual system. Proc. R. Soc. Lond. B **208**, 57–71 (1980)

Hausen, K., Wolburg-Buchholz, K., Ribi, W. A.: The synaptic organization of visual interneurons in the lobula-complex of flies. Cell Tissue Res. **208**, 371–387 (1980)

Hengstenberg, R., Hengstenberg, B.: Intracellular staining of insect neurons with procion yellow. In: Experimental Entomology: Neuroanatomical Techniques (eds. T. A. Miller, N. J. Strausfeld) pp 307–324. New York–Heidelberg–Berlin: Springer 1980

Hengstenberg, R.: Spike responses of "non-spiking" visual interneurons. Nature **270**, 338–340 (1977)

Hertel, H.: Chromatic properties of identified interneurons in the optic lobes of the bee. J. Comp. Physiol. **137**, 215–232 (1980)

Horn, G., Rowell, C. H. F.: Medium and long-term changes in the behaviour of visual neurones in the tritocerebrum of locusts. J. Exp. Biol. **49**, 143–169 (1968)

Järvilehto, M., Moring, J.: Spectral and polarization sensitivity of identified retinal cells of the fly. In: Neural principles in vision (eds. F. Zettler, R. Weiler), pp. 214–226. Berlin-Heidelberg-New York: Springer 1976

Järvilehto, M., Zettler, F.: Electrophysiological-histological studies on some functional properties of visual cells and second order neurons of an insect retina. Z. Zellforsch. **136**, 291–306 (1973)

Kampa, E. M.: The euphausiid eye – a re-evaluation. Vision Res. **5**, 475–481 (1965)

Kennedy, D., Bruno, M. S.: The spectral sensitivity of crayfish and lobster vision. J. Gen. Physiol. **44**, 1089–1102 (1961)

Kien, J.: A preliminary report on cobalt sulphide staining of locust visual interneurones through extracellular electrodes. Brain Res. **109**, 158–164 (1976)

Kien, J., Menzel, R.: Chromatic properties of interneurons in the optic lobes of the bee. 1. Broad band neurons. J. Comp. Physiol. **113**, 17–34 (1977)

King, D. G., Wyman, R. J.: Anatomy of the giant fibre pathway in *Drosophila*. I. Three thoracic components of the pathway. J. Neurocytol. (in press) 1980

Kirschfeld, K.: Das neurale Superpositionsauge. Fortschr. Zool. **21**, 229–257 (1973)

Kirschfeld, K.: Die Projektion der optischen Umwelt auf das Raster der Rhabdomere im Komplexauge von *Musca*. Exp. Brain Res. **3**, 248–270 (1967)

Kirschfeld, K., Franceschini, N.: Ein Mechanismus zur Steuerung des Lichtflusses in den Rhabdomeren des Komplexauge von *Musca*. Kybernetik **6**, 13–22 (1969)

Kirschfeld, K., Franceschini, N.: Optische Eigenschaften der Ommatidien im Komplexauge von *Musca*. Kybernetik **5**, 47–52 (1968)

Kleinholz, L. H.: Pigmentary effectors. In: The physiology of Crustacea (ed. T. H. Waterman), pp. 133–169. New York-London: Academic Press 1961

Krebs, W.: The fine structure of the retinula of the compound eye of *Astacus fluviatilis*. Z. Zellforsch. **133**, 399–414 (1972)

Kunze, P.: Eye glow in the moth and superposition theory. Nature (Lond) **223**, 1172–1174 (1969)

Kunze, P.: Comparative studies of arthropod superposition eyes. Z. vergl. Physiol. **76**, 347–357 (1972)

Land, M. F., Burton, F. A., Meyer-Rochow, V. B.: The optical geometry of Euphausiid eyes. J. Comp. Physiol. **130**, 49–62 (1979)

Langer, H., Schneider, L.: Zur Struktur und Funktion offener Rhabdome in Facettenaugen. Zool. Anz. Suppl. **33**, 494–321 (1970)

Laughlin, S.B.: Neural integration in the first optic neuropile of dragonflies. I. Signal amplification in dark-adapted second order neurons. J. Comp. Physiol. **84**, 335–355 (1973)

Laughlin, S.B.: Neural integration in the first optic neuropile of dragonflies. III. The transfer of angular information. J. Comp. Physiol. **92**, 377–396 (1974)

Laughlin, S. B.: The function of the lamina ganglionaris. In: The compound eye and vision of insects (ed. G. A. Horridge), pp. 341–358. Oxford: Clarendon Press 1975

Laughlin, S. B.: Neural integration in the first optic neuropile of dragonflies. J. Comp. Physiol. **112**, 199–211 (1976a)

Laughlin, S. B.: Adaptations of the dragonfly retina for contrast detection and the elucidation of neural principles in the peripheral visual system. In: Neural principles in vision (eds. F. Zettler, R. Weiler), pp. 175–193. Berlin-Heidelberg-New York: Springer 1976b

Laughlin, S. B., Hardie, R. C.: Common strategies for light adaptation in the peripheral visual systems of fly and dragonfly. J. Comp. Physiol. **128**, 319–340 (1978)

Leder, H.: Untersuchungen über den feineren Bau des Nervensystems der Cladoceren. Arb. Zool. Inst. Wien u. Triest **20**, 297–392 (1915)

Leggett, L. M. W.: Polarized light sensitive interneurons in a swimming crab. Nature **262**, 709–711 (1976)

Levine, J. D.: Giant neuron input in mutant and wild type *Drosophila*. J. Comp. Physiol. **93**, 265–285 (1974)

Levine, J. D., Tracy, D.: Structure and function of the giant motorneuron of *Drosophila melanogaster*. J. Morph. **140**, 153–158 (1973)

Macagno, E. R.: Mechanism for the formation of synaptic projections in the arthropod visual system. Nature **275**, 318–320 (1978)

Macagno, E. R., Levinthal, C.: Computer reconstruction of the cellular architecture of the *Daphnia magna* optic ganglion. In: 33rd Ann. Proc. Electron Microscopy Soc. Am., Las Vegas, Nevada (ed. G. W. Bailey), pp. 284–285 (1975)

Macagno, E. R., Lopresti, V., Levinthal, C.: Structure and development of neural connections in isogenic organisms: Variations and similarities in the optic system of *Daphnia magna*. Proc. Natl. Acad. Sci. U.S.A. **70**, 57–61 (1973)

Meffert, P., Smola, U.: Electrophysiological measurements of spectral sensitivity of central visual cells in eye of blowfly. Nature **260**, 342–344 (1976)

Meinertzhagen, I. A.: The first and second neural projections of the insect eye. Ph.D. Thesis, University of St. Andrews, Scotland 1971

Meinertzhagen, I. A.: Development of the compound eye and optic lobe of insects. In: Developmental neurobiology of arthropods (ed. D. Young). Cambridge: Univ. Press 1973

Meinertzhagen, I. A.: The organization of perpendicular fibre pathways in the insect optic lobe. Phil. Trans. R. Soc. Lond B **274**, 555–596 (1976)

Mellon, De F.: Central and peripheral features of crayfish oculomotor organization. In: Identified neurons and behaviour of arthropods (ed. G. Hoyle). New York: Plenum 1977

Menzel, R., Blakers, M.: Colour receptors in the bee eye-morphology and spectral sensitivity. J. Comp. Physiol. **108**, 11–33 (1976)

Meyer, E. P.: Golgi-EM-study of first and second order neurons in the visual system of *Cataglyphis bicolor* Fabricius (Hymenoptera, Formicidae). Zoomorphologie **92**, 115–139 (1979)

Meyer-Rochow, V. B.: Axonal wiring and polarization sensitivity in the eye of the rock lobster. Nature **254**, 522–523 (1975)

Meyer-Rochow, V. B.: The eyes of mesopelagic crustaceans II. *Streetsia challengeri* (Amphipoda). Cell Tissue Res. **186**, 337–350 (1978a)

Meyer-Rochow, V. B.: The eyes of mesopelagic crustaceans. III. *Thysanopoda tricuspidata* (Euphausiacea). Cell Tissue Res. **195**, 59–79 (1978b)

Meyer-Rochow, V. B., Nässel, D. R.: Crustacean eyes and polarization sensitivity. Vision Res. **17**, 1239–1240 (1977)

Mimura, M.: Movement discrimination by the visual system of flies. Z. Vergl. Physiol. **73**, 105–138 (1971)

Muller, K. J.: Photoreceptors in the crayfish compound eye: electrical interactions between cells as related to polarized light sensitivity. J. Physiol. (Lond) **232**, 573–595 (1973)

Nässel, D. R.: The organization of the lamina ganglionaris of the prawn *Pandalus borealis* (Kröyer). Cell Tissue Res. **163**, 445–465 (1975)

Nässel, D. R.: The retina and retinal projection on the lamina ganglionaris of the crayfish *Pacifastacus leniusculus* (Dana). J. Comp. Neurol. **167**, 341–360 (1976a)

Nässel, D. R.: The fine structure of photoreceptor terminals in the compound eye of *Pandalus borealis* (Crustacea). Acta Zool. (Stockh.) **57**, 153–160 (1976b)

Nässel, D. R.: Types and arrangements of neurons in the crayfish optic lamina. Cell Tissue Res. **179**, 45–75 (1977a)

Nässel, D. R.: Neural connectivity patterns in the compound eyes of crustaceans. Thesis, Lund (1977b)

Nässel, D. R.: Projections and arrangements of relay neurons and associated elements in the crayfish visual system: a cobalt and Golgi study. (in preparation, 1980)

Nässel, D. R., Strausfeld, N. J.: The LTDN: a direct pathway from the optic lobes to thoracic ganglia (in preparation 1980)

Nässel, D. R., Waterman, T. H.: Golgi EM evidence for visual information channelling in the crayfish lamina ganglionaris. Brain Res. **130**, 556–563 (1977)

Nässel, D. R., Berriman, J. A., Seyan, H. S.: Cytochrome C as a high resolution marker for light and electronmicroscopy. Brain. Res. (in press, 1980)

Nässel, D. R., Elofsson, R., Odselius, R.: Neural connectivity patterns in the compound eyes of *Artemia salina* and *Daphnia magna* (Crustacea: Branchiopoda). Cell Tissue Res. **190**, 435–457 (1978)

Nässel, D. R.: Transneuronal labelling with horseradish peroxidase in the visual system of the housefly. Brain Res. (in press 1980)

Nilsson, H. L.: The fine structure of the compound eye of shallow-water Asselotes, *Jaera albifrons* Leach and *Asellus aquaticus* L. (Crustacea: Isopoda). Acta Zool. (Stockh) **59**, 69–84 (1978)

Nosaki, H.: Electrophysiological study of color encoding in the compound eye of crayfish, *Procambarus clarkii*. Z. Vergl. Physiol. **64**, 318–323 (1969)

Ohly, K. P.: The neurons of the first synaptic region of the optic neuropil of the firefly, *Phausis splendidula* L. Coleoptera. Cell Tissue Res. **158**, 89–109 (1975)

O'Shea, M.: Two sites of axonal spike initiation in a bimodal interneuron. Brain Res. **96**, 93–98 (1975)

O'Shea, M., Rowell, C. H. F.: Protection from habituation by lateral inhibition. Nature **254**, 53–55 (1975a)

O'Shea, M., Rowell, C. H. F.: A spike-transmitting electrical synapse between visual interneurons in the locust movement detector system. J. Comp. Physiol. **97**, 143–158 (1975 b)

O'Shea, M., Rowell, C. H. F.: The neuronal basis of a sensory analyser, the acridid movement detector system. II. Response decrement, convergence, and the nature of the excitatory afferents to the fanlike dendrites of the LGMD. J. Exp. Biol. **65**, 289–308 (1976)

O'Shea, M., Rowell, C. H. F., Williams, J. L. D.: The anatomy of a locust visual interneurone; the descending contralateral movement detector. J. Exp. Biol. **60**, 1–12 (1974)

O'Shea, M., Williams, J. L. D.: The anatomy and output connection of a locust visual interneurone; the lobula giant movement detector (LGMD) neurone. J. Comp. Physiol. **91**, 257–266 (1974)

Palka, J.: Discrimination between movements of eye and object by visual interneurones of crickets. J. Exp. Biol. **50**, 723–732 (1969)

Parker, G. H.: The retina and optic ganglia in decapods, especially in *Astacus*. Mitt. Zool. Stat. Neapel **12**, 1–73 (1897)

Parker, G. H.: The movements of retinal pigment. Ergeb. Biol. **9**, 239–291 (1932)

Pearson, K. G., Heitler, W. J., Steeves, J. D.: Triggering of locust jump by multimodal inhibitory interneurons. J. Neurophysiol **43**, 257–278 (1980)

Pflugfelder, O.: Vergleichende anatomische, experimentelle und embryologische Untersuchungen über das Nervensystem und die Sinnesorgane der Rhynchoten. Zoologica **34**, 1–102 (1937)

Pierantoni, R.: Su un tratto nervoso nel cervello della Musca. In: Atti della prima riunora Scientifica plenaria (Camogli, dicembre 1973). Soc. Ital. Biofis. Pura Applicata 1973, pp. 231–249

Pierantoni, R.: An observation on the giant fiber posterior optic tract in the fly. Biokybernetik (Leipzig) **5**, 157–163 (1974)

Pierantoni, R.: A look into the cockpit of the fly. The architecture of the lobula plate. Cell Tiss. Res. **171**, 101–122 (1976)

Retzius, G.: Zur Kenntnis des Nervensystems der Daphniden. Biol. Unters. N.F. **13**, 107–116 (1906)

Ribi, W. A.: The neurons of the first optic ganglion of the bee, *Apis mellifera*. Advances in Anatomy **50**(4), 1–43. Berlin-Heidelberg-New York: Springer 1975 a

Ribi, W. A.: The first optic ganglion of the bee. I. Correlation between visual cell types and their terminals in the lamina and medulla. Cell Tiss. Res. **165**, 103–111 (1975 b)

Ribi, W. A.: The first optic ganglion of the bee. II. Topographical relationships of second order neurons within a cartridge and two groups of cartridges. Cell Tiss. Res. **171**, 359–373 (1976)

Ribi, W. A.: Fine structure of the first optic ganglion (lamina) of the cockroach *Periplaneta americana*. Tiss. Cell **9**, 57–72 (1977)

Ribi, W. A.: The first optic ganglion of the bee. III. Regional comparisons of the morphology of photoreceptor-cell axons. Cell Tiss. Res. **200**, 345–357 (1979)

Röhlich, P., Törö, I.: Fine structure of the compound eye of *Daphnia* in normal, dark and strongly lightadapted state. In: The structure of the eye. II. Symp. (ed. J. W. Rohen). Stuttgart: Schattauer 1965

Rowell, C. H. F.: The orthopteran descending movement detector (DMD) neurons: A characterisation and review. Z. Vergl. Physiol. **73**, 167–194 (1971)

Rowell, C. H. F., Horn, G.: Dishabituation and arousal in the response of single nerve cells in an insect brain. J. Exp. Biol. **49**, 171–183 (1968)

Rowell, C. H. F., O'Shea, M., Williams, J. L. D.: The neuronal basis of a sensory analyser, the acridid movement detector system. IV. The preference for small field stimuli. J. Exp. Biol. **68**, 157–185 (1977)

Rutherford, D. J., Horridge, G. A.: The rhabdom of the lobster eye. Quart. J. Micr. Sci. **106**, 119–130 (1965)

Sandeman, D. C.: Compensatory eye movements in crabs. In: Identified neurons and behaviour of arthropods. (ed. G. Hoyle). New York: Plenum 1977

Schönenberger, N.: The fine structure of the compound eye of *Squilla mantis* (Crustacea, Stomatopoda). Cell Tiss. Res. **176**, 205–233 (1977)

Scholes, J.: The electrical response of the retinal receptors and the lamina in the visual system of the fly *Musca*. Kybernetik **6**, 149–162 (1969)

Shaw, S. R.: Polarized light responses from crab retinula cells. Nature **211**, 92–93 (1966)

Shaw, S. R.: Sense-cell structure and interspecies comparisons of polarized-light absorptions in arthropod compound eyes. Vision Res. **9**, 1031–1040 (1969)

Shimozawa, T., Takeda, T., Yamaguchi, T.: Response entrainment and memory of temporal pattern by movement fibres in crayfish visual system. J. Comp. Physiol. **114**, 267–287 (1977)

Shivers, R. R.: Fine structure of crayfish optic ganglia. Univ. of Kansas Sci. Bull. **47**, 677–733 (1967)

Smola, U., Meffert, P.: The spectral sensitivity of the visual cells R 7 and R 8 in the eye of the blowfly *Calliphora erythrocephala*. J. Comp. Physiol. **133**, 41–52 (1979)

Soohoo, S. L., Bishop, L. G.: Intensity and motion responses of giant vertical neurons of the fly eye. J. Neurobiol. **11**, 159–178 (1980)

Stark, W. S., Ivanyshyn, A. M., Hu, K. G.: Spectral sensitivities and photopigments in adaptation of fly receptors. Naturwissenschaften **63**, 513–518 (1976)

Stark, W. S., Ivanyshyn, A. M., Greenberg, R. M.: Sensitivity and photopigments of R 1–R 6, a two peaked photoreceptor in *Drosophila, Calliphora,* and *Musca.* J. Comp. Physiol. **121**, 289–305 (1977)

Stewart, W. W.: Functional connections between cells as revealed by dye-coupling with a highly fluorescent napthalamide tracer. Cell **14**, 741–759 (1978)

Stowe, S.: The retina-lamina projection in the crab *Leptograpsus variegatus.* Cell Tissue Res. **185**, 515–526 (1977)

Stowe, S., Ribi, W. A., Sandeman, D. C.: The organisation of the lamina ganglionaris of the crabs *Scylla serrata* and *Leptograpsus variegatus.* Cell Tiss. Res. **178**, 517–532 (1977)

Strausfeld, N. J.: Golgi studies on insects. Part II. The optic lobes of diptera. Phil. Trans. Soc. B **258**, 175–223 (1970)

Strausfeld, N. J.: The organization of the insect visual system (light microscopy). I. Projections and arrangements of neurons in the lamina ganglionaris of diptera. Z. Zellforsch. **121**, 377–441 (1971 a)

Strausfeld, N. J.: The organisation of the insect visual system (light microscopy). II. The projection of fibres across the first optic chiasma. Z. Zellforsch. **121**, 442–454 (1971 b)

Strausfeld, N. J.: Mosaic organizations, layers, and visual pathways in the insect brain. In: Neural principles in vision (eds. F. Zettler, R. Weiler), pp. 245–279. Berlin-Heidelberg-New York: Springer 1976 a

Strausfeld, N. J.: Atlas of an insect brain. Berlin-Heidelberg-New York: Springer 1976 b

Strausfeld, N. J.: The representation of a receptor map within retinotopic neuropil of the fly. Verh. Dtsch. Zool. Ges. 1979, 167–179 (1979)

Strausfeld, N. J.: Male and female visual neurones in dipterous insects. Nature **283**, 381–383 (1980)

Strausfeld, N. J., Bacon, J.: Descending multimodal neurons from fly brains: Cobalt and Lucifer yellow analysis of their structural organization (in preparation, 1980)

Strausfeld, N. J., Blest, A. D.: Golgi studies on insects. Part I. The optic lobes of Lepidoptera. Phil. Trans. R. Soc. (Lond.) B **258**, 81–134 (1970)

Strausfeld, N. J., Braitenberg, V.: The compound eye of the fly *(Musca domestica):* connections between the cartridges of the lamina ganglionaris. Z. Vergl. Physiol. **70**, 95–104 (1970)

Strausfeld, N. J., Campos-Ortega, J. A.: Some interrelationships between the first and second synaptic regions of the fly's *(Musca domestica)* visual system. In: Information processing in the visual system of arthropods (ed. R. Wehner). Berlin-Heidelberg-New York: Springer 1972

Strausfeld, N. J., Campos-Ortega, J. A.: The L 4 monopolar neurone: a substrate for lateral interaction in the visual system of the fly *Musca domestica.* Brain Res **59**, 97–117 (1973 a)

Strausfeld, N. J., Campos-Ortega, J. A.: L 3, the 3 rd 2 nd order neuron of the 1 st visual ganglion in the "neural superposition" eye of *Musca domestica.* Z. Zellforsch. **139**, 397–403 (1973 b)

Strausfeld, N. J., Campos-Ortega, J. A.: Vision in insects: pathways possibly underlying neural adaptation and lateral inhibition. Science **195**, 894–897 (1977)

Strausfeld, N. J., Hausen, K.: The resolution of neuronal assemblies after cobalt-injection into neuropil. Proc. R. Soc. Lond. B **199**, 463–476 (1977)

Strausfeld, N. J., Obermayer, M.: Resolution of intraneuronal and transsynaptic migration of cobalt in the insect visual and nervous systems. J. Comp. Physiol. **110**, 1–12 (1976)

Strausfeld, N. J., Singh, R. N.: Peripheral and central nervous system projections in normal and mutant (bithorax) *Drosophila melanogaster.* In: Development and behaviour of *Drosophila melanogaster* (eds. O. Siddiqi, P. Babu, L. Hall). New York: Plenum Publ. Corp. 1980

Trevino, D. L., Larimer, J. L.: The response of one class of neurons in the optic tract of crayfish *(Procambarus)* to monochromatic light. Z. Vergl. Physiol. **69**, 139–149 (1970)

Trujillo-Cenóz, O., Melamed, J.: Electron microscope observations on the peripheral and intermediate retinas of Dipterans. In: The functional organization of the compound eye. Symp. Wenner-Gren Center (1965) (ed. C. G. Bernhard). London: Pergamon Press 1966

Trujillo-Cenóz, O., Melamed, J.: Light- and electronmicroscope study of one of the systems of centrifugal fibres found in the lamina of muscoid flies. Z. Zellforsch. **110**, 336–349 (1970)

Trujillo-Cenóz, O.: Some aspects of the structural organization of the intermediate retina of Dipterans. J. Ultrastruct. Res. **13**, 1–33 (1965)

Tyrer, N. M., Altman, J. S.: Motor and sensory flight neurones in a locust demonstrated using cobalt chloride. J. Comp. Neurol. **157**, 117–138 (1974)

Tyrer, N. M., Bacon, J., Davies, C. A.: Primary sensory hair projections from the wind-sensitive hairs of the locust *Schistocerca gregaria*. Cell Tiss. Res. **203**, 79–92 (1979)

Vigier, P.: Sur les terminations photoréceptrices dans les yeux composés des Muscides. C.R. Acad. Sci. (Paris) **145**, 532–536 (1907a)

Vigier, P.: Sur la réception de l'exitant lumineux dans les yeux composés des insectes, en particulier chez les muscides. C.R. Acad. Sci. (Paris) **145**, 633–636 (1907b)

Vigier, P.: Sur l'existence réelle et le rôle des neurones. La neurone perioptique des Diptères. C.R. Soc. Biol. (Paris) **64**, 959–961 (1908)

Vigier, P.: Mécanisme de la synthèse des impressions lumineuses recueilles par les yeux composés des Diptères. C.R. Acad. Sci. (Paris) **148**, 1221–1223 (1909)

Wachmann, E.: Vergleichende Analyse der feinstrukturellen Organisation offener Rhabdome in den Augen der Cucujiformia (Insecta, Coleoptera) unter besonderer Berücksichtigung der Chrysomelidae. Zoomorphologie **88**, 95–131 (1977)

Walcott, B.: Unit studies on light-adaptation in the retina of the crayfish, *Cherax destructor*. J. Comp. Physiol. **94**, 207–218 (1974)

Wald, G.: Visual pigments of crayfish. Nature (Lond.) **215**, 1131–1133 (1967)

Wald, G.: Single and multiple visual systems in arthropods. J. Gen. Physiol. **51**, 125–156 (1968)

Wald, G., Hubbard, R.: Visual pigment of a decapod crustacean: the lobster. Nature **180**, 278–280 (1957)

Waterman, T. H.: Polarotaxis and primary photoreceptor events in Crustacea. In: The functional organisation of the compound eye (ed. C. G. Bernhard). Oxford-New York: Pergamon Press 1966

Waterman, T. H.: The bridge between visual input and central programming in crustaceans. In: Identified neurons and behaviour of arthropods (ed. G. Hoyle). New York: Plenum 1977

Waterman, T. H.: Polarization sensitivity. In: Handbook of sensory physiology, Vol. VII/6B (ed. H. Autrum). Berlin-Heidelberg-New York: Springer 1980

Waterman, T. H., Fernández, H. R.: E-vector and wavelength discrimination by retinular cells of the crayfish *Procambarus*. Z. Vergl. Physiol. **68**, 154–174 (1970)

Waterman, T. H., Horch, K. W.: Mechanism of polarized light perception. Science **154**, 467–475 (1966)

Waterman, T. H., Wiersma, C. A. G., Bush, B. M. H.: Afferent visual responses in the optic nerve of the crab, *Podophthalmus*. J. Cell. Comp. Physiol. **63**, 135–155 (1964)

Wiersma, C. A. G.: Visual central processing in crustaceans. In : Invertebrate nervous systems (ed. C. A. G. Wiersma). Chicago: University of Chicago Press 1967

Wiersma, C. A. G., Yamaguchi, T.: The neuronal components of the optic nerve of the crayfish as studied by single unit analysis. J. Comp. Neurol. **128**, 333–358 (1966)

Wolburg-Buchholz, K.: The superposition eye of *Cloëon dipterum:* The organization of the lamina ganglionaris. Cell Tissue Res. **177**, 9–28 (1977)

Wolburg-Buchholz, K.: The organisation of the lamina ganglionaris of the hemipteran insects *Notonecta glauca, Corixa punctata, Gerris lacustris*. Cell Tiss. Res. **197**, 39–59 (1979)

Wolff, J. R., Güldner, F. H.: Über die Ultrastruktur des „Nervus opticus" und des Ganglion opticum I von *Daphnia pulex*. Z. Zellforsch. **103**, 526–543 (1970)

Woodcock, A. E. R., Goldsmith, T. H.: Spectral response of sustaining fibres in the optic tracts of crayfish *(Procambarus)*. Z. Vergl. Physiol. **69**, 117–133 (1970)

Yamaguchi, T.: The mechanism of polarized light perception and its visual processing in the optic tract of the crayfish. Zool. Mag. (Japan) **76**, 443 (abstr. in Japanese) (1967)

Yamaguchi, T., Katagiri, Y., Ochi, K.: Polarized light responses from retinular cells and sustaining fibres of the *Mantis* shrimp. Biol. J. Okayama Univ. **17**, 61–66 (1976)

York, B., Wiersma, C. A. G.: Visual processing in the rock lobster (Crustacea). Progr. Neurobiol. **5**, 127–166 (1975)

Zeil, J.: A new kind of neural superposition eye: the compound eye of male Bibionidae. Nature **278**, 249–250 (1979)

Zettler, F., Järvilehto, M.: Lateral inhibition in an insect eye. Z. Vergl. Physiol. **76**, 233–244 (1972)

Chapter 2

Neural Principles in the Peripheral Visual Systems of Invertebrates

S. Laughlin, Canberra, Australia

With 34 Figures and 3 Tables

Contents

A. Introduction

"Everything in the vertebrate eye means something"
G. L. WALLS, preface to The Vertebrate Eye and its Adaptive Radiation,
1942

Neural principles are biological principles, concerning the organisation of cellular components into cohesive systems, contributing to the development, maintenance and reproduction of the organism (and its genes). For a visual system, these principles relate to the cellular structures that assimilate and process optical information from the environment, to help an animal maintain a favourable position within its surroundings. Every information transferring structure in the visual system, from the molecular level of rhodopsins and membrane conductance channels, through the subcellular level of synapses, to the cellular and multicellular levels of specified neuronal geometry and contacts, is devoted to one end: the generation of visually mediated behaviour. This then is the major theme of this review, the adaptation of structure to function in the visual systems of invertebrates.

A major advantage of this functional approach is that descriptions, whether they be anatomical accounts or intricate photoreceptor transfer functions, are converted into an understanding of the visual system. We not only see what happens but appreciate why it happens in the way it does. There will be wrong and misleading functional interpretations, just as there are erroneous descriptions; the most important caveat is that description should determine functional interpretation, and not the other way around.

The field is rich and diverse and I have had to restrict the review to identified receptors and first order interneurons in anatomically defined systems. I have not dealt with molluscs and have not considered the principles of generalisation, command and decision exhibited by higher order interneurons in the insect optic lobe (e.g., HAUSEN, 1976; ROWELL, 1971; ROWELL et al., 1977). A brief outline may assist the reader to locate points of interest within the review and impose some logic upon its structure. The barnacle ocelli are presented as examples of systems where definitive biophysical measurements reveal that single receptors have complex membrane properties and individual regions of the cell membrane are tailored for different aspects of function. Similar experiments in the locust ocellus present the same picture of complexity in an interneuron, and this intricacy presents some challenging general problems for correlating conductance changes with anatomically identified synapses. The gap between response and wiring diagram is still large. The study of ocellar neuron number raises the important question of specificity and evolutionary plasticity in the nervous system. *Limulus* lateral eye is given as a paradigm for the investigation of sensory systems, where the classical phenomena of lateral and self-inhibition are related to cellular mechanisms, and to the processing of the visual signal. Insect and crustacean compound eyes are complicated and sophisticated visual systems whose peripheral structure is well enough defined to see optical information passing through the optic lobes as a succession of neural images, generated in arrays of receptors and interneurons. Neural image quality is determined by the limitations imposed by transduction and synaptic transfer and both receptors and interneurons operate in ways which minimise these constraints. These principles of operation are shared with many of the neurons reviewed in previous sections, and with the analogous receptors and neurons of the vertebrate eye. In the last section these similarities are presented as a list of principles which assist in the efficient processing of visual information in the periphery. One must conclude that the neural principles of invertebrate visual systems are often the principles of vision in general.

In all cases I have attempted to present a complete description of the cellular operations in each visual system so that one can read each section on its own, and gain some idea about how each visual system works. That is what principles are all about.

B. Barnacle Eyes and Their Shadow Reflex

I. Introduction

The adult barnacle plants its castle firmly in one spot and from the turret sweeps up passing organisms and detritus. In view of these sessile habits it is not surprising that the barnacle's nervous system is a reduced version of its larval predecessor (Bullock and Horridge, 1965, p. 1175 ff). Similarly the barnacle does not appear to look closely at what it eats, or whom it mates with, and its visual system is reduced to three simple ocelli and a single paired ganglion (Fig. 1).

The only visual behaviour observed so far is a simple shadow reflex, first recorded in the early nineteenth century (see Gwilliam and Millecchia, 1975). When relatively large objects pass over barnacles they cease feeding and withdraw their cirri into the safety of their shells. The effective stimulus is the passage of a shadow over the barnacle and Fales (1928) showed by surgical ablation, that the response was mediated by ocelli which developed from the median eye of the nauplius larva.

Recent interest in the barnacle visual system stems from a series of studies, initiated by Gwilliam (1963), with the aim of deriving a physiological description of a simple behavioural act. Gwilliam's discovery of the prominent photoresponse of the ocelli, and the conduction of the visual signal over several millimetres of ocellar nerve, without the intervention of action potentials, together with Fahren-

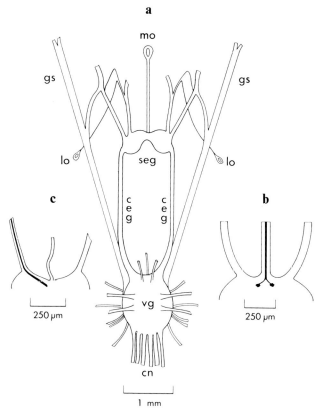

Fig. 1 a–c. The parts of the barnacle nervous system participating in the shadow reflex. **a** The reflex pathway showing the lateral *(lo)* and medial *(mo)* ocelli sending nerves to the sensory supra-oesophageal ganglion *(seg)*, which in turn connects with motoneurons within the ventral ganglion *(vg)* via the paired supra-oesophageal connectives *(ceg)*. cn = cirral nerves; gs = great splanchnic nerve. (After GWILLIAM and MILLECCHIA, 1975). **b** The paired terminals of a single medial ocellar photoreceptor as revealed by cobalt diffusion into single axons (HUDSPETH and STUART, 1977). **c** The terminal of a single photoreceptor axon from the lateral ocellus in the supra-oesophageal ganglion, as revealed by Procion Yellow injection of a single cell (SHAW, 1972)

BACH'S (1965) demonstration that the photoreceptor cells are large enough to be amenable to the most sophisticated techniques of intracellular recording, has stimulated a number of investigations of transduction and signal transmission within the barnacle ocellus. As a consequence of this work, performed with an exactitude that is only possible when working with large, identified single cells, several important processes relevant to the electrotonic processing of small signals within the nervous system have been described.

II. Reflex Pathway

The three ocelli each send their own ocellar nerve to the supra-oesophageal ganglion and this connects to the ventral ganglion by a pair of circumoesophageal connectives (Fig. 1). Within the context of the shadow reflex the supra-oesophageal ganglion can be regarded as sensory. It receives graded potential signals from the ocelli, whose amplitude depends upon intensity. Consequently these signals carry information about intensity increments and decrements. By comparison, the spiking units recorded from the connectives respond only to the decrements. Thus the supra-oesophageal ganglion is the site of an "off" selective neural mechanism and it is this filter which gives the reflex its specific sensitivity to shadow. Any one of the three ocelli can produce a full sized off response in the connective (Gwilliam, 1963, 1965).

The ventral ganglion's role in the reflex is principally motor. It contains the neurons which innervate the relevant musculature and receive the filtered sensory input from the supra-oesophageal ganglion. This input acts upon the motor neurons through unspecified pathways, to interrupt feeding rhythms, and bring about cirriped withdrawal and closure of the operculum (Gwilliam, 1976). An intrinsic oscillator system within the ganglion drives the motor neurons to produce the appropriately timed bursts of impulses, corresponding to the feeding cycle. Shadowing of the ocelli interrupts the rhythmical output of motoneurons, independent from their phase in the cycle, and motoneurons responsible for withdrawal of the cirri are stimulated, while extensor neurons are inhibited (Gwilliam, 1976). We will now examine the sensory mechanisms in more detail, starting with the necessary account of structure, and then moving on to the analysis of signal generation and transmission within photoreceptors, and finally look at the postsynaptic responses in the supra-oesophageal ganglion.

III. Structure of the Ocelli and the Supra-oesophageal Ganglion

Each ocellus contains a small number of photoreceptors, embedded in glial folds and encased by a tough fibrous sheath (Fahrenbach, 1965; Krebs and Schaten, 1976). The number of cells in each ocellus, and their size, depends upon whether the ocellus is lateral or medial and upon the species (Table 1). There is even a suggestion that, within the medial ocellus, the number of photoreceptors varies between individuals from six to nine (Millecchia and Gwilliam, 1972). Given the large size of the photoreceptor axons (Table 1) this variability could easily be studied in greater detail by making axon counts in the ocellar nerve.

The ocellar photoreceptors have large ovoid cell bodies, bearing numerous processes covered in microvilli which are, through comparison with the microvilli on insect rhabdomeres, thought to be the site of phototransduction (Fahrenbach, 1965). The optical pathway for light entering the ocelli in the intact animal is poorly defined. In *Balanus eburneus* and *B. amphitrite* the lateral ocelli are backed by a reflective tapetum and light enters through the shell which acts as an efficient diffuser, probably eliminating directional sensitivity (Shaw, 1972). However, this supposed lack of directional sensitivity ought to be confirmed behaviourally. In the median ocelli examined, there appears to be no tapetum, and light enters through the open shell (Gwilliam and Millecchia, 1975).

Table 1. The complement of photoreceptors in barnacle ocelli and their dimensions

Species	Ocellus	No. of receptors	Cell body dia. μm	Axon dia. μm	Axon length mm	Reference
Balanus carosius	Median	6–9	30	10–12	2.5–3.5	GWILLIAM and MILLECCHIA (1975)
Balanus nubilis	Median	4	40–70	25	8–10	HUDSPETH and STUART (1977)
Balanus amphitrite	Lateral	3	100	10–15	—	FAHRENBACH (1965)
Balanus eburneus	Lateral	3	100	10–15	8–10	SHAW (1972)

Every ocellar photoreceptor sends a fat axon to the supra-oesophageal ganglion, a distance of 2.5–10 mm, depending upon the species and the ocellus (Table 1). In those cases where the anatomy of the ocellar photoreceptors has been investigated by intracellular dye injection, the receptor axons have terminated within the supra-oesophageal ganglion. The median ocellar photoreceptors bifurcate shortly after entering the ganglion and form small symmetrically placed dendritic trees in each side (Fig. 1) (MILLECCHIA and GWILLIAM, 1972; HUDSPETH and STUART, 1977). The lateral ocelli terminate in a simple club ending close to the midline in their half of the ganglion (Fig. 1) (SHAW, 1972). In the giant Pacific barnacle, *B. nubilis*, the terminal branches of the photoreceptor axons have been examined by electron microscopy (HUDSPETH and STUART, 1977). These branches are 1–3 μm in diameter and make what appear to be chemical synapses, with *pairs* of fine (0.5 μm) postsynaptic processes. No postsynaptic cells have been identified, nor have the off sensitive cells leaving the ganglion via the circumoesophageal connective. This is partly because the cells of the supra-oesophageal ganglion are both numerous and small.

IV. Photoreceptor Response

In darkness the barnacle photoreceptor has a resting potential lying within the range -35 to -65 mV (BROWN et al., 1970; SHAW, 1972; HUDSPETH et al., 1977). The extent to which this surprising variability can be attributed to damage by recording electrodes is not known. At low intensities the response to light is a sustained depolarisation, showing no adaptation (Fig. 2), but fluctuating randomly in amplitude. By comparison with other rhabdomeric photoreceptors these fluctuations indicate that single photon absorptions bring about sizeable conductance changes at the photoreceptor membrane. However, discrete depolarising waves or quantum bumps, corresponding to the absorption of single photons (LILLYWHITE, 1977), have not been seen in barnacle photoreceptors although they are present in the retinula cells of *Limulus* and locust compound eyes (YEANDLE, 1958; SCHOLES, 1964). It is of interest that the potential fluctuations are far more pronounced in median ocellar photoreceptors (HUDSPETH and STUART, 1977) than in lateral photoreceptors (SHAW, 1972). The median photoreceptor response rises more rapidly

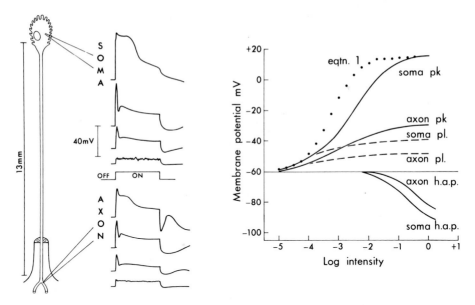

Fig. 2. The receptor potentials and intensity/response functions of the medial photoreceptor of *Balanus nubilis*, recorded in the soma where transduction takes place, and in the axon, close to its terminals in the supra-oesophageal ganglion. The decrement of receptor potential during transmission is greater for depolarisations than for hyperpolarisations. The V/log I curve for peak responses in the soma is compared with that predicted from self-shunting [Eq. (B.1)]. The recordings of receptor potential were made in different preparations (taken from Hudspeth and Stuart, 1977). The V/log I curves are from a simultaneous recording in the axon and soma of a single cell. pk = peak response; pl = steady state plateau response; $h.a.p.$ = hyperpolarising after potential (Hudspeth et al., 1977)

to a peak than the lateral response, which tends to confirm Krischer's finding (1971), from extracellular measurements of receptor current, that median ocelli have a larger voltage gain and faster response than the lateral. This finding does not fit in with comparative observations on the photoreceptors of a variety of insects and crustaceans (Table 2, Sect. E.II) where large responses to single photons correlate with the slowness of waveform. The lateral photoreceptors are electrically coupled, whereas the median are not (Shaw, 1972; Hudspeth and Stuart, 1977), and the low pass filter characteristics of coupling networks may account for the smoothing of responses (S.R.Shaw, personal communication).

The voltage amplitude of response increases as a function of intensity and this relationship can be presented in the form of V/log I curve (Fig. 2). When response amplitude approaches 20% maximal, clear adaptation effects can be observed from the decrease in response to a sustained stimulus, and these become more pronounced as intensity rises (Fig. 2). At least three aspects of adaptation have been remarked upon, the rapid decrease of receptor potential from peak to plateau, the steady decay of the plateau over several seconds and a pronounced hyperpolarisation which follows the peak (Fig. 2) and can, in some cases, hyperpolarise the cell beyond the resting potential (Hanani and Shaw, 1977). The actual number of interlocking processes producing this transient response has not been demonstrated.

Finally, as with other rhabdomeric photoreceptors, light adaptation increases the speed of response (e.g., Fig. 21) (see review by FUORTES and O'BRYAN, 1972a).

One should examine closely the receptor's responses to intensity decrements to define their role in the shadow reflex. Unfortunately dimming responses have not been analysed in detail in the functional range for the reflex (I take this to be an intensity decrement of not more than 1 log unit, applied to a light adapted cell). By comparison with insect retinula cells (LAUGHLIN and HARDIE, 1978) we can expect a small hyperpolarisation, not dropping below the resting potential, followed by a repolarisation to a lower plateau response level. However, most investigations have examined the complex after-potentials following short and exceedingly bright flashes delivered to a dark-adapted photoreceptor. If a light, which produced a response in the range of 50%–100% maximum, is turned off, a slow hyperpolarising afterpotential is seen (Fig. 2). The depression of membrane potential below the normal resting level is thought to result from the activation of an electrogenic sodium pump (KOIKE et al., 1971) and a delayed increase in potassium conductance (unpublished results of D.R.EDGINGTON, cited by HUDSPETH and STUART, 1977). Blinding flashes, 1 log unit or more in excess of saturating intensity, produce afterdepolarisations whose waveform and duration depend upon the intensity of illumination and adaptation state of the cell (HOCHSTEIN et al., 1973). Although positive afterpotentials are useful tools for the study of transduction, they must rarely impinge upon the everyday life of the barnacle.

V. Ionic Basis of the Photoreceptor Responses

A detailed and critical review of the photochemical and membrane events constituting transduction lies outside the scope of this review (see FUORTES and O'BRYAN, 1972a), however, an understanding of basic receptor mechanisms is valuable for the discussion of photoreceptor function in other arthropod eyes. The barnacle photoreceptor has proved a convenient preparation for the analysis of transduction because, by virtue of its large size, voltage clamp techniques can be used to derive the membrane conductance changes underlying voltage responses (BROWN et al., 1970).

The depolarising receptor potential results from an inward light induced photocurrent which is, at low intensities, proportional to light intensity. At high intensities the current is time dependent and an initial surge is followed by a lower steady state current. This reduction in current is partly responsible for the accompanying adaptation in voltage response. Ionic substitution in the external medium suggests that sodium ions carry most of the inward current, but reveal an appreciable inward calcium current. This calcium influx is more pronounced in barnacle photoreceptors than in *Limulus* ventral eye photoreceptors (BROWN and BLINKS, 1974), but in both cases an increase in intracellular free calcium concentration correlates with the reduction of net inward photocurrent. There is now a considerable body of evidence suggesting that in barnacle, *Limulus* and bee photoreceptors (LISMAN and BROWN, 1972; BAUMANN, 1975) a major component of light adaptation is produced by intracellular calcium reducing the inward sodium current

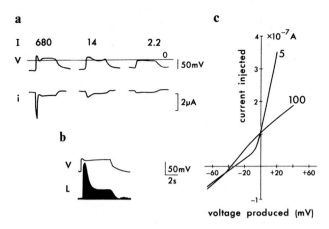

Fig. 3a–c. Electrical properties of the barnacle photoreceptor somata. **a** The voltage response *(V)* of a single photoreceptor illuminated at three different intensities *(I,* given in arbitrary units) with the corresponding current *(i)* required to voltage clamp the photoreceptor at resting potential. The influx of current induced by light changes considerably as a function of time, and intensity, in the absence of any change in membrane potential. **b** Calcium influx during a saturating response to light *(V),* as monitored by the calcium induced luminescence *(L)* of the protein aequorin, previously injected into the receptor (after BROWN and BLINKS, 1974). **c** The membrane potentials recorded 5 and 100 ms after the onset of an applied constant current. Input resistance depends upon both voltage and time, but in the steady state condition the receptor is approximately ohmic within the functionally relevant range of −60 to 0 mV (after BROWN et al., 1970)

(BROWN et al., 1970), probably by reducing the duration and amplitude of membrane conductance events initiated by single photons (LISMAN and BROWN, 1975; LISMAN, 1976). Finally, in barnacle the calcium influx must be triggered either via photoproducts of pigment isomerisation, or by sodium ion influx because voltage clamping the membrane at resting potential does not prevent calcium influx (BROWN and BLINKS, 1974).

At this stage it would be convenient to conclude that a light induced sodium conductance, proportional to intensity, produces a depolarisation of the cell membrane. One can predict (see Sect. E.II.3.b) that for this system, the relationship between intensity and amplitude follow a hyperbolic function of the form

$$V/V_{\max} = \frac{R \cdot I}{R \cdot I + 1} \tag{B.1}$$

where V is the voltage response to intensity I, $V_{\max}$ the maximum saturated response amplitude and R the range sensitivity factor, equals the reciprocal of the intensity required to give a response of 50% $V_{\max}$ (LIPETZ, 1971). Clearly this is not the case (Fig. 2) and several complicating factors have been found. First, the passive (light insensitive) membrane properties of the cell soma are dominated by voltage dependent potassium conductance channels. As a consequence, the membrane's response to step depolarisations and hyperpolarisations is far from simple (Fig. 3), because the membrane resistance changes transiently, before adopting a stable steady state value. Both the transient changes and the final steady state depend upon membrane potential (Fig. 3). Second, the membrane is rectifying in the steady state condition, showing a greater electrical resistance to hyperpolarisations than to depolarisations. Not only are these passive properties of the membrane both time and voltage dependent but so are the light induced conductance changes (BROWN et al., 1970). The roles played by these voltage dependencies in shaping the response have not been established, for no attempt has been made to reconstruct the response from a knowledge of the time and voltage dependent behaviour of the conductances (as done for the action potential by HODGKIN and HUXLEY, 1952). However, the rectification shown by the passive membrane could contribute a little to the flattening of the $V/\log I$ curve (Fig. 2).

In barnacle photoreceptors at least, there is a final complication – the ionic species contributing to the net light induced current have not been fully identified. In *Limulus* ventral eye, voltage clamp studies demonstrate that the reversal potential of the light induced response follows the external sodium concentration, as predicted for a change in sodium conductance alone (Nernst equation). A small discrepancy probably results from a contribution by a light activated potassium conductance (BROWN and MOTE, 1974). Even in the absence of external calcium, barnacle photoreceptors have a reversal potential that is only half as sensitive to external sodium concentration as it should be (BROWN et al., 1970). Although there is some suggestion that a light induced potassium conductance is responsible for the hyperpolarising dip in receptor potential which follows the peak response (HANANI and SHAW, 1977) this has not been related directly to the reversal potential for the light response. It is possible that, because the microvilli are deeply embedded within the body of the lateral ocellus (KREBS and SCHATEN, 1976), sodium concentration cannot be reliably manipulated around the site of transduction and, as a consequence of sodium extrusion into the extracellular space by pumps, there is a degree of regulation of extracellular sodium concentration (KREBS et al., 1975).

In conclusion, one can see that although the basic principles of the transduction process are straightforward the receptor photocurrent is acted upon by a number of voltage dependent processes. It is not possible to decide between these complicating factors being the unwanted by-products of conductance channel operation, or these effects having evolved for a useful purpose. As we will see in subsequent sections the neural membrane is a multicomponent system capable of great functional plasticity. Consequently it would be unwise to reject a functional argument out of hand.

VI. Passive Propagation of Graded Potentials

The receptors and interneurons of several sensory systems fail to produce action potentials, and they transmit messages as continuous modulations of membrane potential. To distinguish these signals from action potentials, which are rapid in time course and have a unitary amplitude, these potentials are known as *slow* or *graded potentials*. Graded potentials can propagate over distances of a millimetre or more, in fine axons that are less than 5 μm in diameter (e.g., the lamina-medulla projection of the fly compound eye, ZETTLER and JÄRVILEHTO, 1973). It is a simple matter to show that if these axons had the same specific membrane resistance as is commonly found in spiking membranes (e.g., 1 kΩ cm^{-2} for squid giant axons, KATZ, 1966) then most of the signal would not propagate over these distances, but would leak away into the extracellular space. Consequently, it has been proposed that active booster mechanisms assist in the transmission of graded potentials (ZETTLER and JÄRVILEHTO, 1973) and that these mechanisms use voltage sensitive conductance channels within the membrane to amplify the signal as it passes down the axon. A voltage dependent regenerative mechanism has recently been found in vertebrate rods (WERBLIN, 1975), but propagation is not really a problem in these vertebrate photoreceptors. As an alternative it has been suggested that graded potential propagation over long distances is strictly passive, and that signal decrement (presumably at low frequencies or steady state) is prevented by having an axon membrane which is a better insulator than the squid archetype (e. g., IOANNIDES and WALCOTT, 1971; MILLECCHIA and GWILLIAM, 1972; WILSON, 1978 b). To distinguish between active and passive propagation processes one needs to determine spatial signal decrement as a function of signal strength and distance of propagation, derive the cable characteristics of the axon and test for the presence of voltage dependent conductance channels. Such experiments require one to manipulate the ionic environment of cells, and examine the membrane properties of single axons by simultaneously inserting two electrodes. These types of measurement are notoriously difficult to perform on small cells embedded deep within a large nerve tract, and for this reason the question of active versus passive propagation of graded potentials has still not been satisfactorily resolved in the insect compound eye (see Sect. E.III.4). The barnacle ocellus is an ideal preparation in which to discover the mechanisms by which graded potentials propagate over long distances (SHAW, 1972). The cells are large, the axons long and identifiable and the early work of GWILLIAM (1963, 1965) suggested that graded signals propagate effectively over several millimeters.

SHAW (1972) examined the propagation of receptor potential along the nerve of lateral ocellus of the Atlantic barnacle, *Balanus eburneus*. Intracellular recordings made from the receptor terminals in the supraoesophageal ganglion showed that slow signals, which propagate 8–9 mm, only decrease in amplitude by two-thirds. If the axon conformed to the squid archetype then the decrement would be a millionfold or more. Nonetheless, no trace of an active booster mechanism is found. The extracellular field potential decays exponentially along the length of the axons, whereas for an active mechanism, one would expect the field to be spatially and temporally complex and to reveal current sources and sinks. Moreover, hyperpolarisations and depolarisations produce identical fields, and no threshold effects are found.

More recently SHAW's findings have been confirmed and extended in the median ocellus of the giant Pacific barnacle *B. nubilis* (HUDSPETH et al., 1977). In this preparation the individual axons can be seen under a dissecting microscope, and two electrodes can be routinely inserted into different portions of a single axon. When propagating over a length of 9 mm, depolarising signals decrement by one-half, whereas hyperpolarisations below resting potential decrement by one-third (Fig. 2). This is because the axon membrane shows an appreciable rectification, similar to that observed in the soma. A depolarising signal travelling along the cell is changed little if a section of the axon through which it passes is immersed in solutions containing either no sodium, no calcium or no ions at all (sucrose gap). Thus none of the common physiologically active ions are required for propagation. Similar treatments applied to the terminals rule out the existence of a voltage booster at the proximal end of the cell. Clearly barnacle ocellar photoreceptors have no use for active propagation and yet signals propagate for distances of up to 1 cm along axons that are only 10–20 µm in diameter.

Such effective propagation must result from the axon being extremely well insulated. FAHRENBACH (1965) made the worthwhile suggestion that the folds of glia he observed sheathing the axons, acted as insulators but SHAW (1972) disproved this by demonstrating that the glial envelope is permeable to Procion Yellow. That the naked axon membrane is the insulator has been confirmed by measurements of the capacitance of the intact axon and sheath, which approximately equals that of "normal" membranes (HUDSPETH et al., 1977). Consequently the axonal membrane itself must have a high resistance, and the application of cable equations to response decrements suggest values for the specific membrane resistance of more than one hundred times that of squid [57–170 kΩ cm^{-2}, B. eburneus (SHAW, 1972); 196 kΩ cm^{-2}, B. nubilis (HUDSPETH ct al., 1977)]. The higher values for B. nubilis have been confirmed by estimating the specific membrane resistance from values of time constant and input resistance (157 kΩ cm^{-2} and 342 kΩ cm^{-2}, respectively). HUDSPETH and co-workers suggest that the lower values obtained by SHAW result from his measurements being made at the peak of the depolarising receptor potential, where rectification effects have reduced the membrane resistance.

One must conclude from both these studies that graded potentials can propagate over considerable distances by virtue of a specialised axonal membrane with excellent insulating properties. The price of such a good steady state signal transmission is a poor frequency response, but because the photoreceptor response itself is slow in time course only high frequency noise will be attenuated and this could well be advantageous (SHAW, 1972). If the membranes of cells can assume a number of properties then it is worth asking why the squid axon is so leaky. One might suggest that a low resistance is required to give the membrane the good frequency response required for spike propagation, or that leakiness is a property of voltage sensitive conductance channels. But to return to the shadow reflex, a picture is emerging of the first component, the ocellar photoreceptor, which is highly specialised for transduction and for conduction of the signal along the ocellar nerve. Examination of synaptic transmission processes suggests that this specialisation extends to the very terminals of the receptor themselves.

VII. Specialisations at the Presynaptic Terminal

Aside from the transmission of the intensity signal as a graded potential, barnacle ocellus shares another property in common with other arthropod and vertebrate visual systems. Extremely small receptor signals are transmitted across the first synapse to produce interneuronal or behavioural responses (SHAW, 1972). The off spikes recorded in the circumoesophageal connective are sensitive to diminution of receptor potential and respond reliably to signals in the receptor somata of

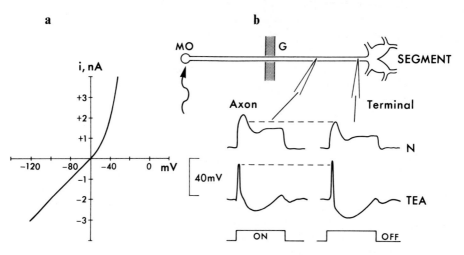

Fig. 4 a, b. The electrical properties of the axon terminals of barnacle photoreceptor. **a** The steady state current/voltage relationships of the axon showing the pronounced fall in input resistance that occurs with depolarisation from resting potential (HUDSPETH et al., 1977). **b** The regenerative calcium spike revealed by application of TEA to the terminal portion of the axon. The receptor potential decrements in passage from axon to terminal under normal conditions *(N)*. With TEA (tetraethylammonium) a calcium spike is triggered by depolarisation. The spike's larger amplitude in the terminals suggests that the active calcium conductances are localised in this region. Stimulus duration = 1.0 s (ROSS and STUART, 1978)

about 0.3 mV (SHAW, 1972). This sensitivity compares favourably with 100 μV threshold signals in fly photoreceptors (Sect. E.II.10) although it is far in excess of the 10 μV threshold calculated for turtle cones (FAIN et al., 1977a).

Recently it has been discovered that the terminals of barnacle photoreceptors have, in their membrane, voltage sensitive calcium conductance channels which could be of importance for increasing the sensitivity of the first synapse (ROSS and STUART, 1978). When the potassium channels of the axon's terminal membrane are blocked by the application of TEA or 4-AP then a regenerative action potential is triggered by small depolarisations (Fig. 4). Both the threshold and the peak amplitude of the action potential are sensitive to extracellular calcium ion concentration, and barium and strontium can be substituted for calcium, whereas cobalt, manganese and lanthanum block the spike. This evidence suggests that the spike results from voltage sensitive calcium channels, similar to those found in several membranes, including barnacle muscle fibres, as reviewed by HAGIWARA (1973). As in squid giant axon, the regenerative activity is normally masked by potassium conductance. These experiments lead ROSS and STUART (1978) to propose that at least two types of voltage sensitive potassium channels occur in the terminal membrane, channels which are sensitive to blockage by TEA and ones which are not. The TEA insensitive channels appear to produce the pronounced undershoot which follows a calcium spike (Fig. 4). Finally they were able to show that the calcium spike is generated in the terminals because it decrements as it travels towards the soma, and application of TEA to axon or soma fails to potentiate a regenerative component.

Clearly the barnacle terminal membrane is also specialised so that depolarisation promotes a calcium influx, which incidentally will boost depolarising signals slightly. Ross and STUART suggest that this calcium conductance makes the receptor synapses extremely sensitive to small depolarisations because in many synapses calcium influx promotes transmitter release (KUFFLER and NICHOLLS, 1976). They also suggest that in the normal terminal this calcium conductance is opposed by potassium conductance, and that this antagonism allows the synapse to produce graded, rather than all or none, responses. It is interesting to note, that if the voltage sensitive potassium conductance is delayed *or*, if there is an inactivation of the calcium channels by prolonged depolarisation, then the synapse has a high pass filter built into it, which only responds to transient signals. Such a high pass system is extremely useful for light adaptation (Sects. D.V.3 and E.III.5). There is at present one outstanding difficulty in the interpretation of the role played by these calcium conductance channels – as reviewed in the following section the postsynaptic response has not been identified and as a consequence the actual signal transmitted across the receptor → first order cell synapse is a matter for further investigation.

VIII. Neurons of the Supra-oesophageal Ganglion

The sensitive off response from neurons leaving the supra-oesophageal ganglion for the ventral ganglion is produced by neural circuits at this level, and in two studies (MILLECCHIA and GWILLIAM, 1972; OZAWA et al., 1976) these have been examined by recording intracellularly from neurons which produce off spikes. In both cases the neurons were not anatomically identified but were impaled close to the terminations of axons from the median ocellus. The neurons hyperpolarised when the ocelli were illuminated and produced a larger transient depolarisation on dimming, which triggered a group of action potentials.

MILLECCHIA and GWILLIAM applied the GABA antagonist, picrotoxin, to the ganglion and found that it abolished off spike activity. Consequently they suggest that the receptors produce a hyperpolarising transmitter, GABA, and that on dimming, spikes are produced by a postinhibitory rebound. The results of OZAWA et al. (1976) are more complex. To begin with they claim that their cells are fundamentally different from those found by MILLECCHIA and GWILLIAM, because at brightest illuminations they produce an on as well as an off spike. However, it is possible that their cell types are really the same, and that the high intensity on spike is triggered by the transient hyperpolarisation produced during the fast phase of photoreceptor light adaptation (Fig. 2). They show that the cell receives collateral inputs because antidromic stimulation through the connective induces delayed bursts of IPSPs, while in darkness the membrane is constantly bombarded by synaptic input.

Their analysis of the response mechanism using current clamp and sodium free solutions suggested to OZAWA et al. (1976) that both the hyperpolarising light response and the dimming depolarisation are produced through changes in sodium conductance. Application of calcium free solutions reversibly blocked all responses and led to a reduction in membrane resting potential, also seen in sodium free solution. On the basis of this evidence OZAWA et al. propose that in darkness an un-

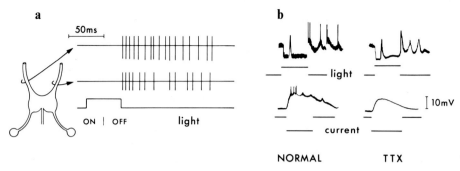

Fig. 5 a, b. Interneuron responses correlated with the dimming of barnacle ocelli. **a** Extracellular responses recorded simultaneously from both supra-oesophageal connectives in response to a brief illumination of *one* lateral ocellus (after SHAW, 1972). **b** Intracellular recordings from an unidentified interneuron in the supraoesophageal ganglion which produces spikes at light off, or when the ocellar nerve terminals are hyperpolarised with current. Application of TTX (tetrodotoxin) eliminates action potentials but does not abolish the graded responses, confirming that graded potentials predominate in signal transmission to this level. Light stimulus duration = 1.0 s; current pulse = 100 ms (after OZAWA et al., 1976)

identified presynaptic cell releases a transmitter which activates sodium conductance. During light this input is inhibited but presumably it is strongly excited at light off. Thus the circuits responsible for producing an off response probably lie between or alongside, the receptor and this neuron.

The inconclusiveness of these preliminary experiments highlights the difficulties that confront any investigator who attempts to deduce presynaptic mechanisms from manipulation of the postsynaptic response. Moreover, because synaptic responses found in another nervous system are often used as models, such deductions become increasingly dubious as the known repertoire of synapses increases (see Sect. C.III.2).

The barnacle photoreceptor terminals are readily accessible and there is hope, that following identification and characterisation of the actual postsynaptic first order interneurons, considerable advances can be made in analysing two fundamental visual processes. The first is the reliable transmission of small signals across synapses, and the second the discovery of neural circuitry capable of generating transient off responses. A thorough understanding of this latter mechanism could provide us with principles applicable to problems of light adaptation and movement detection in more complex visual systems.

IX. Principles Derived from the Analysis of the Shadow Reflex

The most obvious principles learnt from the barnacle ocellus relate to the mechanisms of phototransduction, the passive propagation of small signals over long distances and the passage of small signals across synapses. However, this preparation has another lesson to teach us. It shows that when penetrating experiments can be performed upon single cells, these neurons are found to have surprisingly complex properties. Furthermore, if one understands a little of the behavioural significance of neural function, then some of these complexities can be seen to be of obvious functional significance.

The additional principle to be learnt from the exacting biophysical analysis of ocellar photoreceptors is that the morphological specialisation of neurons is not confined to axon and dendritic form, nor to the specificity of synapses. Large areas of membrane can be divided into domains with differing properties. In barnacle photoreceptors a part of the soma surface is involved with transduction, containing photopigment and light activated sodium channels. The length of the axonal membrane is adapted to have a high resistance and so prevent current leakage during passive propagation of the receptor potential to the terminal. In the terminal area, voltage sensitive calcium channels are found, with properties unlike the voltage insensitive calcium channels of the soma, together with two types of voltage sensitive potassium channels. These are thought to assist in regulating the presynaptic response. Moreover, careful measurements reveal that several types of simple conductance channel have complex time and voltage dependent properties. Thus the simple barnacle photoreceptor is really a multicomponent system, tailored for its specific functions. That a single component of the nervous system can be so complex is truly a sobering thought for those who probe into networks of greater anatomical complexity.

C. Insect Ocelli

I. Introduction

In addition to their compound eyes, many insects possess two or three simple lens eyes mounted frontally and dorsally upon their head capsules. These ocelli usually have a large aperture and a poor image forming capacity. A variety of behavioural and neurophysiological experiments have implicated ocelli in almost every conceivable visual function, except the ones associated with complex form vision. These have been eliminated by the demonstrated failure of a few ocelli to form an adequate image, either optical or neural.

Detailed accounts of ocellar functions are presented elsewhere (this Handbook, volume, VII/6C, Chap. 3) and this review concentrates upon some recent findings from the ocelli of locust and dragonfly where, by carefully employing a combination of anatomical and physiological techniques with skill and rigour, a small group of investigators have been justly rewarded with a crop of general principles, that are certainly applicable to insect compound eyes and could extend to nervous systems in general. Some other principles, although not initially discovered in the ocellus, are shown here with clarity and will be discussed so that they need not overburden the later discussion of the compound eye. We will start by examining the anatomical basis for ocellar function, proceed to the detailed examination of single cell responses and interactions and then attempt to place these results within a behavioural context.

II. Anatomy of Locust and Dragonfly Ocelli

1. General Structure

In the species of locusts and dragonflies that have been examined, each animal has three ocelli, mounted between the compound eyes. Each ocellus consists of a thick lens, lying in front of a cup of receptors, which is in turn backed by a reflective tapetum, and a layer of ocellar neuropile. The receptors lie well in front of the focal plane of the lens so that the spatial resolving power must be comparatively poor. The ocellar photoreceptors resemble their counterparts in the compound eye, each being a single elongated cell, bearing an array of microvilli packed into a rhabdomere, which is itself a part of a well organised fused rhabdom (CHAPPELL and DOWLING, 1972; L.GOODMAN, 1970). Each receptor sends a single axon through the tapetum to synapse and usually terminate in the underlying ocellar neuropile.

A small number of ocellar interneurons leave the ocellar neuropile for the brain, where their cell bodies are situated. The majority of these first order cells are thought to be efferent in function, processing receptors' signals and transmitting a transformed version centrally. Although 500–1,500 receptors terminate in each ocellar neuropile, only 25–30 first order cells run in each ocellar nerve to the brain. Thus the ocellar pathway shows a high degree of convergence and this is another reason for supposing that the ocelli have poor spatial resolving power.

The first order ocellar fibres are classified on their axon diameters into two groups, large (diameter 10–20 µm) and small (diameter 0.5–2.0 µm). In both locust and dragonfly the small fibres greatly outnumber the large, for example in dragonfly median ocellus 2 or 3 large fibres and 25–30 small fibres are reported (DOWLING and CHAPPELL, 1972), but it is only in locust that the complement of ocellar neurons has been analysed in detail. The findings from this thorough search for ocellar neurons are of some importance, both as a necessary basis for further analysis of ocellar function, and as a fascinating example of cell identity, determinancy and plasticity within a nervous system. It is primarily for these latter reasons that we will now examine the complement of ocellar neurons in more detail.

2. Identity and Complement of Ocellar Photoreceptors and Neurons

At present there is little data on the number and identity of ocellar photoreceptors. Existing studies (CAJAL, 1918; L.GOODMAN, 1975) suggest that the ocellar photoreceptors can be divided into three anatomical classes, from their axonal projections. The group I and group II photoreceptors terminate within the ocellar neuropile, the group II fibres project deeper and branch at their ends (L.GOODMAN, 1975). A small number of group III receptors are also reported by both authors, lying close to the rim of ocellar cup and projecting axons into the ocellar nerve. The contribution of this projection in the adult could well bear further analysis. It might be of morphogenetic, rather than integrative, significance because MOBBS (1976) shows that developing receptors in early instars project their axons into the brain, presumably to establish a pathway for the peripheral outgrowth of first or-

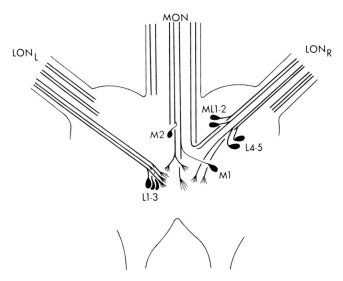

Fig. 6. The complement of 17 L-cells regularly found in the lateral (*LON*$_R$, *LON*$_L$) and median (*MON*) ocellar nerves of locust. With the exception of the median neuron *M2*, all cells are replicated on both sides of the brain. For clarity the cell bodies and central terminals of one set of lateral homologues have been omitted. Note the clustering of cell bodies in groups of two or three (after C.GOODMAN, 1974)

der fibres, and the photoreceptors at the outer rim of the ocellar cup are the last to differentiate.

A definitive study of the ocellar projections within five species of Acridid grasshopper has probably accounted for all the first order ocellar neurons (C.GOODMAN, 1976; C.GOODMAN and WILLIAMS, 1976). Such completeness has proved possible because the total number of neurons is relatively small; they are situated in separate ocellar nerves, each of which can be back-filled with cobalt chloride; and their neurons have their cell bodies and terminals situated in various parts of the brain according to an establishable pattern. Thus each neuron can be recognised, either as an individual identified cell or as a member of an identified cluster. The neurons within a cluster are sufficiently similar for them to be indistinguishable from the others, when viewed in isolation, and the number of cells within a cluster is usually constant.

There are 17 large neurons (Fig. 6) contributing to the neuropiles of the three locust ocelli; 3 individual identified cells and 14 others arranged among 6 clusters according to a regular pattern (C.GOODMAN, 1976). All have cell bodies located centrally around the ocellar tracts. Two pairs of cells, ML 1–2$_R$ and ML 1–2$_L$, have axons running in two ocellar nerves, a lateral and the medial. While producing large dendritic trees at both terminations in the ocellar neuropiles, they fail to produce dendrites centrally (Fig. 6). Thus these two sets of ML cells provide a direct peripheral link between ocellar neuropiles, indicating that for some functions the three ocellar neuropiles must be regarded as an integrated unit. The remaining 13 large cells appear to be afferent, having large peripheral arborisations in one ocellar neuropile, receiving synaptic input from receptors, and a well defined central terminal. All these large cells project to the same area of the brain, the posterior neuropile, where three pairs of postsynaptic cells have been identified by the transynaptic passage of cobalt ions (C.Goodman, 1976). These second order cells project down either the ipsilateral, or contralateral, connective of the ventral nerve cord.

A total of 61 small ocellar neurons have been identified (C.Goodman and Williams, 1976) and these show the same constancy in number and position as the larger cells. Each small cell has a central soma and terminal, and these are distributed over a much wider area of the brain than those of the large cells. Thus small cells project to six major neuropile areas, the posterior neuropile, the ocellar tract, the protocerebral bridge, the ventral bridge, the tritocerebral crotch, the calyces of the mushroom bodies, the antenno-glomerular tracts and the lobula.

This careful account of ocellar neurons provides us with both the information on ocellar projections needed to suggest what ocelli might do, and the exact identification of cells required to see how it is done. C.Goodman and Williams (1976) point out that the large and small ocellar neurons represent two different types of anatomical system. The large fibres are a pathway of extreme convergence; the cells collecting inputs from many receptors and channelling them to a small area of the brain. This convergent system feeds into an area where many of the large descending interneurons of the ventral nerve cord integrate a part of their input, with dendrites in close proximity to the large output neurons of the optic lobes and antennal neuropiles. Thus the ocelli can participate in the formulation of multimodal inputs to this fast conducting system (C.Goodman, 1976). Moreover, the ocelli have a very direct line to the motor centres. The large first and second order neurons place the site of transduction three synapses removed from dendrites, within the motor neuropiles of the thoracic ganglia. Consequently ocellar inputs could participate in rapid visuo-motor reflexes (see Sect. C.IV).

The small ocellar neurons are, by comparison with the large cells, a highly divergent system, connecting small areas of ocellar neuropile with several central regions. This suggests that ocellar inputs can influence the processing of information in other modalities and vice versa. A limited comparison with some other insect orders shows that this dual pattern of ocellar connectivity is by no means restricted to locust. In the fly the ocellar neuropiles, although fused together, have 12 large neurons which project to the posterior slope (the equivalent of the posterior neuropile) and terminate close to the giant neurons of the lobular plate (Strausfeld, 1976a). In crickets a number of small fibres connect the medulla with the ocellar tract (Honegger and Schürmann, 1975).

3. Determination of Ocellar Neurons

The intensive study of ocellar neurons demonstrates two important principles of neuronal determination. The first principle is now a common place in the study of invertebrate nervous systems: assemblies of neurons show a structural constancy from animal to animal, which indicates that each cell is developmentally specified to fulfil a given function.

The second principle is novel: the first order ocellar neurons show variations in structure and number which are compatible with a neural network evolving under natural selection. By diffusing cobalt solution into the cut ends of the two lateral ocellar nerves it is possible to routinely stain 14 of the 17 large ocellar first order neurons (C.GOODMAN, 1974, 1977). This permits one to examine variations in structure and number of ocellar neurons in a large number of individuals. By looking at over 450 animals C.GOODMAN has been able to describe forms of variability in some detail and test the degree to which it is under genetic control.

There are two general types of variation of structure among the homologous ocellar neurons of different individuals. The minor structural variations affect the branching patterns of dendritic trees and similar small changes are seen in insect motoneurons (ILES, 1972) or in interneurons such as the locust DCMD (O'SHEA et al., 1974). Perhaps such small perturbations reflect a complicated sequence of cell interactions, specifying the establishment of correct neuronal interconnections. The major structural variations are more dramatic. The axons of identified ocellar neurons are misdirected and either invade the wrong ocellus, or run centrally to the incorrect neuropile area, or project to the wrong side of the brain (C.GOODMAN, 1974).

Two types of variation in numbers of identified ocellar neurons are found, duplications and deletions (C.GOODMAN, 1977). In duplications, an identified cluster of neurons contains an extra neuron, identical (within the limits of the anatomical techniques applied) to its fellows. In deletions, one cell of a cluster is missing. Because the majority of large ocellar neurons are accounted for in each preparation, one can be confident that deletions and duplications are genuine changes in ocellar neuron complement and not the transfer of a neuron from one cluster to another.

Duplications and deletions are strongly influenced by parentage and must be subject to a degree of genetic control. In two laboratory populations, each initiated from a small number of individuals, the frequencies of duplications were 10/45 and 15/45. In each population the majority of duplications occurred in one cluster, but the cluster favoured was different for each population. The same pattern of family specific duplications was seen in a comparison between the ocellar neurons of offspring reared from different clutches of eggs, each layed by different mated pairs. The influence of genotype upon the identity and frequency of duplications was further investigated by examining isogenic clones of locusts, produced through parthenogenesis (C.GOODMAN, 1977). As expected, the variability between clones exceeds the variations between the isogenic members of any one clone. However, variability still exists within clones. A particular duplication is never seen in more than half the individuals of a clone and, in single animals, duplications can occur in a cluster of neurons on one side of the brain without affecting the contralateral homologues. Thus the genetic factors, inferred from these experiments, express themselves against a "noisy" background of other determinants. It is interesting to note that, with 14 out of 17 cells occurring in clusters, duplications could have played an important role on the evolution of ocellar first order fibres, and deletions might result from a failure to duplicate.

CORY GOODMAN's findings from locust ocellus are of considerable importance for our understanding of the development and evolution of nervous systems. The variability of ocellar neurons takes its place among a growing body of evidence on abnormalities in other invertebrate nervous systems (concisely reviewed by PALKA, 1977). Studies of these naturally occurring, and experimentally produced, "mistakes" can throw a great deal of light on developmental processes, and the association of abnormalities with genetic factors is a significant advance in this field. Perhaps of more general interest, the occurrence of duplications gives us our first glimpse of the genetically based variability which must underly the evolution of nervous systems.

Although the diversity of form and function among nervous systems eloquently expresses their evolutionary plasticity, we have until recently only seen the "fossil record" of such changes, beautifully preserved as homologies between ganglia, single neurons or in ontogeny. Perhaps neuron duplications are a major source of phenotypic variability, capable of being stabilised by selective pressures. As C.Goodman (1977) points out, neuronal duplications could be equivalent to the gene duplications that have occurred during the evolution of proteins, notably hae-moglobins. It has been suggested (Ohno, 1970) that gene duplications promote evolutionary change, by introducing redundancy into the genotype. Similarly, neuron duplications generate redundancy within the nervous system and could make it more tolerant of structural change. If every neuron were to carry out a unique and necessary function, then the probability that a change in connectivity would be deleterious, rather than beneficial, must be high. When a duplicate is made, one cell can sustain normal function while its partner can generate novel contacts. This allows new connections to be generated without necessarily elimi-nating existing patterns. Alternative means of creating redundancy in the nervous system are discussed in connection with the insect lamina (see Sect. E.III.1.e).

Until recently redundant neurons were usually considered as reserves, duplicat-ing pathways to guard against damage (e.g., Kuffler and Nicholls, 1976, pp. 373–376) or as potential recruits for the formation of completely new pathways. With many individual neurons readily identifiable, such redundancy was not gen-erally considered among invertebrates. The analysis of neural constancy in the locust ocellus raises the possibility that some form of neuron redundancy is an essential requirement for long term survival through evolution. By comparison it has been suggested for vertebrates that the overproduction of motoneurons during development, manifested by a later widespread cell death, represents a mechanism that "allows a fairly wide range of variation within its innervation field" (Cowan, 1973) and this redundancy has now been interpreted in an evolutionary context (Katz and Lasek, 1978). However, the verification of such redundancy arguments awaits the observation of redundant neurons producing novel contacts, that are themselves genetically stabilised. Could this be the misplaced axons observed in locust ocellus?

Having entered into a new field we must now return to the function of ocellar neurons, and assume once more, as most physiologists do, that all experimental animals are identical. To ensure that this assumption remains unscathed for several pages we will now examine an area of great complexity, where the normal pheno-type is still far from being established at a quantitative level, namely the synaptol-ogy and connectivity of the ocellar neuropile.

4. A Wiring Diagram for the Ocellus

A thorough account of the anatomical connections between identified neurons is absolutely necessary for unravelling the means by which neuropiles integrate their many inputs. To derive a wiring diagram one ideally begins by identifying the neurons in the system, and then proceeds to analyse their connectivity pattern using techniques which combine the ability of the electron microscope to resolve single synapses with the identification of single cells through selective staining procedures (e.g., STRAUSFELD and CAMPOS-ORTEGA, 1973a) or serial reconstructions (e.g., TRUJILLO-CENÓZ, 1965; ARMETT-KIBEL et al., 1977). A classic analysis of this type has been performed upon the fly lamina, giving us a wiring diagram of unprecedented completeness (see Sect. E.III; Chap. 1 of this volume). Although the merits of such anatomical wiring diagrams are self-evident, they are also deficient in many respects. The ocellar wiring diagram is both incomplete and rudimentary when compared to the marvellous complexity and order of the lamina, but it does provide a better example of the deficiencies inherent in *all* wiring diagrams constructed using existing anatomical techniques. There are two reasons for this. First, it is simpler to explain the inherent shortcomings of a rudimentary circuit, than a complex one. There are fewer names and connections to discuss when giving practical examples. The second reason is more important. Work has just begun in examining ocellar neurons with electrophysiological and pharmacological techniques that are designed to explain the membrane voltage response in terms of the synaptic inputs. Such probing techniques have not been applied to lamina interneurons, consequently the failure of physiologists and anatomists to meet at the synapse is not apparent.

a) Investigation of Ocellar Connectivity

In locust, at least, we now have the catalogue of identified neurons, which is a necessary prerequisite for assembling a wiring diagram (C.GOODMAN, 1976). However, this data was not available at the time when the major investigations of ocellar synaptology were undertaken. Ocellar connectivity patterns were analysed by examining random thin sections, or small numbers of serial sections under the electron microscope, and finding synaptic sites. The pre- and postsynaptic cells involved were then identified, either from the fibre diameter and position, or from their staining properties and organelle content. Such techniques are less reliable than complete serial sectioning (probably impractical for this preparation) and Golgi-EM techniques, as discussed by STELL (1972). The particular problem is that the ocellar neuropile shows little of the structural regularity seen in the lamina, and many of the dendrites are too tenuous to be identified. However, results from the locust ocellar neuropile (L.GOODMAN, 1975) are in substantial agreement with the findings from dragonfly ocellus (DOWLING and CHAPPELL, 1972), and the ocelli of bee and fleshfly (TOH and KUWABARA, 1974, 1975). One striking similarity is that the majority of synapses made by photoreceptors contain a dense presynaptic specialisation and are, at least in locust and dragonfly, dyads, with one presynaptic element opposed to two postsynaptic elements (Fig. 7). Because similar dyad and triad synapses are common to many invertebrate and vertebrate sensory systems it is worth discussing them in greater detail before proceeding with a discussion of connectivity.

b) Properties of Dyads and Triads

The majority of dyad synapses within the ocellus take the form of receptor$\diagdown^{\nearrow \text{receptor}}_{\searrow \text{large first order}}$. The presynaptic terminal contains a prominent, densely staining body, resembling a button in the dragonfly (DOWLING and CHAPPELL, 1972; cf. ARMETT-KIBEL et al., 1977), a ribbon in the locust ocellus (L. GOODMAN, 1975) and, when described in three dimensions from serial reconstructions, a small table in the housefly ocellus (TOH and KUWABARA, 1975). In fly and dragonfly similar presynaptic structures occur in the triads and tetrads formed by the photoreceptors of the compound eyes (BURKHARDT and BRAITEN-BERG, 1976). Triads are a prominent feature of the vertebrate retina, typically with a receptor presynaptic to a central bipolar cell element and two flanking horizontal cell processes (STELL, 1972; RODIECK, 1973). Again a presynaptic inclusion, the ribbon, is a characteristic of the presynaptic terminal.

Are there common functional principles underlying the similarities between the photoreceptor synapses of invertebrate and vertebrate visual systems? Presynaptic ribbons are prominent features of hair cells in the acoustico-lateralis systems of vertebrates, and on this comparative evidence it has been proposed that ribbons are associated with the ability to transmit small amplitude signals (FAIN et al., 1976). However, in insects, although the photoreceptor synapses are very sensitive, presynaptic bodies are also found in many sensory and motor systems and the shape of the body tends to be a characteristic of the species examined (STRAUSFELD, 1976a, pp. 11–12). The correlation with high sensitivity is further weakened by the recent demonstration that ribbons occur in photoreceptor → "on-centre" bipolar synapses, but not in photoreceptor → "off-centre" bipolar synapses (STELL et al., 1977). Thus, although ribbons probably play an important role in organising vesicles prior to release, and are equivalent to the smaller bars seen in most vertebrate synapses (GRAY and PEASE, 1971), their functional significance remains enigmatic.

Wherever they are found one is tempted to suppose that a dyad, triad or tetrad is superior to two or more conventional synapses used in parallel to make the equivalent connections. Three possible advantages are considered here. First, the formation of dyads, triads or tetrads could ensure that the different classes of postsynaptic element received equal strength inputs, despite inherent variability in the number of synapses formed during development. This would ensure that the strengths of signals were correctly balanced. A second advantage is that synaptic noise, generated presynaptically through the random nature of transmitter release (KATZ, 1966), and unique to each presynaptic site, is introduced into more than one pathway. If one member of the dyad or triad is used to control the signal level in another, through inhibition, the synaptic noise components in both neurons will correlate, and subtract. If two parallel synapses were used to distribute the receptor signal to the two synaptic pathways the noise would be uncorrelated and add.

A third and attractive possibility, is for one or more of the postsynaptic elements in the dyad, triad or tetrad, to modulate the signal transferred from the photoreceptor to the other postsynaptic elements. In vertebrate retina the horizontal cell processes, which are thought to mediate lateral inhibition of bipolar cells, are strategically placed within the triad to regulate photoreceptor output. Two alternatives have been proposed whereby current flow from the horizontal cells opposes the receptor signal. Either the current repolarises the photoreceptor terminal by flowing into the receptor terminals (BYZOV et al., 1977; BYZOV and GOLUBTSOV, 1978) or the horizontal cells repolarise the presynaptic membrane by hyperpolarising the synaptic cleft. The proposal for a control of synaptic output through ex-

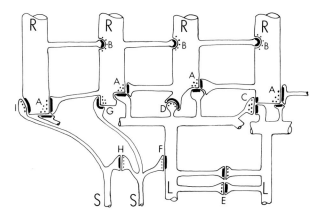

Fig. 7. A summary of the synaptic connections observed in insect ocelli from random EM sections of the neuropile. The connections A–H are described in the text

tracellular field potential, is similar to the function proposed for the passive depolarisation of the insect lamina by current flow from photoreceptor terminals (see Sect. E.III.4). Aside from the basic economy of such electrical field effects, the control of receptor output by one or more members of a triad has the advantage of adding a new level of processing to the system, without introducing additional neurons. Each dyad or triad is equivalent to an interneuron, in the sense that two or more *independent* inputs are combined together to produce an output.

c) Synaptic Connections of Ocellar Receptors and Neurons

The synaptic connections found in the ocellar neuropiles of locusts, dragonfly, fleshfly and bee are summarised in Fig. 7. Note that because the individual interneurons could not be identified at the time these studies of synaptology were undertaken, the connections are only interpretable at the level of the major cell types – photoreceptors, large first order neurons (L-cells) and small first order neurons (S-cells). In all four animals the most commonly observed synapses are made by receptors upon the large first order cells (Fig. 7) (A). In locust and dragonfly the majority of these connections are dyads, receptor$\diagup^{\text{receptor}}_{\diagdown \text{L-cell}}$ but these were not reported from fleshfly. In locust, the receptors are also interconnected via reciprocal "peg synapses" (B) (L. GOODMAN, 1975). All other synaptic contacts are observed less frequently. As well as being postsynaptic to receptors, the large cells are presynaptic to receptors and other large cells, generally via dyads, L-cell$\diagup^{\text{receptor}}_{\diagdown \text{L-cell}}$ (C). Large cells in locust ocellus also make "bulb" synapses (L. GOODMAN, 1975) with receptor endings (D) and make conventional synapses with other large fibres in the optic tract (E).

The interconnection of small ocellar neurons is difficult to resolve, particularly since this "group" is a motley crew of separate individuals. In dragonfly ocellus no small cell connections were observed, and in locust they have only been described as presynaptic to large cells.(F). However, in fleshfly and bee, where more serial sections were examined, the number of small first order cell connections found is much larger, being not only postsynaptic to receptors (G) but presynaptic to all cell types, including other small neurons (F, H, I).

d) Interpretation of Anatomical Wiring Diagrams

The wiring diagram for the locust ocellus (Fig. 7) illustrates many of the shortcomings inherent in anatomical results. These inadequacies can be demonstrated by discussing exactly what the description of cell types, positions and synaptic contacts can and cannot tell us. As pointed out above, the complete identification of ocellar neurons defines the ocellar system and tells us those parts of the brain which receive an ocellar input. A detailed analysis of cell shape and position excludes the possibility of direct interaction between cells, whereas when cells come into close proximity it is feasible for them to interact, either synaptically or through field potentials, or both (e.g., photoreceptors and first order cells of the compound eye).

Cells must interact electrically at points where synapses are observed, and where the synapse is chemical, the direction of transmission is indicated by the presence of vesicles at the presynaptic site. The existing anatomical techniques provide little indication of when a synapse is active and what its postsynaptic effect on membrane potential will be. Although the shape and staining properties of synaptic vesicles have been correlated with specific transmitters in crayfish neurons (Tisdale and Nakajima, 1976), and consistent differences between the vesicles in ocellar receptors and in first order neurons have been observed in locust (L. Goodman, 1975) and fleshfly (Toh and Kuwabara, 1975), it is illogical to assign these structures a postsynaptic response on this basis. The postsynaptic conductance changes determine response polarity, and ultrastructural correlates of this property have not been identified (Palay and Chan-Palay, 1976). Consequently we cannot tell, for example, whether the many serial and reciprocal connections made between ocellar photoreceptors are inhibitory or excitatory. Furthermore, the voltage generated by a postsynaptic conductance change depends upon many factors such as the shape of the neuron and its membrane resistance properties at the time of activation. Thus only crude estimates of synaptic efficacy can be made from anatomical data. For example, because the receptor$\begin{smallmatrix}\nearrow\text{receptor}\\\searrow\text{large first order}\end{smallmatrix}$ dyads seem to outnumber all other synapses in the ocellar neuropile, receptors must be the major input to large first order fibres, and the major synaptic inputs to receptors themselves.

The ocellus is also a good example of a neural system in which anatomical data fail to demonstrate the direction in which information travels through interneurons as electrical signals. If neurons have to communicate electrically over distances which are several times their axonal length constant then regenerative action potentials (spikes) must be used. Such communication is essentially a one way process because when two action potentials collide "head-on" each fails to propagate through the area of inactivated membrane that follows the other. The essential polarity of spiking neurons is usually expressed by the preponderance of postsynaptic sites on the membrane at one end of the cell, and presynaptic sites at the other. However, the large first order neurons do not propagate regenerative action potentials along their axon (Sect. C.III.1), because, as in barnacle photoreceptors, the axonal length constant permits the transmission of slow graded potentials from one end of the cell to the other, with little decrement. It follows that central synaptic inputs to these neurons are equally able to change the membrane potential in the peripheral ocellar dendrites. In this case information has been transferred centrifugally. Thus for non-spiking interneurons it is probably better to abandon the rigid classification of centripetal or centrifugal, and instead regard each neuron as an omnidirectional component, exhibiting a directional bias imposed by the sequential processing of information in successive neuropile areas. In these terms the primary function of large first order ocellar neurons is to transmit information from peripheral receptors to the brain.

Doubts must be expressed about the proposed centrifugal function of the small ocellar first order neurons (TOH and KUWABARA, 1975). If the long thin axons of these interneurons provide a means of electrical communication between the central and peripheral dendritic fields then this must be accomplished by means of action potentials. However, in those cases where the anatomical data indicate pre- and postsynaptic sites on both the peripheral and central dendrites of some neurons in the fly ocellus (TOH and KUWABARA, 1975), then these dendritic fields could equally well function as self-contained components, receiving no input through the axon. The possibility that separate dendritic areas can act essentially as electrically independent interneurons has been raised in the cases of crayfish (MULLONEY and SELVERSTON, 1972) and locust (TYRER and ALTMAN, 1974) motoneurons. A similar situation could also occur in "short axon" horizontal cells of vertebrate retinae, where two dendritic radiations are separated by a thin axon of up to 1 mm in length (BOYCOTT, 1974; GALLEGO, 1976). Consequently, until it is shown that a small ocellar neuron makes only pre- or only postsynaptic junctions at the appropriate ends, the proposed centrifugal function of these neurons is in doubt. It has been reported that the small ocellar neurons terminating at the base of the ocellar neuropile are exclusively presynaptic to large ocellar first order cells (L.GOODMAN, 1975), and if this is so a centrifugal function has been established.

Thus the existing wiring diagram of the ocellar neuropiles demonstrates many of the deficiencies inherent in the anatomical data gathered by existing techniques. Some of these shortcomings will be resolved in the next section, where the intracellular responses of receptors and large first order neurons are discussed, but as we shall see, equally serious deficiencies in electrophysiological and pharmacological techniques still prevent us from discovering the role played by ocellar synapses in the integration of the receptor input. There is, however, one outstanding problem that could be resolved, namely in locust: how do the synapses of the medio-lateral cells linking the lateral and medial ocellar neuropiles differ from those of the other large fibres?

III. The Responses of Ocellar Neurons

The early studies of electrical activity in the ocellus found a pronounced dark discharge of action potentials in the ocellar nerve, which was inhibited by light (HOYLE, 1955; AUTRUM and METSCHL, 1963). By an ingenious analysis of extracel-

lular potentials RUCK (1961) concluded that there were four components in the ocellar response to light. These were
1) A slow depolarisation of the receptors.
2) A rapid spike-like depolarisation of the receptors, induced by the slow potential.
3) A strong hyperpolarisation, postsynaptic to the receptors.
4) A spike discharge which RUCK suggested was inhibited by the hyperpolarising component 3.

The first three components have been measured using intracellular techniques, confirming RUCK's findings; however, their relationship to action potential discharge in the ocellar nerve is still an open question. The necessary intracellular recordings were first made by CHAPPELL and DOWLING (1972) in the dragonfly ocellus and their findings were confirmed in locust ocelli (PATTERSON and GOODMAN, 1974).

1. Intracellular Responses from the Ocellus

a) Response of Ocellar Photoreceptors

Illumination of the ocellus evokes a depolarising response typical of retinula cells (Fig. 8), and the relationship between depolarisation and intensity follows the familiar sigmoidal $V/ \text{Log } I$ curve. The rise and fall of the responses of dragonfly photoreceptors is far more rapid than that of their counterparts in the locust and this same difference is exhibited by photoreceptors of the compound eyes. The ocellar photoreceptors of dragonfly show two properties that have yet to be found in locust ocellus. The first is a large spike response (RUCK's phase 2) superimposed upon the rising phase of the receptor potential. It appears to be an action potential, lasting 2 ms and sensitive to TTX, and is similar to potentials recorded in the photoreceptors of drone bees but not workers (BAUMANN, 1968; SHAW, 1969a). The second property is a pronounced biphasic afterpotential, following light off (Fig. 8). Similar transients of smaller amplitude have been described in the dragonfly compound eye (AUTRUM and KOLB, 1972) and in both cases the potential is thought to be generated by synaptic interactions at the photoreceptor axon terminals. Synaptic interactions between receptors, which the anatomical evidence suggests is strong, may well explain the pronounced wavelength dependent distortion of the $V/\log I$ curves of dragonfly ocellar photoreceptors (Fig. 9), although the interaction of separate photopigment systems within the same receptor cannot be ruled out, on present evidence (CHAPPELL and DEVOE, 1975).

b) Response of Large Ocellar Neurons

The most stable intracellular recordings from the ocellar nerve are of hyperpolarising potentials, of up to 30 mV amplitude, similar in waveform to RUCK's phase 3. It is assumed that these responses emanate from large ocellar neurons (L-cells), because these have the largest axons. This assumption has been validated by one successful cobalt dye injection (WILSON, 1978a). The ocellar hyperpolarising potentials (Fig. 8) are remarkably similar to those recorded from the analogous

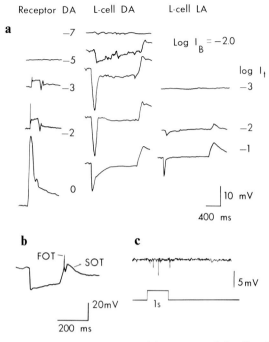

Fig. 8a–c. The responses of ocellar photoreceptors and the postsynaptic L-cells to illumination. **a** Dark-adapted photoreceptor, and dark and light-adapted L-cell responses, to brief flashes. Recordings from dragonfly ocellus, stimulus intensity in log units (after CHAPPELL and DOWLING, 1972). **b** Intracellular responses of a locust L-cell to a 200 ms light flash, illustrating the slow (SOT) and fast (FOT) off transients (WILSON, 1978b). **c** Discrete hyperpolarisations recorded in a fully dark-adapted L-cell during 1 s of dim illumination. (WILSON, 1978a)

first order neurons of the compound eye (Fig. 28), the large monopolar cells (AU-TRUM et al., 1970). In darkness, or in the presence of a sustained background illumination, the membrane potential fluctuates randomly by about 3 mV (PATTERSON and GOODMAN, 1974; WILSON, 1978a). Very dim illumination produces discrete hyperpolarising potentials (WILSON, 1978a, 1978c), similar to those recorded from the locust lamina (SHAW, 1968a). In locust ocellus the mean discrete potential amplitude is about 3 mV, and although their apparently spontaneous production in total darkness is rather perplexing, the statistical properties of light induced events suggest that they arc correlated with single photon absorptions in the receptors (WILSON, 1978c). With increasing stimulus intensity, these unitary events appear to fuse, to produce a noisy hyperpolarisation. At all but the lowest intensities, this hyperpolarising response is strongly phasic, with a pronounced hyperpolarising on transient, a sustained plateau hyperpolarisation, and a depolarising off transient (Fig. 8). This off transient is itself biphasic (Fig. 8), consisting of one or more fast off transients (FOTs), which resemble attenuated action potentials, and a longer lasting depolarising wave, the slow off transient (SOT) (WILSON, 1978a, b). L-cell transients are produced when the transducer input shows no phasic behaviour, consequently they must be produced either at the receptor terminal or at the level of the L-cell membrane, or both (CHAPPELL and DOWLING, 1972).

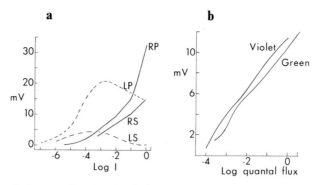

Fig. 9a, b. Intensity/response functions for dark-adapted photoreceptors and L-cells of the dragonfly ocellus. **a** Amplitudes of peak and steady state receptor responses (*RP* and *RS* respectively), compared with corresponding responses of L-cells. Note the interneuron's higher sensitivity, narrower dynamic range, and greater powers of adaptation (after Chappell and Dowling, 1970). **b** The dependence of photoreceptor intensity/response functions upon the colour of stimulus suggests chromatic interactions among receptors (after Chappell and DeVoe, 1975)

Inversion of the light induced signal suggests that the receptor → L-cell synapses are hyperpolarising and chemical, but the long synaptic delay of 10–20 ms (Chappell and Dowling, 1972; Patterson and Goodman, 1974) requires further explanation, because for lamina monopolar cells the value is about 2 ms (Järvilehto and Zettler, 1971; Laughlin, 1973). A comparison of receptor and L-cell intensity/response functions (Fig. 9) shows that considerable amplification takes place (Chappell and Dowling, 1972). It is suggested that this results from the large number of receptors converging onto a single postsynaptic L-cell, and the many synapses formed by each receptor (Patterson and Goodman, 1974). Again, amplification is also seen in the insect lamina where similar amplifier mechanisms were proposed (Laughlin, 1973).

When subject to a sustained background illumination, the ocellar photoreceptors, like those of *Limulus* and insect compound eye (Fig. 18) maintain a steady state level of depolarising receptor potential, whereas the corresponding L-cell hyperpolarisation often adapts to negligible proportions (e.g. Fig. 8). However, the L-cell remains sensitive to small intensity increments, superimposed upon the background (Fig. 8), as do *Limulus* eccentric cells (see Sect. D), and the large monopolar cells of the insect lamina (see Sect. E.III). Dowling and Chappell (1972) suggest that, as in the vertebrate retina (Werblin and Dowling, 1969), the transient responses generated at the first synapse in the visual system play an important role in accentuating small contrast changes.

These intracellular recordings suggest that communication between receptors and L-cells is largely by means of graded potentials. Chappell and Dowling (1972) confirmed this by applying TTX so as to abolish spike activity. This treatment failed to produce a noticeable change in the L-cell response, aside from the blocking of the off spike. Seeing that the receptors often produce an action potential at light on and that this must generate considerable presynaptic current, it is difficult to imagine that receptor spikes have no effect. Is it possible that receptor spikes generate the discrete hyperpolarisations in L-cells?

The L-cells are between 1 and 3 mm long and the graded potential is conducted passively to the central terminal. Simultaneous intracellular recordings in two parts of the L-cell axon show that there is an appreciable signal decrement and conduction is undoubtedly passive (WILSON, 1978 b). The specific axonal resistance is difficult to estimate with certainty because the L-cell cable is shunted by synapses at both ends, however, it probably lies within the range of 2–5 $k\Omega \cdot cm^{-2}$ (WILSON, 1978 b). This value is much less than that estimated for barnacle photoreceptors axon (Sect. B.VI), and the lower value probably enables L-cells to transmit rapid modulations more readily. This possible trade off between length constant and time constant, in graded potential neurons, is an interesting topic for further investigation.

2. Mechanisms Generating the Response of Ocellar Neurons

Three characteristics of ocellar responses, communication via graded potentials, transient enhancement of intensity changes and automatic gain setting to different backgrounds, are similar to the properties of analogous peripheral neurons in the vertebrate (WERBLIN and DOWLING, 1969) and insect retinae (see Sect. E.III). Because of their large size the L-neurons are more amenable to biophysical analysis and this is one reason why the synaptic and membrane responses underlying their response have been analysed in some detail. Two types of analysis have been employed, the measurement of conductance changes associated with L-cell responses (WILSON, 1978 b), and interference with synaptic activity, either generally with cobalt ions (WILSON, 1978 c), or a little less generally with specific pharmacological agents (KLINGMAN and CHAPPELL, 1978). It cannot be said that the ocellar neuropile is yielding its secrets readily.

a) Membrane Conductances and Responses

WILSON (1978 b) succeeded in penetrating single L-cells with two independently controlled microelectrodes, thus allowing for the simultaneous injection of constant current (current clamp) and the accurate measurement of membrane potential. These technically exacting experiments have allowed him to measure the conductance changes associated with the L-cell response, but these findings are subject to the constraints imposed by the unknown geometry and membrane properties of the peripheral and central L-cell dendrites. He was also able to drive the L-cell membrane passively, and so search for feed-back loops. As is often the case when precise measurements are made, the system turns out to be unexpectedly complicated.

In no state can the membrane be called inactive, for even in darkness the voltage noise suggests a steady bombardment by synaptic input (CHAPPELL and DOWLING, 1972; KLINGMAN and CHAPPELL, 1978). The exact dark resting potential of the membrane is difficult to determine, but lies within the range of -20 to -40 mV. In darkness the membrane is rectifying, its conductance decreasing as it is hyperpolarised (Fig. 10). If the level of hyperpolarisation is pushed just beyond the normal level of saturated response, 30–40 mV below resting potential, a second slow conductance change takes place. Over a period of about 1 s the membrane

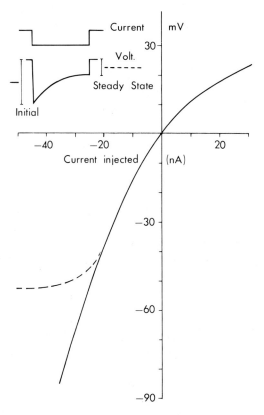

Fig. 10. The time and voltage dependencies of the locust L-cell membrane in darkness. The *inset* shows the voltage response to a strong hyperpolarising current injected through a second electrode. Note the delayed conductance increase. The plot of voltage change vs. applied current reveals that this time dependency is only shown for hyperpolarisations of more than − 50 mV. Conductance drops sharply with depolarising pulses (after WILSON, 1978 b)

conductance rises, so lessening the hyperpolarising effect of applied current (Fig. 10).

When the ocellus is illuminated, the L-cell membrane shows similar rectifying properties. The conductance decrease accompanying the hyperpolarising response can only be measured when the stimulus is powerful enough to saturate. It is suggested that with smaller responses, a superimposed conductance increase, perhaps associated with the normal rectification, obscures the conductance decrease generating the hyperpolarisation (WILSON, 1978 b). The reversal potential for the response is about 40 mV below dark resting potential, indicating that either potassium and/or chloride ion permeability is increased.

What causes the cut back in hyperpolarising on response, from peak to plateau? Both peak and plateau hyperpolarisation have the same reversal potential, and measurement of response amplitude under current clamp suggests that the conductance is reduced during the plateau. These findings indicate that the cut back results from a decreased level of input from the receptors. The slow conductance change, observed with the dark membrane, probably plays little role in adaptation, because it can only be elicited when the membrane is driven beyond saturation. To see if the cut back resulted from a negative feed-back to receptors, driven by L-cell hyperpolarisation, WILSON (1978 b) hyperpolarised the L-cell and measured the intensity/response function. Within the normal range of hyperpolarisations there was no decrease in sensitivity. Furthermore, when the membrane was hyperpolarised beyond the reversal potential of the light induced on response, both on and off transients were still clearly visible. This observation argues convincingly that neither the on transient, nor the slow off transients, are formed by feed-back from a single L-cell's response. Two further observations endorse the insignificance of feed-back. During light adaptation the L-cell response adapts back to the dark resting potential, and in some L-cells the on transient and plateau components of the response have different spectral sensitivities (WILSON, 1978 a).

The origins of FOT and SOT were also investigated. The FOT spike was elicited whenever the membrane was released from hyperpolarisation, either by extinguishing a light, or by switching off an applied current. The spike was always largest when recorded by the electrode closest to the brain, and often could not be seen at all in the more distal electrode, even when clearly visible in the proximal one. This indicates that the FOT is produced at a patch of spiking membrane, restricted to a region near the central terminal. Whether the spike is triggered there by special off selective circuits, or simply results from the abolition of sodium inactivation during hyperpolarisation, remains to be seen. By comparison, the slower depolarising off transient cannot be produced by current injection into the L-cell and is not abolished by hyperpolarisation of the L-cell beyond the reversal potential. Thus the transient conductance increase producing this response is the final expression of a set of neural interactions in which a single L-cell plays a minor role.

In summary, the conductance measurements (WILSON, 1978 b) show that the L-cell membrane is rather complex, containing both active and passive membrane. Furthermore the evidence is strongly in favour of the on and off transients being generated by circuits that shape the L-cell response, without reference to the actual level of signal within the single L-cell – that is to say that feed-back from one L-cell is insignificant.

b) Techniques Which Affect Synapses

A hallmark of a chemical synapse is the granularity of response, resulting from quantal transmitter release (KATZ, 1966). By interfering with transmitter release it is possible to show that the membrane noise seen in L-cells, in complete darkness, results from synaptic activity (WILSON, 1978 c). Cobalt ions are a potent calcium antagonist in low concentrations, and are far more effective than magnesium ions in depressing transmitter release at synapses. Application of cobalt ions to the ocellar neuropile decreases the amplitude of dark noise and reduces the size of the discrete hyperpolarising potentials seen at low intensities, thus eliminating the possibility that discrete potentials are single pockets of transmitter, so adding weight to the idea that they are quantal absorptions in the receptor (WILSON, 1978 c). It will be interesting to see whether the more sophisticated methods of analysing synaptic noise, to reveal the shape and size of underlying unitary conductance events (STEVENS, 1977), can be used to good effect with polysynaptic processes.

KLINGMAN and CHAPPELL (1978) used specific pharmacological agents to dissect the L-cell response. Curare blocks all transmission and abolishes dark noise, consequently they propose that acetylcholine is the transmitter released by receptors, to hyperpolarise L-cells, and that this transmitter is required to produce dark noise. Two GABA antagonists, picrotoxin and bicuculline, abolish the SOT, but have a less well defined effect upon the hyperpolarising response. In the doses used, picrotoxin had no effect, whereas bicuculline decreased membrane noise levels, and the sensitivity of the L-cell to illumination of the receptors. Finally, application of GABA increases the on transient amplitude and the noise level, while prolonging the SOT.

These results led KLINGMAN and CHAPPELL (1978) to suggest that there is a GABA mediated positive feed-back, from L-cell to receptor. GABA could be released by L-cells to depolarise the receptor terminals, and so promote receptor input, even in darkness. When the L-cell is hyperpolarised, this feed-back excitation would be reduced, and if a delay were involved, on and off transients would result. Such a GABA mediated excitation of the receptors certainly explains why bicuculline decreases L-cell sensitivity while GABA increases it. However, one would expect that breaking the proposed feed-back loop with bicuculline would abolish the on transient, as well as the off, and a clear effect of this type is not observed. Moreover, as the authors point out, GABA blockers should decrease the level of dark hyperpolarisation, but a significant depolarisation of L-cell resting potential has not been seen. Finally, the recent conductance measurements (WILSON, 1978b, see above) show that the off transient is associated with the activation of depolarising synapses, rather than with the inactivation of hyperpolarising input, evidence which again conflicts with the GABA feed-back hypothesis.

If the simple feed-back hypothesis is insufficient, then any alternative hypothesis must be far more complicated. Although GABA certainly potentiates the L-cell response, there are at least seven anatomical classes of synapses (Fig. 7), which feed onto L-cells or receptors and it is unlikely that each anatomical type uses a unique transmitter. Consequently any one pharmacological agent might act at several sites, so that the molecular scalpel of pharmacological dissection cuts the network at several points, obscuring both the location and the effect of each.

c) Mechanisms Producing L-Cell Transients – a Paradigmatic Problem

The on and off transients are the most important feature of the L-cell response, resembling as they do the transient responses typical of the first synapses of other visual systems (e.g. barnacle, Sect. B.VIII; arthropod compound eye, Sect. E.III.2; lower vertebrates, WERBLIN and DOWLING, 1969). Yet, despite rigorous analysis the mechanisms producing them are unaccounted for. There are two reasons for this. The on and off transients are produced by transient conductance changes which are not affected by one L-cell's membrane potential, so that the circuits generating these transients are inaccessible to an electrode placed in a single neuron. In addition, the anatomical data suggest many alternative pathways capable of mediating transients. It is not surprising then that pharmacological analysis is ineffective, for despite its molecular specificity the available techniques act at unknown locations. These technical shortcomings are in no way a criticism of the investigators who have worked in this area, in fact the converse is true. It is only because they have pushed back the frontiers to the point where it is the techniques themselves that are insufficient, rather than the skill with which they are practised, that we see the severe methodological problems. Nor are these methodological problems unique to the ocellus. Ideally, an analysis of neuronal interactions would describe each neuron's response in terms of its passive membrane properties, its geometry, the synaptic inputs from other neurons and other local changes, such as extracellular field potentials, short and long term changes in synaptic excitability and hormone levels. Such local changes are simply not measured in the majority of studies, but all of them might be necessary for an adequate description of a synapse's input-output function. Furthermore, the techniques that are used suffer from the disability of simultaneously measuring, or influencing, several sets of variables. Thus the intracellular electrode sees all membrane conductance changes, summed together at one point according to the cells geometry. The potential it measures may not be the local transmembrane potential at many of the synapses involved, either because of electrotonic conduction through the cell, or because of local extracellular field potentials at distant synapses. Similarly, the pharmacological agents lump together all synapses with the same transmitter, irrespective of their position in the wiring diagram. If histochemical techniques can be used to identify the transmitters at known synaptic locations, then it may prove possible, in fortunate cases, to piece together the individual contributions of other interneurons to a cell's response. Nonetheless, the difficulties of assigning a physiological role to an identified synapse are considerable, and will continue to tax us for some time.

IV. The Function of the Ocellar Neurons

Electrophysiological analysis shows that the synapses of the ocellar neuropile produce a response in L-cells which is extremely sensitive to small changes of intensity. Two properties of the L-cell membrane further shape the response. The rectifying properties of the L-cell enhance hyperpolarising responses, while the off spike emphasises intensity decrements. It is impossible to assess the significance of L-cell response without reference to the behavioural function of this pathway (WILSON, 1978a). As suggested at the beginning of this chapter, this point is unresolved, but the examination of L-cell performance has produced an attractive theory which suggests that the ocellus is used for the rapid visual stabilisation of flight (WILSON, 1978a).

Assuming that the ocelli are eyes, one can gain clues to their function by finding out what they are best designed to look at. This essentially requires that one quantifies the response to light intensity, and the response's dependence upon light's spatial, temporal, and chromatic distribution. The dark adapted L-neurons are five times more sensitive to a point source than the equivalent cells of the compound eye, the large monopolar cells. With respect to an extended source they are 5,000 times more sensitive because of their large fields of view. Thus the ocellar neurons can generate healthy responses on moonlit nights (WILSON, 1978a). In these measurements the sensitivity is defined in terms of the energy required to produce a certain level of voltage response (range sensitivity). The recorded responses appear sufficiently noise free to suggest that at these low intensities, the ocellus collects statistically significant numbers of photons. Quantum capture is doubtless aided by the presence of a tapetum, which increases the mean optical path length through the receptor layer. However, a precise measure of ocellus quantum capture efficiency would greatly assist in the assessment of low light level performance and would help account for the origin of the discrete hyperpolarising potentials.

The ocellus appears to be specially constructed to have a very broad angular sensitivity, and so blur out spatial detail. Aside from the L-cells receiving inputs from many ocellar photoreceptors, the lens is defocussed. Moreover, the tapetum reflects rays through the receptor layer and the receptors are organised more as a system of baffles to collect light propagating sideways in the retina than as a series of light columns arranged to ensure that spatial coherence is maintained (WILSON, 1978 a). This combination of factors results in the L-cells having receptive fields of 140° diameter and a half-width (measured at the 50% level) of about 100°. This field of view is not restricted by closure of the radial pupil during light adaptation. The three ocelli are arranged so that the centres of their visual fields are horizontally aligned and the angle between them is about 50–60° (WILSON, 1978 a).

Locust ocelli are predominantly UV sensitive, with a secondary sensitivity peak in the green, at 500 nm, of between 0.3% and 48%, (depending upon the particular L-cell being examined). One median L-cell showed spectral opponency. The delayed inhibition, generating the cut back from on peak to plateau, was greater with green light than when using UV (WILSON, 1978 a). Dragonfly ocellus is, judging from the photoreceptors, also predominantly UV sensitive and there is an inhibitory interaction between green and UV pigment systems in the photoreceptors (CHAPPELL and DeVOE, 1975). Results from both locust and dragonfly indicate that it is possible for these animals to use the ocelli for colour vision (e.g. assessing the chromaticity of skylight to normalise colour assessment by the compound eyes).

The net result of these measurements is a perplexing mixture of properties. L-cells combine sensitive high pass filter characteristics, for intensity measurement, with extreme low pass filter properties, for spatial resolution. WILSON (1978 a) has resolved this paradox by suggesting that the ocelli are used to monitor rapid movements of the largest object a locust is likely to look at, the earth's surface. All three ocelli are directed horizontally so that either pitch or roll of the body in flight, will change the proportion of the ocellar visual fields filled by the sky, and so alter the level of light within them. The UV sensitivity provides high contrast between sky and earth. Irregularities in the horizon will either not be resolved by the ocelli, or will be removed by adaptation in the L-cell response. Thus, a depolarisation or hyperpolarisation of the L-neuron signals that the appropriate ocellus has either dipped or risen, relative to the horizon. WILSON calculates that a 17° change in inclination produces a 5 mV signal in the dark-adapted system. The ocelli then are suited to detect the large changes in inclination that might occur during flight in turbulent conditions. The compound eyes could, by virtue of their superior angular acuity, monitor the position of the horizon more accurately, and this suggests that speed of response may be the vital factor in ocellar performance. Certainly the large diameter of L-cells and M-cells, and the direct projection of this latter cell type to thoracic motor centres, reinforces this view, as does the observation that ocelli are often associated with the capability to fly. However, the wide distribution of small ocellar fibres in the brain (Sect. II.2), and the observed spectral opponency in ocelli, serves to remind us that flight stabilisation is probably just one function. It is, however, an attractive hypothesis worthy of direct behavioural testing.

D. The Compound Eye of Limulus

I. Introduction

The horseshoe crab, *Limulus*, has a pair of lateral compound eyes, a pair of dorsal ocelli, a median rudimentary eye and a ventral eye close to the anterior margin of the mouth (FAHRENBACH, 1975). The giant photoreceptors of the ocelli, median eyes and ventral eyes are favoured preparations for studying transduction, but it is only in the lateral eyes that the projections and interactions of photoreceptors and interneurons, and the resulting integration of their visual signals, have been studied. The results gained from this ancient animal by HARTLINE and his colleagues (RATLIFF and HARTLINE, 1974) have become a classic of sensory neurophysiology. This group looked at the fundamental processes of visual function, rather than the peculiar zoology of *Limulus*, and chose this preparation because its structure and function were simple enough to be described in detail by the available techniques. The benefits of their approach and the rewards of working with a tractable system are summarised by HARTLINE in his Nobel lecture (HARTLINE, 1969). Among the important findings from *Limulus* lateral eye were some of the first extracellular recordings from single visual neurons, the discovery of the logarithmic transform of intensity to spike frequency (a neural correlate of the WEBER-FECHNER relationship), the demonstration of reciprocity between intensity and flash duration (a correlate of BLOCH's law of temporal summation), the determination of photoreceptor spectral sensitivity and the first intracellular recordings of photoreceptor potential. *Limulus* has also given us our first glimpse of single photon responses (quantum bumps) at the receptor level (FUORTES and YEANDLE, 1964). Finally there is HARTLINE's description of an important general class of neural interactions, lateral inhibition, and the analysis of this and other neural processes at the cellular level, to produce a comprehensive account of sensory coding by *Limulus* eccentric cells. These impressive findings have been reviewed in this Handbook by two of the principal investigators (HARTLINE and RATLIFF, 1972) but *Limulus* lateral eye will be discussed here for four reasons. First, no review of neural principles in visual systems would be complete without a discussion of lateral inhibition, and *Limulus* provides a suitable context. Second, the methods employed to analyse *Limulus* lateral eye, are a paradigm for investigations of sensory neurophysiology. Analysis began with the simple unambiguous observation of single cells' responses and the direct determination of cell-cell interactions between identified ommatidia (e.g., HARTLINE and RATLIFF, 1958). It then progressed, via a dissection of the cellular and synaptic mechanisms involved, to a satisfactory description of the dynamic response using linear systems analysis. A third reason for a review is that several important papers have been published since 1972. Finally, HARTLINE's Rockefeller group has tended to present *Limulus* lateral eye as an exemplary sensory system and, wherever possible, this review will try to discuss an arthropod compound eye.

II. The Structure of *Limulus* Lateral Eye

Only the basic structure will be reviewed here and readers are referred to the excellent review by FAHRENBACH (1975) for a comprehensive account. The adult lateral eye consists of approximately 850 ommatidia, each composed of a corneal cone, and 10–15 photoreceptors surrounded by a thick sheath of pigment cells. Every corneal cone corresponds to a single facet on the surface of the eye and transmits light incident upon the facet surface to the underlying cup of photoreceptors (Fig. 11). The shape and high refractive index of the corneal cone suggests that off-axis light is funnelled to the receptors by internal reflection at the edge of the cone so that it acts as an optimum light concentrator, similar to the collectors used for high sensitivity radiometers (LEVI-SETTI et al., 1975).

The photoreceptors are arranged radially around a central rhabdom. Each receptor bears a large number of microvilli which, as in other rhabdomeric photoreceptors, are thought to be the site of transduction. In cross section the rhabdom has the shape of a wheel with a number of radial spokes (Fig. 11). Along the central axis of the ommatidium runs the dendrite of the eccentric cell, which contains many mitochondria but projects relatively few microvilli. This modified photoreceptor appears, from present evidence, to be the principal channel for the transmission of information from the retina to the brain.

On their way to the optic lobe the eccentric cell axons branch and synapse in a lateral plexus. Although it is within this plexus that the much studied processes of lateral and self-inhibition take place, the anatomical basis for these interactions is still poorly defined, partly because the plexus has a diffuse and relatively disorganised structure. The axons from the receptors and eccentric cells of a single ommatidium run towards the optic lobe as a bundle. Directly beneath the ommatidia, and for a depth of about 500 μm, skeins of axon branches pass horizontally between bundles forming a lateral network between ommatidia. In this plexus all axons are extremely fine, the retinula axons being less than 1 μm in diameter, the eccentric cell axons 2.5 μm and the majority of lateral processes less than 2 μm (FAHRENBACH, 1975).

Both the analysis of eccentric cell collateral projections by serial EM sectioning of the neuropile (GUR et al., 1972) and by intracellular dye injection of Procion yellow (SCHWARTZ, 1971) shows that many of the eccentric cell collaterals fail to project beyond the area of neuropile immediately surrounding their own vertical column. Synapses are observed between collaterals of the same eccentric cell and these are presumed to mediate self-inhibition (see below). Only in the dye injected prep-

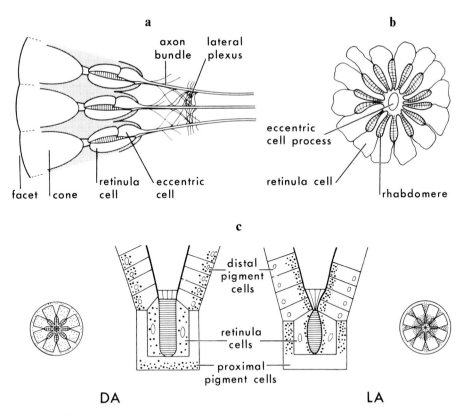

Fig. 11 a–c. The basic structure of *Limulus* compound eye. **a** The ommatidia and the lateral plexus. **b** A cross section through the receptors of a single ommatidium, distal to the eccentric cell body. **c** Changes in ommatidial aperture and the disposition of screening pigment granules in light *(LA)* and dark *(DA)* adapted retinae (after FAHRENBACH, 1975)

aration have eccentric cell collaterals been traced as far as the adjacent columns of descending axons. There is, as yet, no *anatomical* evidence for or against lateral projections to the more distant ommatidia. In the dense neuropile surrounding each column many reciprocal and dyad chemical synapses are found (WHITEHEAD and PURPLE, 1970; GUR et al., 1972).

In addition to the eccentric cells, two other identified axon types run within the vertical strands of the lateral plexus. The retinula cell axons pass through the plexus, presumably to the lamina but their role in vision has not been established. A total of about ten efferent neurons run from the brain to terminate among the pigment cells of each retina, forming "synaptoid" neurosecretory endings (FAHRENBACH, 1975). These centrifugal fibres may play a profound role in the diurnal regulation of sensitivity (BARLOW et al., 1977).

The organisation of the optic ganglia of *Limulus* has received little attention. The first optic ganglion, the lamina, resembles its insect namesake (SNODDERLEY, 1971), with ommatidial axons projecting retinotopically to lamina cartridges and some throughgoing receptor axons forming a brush of dendrites, and then passing on to the next neuropile. First order visual interneurons, similar in shape to the insect monopolar cells, project beside the long visual fibres across a chiasm to the second optic neuropile, called by analogy with the insects, the medulla. This contains seven layers of neuropile and its fibres project centrally to the contralateral medulla, the central body, the circumoesophageal connectives and the corpora pedunculata. Thus the medulla complex may be equivalent to both medulla and lobula of insect optic lobe.

III. Photoreceptor Response

Limulus photoreceptors respond to illumination with a depolarising potential (HARTLINE et al., 1952) which has since proved typical of rhabdomeric photoreceptors. At low intensities, the response consists of a series of discrete depolarising waves whose rate of occurrence follows Poisson statistics, with a mean proportional to light intensity (YEANDLE, 1958; FUORTES and YEANDLE, 1964). The ionic mechanisms of transduction, and the generation of discrete waves in *Limulus* photoreceptors were reviewed in this Handbook in 1972 (FUORTES and O'BRYAN, 1972a, b). The discrete waves (quantum bumps) are probably responses to single photons. These bumps sum to produce the larger sustained responses, but become smaller and briefer at high intensities, to prevent saturation (DODGE et al., 1968). The ionic mechanisms generating the receptor potential are similar to those investigated in barnacle photoreceptors (Sect. B.V). FUORTES and O'BRYAN pointed out that there were several unexplained properties of discrete waves. First, it was not possible to state categorically that one photon produced one bump because the quantum efficiency of the process was not known. In all experiments the ratio of photons to bumps was so high that other transduction processes, such as internal transmitter release could produce the Poisson statistics (FUORTES and YEANDLE, 1964). Second, there were two classes of bumps, large fast bumps, never more than 20 mV in amplitude, and smaller slow bumps. Finally, DOWLING, working with the eye excised from young animals, recorded anomalous giant bumps of up to 60 mV amplitude (DOWLING, 1968). More recent experiments have either resolved these points or suggested further reasonable explanations. Similar discrete waves occur in the photoreceptors of locust (SCHOLES, 1964) and it is possible to determine their quantum efficiency with a precision that gives an unambiguous result – one absorbed photon produces one bump and no more (Sect. E.II.3.a) (LILLYWHITE, 1977). Again, as in *Limulus*, two types of bump are seen, large fast, and slow small. The small bumps recorded in one cell are large bumps generated in neighbouring receptors (LILLYWHITE, 1978a), which are electrically coupled to the cell under observation (SHAW, 1969b). Thus one can argue by precedent, that in *Limulus*, one large bump is produced by one photon, as is usually *assumed*, and the small slow bumps are generated in neighbouring receptors, for in *Limulus* too, the photoreceptors of one ommatidium are electrically coupled (SMITH and BAUMANN, 1969).

The explanation for DOWLING's giant bumps is quite remarkable. The experiments reviewed by HARTLINE and RATLIFF (1972) and FUORTES and O'BRYAN (1972a, b) were carried out on eyes that were excised from the animal, and placed in an organ bath. In the intact animal, the sensitivity of the eye is one hundred thousand times greater (BARLOW and KAPLAN, 1977; KAPLAN and BARLOW, 1975). This sensitivity increase is achieved by the retinula cells producing giant bumps (BARLOW and KAPLAN, 1977). Recordings made in situ, from the intact eyes of healthy animals show that the dark adapted photoreceptors produce two types of response. The large potential fluctuations (LPFs) are 30–80 mV amplitude, and appear to be regenerative events, triggered from small potential fluctuations (SPFs) of less than 20 mV amplitude (BARLOW and KAPLAN, 1977). Thus the LPFs are DOWLING's giant bumps and, to confuse matters, the SPFs are the commonly observed large bumps. The LPFs are abolished by light adaptation, or cutting off the blood supply, and in these cases results typical of the excised eye are obtained. Thus the dark adapted photoreceptors operate in a regenerative mode, which is inactivated by light adaptation, presumably to prevent receptor saturation. The processes controlling or producing LPFs have not yet been examined. However, KAPLAN and BARLOW's findings demonstrate the perils of working with excised preparations. It always pays to minimise trauma.

IV. Integration by the Eccentric Cell

1. Impulse Generation in the Eccentric Cell

The eccentric cell is, judging by the poorly developed microvilli, and its position in the ommatidium, a specialised photoreceptor. Its particular function is to integrate receptor input and then transmit the resulting signal to the brain. To this end it shows three specialisations, electrical coupling to receptors, collateral dendrites making synaptic contacts in the lateral plexus and an active (spiking) axon membrane (Figs. 11 and 12). Simultaneous intracellular recordings from retinula cells and the eccentric cell show that they are linked by rectifying electrical contacts (SMITH and BAUMANN, 1969). Thus the summed receptor potentials from one ommatidium act as the generator potential for spike initiation in the eccentric cell. The failure of this action potential to overshoot, when recorded in the cell body, suggests that the soma of the eccentric cell is passive, and that impulse initiation occurs some hundreds of microns away, in the lateral plexus (PURPLE and DODGE, 1965). The rectifying electrical synapse effectively prevents the action potential from depolarising the receptors, and in doing so, corrupting the information in the receptor input.

2. Self-Inhibition

If current is injected into an eccentric cell, the initial high rate of action potential discharge declines with a time constant of about 0.5 s. It was suggested that this resulted from a feed-back inhibition generated by the self-same eccentric cell (STEVENS, 1964). This hypothesis was confirmed by direct intracellular measurements (PURPLE and DODGE, 1965). A hyperpolarisation of several millivolts amplitude and about 0.5 s duration follows each action potential, and it is accompanied

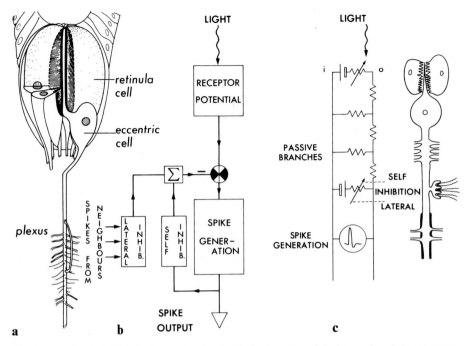

Fig. 12. a Anatomical, **b** block diagram, and **c** electrical schematics of the interactions between receptors and eccentric cells of *Limulus*, showing the relationship between transduction, self-inhibition, lateral inhibition, and spike coding; i = inside; o = outside of cell (from Ratliff et al., 1963; Knight et al., 1970; Purple and Dodge, 1965)

by a conductance increase. During high frequency action potential discharges these inhibitory pulses sum to produce a large sustained hyperpolarisation. Self-inhibition is probably generated synaptically, perhaps by those eccentric cell collaterals which synapse back onto their own cell (Schwartz, 1971).

3. Lateral Inhibition – Mechanisms

Action potentials discharged by one eccentric cell inhibit the discharge of those nearby (Fig. 14). The effects of this lateral inhibition are discussed below and only the synaptic mechanisms are discussed here. The direct effect of lateral inhibition upon the membrane of the eccentric cell has been established by intracellular recordings from the eccentric cell (Purple and Dodge, 1965). The strong inhibition invoked by stimulating many surrounding ommatidia hyperpolarises the eccentric cell and, like self-inhibition, this is associated with an increase in membrane conductance. However, the shape of the Ipsp produced by one action potential's worth of inhibition (literally its impulse response function) has proved difficult to establish because the lateral inhibitory input from a single cell is very weak. By stimulating groups of adjacent eccentric cells antidromically, so that several impulses worth of lateral inhibition arrived simultaneously at the intracellular recording site, and by using poststimulus averaging techniques (Knight et al., 1970), the lateral inhibitory input was found to be biphasic (Fig. 15). A 100 ms wave of lateral excitation precedes a slower, longer wave of lateral inhibition. With one exception (TOMITA et al., 1960), the initial wave of excitation has not been observed when lateral effects are monitored from the discharge rate of a constantly illuminated cell (e.g. Fig. 13). The excitation is clearly indicated when sinusoidal stimuli are used to probe the dynamics of responses (Sect. IV.6; KNIGHT et al., 1970) and its major effect is to delay the onset of inhibition (HARTLINE and RATLIFF, 1972).

The synaptic mechanisms responsible for this diphasic response have not been established. There are precedents from *Aplysia* neurons and from mudpuppy heart sympathetic ganglion cells for single postsynaptic sites producing a biphasic postsynaptic response (WACHTEL and KANDEL, 1971; HARTZELL et al., 1977), but interactions within the tight knot of neuropile surrounding each eccentric cell cannot be ruled out. The application of neurotransmitter agonists, and antagonists to the lateral plexus has done little to clarify the synaptic processes resident there (FAHRENBACH, 1975).

4. Qualitative Effects of Inhibition

Inhibition generates transient patterns of eccentric cell response to stimuli that are sustained in either space or time. The temporal transients are characteristic of single ommatidia illuminated with prolonged flashes. A step increment of intensity generates a transient high rate of activity which then subsides to a lower steady state rate, while dimming produces an inverse response (Fig. 13). Because stimulation of a single facet produces a transient response, self-inhibition must be responsible (providing that intensity increments are sufficiently small to cause negligible receptor adaptation). When several ommatidia are illuminated simultaneously the transient response is more pronounced because the steady state activity is further depressed by lateral inhibition (Fig. 13). However, lateral inhibition acts later than self-inhibition (Fig. 13), as expected from its biphasic impulse response.

Spatial transients are seen in steady state responses, when an array of eccentric cells monitors the presence of a sharp edge (Fig. 13). The transient is usually measured by recording the response from one ommatidium, and moving the pattern past it in steps of one interommatidial angle, so that this one cell successively assumes all the steady state response levels of the members of the array. The transient is produced because the cells close to the edge receive inhibition from areas of dissimilar intensity. On the bright side of the edge, the activity is comparatively high because the inhibition coming from the dark side is relatively weak. Conversely, cells on the dark side are throttled by the strong inhibition from the illuminated side. The decay of the transient away from the edge depends upon the extent of the inhibitory field. The theoretical analysis of spatial transients (BARLOW and QUARLES, 1975) confirms the intuitive notion that the width of the spatial transient equals the maximum extent of lateral inhibition. The exact profile of the transient is insensitive to the rate at which inhibition decays with separation between points (the shape of the curves in Fig. 14) because inhibitory strength is dominated by the area of overlap between the edge and the inhibitory field.

The roles played by spatial and temporal transients in processing the retinal image are discussed later (Sect. D.V). We must first examine self and lateral inhibition quantitatively, in order that their effects can be more precisely appreciated.

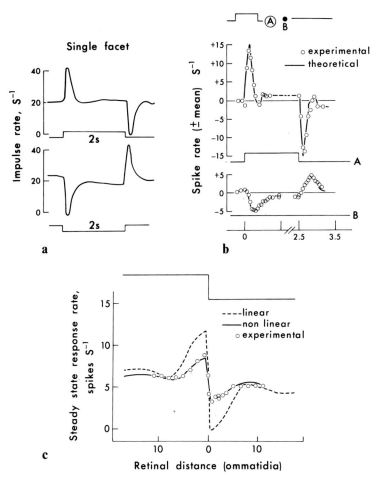

Fig. 13a–c. Inhibition and the generation of spatial and temporal transients in the *Limulus* eccentric cell response. **a** When the illumination of a single facet is changed by a factor of 2, self-inhibition generates temporal response transients (after RATLIFF et al., 1963). **b** When several ommatidia are stimulated, lateral inhibition enhances transient responses. Ommatidium A is in a large patch of retina whose illumination is inhibiting the response of ommatidium B to a small spot of constant intensity. When the intensity at A is increased, the discharge of B is transiently depressed by lateral inhibition, acting with a delay and slower time constant than self-inhibition (after RATLIFF et al., 1974). **c** Lateral inhibition generates spatial transients (MACH bands) at either side of an edge. Measured steady-state responses are compared with the response profiles predicted from the measured dependence of lateral inhibitory coefficient upon retinal separation (BARLOW, 1969) using the linear [Eq. (D.4)] or non-linear [Eq. (D.5)] HARTLINE-RATLIFF equation (BARLOW and QUARLES, 1975)

5. Analysis of the Steady State Eccentric Cell Response

By stimulating single ommatidia and recording from their eccentric cells the responses and the interactions between pairs or groups of ommatidia were observed directly. Providing that the mean level of *response* is low the effects of lateral inhibition can be predicted by a set of simultaneous linear equations (HARTLINE and

RATLIFF, 1957). Thus for two ommatidia, 1 and 2, the net response rates r_1 and r_2 are given by

$$r_1 = e_1 - k_{1,2}(r_2 - r_2^0), \qquad (D.1)$$

$$r_2 = e_2 - k_{2,1}(r_1 - r_1^0), \qquad (D.2)$$

where e_1 and e_2 are the net excitations of 1 and 2 when each is stimulated alone, $k_{1,2}$ and $k_{2,1}$ are the inhibitory coefficients for inhibition of 1 by 2, and 2 by 1 respectively, and r^0 is the threshold for inhibition by each unit. Additional experiments showed that inhibition from many ommatidia sums linearly upon each eccentric cell (HARTLINE and RATLIFF, 1958) so that when n ommatidia are illuminated, the response of each is determined from n simultaneous equations of the form

$$r_x = e_x - \sum_{y=1, y \neq x}^{y=n} k_{x,y}(r_y - r_y^0). \qquad (D.3)$$

Note that in this formulation of the HARTLINE-RATLIFF equations the excitation term for a single ommatidium e_x includes the effects of self-inhibition. For completeness the equations have been rewritten so that

$$r_x = e_x - k_x r_x - \sum_{y=1, y \neq x}^{y=n} k_{x,y}(r_y - r_y^0), \qquad (D.4)$$

where k_x is the self-inhibition coefficient, and e_x the excitation from the receptor cells; k_x can be determined directly by intracellular current injection or inferred, either from the dynamic analysis (Sect. IV.6), or by assuming that the self-inhibitory effects at the peak of the on transient are negligible so that this peak discharge represents e_x, the excitatory input from the retinula cells.

Note that the inhibition derived from any one ommatidium is proportional to its spike output r_x and not to its uninhibited excitation e_x. Thus inhibition is recurrent. The output of an eccentric cell is fed back to inhibit its neighbour. The alternative configuration is forward inhibition, where the input to each ommatidium is used to regulate the response of neighbours. The classic test for recurrent inhibition is to search for disinhibition. If two separate groups of ommatidia are illuminated, then the switching on of a third spot close to the first group, but far from the other, will increase the spike rate in the distant second group because it inhibits the spike rate in the nearer first group, and so throttles their inhibitory influence (Fig. 14a).

The biophysical analysis of the eccentric cell membrane response provides an explanation for the linearity of the steady state response. First, the steady state eccentric cell spike rate is proportional to the receptor and eccentric cell depolarisation (FUORTES, 1958; BARLOW and KAPLAN, 1977). Second, the lateral inhibitory currents produced by the inhibitory synapses are proportional to the mean rate of impulse arrivals at the inhibitory synapse. This is because, at low spike rates, the number of conductance channels activated by inhibitory synapses is small enough for their voltage effects to sum linearly, and each action potential probably produces, on average, the same amount of transmitter (HARTLINE and RATLIFF, 1972).

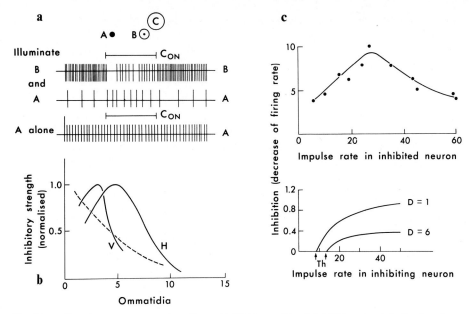

Fig. 14 a–c. Four important properties of lateral inhibition. **a** The disinhibition that is indicative of recurrent inhibition. Ommatidia at *A* and *B* are continuously illuminated. By inhibiting B, the additional illumination of C generates an increase in firing rate at A. If B is not illuminated then C has no effect on A (after HARTLINE and RATLIFF, 1972). **b** The dependence of inhibitory strength upon retinal separation, as measured by BARLOW (1969) in the horizontal and vertical planes (H and V) and by JOHNSTON and WACHTEL (1976) ----. See text for different methods. **c** The two known forms of non-linearity associated with lateral inhibition. *Upper graph*, inhibition depends upon discharge rate in the *inhibited* cell (after BARLOW and LANGE, 1974; see also Eq. (D.5). *Lower graph*, the strength of inhibition increases non-linearly with the discharge rate in the *inhibiting* cell. The inhibition of one cell by another saturates at a value which decreases with increasing retinal separation, D (expressed here in ommatidia) (after JOHNSTON and WACHTEL, 1976)

At higher spike rates a non-linearity appears in the steady state eccentric cell response (BARLOW and LANGE, 1974). The retinula cells sufficiently depolarise the eccentric cell membrane to significantly increase the EMF driving current out of the cell, through the inhibitory synapses. This potentiation of inhibition is seen when the level of excitation elicits between 10 and 30 spikes s^{-1} in the steady state. At these discharge rates the effect of lateral inhibition is proportional to spike rate within the inhibited neuron. A more comprehensive non-linear steady state equation (BARLOW and LANGE, 1974) is

$$r_x = e_x - k_x r_x - (1 + a r_x) \sum_{y=1, y \neq x}^{y=n} k_{x,y}(r_y - r_y^0). \qquad (D.5)$$

At discharge rates of 30–60 s^{-1} the effect of lateral inhibition again decreases (Fig. 14c) for reasons that are unknown and unaccounted for in Eq. D.5. The validity of this non-linear correction has been established by analysing steady state response at borders of extremely high contrast, where the mean steady state discharge rates are amplified by spatial transients. Under these conditions the simple linear formulation cannot describe the spatial response pattern but the non-linear correction copes admirably (Fig. 13c). A second non-linearity, linking the presynaptic impulse rate and the postsynaptic inhibitory response, is described in Sect. D.IV.7.

However, the linear HARTLINE-RATLIFF relationship still proves useful for predicting responses to small intensity changes which produce small changes in discharge rate. The lasting value of HARTLINE and RATLIFF's initial description stems from two facts. First the system is amenable to piecewise linearisation and secondly, the HARTLINE and RATLIFF equations analysed the lateral inhibitory network at the fundamental level of interactions between single cells.

6. Analysis of the Dynamics of Ommatidial Interactions

To successfully describe the transient response of a complex biological system in terms of the individual contributions of its component parts is often difficult but usually worthwhile (e.g. HODGKIN and HUXLEY, 1952). Such an analysis of the *Limulus* ommatidium is considerably simplified by the fact that the eccentric cell response to a sinusoidally modulating light of low contrast is also a sinusoidal function of the same frequency, relatively uncontaminated by rectification or harmonics (KNIGHT et al., 1970). Thus for *small stimulus fluctuations* about the mean, the system is linear over a wide range of *mean* intensities (BIEDERMAN-THORSON and THORSON, 1971). Under such quasi-linear conditions, the dynamic response can be predicted, either in the time domain, by convolving the impulse response function with the input signal, or in the frequency domain using Fourier analysis. Both approaches have been successfully implemented in the *Limulus* lateral eye (HARTLINE and RATLIFF, 1972; RATLIFF et al., 1974), but because the Fourier analysis is easier to understand, and conceptually the most valuable, it will receive our full attention.

In a linear system the response to two inputs applied simultaneously is the sum of the responses to the two inputs applied alone (the superposition principle). Under these conditions Fourier's Theorem establishes that any complicated input varying as a function of time, can be decomposed into component sinusoidal modulations of specified frequency, amplitude and phase. It follows from superposition that, if we can determine how each part of a system behaves in response to simple sinusoidal inputs, we can compute the overall response of the total system to any stimulus, providing that the system is not forced into a region of non-linear operation.

By applying sinusoidally modulating currents, lights and impulse vollies to receptors and eccentric cells, it has proved possible to describe the dynamic response of these elements in terms of their transfer functions; i.e. the degree to which each component changes the amplitude and shifts the phase of a sinusoidal input expressed as a function of frequency (f) (KNIGHT et al., 1970). The transfer functions, conveniently written as complex numbers that encapsulate both amplitude and phase, are then combined into a single dynamic HARTLINE-RATLIFF equation so that the eccentric cell output, as a function of frequency, $r_x(f)$, is given by

$$r_x(f) = I_x(f) \cdot G(f) - k_s S_x(f) \cdot r_x(f) - L(f) \sum_{y=1, y \neq x}^{y=n} (k_{x,y} r_y(f)), \qquad (D.6)$$

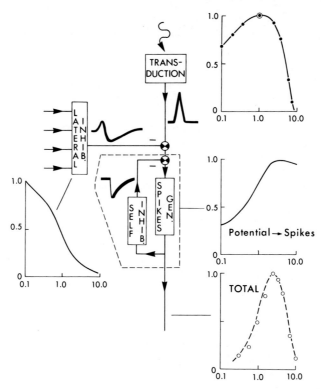

Fig. 15. Frequency responses for the processes of transduction, self-inhibition combined with spike generation (potential→spikes) and lateral inhibition. The phase components are omitted. The overall frequency response of the eccentric cell to a broad light source (TOTAL) can be predicted [Eq.(D.6)] from the component frequency responses (----), and this agrees well with the measured data points. Impulse responses for transduction and lateral and self-inhibition are also included. (Data from KNIGHT et al., 1970)

where $r_x(f)$ and $r_y(f)$ are complex numbers expressing the phase and frequency of the spike outputs of eccentric cells x and y, $I_x(f)$ is the intensity and phase of input light signal as a function of frequency (also a complex number) and $G(f)$, $S_x(f)$, and $L(f)$ are complex numbers expressing the frequency responses of transduction and self and lateral inhibition. Within the bounds of linearity this expression successfully describes the responses of eccentric cells to a number of complicated input patterns (KNIGHT et al., 1970; RATLIFF et al., 1974) (Fig. 13 b). The frequency responses of the components determined from sinusoidal stimulation correspond to the Fourier transforms of their impulse responses (KNIGHT et al., 1970) as determined by other methods and the self-inhibitory and lateral inhibitory coefficients k_x and S_x correspond to those derived from steady state analysis (Fig. 15).

It is interesting to compare the achievements of this piecewise linear analysis with results gained from applying non-linear methods to physiological systems. These non-linear modelling techniques produce an analytic function (Wiener kernels of ascending order) which describe a system's input: output relationship with a high degree of accuracy and under many different conditions (MARMARELIS and

NAKA, 1974; REICHARDT and POGGIO, 1976; FRENCH, 1973). These non-linear methods have proved to be very superior experiments, in which data is collected with maximum efficiency, so that comprehensive input/output functions (including frequency responses) can be measured in a short space of time. By comparison the simple but restricted linear systems analysis has provided us with considerable insight into the working of the *Limulus* ommatidium, simply because each transfer function can be related to physical processes. The transfer function for the receptor relates to the time course of the voltage response to a single photon, and the frequency response for lateral and self-inhibition to the shapes of the individual postsynaptic psps (Fig. 15). The formulation represents each physiological process in a flow chart that relates directly to the measured physiological interactions (Figs. 12 and 14). Each transfer function describes the role its corresponding physiological component plays in determining the output of the eccentric cell. As examples, the high frequency cut off in eccentric cell amplitude response results from the finite duration of photoreceptor responses to single photons, whereas the low frequency roll off is caused by self-inhibition; or when groups of ommatidia are illuminated simultaneously by a sinusoidally flickering light, lateral inhibition boosts the response when its delay is half the period of the input (RATLIFF et al., 1969). Finally, the successful prediction of eccentric cell responses from the transfer functions of the individual components demonstrates that no important class of interaction has been overlooked. Overall, this analysis is a considerable achievement and, until the dry Wiener kernels can be given the flesh and sap of biological processes, they will remain in the domains of instrumentation and mathematical abstraction.

7. Spatial Distribution of Lateral Inhibition

The inhibiting effect of one ommatidium upon another decreases with spatial separation and the precise relationship between inhibitory strength and retinal separation has been investigated by two different means. Because individual inhibitory coefficients are very weak, R.BARLOW (1969) observed the effect of illuminating a group of four ommatidia, upon the steady state response of a single ommatidium to a light constant intensity. By recording simultaneously from one of the four inhibiting ommatidia, BARLOW was able to compute the inhibitory coefficient for this group using the HARTLINE-RATLIFF equations for the *steady state*. This analysis assumes that the four inhibiting ommatidia act as one. It shows that detectable lateral inhibition extends over 30% of the eye's surface and is strongest 3–5 ommatidia away from the test unit (Fig. 14).

JOHNSON and WACHTEL (1976) used a novel technique for determining the spatial dependence of lateral inhibition. The optical isolation of single ommatidia was improved by removing the cornea and stimulating the individual naked ommatidial cups with a light pipe. This light source also contained an extracellular electrode for monitoring the eccentric cell spike rate in the stimulated ommatidium.

This method confirmed BARLOW's finding that the inhibitory field had a radius of 9–10 ommatidia, but it failed to confirm that inhibition is maximum between eccentric cells that are 3–5 ommatidia apart. Instead, the strength of inhibition declined monotonically with separation (Fig. 14). The discrepancy between these two methods has not been resolved by an independent determination. JOHNSON and WACHTEL (1976) also discovered a second non-linearity in the relationship between spike rate and strength of inhibition. The inhibitory input to an ommatidium is only a linear function of spike rate in the *inhibiting* cell for low impulse rates. At higher impulse rates the inhibitory coefficient falls and inhibition saturates (Fig. 14c). In fact the relationship between spike rate and inhibition approximates to the hyperbolic function expected for self-shunting at the postsynaptic membrane [Eq. (B.1)] (MARTIN, 1955). The saturated value of inhibition is a function of distance between inhibited and inhibiting ommatidia and it was strength of saturated input that JOHNSON and WACHTEL (1976) used to estimate the strength of inhibitory interactions within the inhibitory field (Fig. 14b).

The dependence of saturating response amplitude upon distance of separation provides additional evidence for the hypothesis advanced by GUR et al. (1972) that the strength of inhibitory input depended upon the length of the collateral connecting the inhibitory synapse to the axon of the eccentric cell. If one accepts that all inhibitory synapses are, at their postsynaptic site, equally effective then the difference in saturated effect must result from an attenuation during transmission from postsynaptic site to the spike initiated zone. Simple cable attenuation in thin collaterals, with the length of collateral increasing (or its length constant decreasing) as it connects with more distant ommatidia is an attractively simple strategy for regulating the strength of inhibitory inputs to produce the required profile of inhibitory field. If this hypothesis is correct then the self-inhibitory branches will synapse upon the shortest collaterals and distant ommatidia upon the longest (JOHNSON and WACHTEL, 1976).

V. Function of Inhibition in the Lateral Eye

Inhibition produces transient responses. Self-inhibition attenuates those components of the signal from a single ommatidium that change little with the passing of time. Similarly, in the spatial domain, lateral inhibition suppresses the discharge over wide areas of constant illumination and emphasises edges.

What is the value of inhibition? Three general classes of function have been considered, image reconstruction, feature extraction and light adaptation. All are interrelated because they reflect different aspects of the same highpass filter characteristics, but it is convenient to discuss each function separately. Note that because these functions are teleological interpretations of the data, they are not mutually exclusive.

1. Image Reconstruction

a) Fundamental Limitations

The majority of eyes operate by a simple set of optical principles. A well designed optical system directs light to photoreceptors, which transduce the intensity they receive to a receptor potential. Thus the voltages of receptors record the distribution of light intensity in both space and time and these photoreceptor voltage levels can be thought of as a *neural image*. Many eyes sample the spatial distribution of object intensity by constructing a two-dimensional mosaic of receptor outputs, with each receptor looking in a different direction. In vertebrate eyes this spatial mapping is achieved by placing the photoreceptor array in the focal plane of a single lens. In apposition compound eyes, for which *Limulus* provides an example, the mapping is accomplished by an approximately spherical array of ommatidia, each with its own lens and each looking in a different direction (Fig. 11). In both the single lens and compound eyes, the clarity of the neural image is clouded by three inescapable factors. These are:

α) Granularity. The neural image has a distinct graininess because it is composed of many discrete elements, corresponding to the outputs of single photoreceptors. The coarseness of this granularity can be expressed in terms of the number of photoreceptors per unit solid angle of object space. Note that in compound eyes with narrow fused rhabdomes the spatial unit is the ommatidium because the photoreceptors contributing to the rhabdom share the same incident light.

β) Blurring. In an ideal imaging system, the light from a single point in object space should fall entirely within one photoreceptor. In fact this ideal is seldom realised because pupil diffraction, lens aberrations and refractive errors tend to spread the light from one point over several receptors. Consequently sharp edges are smoothed and the image of a point is a diffuse spot (Fig. 16). For an eye with a single lens, blurring is usually described by the point spread function – the distribution across the retina of light from a single point (WESTHEIMER, 1972a). In the apposition compound eye, the corresponding measure of blurring is the angular sensitivity function of the ommatidium. This curve (Fig. 23) gives the relative sensitivity of the ommatidium as a function of the angle of incidence of light and so describes the contamination of the signal in one spatial element by light from a correspondingly wider area of object.

γ) Noise. The amount of information that an array of photoreceptors can capture from the object is greatly reduced by noise. If there were no noise then every photoreceptor could measure infinitesimally small intensity differences with perfect reliability. When noise is present there are random fluctuations in receptor output which do not correspond to equivalent changes in object intensity and the receptor signals are no longer a reliable representation of intensity. The statistical distribution of noise fluctuations defines the probability that a given fluctuation in receptor potential corresponds to a change in input. Alternatively, the noise defines the smallest fluctuation in receptor output that can be attributed to a change in intensity with a specified minimum level of reliability. One can think of the noise dividing the limited response range of a photoreceptor into discrete signal states, just as a ruler is divided into gradations (Fig. 16). This analogy demonstrates that the greater the noise, the fewer the number of different measurements a receptor can make, but this comparison is crude. One can always choose between having many unreliable levels of response, or a few measurements of greater certainty. A better measure of receptor signalling power is derived from information theory (SNYDER et al., 1977a, b; SNYDER, 1979).

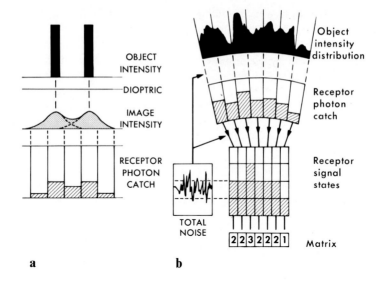

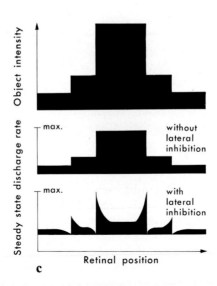

Fig. 16a–c. Three of the principles underlying image processing in the peripheral retina. **a** The dioptric apparatus blurs the image (via the point spread function) and spreads light from one object point to many receptors, so reducing the depth of fluctuation of signal among receptors. **b** The receptor mosaic divides the image into a finite number of elements, each of which can only assume a finite number of reliable output stages, as determined by the noise level. Thus the outputs of receptors or retinotopic neurons can be modelled in terms of matrices, each element assuming one of a limited set of integer values. **c** Lateral inhibition reduces the number of impulses required to transmit image detail, by reducing discharge rates across areas where intensity remains constant. This is equivalent to reducing the redundancy in the final output

Noise is always present in photoreceptors because photons arrive and are absorbed at random, according to Poisson statistics (BARLOW, 1964). The resulting *photon noise* has a variance (power) that equals the mean number of photons absorbed. When the visual signal has an amplitude proportional to intensity the signal to noise ratio (signal amplitude/standard deviation of noise fluctuations) is proportional to the square root of the number of photons absorbed. Consequently the effects of photon noise can only be reduced by absorbing more light. If photon noise is limiting the detection of a signal then the threshold intensity fluctuation should be proportional to the square root of the mean intensity and this relationship is known as the "square root law" (DEVRIES, 1943; ROSE, 1942; BARLOW, 1964). Note that the inverse of this law does not hold. When the threshold follows the square root law this is only proof that the variance of noise limiting detectability is proportional to intensity. If photon noise is to be proven the *only* limiting factor, the constant of proportionality must be found equal to unity, because other sources of noise in the visual system can produce a variance proportional to mean intensity (e.g. transducer noise – Sect. E.II.5). Nonetheless, photon noise is inescapable and, although most pronounced at low intensities, it can limit the resolution of brighter stimuli when they are rapidly moving, brief in duration or of limited spatial extent (BARLOW, 1964; SNYDER et al., 1977a, b; SNYDER, 1979).

The discussion of these fundamental optical limitations to resolving power leads to the concept of the neural image as a matrix of discrete elements, each of which represents the intensity within a certain area of the object. At any one time each of these receptors can assume one of a finite number of response states, and each of these discrete states can be thought of as a shade of grey or grey tone. Noise in the receptors coarsens the gradation between available grey tones. Blurring reduces the range of grey tones that can coexist in adjacent receptors and so washes out contrast from the neural image. The interrelating effects of noise, blurring and receptor granularity upon image quality can be quantified by calculating the number of different grey tone patterns a matrix of photoreceptors can make (SNYDER et al., 1977a, b). If each grey tone is assigned a number, the neural image can be described by a matrix and the effects of blurring handled by matrix algebra (e.g. REICHARDT, 1961). Matrix techniques are being developed for the processing of images by digital computers (FRIEDEN, 1975) and these techniques may prove useful because eyes share a common goal with preprocessing techniques, the extraction of the most reliable image from an imperfect optical image. For analysing eyes, matrix methods have the advantage of being isomorphic to receptor and neural arrays. Each element within the matrix can represent the output of an identified neuron and the interactions between neurons can be dealt with algebraically (e.g. REICHARDT, 1961, for lateral inhibition between eccentric cells). By comparison the fashionable Fourier techniques analyse spatial interactions within a structure which may just be a mathematical abstraction. There is no proof that spatial frequency is actually coded for in the visual system, at the level of single neurons (OCHS, 1979).

It will not have escaped notice that this description of image quality has been confined to a static "snapshot" representation of the object. In most cases the neural image is constantly changing, either through movement within the object or through movement and tremor of the eye. Such changes in neural image are thought necessary for continued perception at a higher level. An optical image that is fixed in one position on the human retina is perceived normally when first presented but the percept fades away within 2–10 s (DITCHBURN, 1973). A similar fading of the stabilised image can be inferred from the orientation behaviour of flies (REICHARDT and POGGIO, 1976). As of yet, we have little understanding of the effects of motion on visual acuity, either in theory or in practice. One factor, the smearing of the neural images of rapidly moving objects across the retina, is dealt with in Sect. E.II.6 together with the possibility of using motion to improve spatial acuity.

b) Image Reconstruction in Limulus

Because of the wide angular separation between individual ommatidia, varying from 2° in the centre of the eye to 10° at the periphery (VON CAMPENHAUSEN, 1967) the lateral eye must have poor spatial resolution. The irregular and rather jumbled lattice of facets support this contention (FRENCH et al., 1977). Moreover each ommatidium accepts light over a wide angle of space so that any image is badly blurred by the broad point spread function. The sensitivity to a point source moved in front of an ommatidium has been measured by recording the eccentric cell discharge (WATERMAN, 1954). The resulting angular sensitivity function has a half-width (width at 50% sensitivity) of 8–10° and this agrees with the gaussian angular sensitivity function of half-width 8°, inferred from the response to edges moved in front of the eye (KIRSCHFELD and REICHARDT, 1964). However, because little image detail is gained by spacing the receptors closer together than half the acceptance angle (Fig. 22) (see also SNYDER, 1979), the acceptance angle of 8° is incompatible with an interommatidial angle of 2°. To resolve this discrepancy it is suggested that the reported acceptance angle is an overestimate, for three reasons. First, WATERMAN (1954) acknowledged that because he was interested in the total extent of the visual field of a single ommatidium, he used a wide stimulus of 8° diameter. This must overestimate the acceptance angle. Second, as found in the praying mantis (ROSSEL, personal communication), acceptance angle probably varies across the eye to match the changing sampling density (interommatidial angle) and these variations have not been taken into account. Finally the pigment movements observed in the ommatidia suggest that the acceptance angle is very wide when dark adapted.

Whatever the angular acceptance function of Limulus photoreceptors is, it removes contrast detail from the retinal image. The idea that lateral inhibition restores this lost detail dates back to Mach's original discussions of the lateral interactions in the human visual system which he inferred from the observation of spatial transients or Mach bands (see RATLIFF, 1965, p. 146 ff.). One basic principle underlying image enhancement through lateral inhibition is simple. Blurring by the optics transfers energy from one object point to several image points, according to the point spread function. If one knows the point spread function then its effects can be counteracted by performing a subtraction upon receptor outputs equal and opposite to the blurring. This correction is essentially lateral inhibition that is equal and opposite to the point spread function. However, this type of restoration is subject to constraints. Lateral inhibition does not allow the system to operate as if it had a perfect optical system that is blur free, rather the image is deblurred within the limits of resolution set by the optics, because lateral inhibition only accentuates differences that are already apparent at the photoreceptor level. In addition, practical application of this method to the digital image processing techniques used in spectroscopy and astronomy shows that these inverse transform methods are very sensitive to noise (FRIEDEN, 1975).

Perhaps this is one reason why lateral inhibition in *Limulus* lateral eye is not powerful enough to deblur the lens aberrations. REICHARDT (1961), using the matrix techniques mentioned above, demonstrated that lateral inhibition could, in principle, deblur the retinal image. However, direct estimation of the spatial frequency response of the eccentric cell array, with and without lateral inhibition and receptor overlap, showed that inhibition is too weak and too widely distributed to function effectively in image restoration (KIRSCHFELD and REICHARDT, 1964). Consequently we must search for other functions for lateral inhibition in the *Limulus* eye.

2. Feature Extraction

By acting as a high pass filter, inhibition extracts the changing components from the retinal intensity signal and rejects the static. As H.B.BARLOW pointed out (1961), high pass filtering greatly increases the efficiency with which information is encoded by an array of neurons. The unchanging components of the intensity signal carry little information because they are, by definition, predictable and their rejection allows the restricted signalling capabilities of the nervous system to be devoted to transmitting more accurately those fluctuating signal components which carry the greatest information. This is illustrated in Fig. 16 where two hypothetical arrays of cells, one with, and one without, lateral inhibition monitor a "top hat" intensity pattern. The system with lateral inhibition expends less action potentials. Furthermore, because lateral inhibition prevents saturation by the background, it allows the retina to monitor the intensity changes at edges with high sensitivity and consequently greater accuracy. We will return to this important concept of optimal coding in the peripheral visual system when considering the insect lamina (Sect. E.III.5).

Nonetheless, in increasing efficiency some less important aspects of the signal must have been rejected. Wherever high pass filtering is used in a visual system, information about absolute energy levels is lost. This is best illustrated by considering the response of a single eccentric cell to intensity signals that modulate in the time domain. The changing components are coded according to the steep intensity response function for transient responses. Thus the entire spike response range is dedicated to 3 or 4 log units of intensity. Because the transient intensity/response functions are shifted by light adaptation (Fig. 17c) (HARTLINE and MACDONALD, 1947) no one transient response can be allotted to an absolute intensity without knowing the steady state plateau response. The steady state function encompasses 11 log units of intensity within the dynamic range of the cells spike output, consequently absolute intensity levels are measured far less accurately than the relative intensity levels.

A second possible filter function for lateral inhibition is as an edge detector. Spatial transients emphasise edges at the expense of gradual changes in object intensities (e.g. Fig. 16). Consequently uniformly illuminated objects tend to be picked out in relief (e.g. RATLIFF, 1965). This hypothesis is attractive but is difficult to assess in relation to the other functions proposed. The edges of small or low contrast objects produce modulations of the same order of magnitude and periodicity as smoother continuous intensity profiles and under these conditions the requirements for the better resolution of "edges" are the same as those for improved image reconstruction through deblurring. The importance of the edge detection concept must be established by showing that edges actually are detected, either by examining central neurons, or by investigating those aspects of visual patterns that are most significant in determining visually mediated behaviour. So far the data from both these areas of investigation is inconclusive, due in no small part to the technical and practical problems confronting workers in these areas (e.g. SNODDERLY, 1971; VON CAMPENHAUSEN, 1967).

In summary, although the case for lateral inhibition as an edge detector is incomplete, it must certainly assist in separating fluctuating signal components from the unchanging, and has, in this sense, a filter function.

3. Inhibition and Light Adaptation

Many eyes operate over a wide intensity range, often in excess of a millionfold, and to achieve this the sensitivity of the visual system is adjusted to suit the level of incident light. It is critical to make the appropriate adjustment, for if the sensitivity is set too low then fine detail cannot be resolved. If the sensitivity is too high then the system saturates with all inputs jammed open at the level of maximum response. To operate at an appropriate sensitivity, which strikes a balance between high sensitivity and the possibility of saturating, eyes use a number of light adaptation mechanisms to reduce sensitivity as intensity rises.

For *Limulus* lateral eye it has been suggested that self and lateral inhibition assist in light adaptation by suppressing the maintained level of eccentric cell discharge (e.g. Figs. 14 and 17) (HARTLINE and RATLIFF, 1972). More recent results suggest that such synaptic inhibition of the eccentric cell is but one of several light adaptation mechanisms so that its role as a sensitivity control cannot be assessed in isolation. To this end we will begin by examining the response of the ommatidium over a wide intensity range, to observe the effects of light adaptation, and then proceed to a discussion of the known mechanisms. The final discussion of light adaptation within a functional framework will demonstrate that eccentric cell function over a wide intensity range is still imperfectly understood, and the specific role of inhibition in light adaptation undefined.

a) Response Range of the Ommatidium

The recent works of KAPLAN and BARLOW show that the single ommatidia of the intact eye operate effectively over an intensity range of 11 log units. This working range equals that of the human visual system yet it is achieved without recourse to scotopic and photopic receptors and complex neural circuitry. The fundamental processes of sensitivity control need not be complicated.

The sensitivity of the dark-adapted eye follows a diurnal rhythm, mediated by afferent activity in the optic nerve (BARLOW et al., 1977), presumably transmitted via the efferent fibres that end among the pigment cells in the receptor layer (Sect. D.II). At night the eccentric cell is 1–2 log units more sensitive than during the day and the sensitivity change correlates with an increase in the amplitude of the ERG (BARLOW et al., 1977). Paradoxically the ever present spontaneous activity of the eccentric cell follows an opposite trend, being highest during the day (2 spikes s^{-1} and lowest at night, 0.3 spike s^{-1}). The origin of this dark discharge remains an enigma but similar rates of spontaneous large potential fluctuation (LPF) are recorded from the receptors. These could be generated either by stray light, thermal photopigment isomerisations or other sources of noise. Given that locust and mantid photoreceptors show very low rates of spontaneous dark bumps (less than 1 per 360 s – LILLYWHITE, 1977) the source of spontaneous activity in the *Limulus* lateral eye remains an open question.

At absolute dark-adapted threshold the eccentric cells and retinula cells might be responding to the absorption of single photons. A regenerative LPF in the receptor triggers an action potential in the eccentric cell (KAPLAN and BARLOW, 1976; BARLOW and KAPLAN, 1977) and LPFs and spikes are correlated with the statistical properties of single photon hits in the following ways.

1) For long dim stimuli the rate of LPF production in photoreceptors is proportional to intensity within the range 0.04–1.7 LPF/s (BARLOW and KAPLAN, 1977).

2) When weak brief (50 ms) flashes are delivered to the eye the probability of response increases slowly with intensity indicating that photon coincidence is not required (these observations are comparable with the classical "frequency seeing" curves used by HECHT and coworkers to show that human rods respond to single photons; HECHT et al., 1942).

3) The number of spikes elicited from an eccentric cell in response to brief flashes is linearly related to light intensity and the probability of getting either 0, 1, 2 or more spikes from a single flash follows the Poisson distribution (KAPLAN and BARLOW, 1976).

Given that LPFs correspond to events which are triggered by single photons, and that one LPF produces an eccentric cell spike, the evidence for photon counting by eccentric cells is good. However, the quantum efficiency of the single ommatidium is extraordinarily low for an eye which is, in other respects such as cone structure, specialised for vision at low intensities. Even after allowing for a measly 10% transmission through the cornea and a paltry 3% absorption by the photopigment the available photons outnumber LPFs and spikes by eight to one (KAPLAN and BARLOW, 1976). Such a low overall quantum efficiency of one in ten thousand has little difficulty in accommodating alternative hypotheses which require photon coincidences to trigger low efficiency random events in the receptors or eccentric cell. Clearly reciprocity tests for photon coincidence (SCHOLES, 1964; REICHARDT et al., 1968; LILLYWHITE, 1978 b) and better calibrations of actual photon catch are required if it is to be established that eccentric cell spikes correlate precisely with the statistical properties of incident photons. Nonetheless, we might, on comparative grounds, accept that this is the case.

For spike rates in excess of 2 s^{-1} the steady state eccentric cell discharge no longer increases in proportion to intensity. Light adaptation has begun and, as in retinal ganglion cells (H.B.BARLOW and LEVICK, 1969), the fall in sensitivity can be

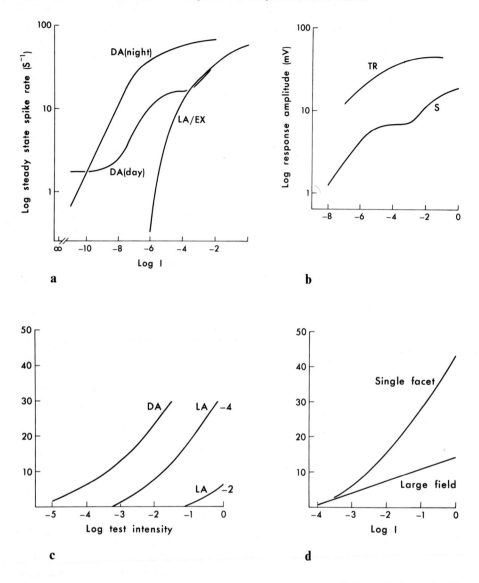

Fig. 17a–d. The intensity/response functions for the transient and steady state responses of *Limulus* eccentric cells and photoreceptors, under different conditions of adaptation or preparative technique. **a** Intensity dependence of the eccentric cell's steady state discharge rate under four different conditions: *DA (night)*, intact eye, dark adapted at night; *DA (day)* intact eye, dark adapted during the day; *LA/EX*, either intact, light adapted eye, or dark adapted, excised eye (after Barlow et al., 1977; Kaplan and Barlow, 1975). **b** Intensity dependence of transient *(TR)* and steady state *(S)* photoreceptor responses in the dark adapted intact eye – time of day not specified (after Barlow and Kaplan, 1977). **c** Transient responses of eccentric cell, excised eye, when dark adapted *(DA)* and light adapted with backgrounds of level indicated. Adapting light was extinguished immediately before testing (after Hartline and McDonald, 1947). **d** Eccentric cell, steady state response, excised eye, with (large field) and without (single facet) the effects of lateral inhibition (after Barlow and Lange, 1974)

expressed as an increase in the quantum/spike ratio. Note that the photoreceptor response is still composed of unitary shot events (DODGE et al., 1968), which suggests that they continue to register the arrival of every photon, thus maintaining a high signal to noise ratio. At intensities in excess of the steady state photon counting range, the eccentric cell response is dominated by its temporal high pass filter characteristics. The quantum/spike ratio, or gain, for high frequencies or peak transient is five times that for the low frequencies or steady state (Figs. 15 and 17).

The intensity/response function for the transient response to a step flash has received little attention since the first study by HARTLINE and McDONALD (1947) which indicates that, as in insect or vertebrate retinae (Sect. E.III.3), the response curves are displaced to higher intensities by light adaptation (Fig. 17). Two lines of evidence suggest that for the eccentric cell, the slopes of the response/log I curves increase with background intensity, as found in the analogous monopolar cells of the insect lamina (LAUGHLIN and HARDIE, 1978; Sect. E.III.3). First, the modulation transfer functions derived at different intensities (BIEDERMAN-THORSON and THORSON, 1971) show that the response to a fixed contrast modulation increases with background. Second, the increment threshold for eccentric cells is not proportional to background (WEBER-FECHNER law); the contrast required to produce a threshold response falling as intensity rises (KAPLAN and BARLOW, 1975).

The shape of the steady state intensity/response function is influenced by the diurnal rhythm. At night it is a monotonic function of reduced dynamic range, but during the day it shows a pronounced hump related to the production of LPFs in receptors (BARLOW et al., 1977; BARLOW and KAPLAN, 1977). However, in deriving this steady state intensity/response function, the ommatidium was maintained in a dark adapted state between test flashes. Under normal conditions, where mean intensity changes less abruptly, the kinks in this curve will be ironed out if they represent minimum energy thresholds for adaptation processes.

b) Light Adaptation Mechanisms

The sensitivity of a visual system can be matched to incident light intensity in two ways. First, photomechanical or photochemical processes regulate the proportion of incident photons contributing to the receptor signal. Second, gain control mechanisms adjust the amplitude and duration of the membrane response corresponding to a single photon hit. This gain control occurs either at the level of transduction or in subsequent neural processing. Both types of process act in *Limulus* lateral eye, but their precise contributions to sensitivity regulation have not been determined.

During light and dark adaptation there are extensive changes in ommatidial structure (Fig. 11) which must regulate both the photon catch and the angular acceptance properties of the rhabdom. Illumination of the dark adapted eye causes pigment to move radially at the base of the corneal lens and the distance between corneal lens and rhabdom to increase. Thus the exit aperture of the cone shrinks, from a structure 70 μm wide and 10 μm deep, to a long tube 5–10 μm wide and 70 μm long. This must both reduce photon flux, and enhance the directional sensitivity of the ommatidium (BEHRENS, 1974). Pigment also moves into the spaces between the rhabdom spokes, the rhabdom diameter decreases and the rhabdomeres decrease in width (BEHRENS, 1974; MILLER and CAWTHON, 1974; BEHRENS and KREBS, 1976). Again these changes will attenuate the photon flux within the rhabdomeres and reduce the effective capture area of the photoreceptors. Rhabdomere shrinkage is accompanied by ultrastructural changes, suggestive of a cycle of photoreceptor membrane assembly and disassembly, similar to that found in spiders (CHAMBERLAIN and BARLOW, 1977; BLEST, 1978; BLEST and DAY, 1978). Although all these changes are directly driven by light, partial light adaptation occurs during the day when the eye is maintained in total darkness (BEHRENS, 1974), and this effect can be reversed by stimulation of the efferent nerves within the optic tract. Consequently these photomechanical responses may be the effectors for the efferent control of sensitivity (BARLOW et al., 1977).

Gain changes occur mainly within the photoreceptors, at the level of transduction. When dark adapted, the unitary response is an LPF of 80 mV amplitude and at least 500 ms duration (BARLOW and KAPLAN, 1977). Shot noise analysis (Sect. E.II.5) of the light adapted response suggest that it is composed of elementary events of 10 µV amplitude and 100 ms duration (DODGE et al., 1968). Given that any transducer noise will cause shot noise analyses to overestimate the voltage response (LAUGHLIN, 1976a; LILLYWHITE and LAUGHLIN, 1979; Sect. E.II.5) the product of unitary response amplitude and duration varies over a 5 log unit range. Providing that in both cases the unitary event represents single photon absorptions, this corresponds to a sensitivity change of the same order of magnitude. The processes controlling the production of LPFs are unknown but when considering unitary events of less than 20 mV (SPFs) the lateral eye photoreceptors are probably similar to those of the ventral eye, in which the decrease in response amplitude during light adaptation is associated with changes in intracellular calcium ion concentration (FEIN and CHARLTON, 1977), as discussed in barnacle photoreceptors (Sect. B.V).

The steady state discharge rate of the eccentric cell is approximately linearly related to steady state mean receptor potential over most of the dynamic range (FUORTES, 1958; BARLOW and KAPLAN, 1977). Thus the receptor sensitivity, itself a function of the voltage gain of the transducer and the photon capture efficiency, dominates the sensitivity of the eccentric cell. This is to be expected because, if the receptors saturate or work at an inappropriately low sensitivity, then image detail is lost (by clipping or by masking by intrinsic noise). This lost image detail cannot be restored by subsequent processing so that in eyes, as in many other sensors, it pays to place one's sensitivity controls on the front end. It follows that one role of lateral and self inhibition in light adaptation is to depress the (receptor cell voltage/eccentric cell spike) ratio to prevent the background steady state signal saturating the eccentric cell response.

c) A Functional Interpretation of Light Adaptation

Light and dark adaptation is accomplished within the *Limulus* ommatidium by several interlocking processes. Several of these mechanisms are similar to processes seen in other compound eyes and all can be interpreted in a functional framework, as devices to capture the highest quality neural image, and present it to higher order neurons in the most reliable and concisely coded form.

The major determinant of sensitivity is the transducer's voltage gain, that is the amplitude of the receptor potential corresponding to the absorption of one additional photon. In the dark adapted ommatidium, gain is certainly high because the smallest response is an LPF of 80 mV amplitude. At higher intensities light adaptation reduces transducer gain to prevent the receptor saturating. A high voltage gain at low intensities would certainly be advantageous. If each LPF corresponded to the absorption of a single photon then the *Limulus* ommatidium would be an accurate photon counter, producing a very large unit pulse for each photon received and so attaining the upper limit of signal to noise ratio. Unfortunately the pleasing prospect of such an excellent performance is still marred by apparent and appalling wastage of photons between incidence on the cornea, and the triggering of an LPF. In the locust compound eye, where it is actually established that single bumps register the arrival of single photons with high efficiency, these events are smaller in amplitude. These photon counts might be rendered less efficient by being lost in noise at a higher level. At least, *Limulus* insures against this loss, by generating the 80 mV LPF.

Just as transducer voltage gain is matched to the level of incident illumination, so is the optical performance of the ommatidium. At lowest intensities, when photons are scarcest, the entrance aperture of the ommatidium is opened up to increase the quantum catch from extended sources. A similar sacrifice of angular sensitivity for photon catch is characteristic of many compound eyes (WALCOTT, 1975). The improved quantum catch actually increases angular resolution at low intensities by reducing the level of photon noise (LAUGHLIN, 1975a) and the strategy of opening up the ommatidial aperture at low intensities is most effective when it is combined with the summation of inputs from many ommatidia in a higher level "neural pool" (SNYDER, 1977; 1979). This pooling strategy probably benefits greatly from the production of large quantum bumps (Sect. E.II.4.a). Finally, in common with crabs (LEGGETT, 1977) and mantids (ROSSELL, 1979) the full opening of the acceptance angle is prevented during daytime (STAVENGA, 1979). It has been suggested (LEGGETT, 1977) that such a diurnal rhythm is advantageous because the slow retinomotor mechanisms for full opening of the acceptance angle take minutes to complete their operations. Consequently an animal which was fully dark-adapted during the day, while burrowing for example, would operate at less than optimum acuity for several minutes after re-emergence into the light.

It is difficult to assign self and lateral inhibition definite roles in light adaptation. Although inhibition undoubtedly increases the intensity range over which the eccentric cell operates, by suppressing the response to sustained illumination (Fig. 17d), the contributions of neural factors have not been separated from sensitivity changes in the receptor (cf. insect lamina, Sect. E.III.3). One can only say that the transients generated by inhibition increase the efficiency of coding, both by reducing redundancy and by lessening the risk of prolonged saturation and so allowing the eccentric cell to retain a high sensitivity to small fluctuations.

Of obvious functional significance is the noise suppression that occurs in the inhibitory network. Noise can be extremely damaging in situations where one signal subtracts from another, because in this same situation the uncorrelated noise fluctuations add. For self-inhibition, the presence of noise fluctuations in the eccentric cell response is less critical, because the noise is fed back onto itself and must be highly correlated, and so subtracts just like the signal. The uncorrelated photon and synaptic noise injected from adjacent ommatidia, via lateral inhibition, can be more disruptive, and this noise is suppressed in three ways. First, and most importantly, lateral inhibition is produced by summing together small contributions from many surrounding ommatidia within a pathway with a long time constant. Consequently the inhibitor has a better signal to noise ratio than the response of any one ommatidium, principally because many more photons contribute to its generation. Second, when photon noise is most pronounced, at low intensities, the strength of lateral inhibition between single ommatidia is reduced because of its dependence upon the spike rate in the inhibited cell (Fig. 14). It would be interesting to see if this decrease in contribution by a single ommatidium was compensated for by an increase in the size of the inhibitory surround and a further fall in photon noise level. Third, the frequency responses of lateral and self-inhibition are adjusted to block noise (SHAPLEY, 1971). Lateral inhibition has the characteristics of a low pass filter while self-inhibition is a high pass filter (Fig. 15). Consequently self-inhibition protects the spike encoder from low frequency noise in the lateral inhibitory network. Although rarely discussed, these self same noise suppressing characteristics are found in other lateral inhibitory networks. It is common for a large surround, driven by many receptors to inhibit a smaller centre (e.g. retinal ganglion cells, rev. RODIECK, 1973). As predicted by SHAPLEY (1971) selective noise filtering has been observed in the vertebrate retina (BAYLOR and FETTIPLACE, 1977). Finally the inhibitory surrounds of some retinal ganglion cells are inactivated when dark adapted (RODIECK, 1973).

4. Function of Lateral Inhibition

Lateral inhibition's role has been assessed with respect to three classes of function, image restoration, feature extraction and light adaptation. For each case the data is far from complete but the present situation can be summarised as follows. For image restoration the measured lateral interactions are too weak to restore much of the contrast blurred out by the optics (KIRSCHFELD and REICHARDT, 1964). For feature extraction, the role of *Limulus*'s lateral inhibitory network as an edge detector has not really been investigated. The *a priori* argument is weak and edge detection can only be established by finding higher order neurons which respond selectively to edges only because there is lateral inhibition. For light adaptation, lateral inhibition suppresses the background signal in the eccentric cell but plays a minor role in adjusting the sensitivity of the eye over the observed intensity range of 10^{11}. This intensity range is accommodated by the photoreceptors and their accessory optical structures. Given this incomplete understanding we can suggest the following hypothesis to guide further investigations. Inhibition's major function is as a fine sensitivity control, acting in series with the coarser controls in photoreceptors. It converts the eccentric cell into a high pass filter and so reduces the level of redundancy within the eccentric cell discharge (H.B.BARLOW, 1961). The reduced discharge rate leaves much of the eccentric cells response range free for signalling intensity increments, as suggested for retinal ganglion cells by BARLOW and LEVICK (1976). Finally, the existence of a negative feed-back reduces the length of time for which the eccentric cell will be saturated by a sudden large intensity increment.

Thus the eccentric cell can monitor intensity fluctuations with higher sensitivity because the risk of prolonged saturation is reduced. These same spatial and temporal
high pass filter characteristics are seen in insect compound eyes, and in the peripheral retina of vertebrates. We will expand upon these functions of lateral and self-
inhibition for optimal coding in connection with a system for which there is a more
comprehensive study of the intensity/response functions, the insect lamina (Sect.
E.III.5). Notwithstanding these uncertainties as to lateral inhibition's precise function in *Limulus*, the principle of lateral inhibition has found widespread application
in other sensory systems, and this is worthy of further discussion.

VI. The Principle of Lateral Inhibition

The discovery of lateral inhibition in *Limulus* was a major turning point in sensory physiology because it realised, in terms of neurons, a set of retinal interactions
first deduced by ERNST MACH from his observations of spatial transients in human
visual perception (the MACH bands). The relationships between MACH's findings
and theories, more recent psychophysical investigations and models, and the uses
of contour enhancement in art, are discussed in RATLIFF's scholarly book, Mach
Bands (1965). Suffice it to say here that MACH clearly foresaw the potential importance of lateral inhibition, writing that

> since every (retinal) point perceives itself, so to speak, as above or below the average of its neigh-
> bours, there results a characteristic type of perception. Whatever is near the mean of the surround be-
> comes effaced. Whatever is above or below is brought into disproportionate prominence. One could
> say that the retina schematises and caricatures. The teleological significance of this process is clear in
> itself. It is an analogue of abstraction and the formation of concepts (MACH, 1868, translated in RATLIFF
> and HARTLINE, 1974, p. 254).

MACH also suggested that the deblurring effects of lateral inhibition could be
analysed using spatial sinusoids and FOURIER analysis. Thus *Limulus* provides the
potent concept of a simple neural network forming an effective filter, capable of
several functions, and the principles of lateral inhibition have found widespread
application among sensory systems.

For example, lateral inhibition is common to many visual systems. In the insect
retina the first order monopolar neurons are subjected to both lateral and self-inhibition (Sect. E.III.4) and this is used to suppress the background signal and enhance changes about the mean intensity level, much as MACH envisaged (LAUGH-
LIN and HARDIE, 1978). In the vertebrate retina the first order bipolar cells are subject to lateral inhibition via horizontal cells (WERBLIN, 1972), and spatially directed
inhibition is also seen in the receptive fields of retinal ganglion cells and cells of the
lateral geniculate and visual cortex (e.g. HUBEL and WIESEL, 1962). Unidirectional
lateral inhibition also provides a basis for movement sensitivity (BARLOW and
LEVICK, 1965), and inhibition between interneurons with differing spectral sensitivities forms the basis of colour opponency (ABRAMOV, 1972; MENZEL, 1979).
The concept of lateral inhibition has also been applied to the auditory system,
where it is proposed that it aids in localising points of maximum displacement in
the cochlea and so enhances pitch discrimination. Similarly, lateral inhibition helps
localise pressure points on the skin (VON BÉKÉSY, 1966). The abdominal stretch re-

ceptors of crayfish exhibit both lateral and self-inhibition and this could assist in localising regions of abdominal flexion that are greater or lesser than average (LIESTØL et al., 1976). The filter properties of lateral inhibitory networks have been the subject of many theoretical models but the outputs of such theoretical systems often appear to be far more complicated than the inputs they are given; the physiologist sees little advance in this area. Through all of the physiological studies runs the most important general principle, that directed neural interactions form the basis of much of brain function. It is for a concrete realisation of this principle and for the development of many of the methods used to study interactions that we owe so much to HARTLINE's Rockefeller group and to *Limulus* lateral eye.

E. The Compound Eyes of Insects and Crustacea

I. Introduction

The compound eyes and optic lobes of the more agile arthropods are sophisticated visual systems, capable of colour vision, perception of plane polarised light, depth perception, pattern recognition and the optomotor, oculomotor and tracking reflexes required for resolving moving objects. When compared with the vertebrate visual systems, the deficiencies of compound eyes are in quality and versatility, rather than competence. A smaller eye must have poorer resolving power (KIRSCHFELD, 1976; SNYDER, 1979) while a smaller brain is restricted in the breadth of its repertoire, but not necessarily in the sophistication of some of its acts (e.g. navigation by bees, VON FRISCH, 1967). Despite their complexities, compound eyes exhibit many of the principles seen in the simpler ocelli and the compound eye of *Limulus*. These principles, relating to cellular adaptation and adaptability, and the tailoring of excitability and connectivity to function, ought to be apparent in all visual systems, yet they are more clearly expressed in compound eyes by virtue of a clearly delineated structure.

Compound eyes are obviously columnar in organisation. The well defined mosaic of receptor units, the ommatidia, is replicated as a matrix of neural subunits, or cartridges, in each of the neuropiles of the optic lobe (STRAUSFELD, 1976b; this Vol. Chap. I). In any one neuropile there is a single cartridge for each ommatidium, which is similar in structure to its neighbours. The precise projection of axons between neuropiles ensures that adjacent cartridges receive inputs that are ultimately derived from receptors looking at adjacent points in space. A retinotopic pattern of projection is common to many visual systems (e.g. frog tectum, JACOBSON, 1970; mammalian cortex, HUBEL and WIESEL, 1977) and suggests that even at higher levels the most frequent neural interactions concern points that are spatially contiguous.

The redundancy within these mosaics of ommatidia and cartridges facilitates the investigation of cellular structure and function in the compound eye. The same types of cell are encountered repeatedly in the one section or electrode track, and the patterns of activity generated in the neuropile in response to an object can be predicted from the responses of cell types, and the interactions between cartridges. An attempt to reconstruct this *neural image* of an object is only worthwhile when one is confidently working with identified neurons in an established mosaic.

The pursuit of the neural image through the retina and the lamina is taken as the theme for this review. The approach emphasises that vision involves the transmutation of *patterns* of energy and activity, from intensity on the retina, through signals in successive neuropiles, to a form related to the patterns of motor activity in muscles. Compound eyes can provide concrete examples of pattern generation and transformation in sophisticated visual systems and emphasise some of the difficulties and uncertainties inherent to their analysis. Thus the retina is considered as an exemplary neural image whose quality can be measured and related to both the input of the visual system, light, and its output, behaviour. At present we can take the lamina as an example of a neural image transformed by cellular interactions, in a situation where the transformed image can again be related to function. The medulla and lobula complexes are not considered. They are examples of an all too common problem, a neural image obscured by complexity and technical difficulties. There are almost 50 neurons making connections in each medulla cartridge (CAMPOS-ORTEGA and STRAUSFELD, 1972) yet only a handful have been both recorded from and identified (DEVOE and OCKLEFORD, 1976). There is doubtless scope in the medulla for complex interactions and perhaps several neural images in parallel. In the output fibres from the optic lobes we can again detect the vaguest glimmerings of neural image. Some of the largest neurons have been characterised both physiologically and anatomically. The results suggest that the neural images displayed among these outputs are mapped onto fresh coordinates. Exact retinotopic projections have been replaced by generalisations, in space and time, such as movement over retinal areas or novelty, and these patterns are displayed in a form that is relevant to the choice and organisation of different behavioural responses.

Before proceeding, it must be emphasised that the cellular approach to a neural image precludes many of the basics of compound eye structure and function, and in particular their structural and functional diversity and the precision and versatility of behavioural performance. Readers are referred to the reviews by HORRIDGE (1978a), GOLDSMITH and BERNARD (1973), REICHARDT (1970), REICHARDT and POGGIO (1976), POGGIO and REICHARDT (1976), LAND (1977) and to other chapters of this handbook.

II. The Photoreceptor Matrix – an Exemplary Neural Image

1. Assessing the Neural Image

The mosaic of receptor potentials within the retina is a vital neural image for it is the substrate for all subsequent visual processes. If we are to grasp the principles by which the visual system operates, it is essential that we understand these neural image qualities. Yet, despite 25 years of intracellular recording from photoreceptors, we lack a comprehensive assessment and measurement of the receptors' neural image. Indeed there is only one account of a receptor mosaic that is complete enough to predict the static pattern of receptor potentials set up on the retina by a stationary object (Rossel, 1979). More analyses of neural image quality within the receptor mosaic should be of as great an importance to explaining vision as the analogous study of optical image quality (Westheimer, 1972a, b). This section will show that the compound eye is extremely suitable material for a fundamental analysis of wider applicability, because these eyes present a unique opportunity not yet found in the vertebrates, through the conjunction of three factors. Intracellular recordings can be made from photoreceptors in a virtually intact retina (Wilson, 1975) and the optical axes of photoreceptors can be mapped for the entire retina (Franceschini, 1975; Beersma et al., 1975; Sherk, 1977, 1978b; Horridge, 1978b). Finally the limitations imposed by the measured neural image quality can be assessed from quantitative measures of visual behaviour (e.g. reviews by Reichardt, 1970; Kirschfeld, 1972; Poggio and Reichardt, 1976; Land, 1977).

The consideration of neural image quality presents fresh perspectives of the adaptation of cellular structure to function in the visual system. Just as many lens systems and photoreceptor mosaics seem engineered to take into account the fundamental optical constraints of aberrations, diffraction and limited quantum catch (Westheimer, 1972a, b; Kirschfeld, 1976; Snyder, 1979), so the matrix of photoreceptors should be designed within the additional constraints imposed by transduction, cellular communication, metabolism and differentiation. To assess design we must describe the limitations – optical, biophysical, biochemical, and ontogenetic – and relate these to image quality.

Unfortunately there is still no established measure of neural image quality and it is debatable that a simple metric measure will apply to a diverse spectrum of compound eyes (e.g. Snyder et al., 1977a; cf. Horridge, 1978b). To assess receptor performance I have used the notion of measurement within a receptor mosaic, as constrained by the total range of signal intensities it can encompass; the size of signals, the rate at which signals can change, and the level of noise (Sect. D.VI.1.a). Measurement is a convenient yardstick, partly because it is related to information (e.g. Snyder et al., 1977b), partly because it is flexible (one can set out to measure different signals) and partly because measurement represents a real limitation to visual function. When a measurement expert, a statistician, cannot detect a pattern within a neural image it is lost to the animal. No amount of "inhibitory sharpening" or "neural template fitting" will restore the lost information. The concept of measurement by photoreceptors has one last and very important advantage. It is directly related to behavioural thresholds for these are often determinations of the entire visual system's overall measuring ability (and the ability to express the measurement behaviourally). As discussed in the last section (E.II.10), correlations with behaviour allow us to test directly what receptors can do for animals. The discussion of the neural image is restricted to moving black and white patterns. The representation of polarisation and colour in parallel images, and their relationship to behaviour are reviewed by Waterman (this Vol.) and Menzel (1979). We will begin by presenting the bones of structure to show that the retina is structurally an integrated organ of several cell types.

2. Structure of the Retina

In most compound eyes the photoreceptors (retinula cells) and their accessory cells are arranged in structural units, the ommatidia. These are replicated across local eye regions to form morphological units with a coarser mosaic than the individual photoreceptors. Each ommatidium usually consists of an area of cornea overlying a cone, a group of photoreceptors and a sheath of pigment cells (Fig. 18). The cone can be formed from cornea, as in firefly and several beetle eyes (HORRIDGE, 1975a), be an extracellular space filled with a gelatinous matrix, as in flies (BOSCHEK, 1971) or, a crystalline structure, formed within the cytoplasm of Semper cells. The cornea, cone, pigment cells and trachea of the compound eye, together with the basement membrane are accessory structures devoted to one end, the adequate function of the photoreceptors. Their accessory functions can be categorised into five general areas – light gathering, receptor maintenance and retinal homeostasis, electrical insulation, structural integrity and developmental determination. The cornea, cone and pigment cells are often specialised to collect and direct light to the photoreceptors, so that these sensory structures have both angular sensitivity, and receive sufficient light to respond. The homeostatic function is all too little explored but divides into at least two components; the maintenance of a satisfactory ionic milieu around the photoreceptors, and the provision of oxygen and metabolites to the receptors to fuel transduction. The energetic requirements of photoreceptors are important because transduction involves considerable amplification of the energy from a single photon. For example, in fly, the light induced oxygen consumption of the retina is 8.9 ml/g/h (HAMDORF and KASCHEF, 1964) and this compares with a consumption by active flight muscle of 480 ml/g/h (SAKTOR, 1965). Tracheoles and pigment cells must play a major role in satisfying photoreceptor energy requirements. The maintenance of an ionic balance around the photoreceptors, in the face of a sustained photocurrent is dealt with in Sect. E.II.3.d (see also SHAW, 1977, 1978a). Little is known of the roles of pigment cells and cone cells in maintaining the structural integrity of the retina and still less of the cellular interactions underlying the differentiation of the retina.

The functional attributes of receptor structure are well understood. In the retina, each photoreceptor (retinula cell) bears a rhabdomere, a long column of densely packed microvilli. Microspectrophotometry shows that rhabdomeres contain the visual pigments, which are generally rhodopsins (HAMDORF, 1979), but in fly there are additional sensitising pigments, probably carotenoids, which are capable of transferring energy to rhodopsin (KIRSCHFELD et al., 1977, 1978). In many compound eyes the rhabdomeres of receptors combine to form a fused rhabdom. In apposition eyes the rhabdom is generally a long cylinder, or prism, running up the centre of the ommatidium for much of its length (Fig. 18). With a typical diameter of 2–5 μm, and a refractive index higher than the surrounding cytoplasm (as a consequence of the high lipid and protein concentration within the rhabdomeres), the rhabdom acts as a waveguide. Thus all contributing receptors have the same field of view (SNYDER, 1979). In flies, the individual rhabdomeres are separated so that each is a light guide with its own optical axis. This open rhabdom structure allows for improved photon capture through neural superposition (Sect. III.1.b). The complex shapes of rhabdoms in many superposition eyes still defy explanation (HORRIDGE, 1975b).

In the vicinity of the rhabdomeres, the cytoplasm of the receptors is rich in organelles. There are often small pigment granules within the photoreceptor that can be moved close to the rhabdom to regulate the light flux within it. There are also many mitochondria, presumably supplying energy for transduction and ionic regulation, and a prolific maze of rough ER and multivesicular bodies involved in the continuous synthesis and degradation of photoreceptive membrane (e.g. WHITE and LORD, 1975; EGUCHI and WATERMAN, 1976).

At the base of the retina the rhabdom terminates and the retinula cell forms an axon which projects through the basement membrane to the photoreceptor's synapses, either in the lamina or in the second optic neuropile, the medulla (Sect. E.III). It is worth observing that no synapses have been seen in the retina although the photoreceptors within one ommatidium can be electrically coupled (Sect. E.II.8.a). Thus the substrate for neural processing, the current generated at the photoreceptive membrane, is left uncorrupted at its source.

3. Relationships Between Intensity and Response

An unequivocal relationship between intensity and response amplitude lies at the heart of transduction, and the representation of the retina's neural image. Intracellular recordings show that, at low intensities, retinula cells produce discrete quantum bumps (Fig. 18). At intermediate light levels the bumps fuse to produce a sustained depolarisation and at still higher intensities the response amplitude is cut back by light adaptation (Fig. 18). Each of these phases will be discussed: the intensity dependence of bumps, the non-linear summation of bumps to generate an intensity/response function, the modification of intensity/response functions by light adaptation and the biophysical basis for non-linearity and adaptation. The general presentation is applicable to the majority of known retinula cells but this does not mean that all rhabdomeric photoreceptors are identical. For example, large slow and regenerative waves, LPFs, have only been found in *Limulus* (Sect. D. VII) while in drone bee retina the receptors produce fast regenerative action potentials that are sensitive to tetrodotoxin (BAUMANN, 1968). The photoreceptor membrane can be tuned up to suit particular functional needs (e.g., barnacle photoreceptors, Sect. B) and the true extent of biophysical diversity among retinula cells is simply not known, but most variations are probably superimposed upon the mechanisms outlined below.

a) Responses to Single Photons – Bumps

Two careful studies of the statistical dependence of bump occurrences on light intensity show that, in locust at least, each bump is produced by the absorption of one photon (SCHOLES, 1964, 1965; LILLYWHITE, 1977). The evidence is as follows. The rate of bump production is proportional to intensity and, as would be expected of photon triggered events, bumps are distributed according to the Poisson statistics (SCHOLES, 1964, 1965; LILLYWHITE, 1977). A bump does not require the coincidence of two or more photons because the number of bumps produced by a flash

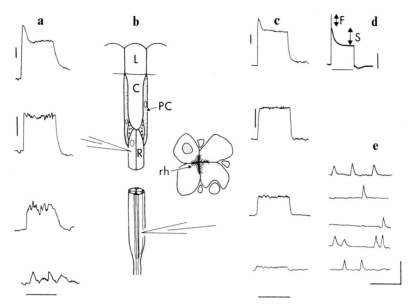

Fig. 18a–e. Responses of photoreceptors (retinula cells) in insect compound eyes. **a** Intracellular recordings from a UV sensitive cell in the retina of the dragonfly *Hemicordulia*, showing responses to
500 ms flashes of increasing intensity (lowest intensity at bottom). **b** Simplified structure of an ommatidium in *Hemicordulia*'s ventral eye region, showing the position of the photoreceptors *(R)* beneath
a dioptric apparatus consisting of a corneal lens *(L)*, a crystalline cone *(C)*, and a sheath of opaque
pigment cells *(P)*. A cross section through the bundle of photoreceptors shows four of them contributing photoreceptive microvilli to the fused rhabdom, which in this ommatidium is 2 µm across and over
700 µm long. **c** Responses from a green sensitive cell in the same retina, to 500 ms flashes. Note that
its responses show less noise than the UV cell in **a**. **d** Fast *(F)* and slow *(S)* phases of light adaptation
during the response of fly retinula cell to an initially saturating flash, of 60 s duration. **e** Quantum
bumps, the proven responses of single photons, by locust retinula cells (LILLYWHITE, 1977). Calibration
bars: **a** and **c** = 10 mV; **d** = 20 mV; **e** = 5 mV, 0.5 s. **a** and **c** from LAUGHLIN (1976a); **b** after LAUGHLIN
and MCGINNESS (1978); **d** from LAUGHLIN and HARDIE (1978); **e** LILLYWHITE and LAUGHLIN (unpublished data)

depends only upon its total energy, and not upon the time over which that energy
is delivered (SCHOLES, 1964). The probability of a bump being produced, by a short
flash, depends upon intensity in the manner that is symptomatic of an event triggered by one photon (SCHOLES, 1964; LILLYWHITE, 1977). Finally, in a rigorous
analysis, where the careful exclusion of stray light had reduced the rate of production of bumps in "total" darkness to an unprecedented low of 12 h^{-1}, there was
no tendency for bumps to cluster together during prolonged dim illumination
(LILLYWHITE, 1977). Thus bumps are produced singly, and share no common ante-
cedent event. With 60% of the photons incident on the cornea generating a bump,
LILLYWHITE concluded that one effective photon produces just one bump, with a
very high efficiency; a finding that is important for understanding both transduction and intensity coding at low intensities. Similar bumps have been recorded
from the photoreceptors of several insect apposition eyes (Table 2) and the dark
bump rate is less than 1 min^{-1} in the fly *Lucilia*, and 10 h^{-1} in the mantid (LILLY-
WHITE, 1977; ROSSEL, 1979). For these species too, bumps are probably single

photon signals. Reports of high dark bump rates, e.g. $8\ s^{-1}$ in *Drosophila* (Wu and Pak, 1975), must now be treated with caution. It is difficult to screen out stray light, and bumps can be produced 20 min after illumination ceases as a part of the positive afterpotential (Horridge and Tsukahara, 1978).

b) The Dark-Adapted Intensity/Response Function

For many species the photoreceptor intensity/response functions have only been measured in the dark-adapted state. A receptor is maintained in darkness and the intensity/response function constructed from the amplitudes of responses to brief, and widely separated flashes of different intensity. Although such stimuli are rarely encountered outside of the laboratory an understanding of the dark-adapted intensity/response function is important, because it clearly demonstrates the non-linear summation of bumps to produce a larger response; i.e. the voltage response to ten photons is considerably less than ten times the response to one (Fig. 19 c). Non-linear summation is a vital part of the overall strategy for light adaptation and the dark-adapted intensity/response functions indicate that it originates from two different properties of the transducer, one of which is an unavoidable constraint.

The first and principal cause of non-linear summation is the self-shunting of membrane conductance channels. Imagine a simple transducer where a single photon activates a fixed number of membrane conductances to produce a bump. The number of active conductances rises in proportion to intensity, and the currents from these channels sum, producing a voltage response across the passive resistance of the cell. However, the total current produced does not vary linearly with the number of conductances activated. The ratio of current to conductance falls, as the total conductance increases because the receptor potential reduces the EMF across the membrane. In other words, the photocurrent induces a voltage across the cell's load resistance which shunts out its own EMF, hence the term self-shunting. As reviewed by Lipetz (1971), self-shunting is a property of all membrane responses generated by conductance channels acting in parallel. It is, therefore, a fundamental and unavoidable constraint to the function of many excitable cells. Self-shunting has been described for the generation of motor end-plate potentials at the postsynaptic membrane of the neuromuscular synapse (Martin, 1955), in Pacinian corpuscles (Loewenstein, 1958) and in the horizontal cells of the vertebrate retina (Naka and Rushton, 1966). In our case of the hypothetical photoreceptor, where the number of light activated channels is proportional to intensity, self-shunting generates a hyperbolic intensity/response function

$$V/V_{max} = R \cdot I/(R \cdot I + 1), \tag{E.1}$$

where V is the receptor potential produced by intensity I, V_{max} the saturated response amplitude – assumed equal to the reversal potential of the response, and R, the range sensitivity, is a constant equalling the reciprocal of the intensity required to produce a response of half maximal. This non-linear hyperbolic intensity/response function is plotted in Figs. 2 and 19 c. It has a similar shape to measured intensity/response functions, but for many receptors the slope of the real function is depressed (e.g. Fig. 19 c). This additional flattening of the curve is a second form of non-linear summation, superimposed upon self-shunting.

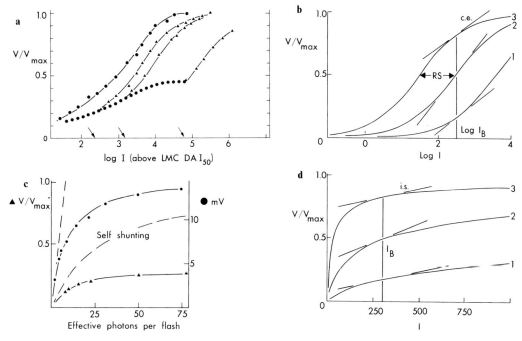

Fig. 19 a–d. Photoreceptor intensity/response functions and the dependence of increment sensitivity, dV/dI, on non-linear summation, range sensitivity and background intensity. **a** Changes in range sensitivity of fly photoreceptor during light adaptation to the backgrounds indicated by *arrows*. (-●-)=dark-adapted transient responses to increments, (-▲ -)=light-adapted transient responses, (● ● ● ●)=steady state response to backgrounds. LMC DA $I_{50}=1.3 \times 10^8$ axial quanta·cm^{-2}·s^{-1} at peak wavelength 484 nm (see Fig. 30). Data from *Calliphora:* LAUGHLIN and HARDIE (1978). **b** Theoretical $V/\log I$ curves, according to Eq. (E.2), with an exponent, $n=0.66$ and three values of range sensitivity, a log unit apart. *c.e.* = contrast efficiency, dV/d (log I). RS=range shift. **c** Non-linear summation of responses illustrated by linear plots of a locust photoreceptor's intensity/response function. Normalised and absolute voltage scales are used. The empirical curves fall far short of those predicted from self-shunting, by using mean bump amplitude to solve Eq. (E.1) for the case of $I=1$ effective photon. Data from LILLYWHITE and LAUGHLIN (1978). **d** Linear plots of the theoretical curves given above, in **b**, demonstrate that for every background intensity, I_B, there is a single value of range sensitivity which gives maximum increment sensitivity about the background *(curve 2)*, and in **b** this curve has the maximum contrast efficiency at log I_B. *i.s.* = increment sensitivity

This second non-linearity could result from a number of factors, including a reduction, with rising intensity, in the number of photons that open conductances. This possibility is unlikely. Shot noise analysis suggests that the number of effective photons rises linearly with intensity over a wide intensity range (DODGE et al., 1968; WU and PAK, 1978) and the reduction is seen when less than ten photons are involved (Fig. 19 c). The additional reduction in response must result from absorbed photons becoming less effective at generating a voltage, either because the ratio of channels to photons, the conductance gain, declines or because antagonistic hyperpolarising conductances are activated. The precise sources of this second source of non-linear summation have not yet been identified, so the phenomenon will be given the general title of "declining photon effectiveness." It is a remarkable observation that this second non-linearity can be approximated by a minor adjustment to the hyperbolic self-shunting formula so that

$$V/V_{max} = (R \cdot I)^n / [(R \cdot I)^n + 1]$$ (E.2)

The exponent, n, is empirical and adopts a range of values among different photoreceptors. It can also vary in the same photoreceptor, with stimulus conditions, but n must be less than one to flatten the curve. For example, $n = 1.0$ in crayfish (Glantz, 1972) and waterbug (Ioannides and Walcott, 1971), is 0.6 in dragonfly [Laughlin, unpublished observation correcting an earlier erroneous estimate of $n = 1.0$ (Laughlin, 1975a)]. In *Drosophila* $n = 0.6$ (Wu and Pak, 1978) and in the hoverfly *Eristalis* $n = 0.4$ for cells R 1–6, and 0.6 for an unidentified cell that is sensitive to longer wavelengths and is believed to be R 8 (Tsukahara and Horridge, 1977b). Moreover, when *Eristalis* R 1–6 are stimulated at long wavelengths, the slope of the $V/\log I$ curve increases and the evidence suggests that there is a depolarising synaptic input from the long wavelength receptor. A similar dependence of $V/\log I$ curve slope on wavelength is seen in some *Calliphora* R 1–6 cells but experiments designed to test for synaptic inputs from other cells, and for local adaptation effects along the length of the rhabdomere, fail to produce a positive result (Hardie, 1978). Vertebrate rods and cones have $V/\log I$ curves of the same form and the slope of the initial transient response is depressed by prolonging the stimulus from 100 ms to 2 s (Normann and Werblin, 1974). There are no reports of this effect in retinula cells.

The drastic total effect of non-linear summation is best illustrated by a linear plot of response versus intensity (Fig. 19c). This data from the locust (Lillywhite and Laughlin, 1979) shows two additional and important properties of non-linear summation. The decline in photon effectiveness begins at intensities where fewer than five photons are absorbed in 4 ms, and the decline is seen in the peak response to extremely brief flashes. Declining photon effectiveness occurs in the most rapid responses to the briefest stimuli. Non-linear summation is not the only factor determining a photoreceptor's response amplitude. At higher intensities light adaptation mechanisms further reduce the size of response.

c) Light-Adapted Intensity/Response Functions

When a photoreceptor is illuminated with a sustained light of sufficient intensity, the receptor potential decays in amplitude, from an initial peak, the transient response, to a stable steady state level (Fig. 18). This adaptation in response results from a reduction in the receptor's sensitivity to light incident upon the cornea, so that the sustained background light has modified the receptor's intensity/response function. The new function, determining the amplitudes of the cell's responses to sudden departures in intensity from the background level, can be derived experimentally by measuring the transient response amplitudes produced by test lights that are superimposed upon the background. All light-adapted intensity/response functions are best presented in absolute terms (Fig. 19a), as plots of the total response amplitude (i.e. measured as deflection from dark resting potential) against total intensity (i.e. the sum of test and adapting lights). Plots of increments (e.g. the incremental response to a test light versus test light intensity) are often used in the vertebrate literature, but can be misleading. Increment curves make a distinction, between photons in the background and test light, that the transducer must find impossible. Increment plots also fail to present responses within the context of a cell's limited dynamic range, yet this fixed response interval is one of the most important constraints. Receptors must either light adapt or reach the limits of their response amplitude and saturate.

Typical dark and light adapted intensity/response functions are correctly plotted (as $V/\log I$ curves) in Fig. 19 a. The steady state response runs along a curve of flattened slope while the transient responses follow a steep function which, on semi-logarithmic coordinates, retains the same sigmoidal shape as the dark adapted transient response curve. The depression in sensitivity, induced by a background, propels the transient curve towards higher intensities. The position of the transient curve, at any one background, defines the range of intensities over which the cell will operate in response to sudden intensity changes. For this reason, the sensitivity parameter defining the position of the curve is called the *range sensitivity*. Similarly, any change in sensitivity induced by an alteration of the background intensity moves the curves along the log intensity axis. This sensitivity change (Fig. 19 b) is called a *range shift* (LAUGHLIN and HARDIE, 1978). These two sensitivity parameters are defined in terms of the reciprocal of the total intensity required to produce a constant absolute response amplitude, at any one background level. Because the $V/\log I$ curves remain parallel during light adaptation the sensitivity change is uniform over the cell's entire dynamic range and the actual criterion voltage amplitude used to define range sensitivity does not change the range shift. A criterion voltage of 50% V_{max} (half maximal response) has been chosen for two reasons. The dark adapted range sensitivity of retinula cells was initially defined in terms of this amplitude because the $V/\log I$ curve has greatest slope at this point and this facilitates the most accurate experimental determination (LAUGHLIN, 1976 a). It happens that when the transient $V/\log I$ curves retain the same shape, the underlying intensity/response function has retained the same analytic form (Eq. E.2). All that is altered is the value of the constant R that multiplies the intensity term, I (Fig. 19 b). By definition this constant is the reciprocal of the intensity required to produce a half maximal response and equals the range sensitivity. Thus there has been a happy, albeit accidental, union between pragmatism and theory. Note that, when $V/\log I$ curves have the same shape, the value of light adapted range sensitivity can be predicted from the amplitude of the steady state response, because this value, in conjunction with the background, defines one point on the intensity/response function and allows for a solution of Eq. (E.2). It follows that with parallel $V/\log I$ curves the decline in response amplitude during light adaptation can be used to predict the range shift; as observed empirically by BADER et al. (1976).

Light-adapted intensity/response functions have been determined for the photoreceptors in drone bees (NAKA and KISHIDA, 1966; BAUMANN, 1968, 1975; BADER et al., 1976), in dragonfly (LAUGHLIN, 1975 b; LAUGHLIN and HARDIE, 1978), in the fly *Calliphora* (DÖRRSCHEIDT-KÄFER, 1972; LAUGHLIN and HARDIE, 1978), in the praying mantis (ROSSELL, 1979) and in the crayfish (GLANTZ, 1968). In all cases the effects of light adaptation are similar. The $V/\log I$ curves shift but keep approximately the same shape, although this critical point requires more exact measurements. Dim backgrounds produce small range shifts (Fig. 32), as expected from the small changes in amplitude during prolonged stimuli (e.g. Fig. 18 a). As background intensity increases, the light adaptation becomes more effective until, at the highest intensities used, the range shift becomes proportional to background intensity. As a consequence, steady state potential remains constant, irrespective of intensity, at about 50% V_{max} (LAUGHLIN and HARDIE, 1978). This observation has only been made in fly and dragonfly, but, with one exception, no other experiment has used backgrounds of sufficient intensity. The one comparable study was made on the photoreceptors of a white eyed mutant *Calliphora*, using a preparation in which the head was cut off (DÖRRSCHEIDT-KÄFER, 1972). It produces a contradictory result. At background intensities greater than those which initially saturate the dark-adapted cell, the amplitude of the steady state response is depressed by further intensity increases, instead of rising or remaining constant (Fig. 19 a). The fall in amplitude is accompanied by a decline in V_{max} and a flattening of the $V/\log I$ curves for the transients. These results suggest that the reversal potential for the response, i.e. the EMF driving the total photocurrent, is declining at high intensities. This decline was not seen in flies with heads attached and left free enough to maintain respiratory pumping movements of the abdomen (LAUGHLIN and HARDIE, 1978). For these latter experiments only a small part of the retina was illuminated whereas in DÖRRSCHEIDT-KÄFER's work the whole retina was flooded with light. Thus it remains to be seen whether a decline in V_{max} and plateau response is the natural response of the fully illuminated eye or the result of an inadequate energy supply.

d) Mechanisms for Light Adaptation

The processes of light and dark adaptation are reviewed by AUTRUM (this Handbook, Vol. VII/6C, Chapt. 1) and a thumbnail sketch is produced here for two reasons. The first is that light adaptation, a major functional attribute of eyes, is brought about by a complex of mechanisms, often resident within different cells of the retina, or within different regions of the same cell. Each mechanism has its own attributes and disadvantages, and we can expect future research to show that the mechanisms are carefully organised within the complex, to ensure clarity of the neural image at different light intensities (e.g. SNYDER, 1979). The available results indicate that the light adaptation complex of the retina is an elegant example of biological adaptation, embracing functions such as optics, cellular and organelle motility, membrane synthesis and degradation and the regulation of transduction. The second reason is that a description of these mechanisms helps one to understand the changes in sensitivity and their influence upon the intensity/response function.

At the level of the photoreceptor potential, the light-adaptation complex of the retina produces one net result: more photons are required at the cornea, from extended sources, to generate the same level of depolarisation. Because the $V/\log I$ curves keep their same sigmoidal shape, to a first approximation (Fig. 18 a), the range shift mechanisms are superimposed upon the non-linear summation of responses. The intensity/response function [Eq. (E.2)] retains its same general form and it is principally the range sensitivity factor R that alters (LAUGHLIN, 1975 a, b).

Two classes of mechanism could be superimposed upon non-linear summation, to produce a range shift. Optical processes can reduce the proportion of incident photons activating the transducer, and transducer amplification control mechanisms can regulate the current and voltage responses produced by each photon (over and above the effects of non-linear summation). Amplification can be regulated by changing the transducer's conductance gain, the ratio of activated depolarising conductances to effective photons, by the production of antagonistic hyperpolarising currents, and by reducing the load resistance across which the current produces the receptor potential. Both amplification and optical mechanisms have a direct effect on range sensitivity. In the theoretical derivation (E.2), the range sensitivity R, is proportional to quantum capture efficiency, conductance gain, and load resistance (SHAW, 1968 b; LAUGHLIN, 1975 a).

As yet no photoreceptor has a measured range shift been dissected into the components due to the different members of the adaptation complex, but there is enough data from studies of individual mechanisms to assess their relative contributions and roles. Take transducer amplification controls first. The voltage clamp techniques used on the large photoreceptors of barnacles and Limulus ventral eye show that during light adaptation the net inward current is reduced (Fig. 3), probably by a calcium mediated mechanism. As a dramatic confirmation, calcium can reduce both the magnitude and the duration of currents produced by single photons (FEIN and CHARLTON, 1977). Such definitive measures of current under voltage clamp have not been possible in insect retina, but observations of similar effects suggest similar mechanisms. The amplitudes and durations of locust retinula bumps are reduced by light adaptation (TSUKAHARA and HORRIDGE, The fast phase (Fig. 18 d) of light adaptation shows the dependence upon calcium and sodium ions seen in Limulus ventral eye, so suggesting that insects use a similar calcium mediated control for light adaptation (BADER et al., 1976). A consideration of energy expenditure suggests that the net inward current should be reduced by dropping the transducer's conductance gain. If every conductance activated requires the discharge of "internal transmitter" (HAMDORF, 1979) and generates an ion flux across the membrane, then adaptation mechanisms using opposing hyperpolarising currents (or membrane resistance shunts) are very wasteful. They actually increase the transmitter and ion flux required to produce a certain level of depolarisation. By comparison, a conductance gain control reduces the ratio of conductances to photons as intensity rises. Finally, the transducer amplification controls are both rapid and effective. A range shift of more than 2 log units is produced in 100–200 ms (BADER et al., 1976; LAUGHLIN and HARDIE, 1978).

The optical mechanisms for light adaptation generate a range shift by altering the quantum capture efficiency with respect to extended sources. In both apposition and superposition eyes one finds three subclasses of mechanism. *Aperture mechanisms* regulate the amount of light reaching the rhabdom by changing the effective cross-sectional area of the rhabdom, or by altering the area of cornea through which light is admitted to a single rhabdom. This usually involves movement of pigment cells or granules around the cone, a widening of the rhabdom, movement of the rhabdom tip and movements of the cone cells (WALCOTT, 1975; see also this Handbook, Vol. VII/6C, Chapt. 1). The increased aperture widens the ommatidium's acceptance angle, either by increasing the level of aberrations associated with a larger corneal aperture or by increasing the angle subtended by the rhabdom. Thus angular sensitivity is sacrificed for increased photon catch (WAL-COTT, 1975; SNYDER, 1979; STAVENGA, 1979). These changes are generally slow to execute. In mantis, the best studied example, the aperture effects widen the acceptance angle (Fig. 23) and increase the sensitivity of the cell to extended sources by 1 log unit (ROSSEL, 1979).

Longitudinal pupil mechanisms attenuate light flux within the rhabdom, by moving small pigment granules close to the rhabdom walls to frustrate the total internal reflection of light (KIRSCHFELD and FRANCESCHINI, 1969). The distances moved by the granules are relatively small so the effect is rapid. In fly, butterfly, bees and wasps an attenuation of 1–2 log units is accomplished in 10–60 s (STA-VENGA, 1979).

The final optical factor is the quantity of unbleached pigment. This can be varied rapidly through bleaching and photoreisomerisation (HAMDORF, 1979), or slowly through metabolic reisomerisation (HAMDORF, 1979) or photoreceptor membrane synthesis and degradation (WHITE and LORD, 1975; EGUCHI and WATERMAN, 1976). As opposed to vertebrate photoreceptors, where large bleaches can occur and *log* sensitivity is proportional to unbleached pigment concentrations, natural bleaches are small in retinula cells, thanks to photoreisomerisation, and sensitivity is directly proportional to concentration (HAMDORF, 1979). Consequently bleaching effects are minor. The role of pigment synthesis and breakdown in increasing rhabdom length and cross-sectional area, and perhaps synthesising a special high gain membrane has not been assessed, although it is undoubtedly important in some species [e.g. in larval mosquito ocelli the rhabdom volume increases threefold during dark adaptation (WHITE and LORD, 1975)].

Another mechanism for light adaptation has been proposed, depletion of extracellular sodium around the site of photocurrent generation (HAMDORF and SCHWEMER, 1975). However, SHAW (1978a) has pointed out that this hypothesis is based upon a gross overestimate of the light induced sodium flux during a saturated response. When more realistic estimates are combined with his own careful measurements of the volume, distribution and accessibility of the extracellular space to small molecules, it becomes clear that no significant sodium depletion takes place, at least in locust retina (SHAW, 1978a). In fact, the presence of small dilations of the extracellular space around the rhabdom suggests that the system is designed to avoid sodium depletion. On *a priori* grounds, discharging the sodium battery is inadvisable, because it restricts the voltage response range of the receptor. One purpose of light adaptation is to adjust sensitivity to avoid saturation and maintain as large a dynamic range as possible, and, with the exception of experiments performed on isolated heads, prolonged light adaptation with initially saturating stimuli does not reduce the maximum response amplitude (e.g. Fig. 19).

In conclusion, a complex of light-adaptation processes produce a range shift in an insect photoreceptor, so modifying its intensity/response function to match the level of incident illumination. Many will argue, quite correctly, that for an understanding of visual performance, an appreciation of range shift is quite unnecessary. What matters to the optic lobe is the voltage fluctuation produced in a receptor by a change in intensity. Consequently incremental plots of intensity/response functions are more appropriate. Unfortunately the vertebrate literature has been confused by the unthinking application of self-shunting equations to both incremental and absolute plots of intensity/response functions, and this situation has only recently been tidied up (NORMANN and PERLMAN, 1979). By avoiding this pitfall we are in a better position to see how both non-linear summation and range shift conspire to determine a receptor's sensitivity to small intensity fluctuations.

4. Responses and Light Measurement

Many photoreceptors operate in two distinctive modes. Bumps give the eye the capability to work as a photon counter, so achieving the upper "photon noise" limit of resolution. At the higher intensities the level of depolarisation depends upon the rate of arrival of photons. Even though one response mode must merge into the other, in a cross-over region, it is convenient to treat the two cases separately. For both modes, the receptor response characteristics will be discussed in terms of their ability to measure light intensity and produce a signal that is appropriate for subsequent processing. It is hoped that this will show that the transducers of photoreceptors are adapted, in the evolutionary sense, to their individual functions so that both the capabilities and constraints of biological amplifiers are put to their best uses.

a) Single Photon Signals

It has never been *conclusively* shown that arthropods use quantum bumps to see things. No one has succeeded in showing that a dimly illuminated test pattern, which produced a defined behavioural response, is only capable of generating a dribble of quantum bumps in single receptors. Nonetheless, there is good evidence to suggest that single bumps are resolved within the optic lobe. Ingenious optomotor experiments (REICHARDT, 1969, 1970) suggested that flies resolve single photon arrivals at very low intensities. Thresholds follow the square root law and also obey reciprocity, i.e. the threshold is determined by the number of photons delivered rather than the time interval over which they were distributed. A brave attempt to measure photoreceptor signals at absolute threshold failed (SCHOLES and REICHARDT, 1969) because quantum bumps were not found (cf. HARDIE, 1979). To gain further support for this behavioural evidence, and to see how efficiently the visual system processes single photon signals, LILLYWHITE and DVORAK (in LILLYWHITE, 1978 b) looked at the absolute threshold of a lobula giant movement detector neuron's response to a flash of light. About one in eight of the photons available to the photoreceptors produced a spike in this fourth order cell. A battery of statistical tests, together with reciprocity experiments, indicated that photon coincidence was not required to trigger a spike. The very existence of quantum bumps in receptors and single photon signals in higher order neurons suggests that the visual system *does* have the capability to derive pattern information from a peppering of photon hits across the retina. But to register a single photon in a higher order cell is but a part of this capability, albeit an important one. How is the pattern read from a splutter of spikes in several cells?

Given that bumps are useful for encoding information at low intensities why are they large in some species, small in others, and sometimes never seen at all (Table 2)? After all, if a fly can use 1 mV bumps why should a locust produce a bump of 5 mV, and *Limulus* the LPF of 80 mV? The question of bump size can be broken into two parts. One must first establish that the observed differences (Table 2) between the bumps of different cells (sometimes in the same retina) are real, rather than artefactual. Bump amplitude is notoriously labile, being susceptible to experimental insult and light adaptation. If differences are not artefacts, one can then look at the functional significance of bump size. Taking the amplitude

Table 2. Amplitudes and durations of quantum bumps in insect retinula cells

Animal	Bump amplitude mV	Bump duration ms	Reference
Locust – isolated head	0.2– 1.2	70	Scholes (1964)
Locust – intact animal	1.0–10.0	80	Lillywhite (1978b)
Cockroach	1.0– 6.0	100	Laughlin (unpubl. obs.)
Mantis	1.0– 3.0	75	Rossel (personal comm.)
Fly, *Calliphora*, R1–6	0.5– 1.3	30	Hardie (1979)
Fly, *Calliphora*, R7	0.7– 3.8	35	Hardie (1979)
Fly, *Musca*, R1–6	1.1– 4.5	45	Hardie (1979)
Fly, *Drosophila*	0.2– 1.0	100	Wu and Pak (1975)

differences first: the mean size of bumps is the purest expression of a photoreceptor's dark adapted voltage gain (expressed as mV/effective photon). The following argument suggests that the observed differences between photoreceptors' voltage gains are neither artefactual, nor are they the *trivial* consequence of factors such as cell size and input resistance. Rather, the dark adapted voltage gain is an important design parameter which is set to a specific value, by natural selection. In the dragonfly *Hemicordulia tau*, the UV cell of the ventral retina has a noisier response than the neighbouring green sensitive cell (Fig. 18) and a simple shot noise analysis (Sect. E.II.5) shows that this noisiness is symptomatic of a higher voltage gain (Laughlin, 1976a). Similarly, in the flies *Calliphora stygia* and *Musca domestica*, the cells R 7 and R 8 have noisier responses than R 1–6 and in this case the higher voltage gain of the noisier cells was confirmed from direct recordings of bump amplitude (Hardie, 1979; see also Table 2). It is quite remarkable that in these three animals, the cells with the higher voltage gains have the more highly tuned spectral sensitivity functions so that they transduce light from a narrower window of the spectrum. When the spectral sensitivities of the high and low gain cells are convolved with the spectral composition of daylight, one finds that the higher voltage gains compensate for this paucity of photons. Consequently in daylight, cells in the same retina operate at almost identical levels of voltage output (Laughlin, 1976a; Hardie, 1979). This matching of receptor outputs in three different eyes suggests that it is important for adjacent receptors to operate with similar voltages, perhaps to avoid the extracellularly mediated electrical inhibition of the weak by the powerful, described by Shaw (1975) (Sect. E.II.8.b). The matching establishes that a receptor's dark-adapted voltage gain is an important design parameter, irrespective of its biophysical basis.

We can now consider the appropriate amplitude for a quantum bump. If bumps are to provide useful single photon signals they must be resolvable amid the intrinsic noise of the optic lobe. Consequently bump amplitude may be an expression of the noise levels encountered by single photon signals during subsequent processing. We have no reason to suppose that a locust's neurons are inevitably noisier than a fly's, and demand bigger bumps in the retina, so the limiting noise level might be set by the circuitry used. One particular processing strategy, area summation or neural pooling (Snyder, 1979), is a potent generator of high intrinsic noise levels. It is also vital for obtaining the best possible spatial resolution at low intensities, when photons are scarce (i.e. when one might wish to use bumps). This is because two areas of the retina can only be judged to have received different levels of illumination if the numbers of photons falling in those two areas are significantly different. Because the signal to noise ratio is, at best, proportional to photon catch, a valid judgment requires that a certain minimum number of photons be recorded in each area. It follows that, as intensity falls, the catches of larger and larger retinal areas must be summed together to achieve a significant photon count. This is why we lose resolution at low intensities (ROSE, 1972). Thus, unless the nervous system sums the single photon signals from many receptors, over a wide retinal area, it cannot produce statistically significant signals at low intensities and much of the available spatial information is lost (rev. SNYDER, 1979; see also PIRENNE, 1967, for an identical proposal for the human retina). This spatial summation exacerbates intrinsic noise by bringing together the inputs from many ommatidia and summing, at one point, the noise levels from each receptor channel. Consequently a summation involving more receptors will be noisier, and will require larger single photon signals for detectability. With intrinsic noise occurring at the photoreceptor's first synapse (Sect. E.III.4) the most effective place to increase the size of a single photon signal is at the transducer. Thus, in most general terms, if quantum bumps are to be equally detectable in summation areas of different sizes, their amplitudes should be proportional to the square root of the number of photoreceptors contributing to each pool.

To support the hypothesis that the voltage gains of dark adapted retinula cells are adjusted to provide detectable quantum bumps, the insects in which large bumps have been most obvious, locust, cockroach, and mantis (Table 2) are active by day and night. In addition they have ommatidia which open up their acceptance angles at low intensities and this is a highly effective way to increase acuity at low intensities *if* it is combined with area summation (rev. SNYDER, 1979). By comparison, the fly which has small bumps (Table 2), and the dragonfly, in which bumps are never observed, change their acceptance angles relatively little upon dark adaptation (HARDIE, 1979; LAUGHLIN, unpublished observations). Thus the size of quantum bumps could be an example of the tailoring of photoreceptor performance to the neural processes employed at higher levels. We will pursue this theme of the optimisation of photoreceptor's intensity/response function by examining the values of range sensitivity that are most advantageous for intensity coding over a wide range of ambient intensities.

b) A Strategy for Signalling at Higher Intensities

Over most of its total working range, the receptor's capacity to signal intensity is dominated by its non-linearity. As intensity rises, light becomes progressively less effective at producing a voltage response (Fig. 19). The dominant compressive effects of the hyperbolic intensity/response function are compounded by the fall of range sensitivity due to light adaptation. These attenuating factors are, in several senses, unavoidable; self-shunting is ubiquitous to conductances operating in parallel on the same membrane, while light adaptation is demanded by the limited response bandwidth of the photoreceptor, as dictated by ionic reversal potentials. In discussing intensity coding, we will begin by formulating the ideal strategy for handling these constraints. We can then assess the function of real receptors against this ideal. The argument shows that the non-linearities of transduction provide an interesting example of a constraint being turned into a virtue by selecting for a different, and more direct advantage.

Before constructing the ideal non-linear photoreceptor, one must define the objects it is to look at. For simplicity we examine the transmission of a "black and white" picture. Surprisingly, there is little information available about the spatial distribution of intensity within black and white visual scenes. By comparison, there are many descriptions of the spectral composition of light in different environments (e.g. WYSZECKI and STILES, 1967; MUNZ and MCFARLAND, 1977), yet the spatial distribution of intensity is to spatial coding, what spectral irradiance is to colour vision. Some key aspects of the intensity signal can be deduced from the way an intensity pattern is generated, and by looking at those parts of the intensity signal that are picked out by higher order neurons.

There are four primary causes for intensity changes within the environment. (1) Luminescent objects produce their own light. (2) The light from the sun comes from one direction. (3) The direction and intensity of sunlight varies throughout the day. (4) Objects reflect and absorb different proportions of the light falling upon them. Which of these determinants is of the most importance? In general, natural luminescent objects are restricted to special purposes, such as celestial navigation and communication. Diurnal intensity changes are of paramount importance because they demand that the visual system works over a wide intensity range, exceeding the span of a single $V/\log I$ curve. These diurnal intensity changes are usually slow and can usually be dealt with by range shift mechanisms (for a possible exception see MUNZ and MACFARLAND, 1977). Uneven illumination of a scene, and in particular areas of highlight and deep shadow, pose a major problem to the visual system. Nonetheless, practical experience suggests that the total intensity range across a visual scene usually falls within a single $V/\log I$ curve. For colour television a dynamic range of 1.6 log units (WIGGIN, 1968) is sufficient for live broadcast, while an analysis of one hundred photographs of outdoor scenes showed that the maximum intensity range was 3 log units, with a mean at 2.2 (COMPTON, 1978).

The greatest amount of detail in a picture is generated by differences within areas of fairly uniform illumination. Reflectance patterns have two qualities of particular relevance to a visual system operating over a wide range of average intensities. First, the intensity of light reflected by objects is proportional to reflectance and to the level of illumination. Consequently, as mean intensity increases, the absolute energy differences between objects widens, yet the relative difference remains constant. Thus contrast, a measure of relative intensity, is one parameter in reflectance patterns that is unaffected by changes in mean intensity. If objects are to look alike at dawn and midday, contrast should be measured, not intensity. The second property of reflectances is that they generate a fairly narrow range of intensity differences, when compared to the overall range of the visual system or of a single $V/\log I$ curve. The blackest Russian soil is only 1.2 log units darker than an adjacent patch of snow (WYSZECKI and STILES, 1967) and these two examples are extremes. Thus at any one mean luminance level, contrast signals occupy a comparatively narrow bandwidth.

That the visual system should have a predilection for small intensity changes within a narrow range is confirmed by recordings from higher order interneurons. As reviewed in Sect. E.III.3, the first order large monopolar cells of the insect retina have an operating range of 1–2 log units as does the locust DCMD (ROWELL et al., 1977) and the sustaining fibre of the crayfish optic tract (GLANTZ, 1971). Thus our ideal photoreceptor should be designed to respond to intensity changes of about 1 log unit, both above and below the background level. This can easily be achieved by sliding the $V/\log I$ curves back and forth, in response to different mean luminance, but what is the most appropriate $V/\log I$ curve for each mean intensity level?

For the optimal measurement of small intensity fluctuations about the mean, one selects the intensity/response function which has greatest slope (dV/dI) as it passes through the mean intensity level. The slope is often called the gain or the sensitivity (e.g. NORMANN and WERBLIN, 1974) but to avoid confusion with other definitions of sensitivity we have redefined (dV/dI) as the *increment sensitivity* (LAUGHLIN and HARDIE, 1978). There is a simple way to select the intensity/response function with the high increment sensitivity: find the $V/\log I$ curve with the greatest slope as it passes through the mean intensity level, for, by the chain rule

$$\frac{dV}{dI} = \frac{dV}{d(\log I)} \cdot \frac{d(\log I)}{dI} = \frac{dV}{d(\log I)} \cdot \frac{1}{I} \tag{E.3}$$

(NORMANN and WERBLIN, 1974). Because the slope of the $V/\log I$ curve is always maximum at 50% V_{max} then the maximum increment sensitivity is obtained by allowing the mean intensity level to generate a half maximal response (Fig. 19 b, d).

By operating a photoreceptor at this maximum possible gain, over a wide range of different mean intensities, one attains the unexpected virtue, contrast normalisation. When operated at half maximum response the slope of the $V/\log I$ curve is always constant. Now, a constant logarithmic intensity increment, $\Delta \log I$, corresponds to a constant contrast increment, and for this reason the slope of the $V/\log I$ curve is called the *contrast efficiency* (LAUGHLIN, 1975 b). By operating with constant contrast efficiency, the receptors have achieved contrast normalisation. Inspection of Eq. (E.3) shows that, when contrast efficiency is constant, the increment sensitivity is inversely proportional to mean (background) intensity as required for signals of equal contrast to look alike at different mean luminances.

It has long been realised that the human visual system can operate according to the principles of contrast constancy. The well known WEBER-FECHNER law states that for much of the intensity range, the minimum discriminable intensity increment, ΔI, is proportional to the background intensity upon which it is superimposed,

$$\text{thus} \quad \Delta I/I = k \,. \tag{E.4}$$

If one assumes, as FECHNER did (BLACKWELL, 1972), that a constant internal signal increment, ΔS, is produced at threshold then

$$\Delta S/\Delta I = I^{-1} \,,$$

$$\therefore S = c \cdot \log I \,. \tag{E.5}$$

This is identical in form to Eq. (E.3) and is equivalent to a log transformation. Note that the log transformation is produced by having many parallel $V/\log I$ curves of equal slope, rather than a single straight line and, in this way, the log transformation does not exceed the bounds imposed by a receptor's finite response range. Log transformations, like the hyperbolic self-shunting relationships of receptors and synapses, are found in many other sensory systems (e.g. LIPETZ, 1971). It may be of some significance then, that a log transformation is produced by taking a self-shunting membrane conductance system, and regulating it to operate about any one mean level of input with maximum gain.

The fact that any given intensity/response function has its maximum slope at the origin, where intensity is zero, can cause confusion. In selecting the operating curve with maximum slope at a particular background intensity, one is not choosing the point of maximum gain on any one function, one is making a compromise. If the range sensitivity is too low then the entire curve is too depressed (curve 3, Fig. 18 d) and if too high (curve 1) the initial slope is so great that non-linear summation has throttled the response by the time the background intensity is reached. The optimum curve (curve 2) is only best for one value of background, holding the middle ground between insensitivity and non-linear summation.

How closely do the photoreceptors of compound eyes approach the ideal of maximum increment sensitivity, and so reap the benefits of contrast constancy? Using sinusoidally modulated stimuli of constant (20%) contrast ZETTLER (1969) showed that *Calliphora* receptors performed an imperfect logarithmic transform over a 4 log unit range of mean luminances. Although intensity changed by a factor of 20,000 the gain only changed by 5,000 so that there was a fivefold increase in increment sensitivity. Similar results have been obtained from *Calliphora* (LEUTSCHER-HAZELHOFF, 1975) and from cricket and locust (PINTER, 1972). In addition, LEUTSCHER-HAZELHOFF showed that voltage modulation is approximately proportional to contrasts of less than 0.3. In all these studies, the reason for the imperfect log transform is clear. At dimmest intensities the receptors operate at the toe of the dark-adapted $V/\log I$ curve, where contrast efficiency is far below optimum. This breakdown in the log transform is inevitable. The position of the dark-adapted $V/\log I$ curve is probably determined by the minimum resolvable response required to see single photons. Unless the early stages of light adaptation increase the sensitivity, the receptor most rapidly approaches its optimum operating range by refraining from light adaptation, and allowing the background to push its voltage response up the dark-adapted intensity/response function.

In fact the available data does suggest that the background rapidly propels the photoreceptors towards their maximum gain. Light adaptation does not produce a range shift until the operating voltage reaches the steep region of the $V/\log I$ curve and from then on range shift becomes progressively more severe, until it reaches proportionality to background increments (LAUGHLIN and HARDIE, 1978). Because contrast efficiency is close to maximum at outputs in the range of 30%–70% V_{max} (Fig. 19) little increment sensitivity is lost by operating within this almost linear region rather than exactly at 50% V_{max}, and the photoreceptor conserves energy by operating closer to resting potential.

To summarise the concepts drawn from the limited amount of data, (almost entirely from insect apposition eyes): the photoreceptors operate with an increment sensitivity close to the maximum imposed by the inevitable constraints of a non-linear intensity/response function and a finite response range. This maximisation of gain is achieved by appropriate adjustments in range sensitivity but also brings about, as a by-product, contrast constancy. Consequently one can suggest that one part of the visual system has acquired this desirable logarithmic transform simply by selecting for maximum gain within the constraints imposed by self-shunting. As a result of this log transform, contrast fluctuations about any one mean luminance generate a profile of responses across the receptor mosaic which is independent of mean illumination, but is elevated or depressed by the steady state plateau response to mean luminance. The accuracy with which intensity can be measured within this profile depends largely on the level of noise.

5. Photoreceptor Noise

Noise is often one of the major constraints to image quality in the receptor mosaic (SNYDER, 1977) (Sect. D.V.1.a), yet, despite its conspicuous presence, receptor noise levels have received comparatively little attention, perhaps because it is often seen as merely interference. Yet, when armed with the appropriate concepts and techniques, noise is rich in information. We will see that it can provide estimates of photon catch, show what single photon signals look like and how they add together. Analysis can also reveal the origins of noise and might even reveal the kinetics of membrane conductances (STEVENS, 1977). Nor is noise of purely biophysical interest. Intrinsic noise is an almost inevitable bugbear in cellular communication, and must always be considered as a determinant of acuity, if only to be dismissed. We will start by looking for the origins of receptor noise, analyse transducer noise as an exemplary form of intrinsic noise, and then assess the effects of receptor noise and the lessons it teaches us.

a) Noise and Its Sources

During the steady response to light, noise rises progressively with mean amplitude, reaches a peak at around 20% V_{max}, and then falls away (Fig. 20a) (see also WU and PAK, 1978). The relative amplitude of receptor noise also varies from species to species (SMOLA and GEMPERLEIN, 1973; SMOLA, 1976) and among different cells from the same retina (LAUGHLIN, 1976a). In some "low noise" receptors, the noise amplitude peak is poorly defined (Fig. 20a). The observation that discrete randomly occurring bumps fuse to produce a ragged receptor potential suggests that photoreceptor noise originates from the random arrival of photons. This hypothesis is supported by the "shot noise" analysis of receptor potentials.

The fundamentals of shot noise analysis are simple. Consider the responses to very brief flashes, in which photons essentially arrive simultaneously, so that the response is made up of a number of photon triggered events of amplitude a, piled one on top of the other. If the mean number of effective photons from a flash is $\bar{N}$, then the mean response amplitude, $\bar{V}$, is given by

$$\bar{V} = \bar{N} \cdot a. \tag{E.6}$$

The variance among responses, s^2 is given by

$$s^2 = a^2 \cdot (\text{variance in photon catch}) = a^2 \cdot \bar{N}. \tag{E.7}$$

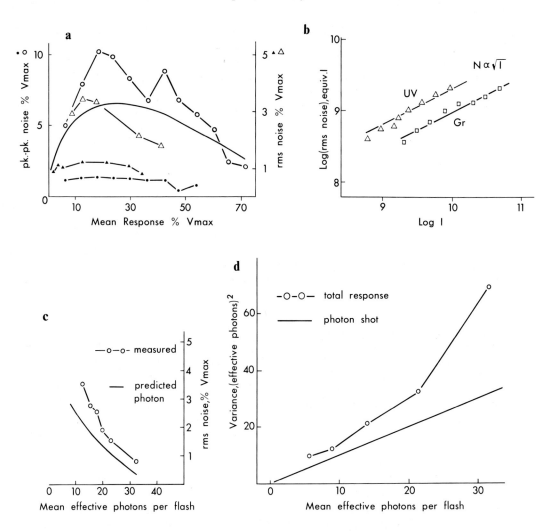

Fig. 20 a–d. The dependence of photoreceptor noise levels on mean response amplitudes, intensities and photon catches. **a** Noise levels as a function of mean response amplitude in cockroach (△) and fly R 1–6 (▲) (from SMOLA, 1976); and in the UV (0) and the green (●) cells of dragonfly retina, shown in Fig. 18 (after LAUGHLIN, 1976a). Where noise is prominent, its amplitude rises initially and then falls. Qualitatively, this is the behaviour expected when, at its source, the variance is proportional to mean intensity but the response amplitude is reduced by non-linear summation; as illustrated by the noise levels (in arbitrary units) expected from a self-shunting motor endplate (——) when the variance among activated conductances is proportional to the mean (adapted from KATZ and MILEDI, 1972). **b** If the effects of non-linear summation are accounted for by expressing noise levels in terms of an equivalent intensity input, the total variance or (r.m.s. noise)², is proportional to intensity (LAUGHLIN, 1976a). **c** When photon noise levels are predicted from the measured quantum capture efficiencies and intensity/response functions of locust photoreceptors, an excess of intrinsic transducer noise is found. **d** Again, when plotted as equivalent intensity, the noise variances are proportional to intensity up to values of 20 photons per flash (LILLYWHITE, 1978b; and LILLYWHITE and LAUGHLIN, 1979)

The average number of photons contributing to the flash response can now be calculated from response amplitudes because, from Eqs. (E.6) and (E.7),

$$\bar{N} = \bar{V}^2/s^2 = (\text{r.m.s. signal: noise})^2 \tag{E.8}$$

and the event amplitude by

$$a = s^2/\bar{V}. \tag{E.9}$$

Note that Eq. (E.8) predicts the photon catch from the signal to noise ratio of the response, no matter what units the signal to noise ratio is expressed in. By comparison Eq. (E.9) should be expressed in units of voltage amplitude.

For the case of a response to a continuous stream of photons the solution is complicated by the random overlap of photon triggered events. Both the mean response level and the variance depend upon event amplitude, duration and waveform. If the events are rectangular pulses of amplitude a, duration t, and occurring at a rate of n per unit time then

$$\bar{V} = n \cdot a \cdot t \tag{E.10}$$

and

$$s^2 = n \cdot a^2 \cdot t \tag{E.11}$$

(KATZ and MILEDI, 1972). The effective duration of an event, and even its time course can be deduced from the noise power spectrum (DODGE et al., 1968) allowing the rate of event occurrence and the amplitude to be derived from the mean and variance of the response (STEVENS, 1977). Note that in both types of shot noise analysis, the derivation depends upon a knowledge of the source of variance, and its relationship to the mean.

Shot noise analysis has produced self-consistent results from invertebrate photoreceptors. Analysing continuous responses, DODGE et al. (1968) and WU and PAK (1978) found that shot event rate was proportional to intensity. Voltage noise amplitude failed to increase continuously with intensity, as predicted by Eq. (E.7), because the non-linear summation effects reduce the gain (Fig. 20a). Similarly, when analysing the responses of *Musca* photoreceptors to brief low energy flashes, KIRSCHFELD (1966) found that, after equating variance and voltage response with the mean, according to Eqs. (E.6) and (E.7), the equivalent photon catches of responses followed the Poisson distribution. In an analysis of noise in dragonfly photoreceptors LAUGHLIN (1976a) corrected for the non-linear summation of responses, by converting every voltage measurement to an equivalent intensity, read off the measured intensity/response function, but made no attempt to derive, and correct for, the shape of individual single photon responses. The response variance, expressed in equivalent intensity units, was proportional to the mean intensity over a 2 log unit range (Fig. 20b). The underlying Poisson nature of the response noise was uncovered by plotting the frequency distribution of the equivalent intensity readings. This study also indicated that the receptors with the poorest signal to noise ratios at low response levels, were receiving fewer photons, and transducing them with a higher voltage gain [Eqs. (E.8) and (E.9)].

Although indicating that the photoreceptor voltage noise derives from the random absorption of photons, the results from all the existing photoreceptor shot noise analyses are inaccurate, because they are based upon the assumption that all noise results from random photon absorptions. KIRSCHFELD (1966) was careful to point out that additional sources of variance will bias the results, leading to an overestimate of event amplitude and an underestimate of event number or rate [Eqs. (E.7) and (E.8)]. Observing that in many photoreceptors, single quantum bumps vary in amplitude and latency, Laughlin (1976a) emphasised that the process of transduction itself is noisy, and this *transducer noise* could introduce significant errors into those physiological and behavioural analyses that assumed that all variance came from photon shot noise.

b) Transducer Noise

To investigate transducer noise one must first account for photon noise. Using locust photoreceptors, where quantum capture efficiencies can be accurately determined from bump counts, Lillywhite and Laughlin (1979) demonstrated that photon shot noise produced but one-half of the total response variance, over an intensity range of at least 2 log units. The receptors show negligible dark noise (Lillywhite, 1977), and the excess variance produced during the response is proportional to the mean photon catch (Fig. 20d). This suggests that the noise is generated during transduction, with each effective photon making its own contribution to the variance. One must conclude that the source of transducer noise causing single quantum bumps to vary in amplitude, latency and duration (e.g. Laughlin, 1976a; Tsukahara and Horridge, 1977a) is active at higher intensities, and makes substantial inroads upon receptor fidelity.

To evaluate previous analyses of both photoreceptor noise, and of behavioural thresholds, Lillywhite and Laughlin (1979) subjected their data to a classical shot noise analysis. Setting aside their direct determinations of quantum capture efficiency, they estimated the apparent mean photon catch from the signal to noise ratio of the response [Eq. (E.8)] and used this to derive an *apparent* quantum capture efficiency. As expected from the excess noise the apparent efficiency was half the actual. The apparent photon catch underlying *each* measured response was derived by first converting response amplitudes to equivalent intensities (photons/flash, at the cornea), via the intensity/response function, and then multiplying this equivalent intensity by the apparent quantum capture efficiency. The distribution of apparent photon catches was, within the limits of their sample size, Poisson. This shows that transducer noise mimics photon noise and so passes undetected by shot noise analysis. Nor would transducer noise be revealed by more sophisticated statistical techniques (Lillywhite, 1978b). It is only by knowing the actual quantum catch that one discovers that transducer noise has halved the apparent quantum capture efficiency.

Why does transducer noise pass undetected? The first reason is trivial. By initially equating the variance with the mean [Eq. (E.7)] a shot noise analysis derives the appropriate correction factor for scaling down all apparent photon catches, so that they fit into a Poisson distribution. The second reason is more profound because, even after scaling the variance to the mean, the distribution could still be wildly different in shape from a Poisson. The distribution looks Poisson, because, at its root, the production of transducer noise follows a Poisson process, the absorption of single photons.

This analysis of transducer noise confirms the earlier suspicion (Laughlin, 1976a) that the usual shot noise analyses (e.g. Dodge et al., 1968; Wu and Pak, 1978) seriously underestimate a photoreceptor's quantum catch and overestimate the event amplitude. It also qualifies the conclusions drawn from observations of threshold intensities proportional to the square root of the background intensity. Adherence to this square root law (Sect. D.V.1.a) is commonly used in vertebrate and invertebrate work as evidence for a photon noise limited response (e.g. REICHARDT, 1970). With the discovery of an alternative noise source which also produces a variance proportional to mean intensity, the square root law is seen for what it really is; an indication that noise variance is proportional to mean intensity! Unless one actually knows the quantum capture efficiency, the effect of photon noise cannot be defined if an intrinsic noise source is present which shows a similar proportionality.

The large amount of variance injected during transduction is rather puzzling, for in all other respects the locust photoreceptor is well adapted to minimise noise. Several possible sources of unnecessary signal fluctuation are avoided (LILLY-WHITE, 1978 a). A single photon produces one bump, no less and no more; the size of this bump does not depend upon the stimulating wavelength; and amplitude is not significantly changed by the position along the length of the cell at which a bump is generated. The levels of dark noise are, by comparison with vertebrate photoreceptors (SIMON and LAMB, 1977), very low, at least in the cell body. Continuous baseline noise is about 15% of mean bump amplitude (LILLYWHITE and LAUGHLIN, 1979) and there are almost no spontaneous dark bumps (LILLYWHITE, 1977). The juxtaposition of amplitude variance with the exclusion of other sources, suggests that this type of transducer noise is unavoidable, perhaps because a biochemical and biophysical amplifier depends upon the random collision of molecules and the activation of small numbers of conductance channels for its function. As a general principle it is worth noting that such noisy transfer characteristics are symptomatic of other transmission elements in the nervous system. At synapses, in particular, individual acetylcholine molecules rain onto the postsynaptic membrane at random, producing shot noise (KATZ and MILEDI, 1972) while quanta of transmitter are released according to binomial or Poisson statistics (KUFFLER and NICHOLLS, 1976). Note that, like transducer noise, these sources of synaptic noise produce a variance proportional to the mean, further weakening the square root law.

c) Effects of Receptor Noise

The effects of noise upon a photoreceptor's signalling capabilities can be assessed in at least two ways. The first is to regard the receptor as an information channel, designed to transmit as many different signals as possible, regardless of their form. The second is to take a practical approach and assess the effect of noise upon a specific resolution task. The information capacity of a single photoreceptor can be computed according to SHANNON's expression

$$C = F \cdot \log_2(1 + \sigma_s^2/\sigma_n^2), \qquad (E.12)$$

where C is the information capacity in bits s^{-1}, F the upper cut off frequency (Hz) of the fastest response, and σ_s^2 and σ_n^2 the variances (powers) of signal and noise respectively. SMOLA and GEMPERLEIN (1973) have spearheaded this type of analysis in the visual system by making the necessary measurements of noise levels and frequency responses in *Calliphora*, and in cockroach retinula cells, and assuming that the signal is a random fluctuation with a restricted contrast range (i.e. the receptor is looking at a random contrast pattern being swept past the eye). At all intensities the receptors of *Calliphora*, and of bees (SMOLA, 1976), outperform cockroach cells, by virtue of their lower noise levels and faster responses. Although the two faster, low gain, receptors definitely perform better at high intensities, one suspects that the cockroach retinula cells, with their higher voltage gains and larger rhabdomere cross-sectional areas, outstrip fly and bee cells at low intensities, where bump counts are important. To take account of this, information capacity should be expressed relative to a photon noise limit, and the formula extended, to include the intrinsic noise levels faced by bumps. Information capacity should prove a useful measure for a receptor's noise-limited performance, for the same reasons that it has helped us to appreciate the principles of optical sampling by photoreceptor arrays (SNYDER et al., 1977 a, b). Information can be used to evaluate trade-offs between different aspects of a signal (e.g. amplitude vs. response speed) without giving undue emphasis to any one signal parameter.

The practical assessments, the effects of noise upon specific resolution tasks, provide a simpler means for evaluating many of the relationships between signal and noise (e.g. SNYDER, 1977; cf. SNYDER et al., 1977 a). For example, how is the rising level of noise in receptors with increasing intensity, affected by the non-linear summation of photoreceptor intensity signals? This question can easily be solved by deriving, from measured noise levels and intensity response functions, the smallest detectable intensity increment as a function of mean intensity. In other words one derives the intensity fluctuation which produces a voltage signal that is a constant proportion of the noise at each intensity. The derivation is very simple if the noise is measured in units of equivalent intensity (Fig. 20 b); one multiplies the r.m.s. noise by a factor equal to the desired signal to noise ratio, and that is the relevant intensity increment. Figure 20 b shows that, as far as the receptor is concerned, non-linear summation has no effect upon increment threshold over a considerable intensity range because both signal and noise are scaled down equally. Detectability follows the square root law, as determined by photon and transducer noise.

Such practical assessments of noise effects can easily be extended to cover additional parameters, such as the effects of intrinsic synaptic noise, and the roles of angular sensitivity and temporal frequency response. The one limitation is that genuine behavioural performance depends upon the processing procedures adopted in the optic lobes. For example, if one sets out to determine the smallest sinusoidal intensity modulation resolvable in a receptor, as might be set up by a moving sinusoidal grating, then over the intensity range considered in the previous example, this will follow the square root law. However, the actual value of the minimum detectable modulation depends upon the filtering procedures adopted in the optic lobes. If the system is simply a level detector, all noise seen in the receptor obscures the modulation. But if the nervous system filters out frequencies that are higher and lower than the intensity modulations, then much of the noise is blocked and resolution is greatly enhanced. Clearly a correlation of receptor signal: noise ratios with behavioural thresholds can help decide the types of filtering that are employed, and show how closely the nervous system approaches a processor ideally adapted for the task in question.

d) Lessons from Receptor Noise

Receptor responses are noisy for two reasons. Photons arrive and are absorbed at random, and the transducer is a noisy amplifier. One suspects that transducer noise is an expression of a general failing among all those biological amplifiers which operate by the collisions of relatively small numbers of molecules or transmitter quanta, and the activation of small populations of conductance channels. For this reason transducer noise might be as inevitable as photon noise. The transducer is the first of several biophysical processes to introduce noise into the visual signal, and its investigation has provided us with three lessons on the analysis of intrinsic noise sources and their effects on visual performance. First, one cannot assess an intrinsic noise source without knowing the level of photon noise. Second, sources of noise can mimic each other when they have common origins; consequently noise sources cannot always be separated by a statistical analysis of their combined effects. Third, by lowering the signal to noise ratio, and by mimicking photon noise, a source of intrinsic noise can degrade the visual signal in such a way that it simply appears as if the number of photons arriving is reduced. It has long been suspected that intrinsic noise sources within the visual system can reduce the apparent quantum efficiency (H.B.BARLOW, 1977) but degradation of this type had never previously been demonstrated. Note again, that all these conclusions depended upon a precise determination of the locust photoreceptor's quantum capture efficiency. Finally, work on receptor noise is far from complete. The noise analysis of transduction processes is progressing to the identification of conductance channels (RICHARD PAYNE, personal communication) and one still has to explore the noise level at the receptor terminal, in the lamina. Furthermore, the effects of transducer noise on continuous, rather than flash, responses, and changes of noise level with light adaptation have not been looked at. We must now leave the investigation of interference and return to distortion of signals by receptors, by examining the imperfect manner in which photoreceptors handle rapid changes in stimulus intensity.

6. Temporal Resolving Power and Neural Image Quality

When an object moves across the retina its spatial details cause voltage fluctuations in the receptor matrix. It follows that the speed with which the transducer responds and modulates the receptor potential, can limit both the resolution of fine detail within moving patterns and the localisation of rapidly moving objects. In fact, receptor response speed should always be considered as a determinant of neural image quality because, as a result of muscle tremor and purposive movement, objects are rarely stationary with respect to the retina. Furthermore, the sensations generated by stationary objects (stabilised retinal images), tend to fade away within a few seconds in both fly (REICHARDT and POGGIO, 1976) and man (DITCHBURN, 1973). We will start the discussion of response speed by examining its measurement and its intensity dependence. We will then look for the biophysical factors controlling photoreceptor response speed and examine the roles that temporal resolving power can play in determining neural image quality.

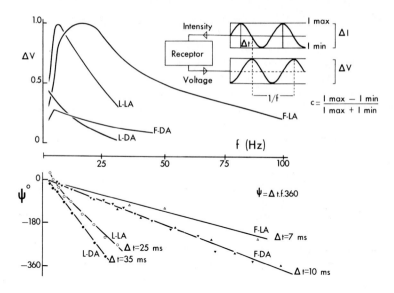

Fig. 21. The temporal resolving powers of fly *(F)* and locust *(L)* photoreceptors in dark *(DA)* and light-adapted *(LA)* states, as expressed by *linear* plots of frequency response. The parameters, stimulus and response modulation frequency, f; intensity modulation, ΔI; voltage modulation, ΔV; phase angle, Ψ; and time lag, Δt; are defined by the *inset*, where the sinusoidal stimulus and response are plotted as functions of time. All voltage modulations are normalised to the maximum amplitude recorded from the light-adapted photoreceptor at the particular value of stimulus contrast, c, that was used. For the locust data $c=0.9$ (PINTER, 1972); for both the fly amplitude curves, and one dark adapted phase curve (▲), $c=0.2$ (ZETTLER, 1969). The other dark adapted phase curve (▼) is from FRENCH and JÄRVILEHTO (1978a) who used a white noise analysis to derive frequency response. The light-adapted phase curve ($c=0.16$) is from GEMPERLEIN and SMOLA (1972a)

a) Measuring Response Speed

Temporal resolution can be described in a number of ways, but the most commonly used measures are the frequency response, the impulse response function, the flicker fusion frequency, and the integration time. Of these parameters the frequency response (Fig. 21) is the most comprehensive and useful, as illustrated by our considerations of the dynamics of *Limulus* photoreceptors (Sect. D.IV.6). This is partly because, as in *Limulus*, the insect photoreceptors' responses to stimuli of low contrast are approximately linear at any one mean intensity (PINTER, 1972; LEUTSCHER-HAZELHOFF, 1975; ECKERT and BISHOP, 1975), so that the frequency response can be used to predict the response to any low contrast input, and partly because the frequency response helps identify the physical processes underlying transduction. Remarkably few photoreceptors have had their frequency responses measured, and with the exception of *Limulus*, the most studied preparations are the compound eyes of muscoid flies (ZETTLER, 1969; GEMPERLEIN and SMOLA, 1972a; McCANN, 1974; ECKERT and BISHOP, 1975; LEUTSCHER-HAZELHOFF, 1975; FRENCH and JÄRVILEHTO, 1978a). The investigations of fly illustrate two important properties of insect photoreceptors. (1) The temporal resolving power is, by comparison with vertebrates (e.g. SIMON and LAMB, 1977), excellent. (2) Resolution improves with light adaptation (Fig. 21).

Take first the dependence of response amplitude upon stimulus frequency (Fig. 21). For the dark-adapted fly photoreceptor the amplitude is maximum at 6 Hz, but a response is still detectable at 50 Hz (ZETTLER, 1969). Light adaptation increases the response speed so that the frequency maximum is shifted to 16 Hz and responses at 150 Hz are resolvable. There is even one account of responses at over 250 Hz (LEUTSCHER-HAZELHOFF, 1975). The pronounced attenuation at low frequencies represents the intervention of light adaptation and emphasises the receptor's high pass filter properties.

The dependence of response phase lag on frequency and intensity is well documented for phase differences of less than one complete cycle (360°). In this phase region the response of the receptor lags behind the stimulus with a constant delay that is reduced by light adaptation (GEMPERLEIN and SMOLA, 1972a) (Fig. 21). A constant time delay is advantageous for monitoring moving stimuli. Were the delay to change significantly with stimulus frequency, the low spatial frequencies in patterns would become separated from the high as they swept across the retina. For phase lags greater than one cycle, there is disagreement between studies, due in no small part to the difficulties in resolving the small amplitudes of the responses produced at high frequencies. Using a white noise analysis, FRENCH and JÄRVILEHTO (1978a) find a clear phase asymptote at 450°, which they take to be indicative of a cascade amplifier with five stages. Averaging an unspecified number of cycles from sinusoidal responses, LEUTSCHER-HAZELHOFF (1975) could find no asymptote. Phase carried on increasing out to 600°. This discrepancy, which is of some importance for modelling of transduction, can only be resolved by a more extensive averaging of responses to high speed sinusoidal stimuli.

The other measures of temporal resolving power are more restricted in their application. The impulse response function is probably the most useful. Being simply the voltage response to a very brief (essentially instantaneous) flash, it is easy to produce experimentally, simple to average, and can be converted into the frequency response by Fourier transformation, providing that the response is small enough to lie in the linear range. Linearity is checked by the superposition of two flashes (LEUTSCHER-HAZELHOFF, 1975). This impulse response method should find wider application, especially for comparative studies where the highest accuracy is less important than the ability to get results quickly from many species.

The flicker fusion frequency is a yet simpler method, and has often been used to study the speed of the ERG response (e.g. AUTRUM, 1950, 1958). Because it uses stimuli of maximum contrast, the responses are usually non-linear and provide little information about the decline of response amplitude with frequency at the more natural lower contrasts. As an additional complicating factor, the actual value of fusion frequency depends upon the signal:noise ratio of the recordings. Consequently, flicker fusion frequency methods should be used with care.

The linear integration time of a photoreceptor is a specialised measure of temporal resolution that is useful, either to simplify the analysis of photon noise (LAUGHLIN, 1976a; SNYDER et al., 1977a; LILLY-WHITE and LAUGHLIN, 1979), or for comparison with the dependence of behavioural thresholds on the intensity and durations of stimuli (WASSERMAN and KONG, 1975). It is the largest time interval within which all incident light is treated by the photoreceptor as if it arrived at the same instant. Strictly speaking this interval must correspond to half the period of the upper cut off frequency. However, it is very difficult to detect small departures from linear temporal summation, because of the non-linear summation of response amplitudes, and the linear integration time is easily overestimated. In dark-adapted locust photoreceptors, the integration time is 20–30 ms (LILLYWHITE, 1978 b) and this compares with an upper cut off frequency of around 30 Hz (PINTER, 1972).

b) Factors Limiting Response Speed

Two classes of mechanism can limit the photoreceptor frequency response; the time course of the conductance changes initiated during transduction, and the impedances (active and passive) through which the resultant current flows. The available evidence suggests that the timing of conductance changes predominates, partly because the roles played by input impedance have received little attention. Both the finite duration of bumps, and their latency scatter, smear out the intensity signal in the time domain and, these two factors are reduced by light adaptation (Sect. E.II.3.c), in keeping with the improved frequency response (Fig. 21).

The Fourier transform of single bumps resembles the frequency response and the photoreceptor frequency response is worsened by cooling (FRENCH and JÄRVILEHTO, 1978 a), suggesting that time resolution is partially limited by the speed of the chemical reactions underlying transduction. The decrease in receptor response amplitude at low frequencies is unaccounted for, but the time course of the response decrement from peak to plateau (Fig. 18) suggests that the rapid phase of light adaptation contributes.

c) Are Changes in Response Speed Useful?

It is difficult to decide, at present, if the slowing down of response speed with dark adaptation is advantageous to the visual system, or is merely the unwanted consequence of increasing the transducer's gain to produce a detectable response to single photons. A decrease in temporal resolving power at lower intensities is found in many eyes, both vertebrate and invertebrate. The slow compound eyes have been associated with a high absolute sensitivity and this can be compared with analogue measuring devices where, at high sensitivity settings, a low pass filter is often used to provide a workable signal to noise ratio (AUTRUM, 1950). However, when one looks at the information recorded by photoreceptors, it is quite clear that a poor frequency response is disadvantageous. Information arrives as photon hits, and the quantity is limited by the number of photons and the accuracy with which their arrival times and probable origins are recorded by receptors. For spatial sampling, a compound eye can sacrifice spatial resolving power to gain more photons, and so increase the information available, but this argument is inapplicable to the time domain. Opening up a photoreceptor's acceptance angle increases the total photon catch, but smearing out photon signals in time does not. The optimum photoreceptor records the arrival time of every photon as accurately as possible, because when the signal is random, low pass filtering reduces signal and noise alike. By this argument, a poor frequency response is unwanted, and simply results from turning up the gain on a biochemical amplifier. A priori justification for the low pass filtering of noisy signals in photoreceptors must consider the aspects of intensity measurement which require a good voltage signal noise ratio in the receptor. For example, the eye may be very inefficient at filtering signals in the frequency

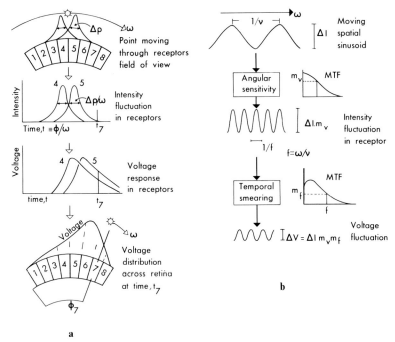

Fig. 22 a, b. The combined effects of spatial blurring and temporal smearing upon the resolution of moving objects by photoreceptor arrays, illustrated in two ways. **a** The voltage response to a moving point source is smeared across the retina. The moving point source generates a transient intensity signal in each receptor, which is transduced to a transient voltage response of longer duration (fluctuations and responses shown for two receptors only: 4 and 5). At any one time, i.e. time t_7, when the object is in front of receptor 7, several photoreceptors are responding to a point source. Based upon SRINIVASAN and BERNARD (1975). $\Delta\varrho =$ acceptance angle; $\omega =$ angular velocity of point source; $\phi_7 =$ angular position of point source at time t_7. **b** Analysis in terms of the response to a sinusoidal contrast grating, moved across the retina. The final modulation in receptors (ΔV) is predicted from the spatial modulation transfer function of the photoreceptor dioptrics, as determined by the angular sensitivity; and the temporal modulation transfer function for the photoreceptors, as determined from the frequency response (Fig. 21). This method is most useful for contrasts so small that the transducer behaves linearly. $\Delta I =$ intensity modulation in pattern, $\nu =$ spatial frequency (cycles per unit angle); $m_\nu =$ modulation transfer at spatial frequency ν; $m_f =$ temporal modulation transfer at frequency f; $\omega =$ angular velocity of grating

domain, for there is absolutely no evidence for any system having a well tuned frequency filter of the type that would be used by an electrical or audio engineer. Without sharp filtering the signal has to be extracted from noise over a wide range of frequencies, and an overall lowering of the receptor frequency response would be advantageous if the signal power is also greater at low frequencies. This second proviso is readily met at low intensities when the temporal modulations generated in receptors by object movement have their high frequency components attenuated by the optical blurring and an increase in receptor aperture. If we are to understand the function of receptors we must understand the range of operations that can be performed upon their outputs.

Whatever one's doubts are about the merits of low pass filtering, a good frequency response is advantageous at high intensities. Arguing from first principles, a high frequency response improves the channel capacity of a photoreceptor, as derived from SHANNON's equation [Eq. (E.12)], by allowing for more signal fluctuations per unit time. This is dramatically illustrated when frequency response data is plotted using a linear frequency ordinate (Fig. 21). In terms of information, the insects with fast compound eyes compensate for a lack of spatial acuity with temporal acuity, as suggested by AUTRUM (1958), but spatial acuity itself is not usually improved. Unless a scanning mechanism (Sect. E.II.7) is employed, spatial acuity is not increased beyond the level dictated by the photoreceptor spacing, and even scanning cannot improve upon the limitations imposed by the receptor angular sensitivity function (KIRSCHFELD, 1976).

The principal advantage of a fast response is that it helps resolve moving objects (SRINIVASAN and BERNARD, 1975). The sluggish responses of receptors smear a moving image across the retina. This type of effect is vividly seen when a small point source, such as flashlight, is waved around in the dark and appears to draw figures in the air with a luminous line. The point source may only be in front of a single receptor for two or three milliseconds, yet the response lasts several times longer and at any instant, the image of the point source is represented in several consecutive points in the retina (Fig. 22). This temporal smearing is similar to the blurring of objects by the optics, but it is the receptor potential which is spread across the retina and not light intensity. The effects of temporal smearing can be analysed by considering the resolution of point sources (SRINIVASAN and BERNARD, 1975), or by considering sinusoidal stimuli and converting every spatial sinusoid via velocity into a temporal intensity modulation and then passing this through the photoreceptor's frequency response (Fig. 22). Alternatively one can use a simple and elegant approximation (conceptual method). The angular sensitivity of the photoreceptor is widened by an amount equal to the product of angular velocity and the half-time of the gaussian approximation of the receptor's impulse response (SNYDER, 1977). Whichever method one uses, a receptor's sluggish response blurs out the spatial detail from moving objects. This goes a long way towards explaining AUTRUM's original observation that the ERGs of the fast flying insects had a better flicker fusion frequency than the slower ones (e.g. fly, cf. locust, Fig. 21).

7. Spatial Resolution

For the photoreceptor mosaic to represent the spatial distribution of intensity, each photoreceptor must have a restricted field of view. This field is described by the angular sensitivity function, which expresses the relative sensitivity of a photoreceptor to light incident from different directions (Fig. 23). The fundamental role played by angular sensitivity has been discussed in Sect. D.V.1. By accepting light from many directions, the receptor's light gathering apparatus blurs the image laid upon the receptor mosaic, and angular sensitivity sets a limit to the smallest resolvable separation of objects (Fig. 23). In compound eyes, the angular sensitivity can be related to the photoreceptor capture area and to the angle between photoreceptors. Thus three of the fundamental optical sampling parameters, blurring, receptor spacing and quantum catch, are often interdependent and the theoretical evaluation of their interactions (SNYDER, 1977; SNYDER et al., 1977 a, b) has allowed us to place the optical sampling characteristics of compound eyes within a functional setting (SNYDER, 1979). We will examine the influence of angular sensitivity on the voltage signal within photoreceptors, and the possible roles that photoreceptors play in limiting spatial resolution.

In the majority of compound eyes examined, the angular sensitivity is a triangular or bell-shaped function (Fig. 23) that is often approximated by a gaussian curve (e.g. GÖTZ, 1964). The width of the function at its half height is defined as the acceptance angle. Because most studies have been made upon apposition eyes, there is insufficient data to relate the shapes of angular sensitivity functions to the different types of optical systems used to gather light within receptors (e.g. Fig. 23).

Angular sensitivity plays an important part in determining spatial acuity, and in doing so interacts with other parameters, principally the receptor response speed, noise level and angular spacing. By blurring the retinal image the angular sensitivity reduces the depth of signal available to the receptors from a contrast pattern – the wider the acceptance angle the shallower the modulation (GÖTZ, 1964; 1965). Modulation amplitude is also influenced by the temporal frequency response. Compared to a stationary object, slow movements *enhance* the depth of modulation in the neural image by avoiding the depressing influence of light adaptation, while too rapid a motion leads to a loss of detail through temporal smearing (Figs. 19 and 21).

How does the depth of voltage modulation within the neural image influence spatial acuity? If detail in an object is to be seen, the corresponding modulations in the neural image must be detectable. At high intensities, when the neural image is relatively noise free, central mechanisms probably determine the minimum detectable voltage modulation. In this case, angular sensitivity and response speed are of great importance because they determine the depth of voltage modulation in the neural image. At low intensities one would guess that the noise within the neural image limits resolution. This hypothesis has not been tested directly at the neural image response level but it has been suggested for the optical image by KIRSCHFELD and WENK (1976). They find that the ability of male simuliid flies to detect overflying females is determined by photon noise at low intensities, and lens diffraction, the upper limit of acceptance angle, at high intensities.

The remaining factor, receptor spacing or granularity (Sect. D.V.1.a), has no direct influence upon the depth of voltage modulation induced in single receptors by moving objects. It determines the angular size of the smallest details that can be mapped unambiguously onto the retinal mosaic and this relationship has been extensively explored both theoretically and experimentally (SNYDER, 1977, 1979; BUCHNER, 1976). The granularity of receptors should be matched to the other quality factors in the neural image because there is little advantage to be gained from placing receptors closer together than the smallest detail that can be resolved, after optical blurring and noise contamination. In addition, as a general principle of economy, one should try to get the most out of the receptors one uses. Receptors are expensive to fuel and maintain, and each ommatidium requires a set of neurons in each of four subsequent neuropiles, to process the information it receives. A simple way to derive the minimum useful receptor density is to look at two-point resolution. For two points to be told apart, three receptors are used, one for each point and one to resolve the gap between (Fig. 23). Consider first the minimum om-

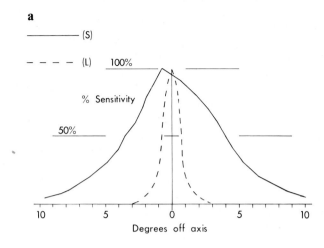

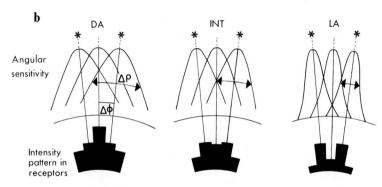

Fig. 23a, b. Spatial resolution in the compound eye. **a** Angular sensitivity functions for two eyes with different optics. S = skipper butterfly, refracting superposition eye, dark adapted (Horridge et al., 1972). L = locust, apposition eye, light adapted (Wilson, 1975). **b** The change of acceptance angle with adaptation, observed in the fovea of the praying mantis (after Rossel, 1979). DA = at fully dark adapted state at night; INT = intermediate state, LA = fully light adapted condition during the day. These functions, together with the measured acceptance angles, are used to illustrate the dependence of two point resolution upon the ratio between the acceptance angle, $\Delta\varrho$, and the interommatidial angle, $\Delta\phi$. Note that when the ratio $\Delta\varrho/\Delta\phi$ is reduced, the contrast transferred from two points is increased. Angular magnification in drawing is $\times 10$

matidial separation dictated by optical blurring, as expressed by the acceptance angle, $\Delta\varrho$. When trying to resolve points separated by less than $\Delta\varrho$ the centre receptor is more strongly stimulated than its neighbours, so the image is of a single larger spot (Fig. 23 b, DA). The gap between points just becomes apparent when the spacing is slightly greater than $\Delta\varrho$ (Fig. 23 b, INT). Consequently the upper limit for receptor spacing is about half the acceptance angle. If noise is present, the trough represented by the middle receptor must be deeper, if the gap between points is to be resolved, and this requires that the receptors are moved further apart (Fig. 23 b LA). Any temporal smearing will also reduce the depth of the trough and, in the presence of noise, force the receptors still wider apart. The conclusion, that acceptance angle determines the maximum density of receptors, was first formulated by considering two point resolution and applying the Rayleigh criterion for diffraction limited resolution, and provided the first indication that the physical size of a compound eye limits acuity by fixing a maximum usable number of ommatidia (KIRSCHFELD, 1976; SNYDER, 1979). The suggestion that receptor noise and blurring through motion demand a wider receptor spacing is more recent, coming largely from the theoretical work of SNYDER and his colleagues (SNYDER, 1979). To support this argument, diurnal dragonflies which hover, have their receptors spaced close to the limit imposed by diffraction, with $\Delta\varrho/\Delta\phi=2$, but dragonflies which hunt at dusk, when photon noise worsens, have their ommatidia spaced further apart (HORRIDGE, 1978b). In some flies the ratio of acceptance angle to interommatidial angle is commonly one or less (KIRSCHFELD, 1976) and this wide spacing has been correlated with the temporal smearing that occurs during rapid turns (SNYDER, 1977). By comparison, the mantis, an animal that hunts during the day from a stationary position has a ratio of $\Delta\varrho/\Delta\phi \simeq 1$ over the entire eye surface, despite extensive changes in the actual values of $\Delta\varrho$ and $\Delta\phi$ (ROSSEL, 1979). This leads one to search for additional advantages for having a very narrow acceptance angle, sampling fine spatial detail that the receptor mosaic cannot represent. ROSSEL (personal communication), suggests that such a narrow acceptance angle helps the mantis to track prey by increasing the size of the voltage fluctuations set up by small objects sweeping across the visual field. Such arguments for improved contrast resolution lead one to an important general point which has yet to be tackled theoretically. All previous theoretical studies of eye design (SNYDER, 1979) have looked at the performance of unit areas of retina or volumes of eye. If one fixes, instead, the number of receptors, then a narrowing of their acceptance angles improves their contrast resolution. Thus a fixed number of receptors is used with greater effectiveness because each receptor receives a wider contrast range. In this sense, the maximisation of available signal power in receptors, first proposed by GÖTZ (1965), can be justified by stipulating economy of ommatidia.

The additional contrast detail obtained by narrowing $\Delta\varrho$ so that $\Delta\varrho/\Delta\phi<2$ brings attendant dangers. The modulations set up by small objects, spatial details smaller than $\Delta\phi$, are still mapped out onto the retina and so appear as if they came from larger ones. These are aliasing errors and they generate spurious outputs, an example of which is the apparent reversal of the direction of moving gratings presented to flies when the stripe width is less than one interommatidial angle (VON GAVEL, 1939; HASSENSTEIN, 1951; GÖTZ, 1964). Although many accounts of optical and electrical sampling techniques warn of the perils of aliasing, insects seem to live quite happily with it (SNYDER, 1979). Either aliasing is tolerable, or insects use special processing strategies at a higher level to suppress it. For example, a conceptually simple, but practically difficult, strategy, is to scan the eye across the object, as suggested by KIRSCHFELD (1976). Imagine that the eye takes a snapshot and then rotates by half an interommatidial angle to take another. The two snapshots combined are now equivalent to a single picture taken by an array with twice as many photoreceptors, and the receptor spacing is effectively halved. Although crab eyes scan, their movement is insufficient to improve the receptor grain in this way (SANDEMAN, 1978) and scanning mechanisms have yet to be demonstrated in insects. However, scanning illustrates a principle; object movement can be used to improve resolution so that movement detection and form vision can, theoretically, be interrelated.

In conclusion, both the acceptance angle, interommatidial angle and photon catch interact to determine the quality of the optical image available in the rhabdomeres. However, a complete study of the receptors should also examine their intensity/response functions and their range sensitivities because, through contrast efficiency, these determine depth of voltage modulations of the neural image. These parameters can then be measured (e.g. ROSSEL, 1979) and placed within a theoretical framework which evaluates their interrelationship against a metric of performance (e.g. smallest resolvable sinusoidal grating, information capacity). The difficulty is to provide a metric that is relevant to the animal in question, which not only assesses the behavioural tasks, and the neural processing underlying visual discrimination, but also takes into account the structural restrictions imposed by ontogeny and the total energy budget of an animal. Despite such an imposing challenge, the recent comparative studies of compound eye design (HORRIDGE, 1977; 1978 b) illustrate that the adaptive radiation of compound eyes is as rich and fascinating as that of vertebrate eyes (WALLS, 1942) and is capable of raising many new questions about eye function.

8. Photoreceptor Interactions

Throughout the preceding accounts of receptor sensitivities, it has been assumed that each photoreceptor is electrically isolated from its neighbours. In fact, in several compound eyes, two types of photoreceptor interaction have been described or inferred; positive electrical coupling by which receptors share their signals, as if they were connected by a low resistance pathway; and inhibitory coupling, related to extracellular field potentials. These interactions, and their significance, will be discussed in turn.

a) Electrical Coupling

By simultaneously impaling two cells in a single *Limulus* ommatidium, passing current into one, and observing the voltage generated in the other, SMITH and BAUMANN (1969) showed that *Limulus* photoreceptors are electrically coupled (Sect. D.III). SHAW (1969 a) performed similar, but technically far more challenging experiments, in the compound eyes of drone bee and locust and found that photoreceptors in single ommatidia are electrically coupled. The stronger coupling of drone cells (ratio of 1.0:0.53, cf. 1.0:0.15 in locust) accounted for their lower PS. The differences in coupling ratios of cells in the same eye could be explained by the difference in distance between cells in the same ommatidium. Some pairs of cells were adjacent to each other, and others were one or two cells removed from each other. At the same time, SCHOLES (1969) found that positive potentials, recorded in the fly lamina, had the waveform expected of photoreceptor axons, but were driven by illumination of any one of the six facets sending axons to a single neurommatidium (Sect. E.III.1.b). This led to the suggestion that the axons of fly photoreceptors are electrically coupled. In support of this hypothesis KIRSCHFELD (1966) had already shown that such lamina potentials had lower noise levels. His shot noise analysis suggested that they represented a photon catch six times greater than that of individual receptors. This improvement in signal to noise ratio was confirmed by GEMPERLEIN and SMOLA (1972b), who presented this as further evidence for the electrical coupling of axons.

These earlier descriptions of coupling were the subject of some debate (e.g. AUTRUM and VON ZWEHL, 1964; SNYDER et al., 1973; LAUGHLIN, 1974a) because the technical difficulties of double recordings raise the possibility of cell damage, and the recording site of lamina positive potentials is ambiguous, but coupling has recently been confirmed. In locusts, LILLYWHITE (1978a) observed that for some cells the normal large quantum bumps were accompanied by more numerous and longer lasting bumps of much smaller amplitudes. Their relative frequencies and polarisation sensitivities suggest that each small bump corresponds to a large bump generated in a nearby receptor. The coupling ratios estimated from the relative amplitudes of large and small bumps, fall within the range of SHAW's direct measurements. For fly photoreceptors RIBI (1978) has found a possible coupling site in the lamina – gap junctions between the six receptor axon terminals in each cartridge. Recordings made from cell bodies in the retina confirm that the receptors converging to a single neurommatidium are coupled, but when recorded at this distance from the axon terminals the interactions appear much weaker than they really are (SHAW, personal communication).

No comparable coupling site has been identified in the retinae of other species, although PERRELET (1970) suggests that the close apposition of microvilli may lead to coupling (see also SNYDER et al., 1973). Electrical coupling via the tips of microvilli was also suggested by MULLER (1973) because his double recordings from crayfish ommatidia showed that coupled cells always had the same PS. In this crustacean rhabdom the cells with parallel microvilli lie opposite each other. MULLER's pairs of cells showed unity coupling ratios and the noise within them correlated strongly. Consequently, in the absence of other controls, one can just as easily conclude that this complete coupling is an artefact caused by the double penetration of a single cell. In the pairs of cells which, judging from their spectral sensitivity or PS must have been different, there was no coupling. The case for coupling via microvilli remains open.

A common observation, that insect and crustacean photoreceptors have broad spectral sensitivities, and low PS, suggests that the electrical coupling of photoreceptors is widespread (SNYDER et al., 1973). It is not universal because some locust photoreceptors showed no small bumps at all (LILLYWHITE, 1978a) and cells such as the UV-PS cells of dragonfly show the spectral sensitivity and PS associated with a single pigment in one rhabdomere (LAUGHLIN, 1976a), despite being located in the distal retina where five cells contribute to the rhabdom (LAUGHLIN and McGINNESS, 1978). Consequently, electrical coupling need not be the inevitable consequence of the close spacing of receptors around the rhabdom. Given that frog rods are interconnected (FAIN et al., 1976), electrical coupling must be a design strategy of some significance. Several suggestions have been made towards this end.

FAIN (1975) proposed that, because electrical coupling diverts single photon signals through many synapses, single photon events in receptors have more chance of being detected. This mechanism only works if regenerative mechanisms in receptors amplify small signals, or if subsequent non-linearities in transmission transmit small signals with a gain greater than for larger ones (Fain et al., 1976; Lillywhite, 1978a). Electrical coupling also improves the signal to noise ratio in receptors (Gemperlein and Smola, 1972b; Smola, 1976) but, because photoreceptors with the same field of view sum their signals postsynaptically, upon lamina interneurons, there is apparently little to be gained by electrical coupling (Laughlin, 1974a). However, Ribi (1978) has suggested that when synaptic transmission is non-linear, there are distinct advantages to be gained from improving the signal to noise ratio before synaptic transmission. By reducing the noise level the range of voltages experienced by the synapse is reduced and this minimises the distortions introduced by non-linearities. It also increases the response range available to the signal. Finally, electrical coupling could prevent an unequal weighting of receptors, resulting from the unequal development and growth of synapses from receptors to common interneurons.

b) Extracellular Interactions

In steady state conditions, the flow of photocurrent into a receptor must be accompanied by an equal current outflow, and a return of this current to its origin, in the extracellular space adjacent to the site of transduction (Fig. 24). The return current will set up a voltage across any resistance barrier that it encounters. These simple facts have long been exploited to measure extracellular ERGs from the retina (e.g. Heisenberg, 1971) but until recently (Shaw, 1975, 1978b) its full significance has not been appreciated or explored. The thorough analysis of extracellular resistance and light induced extracellular potentials shows that, in locust, the retina is isolated from the lamina and the body cavity by a substantial resistance barrier, located just beneath the basement membrane (Shaw, 1975, 1978a). Photocurrent entering the photoreceptors hyperpolarises the surrounding extracellular space because it has to return either across this barrier, or across the membranes of adjacent and less strongly stimulated receptors (Fig. 24). This light induced hyperpolarisation of the retina's extracellular space, relative to the body cavity, has often been observed and can reach an amplitude of at least 10 mV (Mote, 1970a; Muller, 1973). The hyperpolarisation of adjacent and less stimulated photoreceptors was demonstrated directly, by recording from a receptor whose corneal facet was covered by a mask, and strongly illuminating a patch of surrounding ommatidia (Shaw, 1975). A similar hyperpolarisation is seen in the UV cells of worker bee retina, when the surrounding green and blue sensitive receptors are stimulated with longer wavelengths (Menzel and Blakers, 1976).

Menzel and Blakers (1976) suggested that the hyperpolarisation of their UV cell showed that it was inhibited by the longer wavelength receptors. Unfortunately, one cannot assess these extracellularly mediated effects by looking at the retina in isolation. One must analyse the complete circuit for return currents (e.g. Shaw, 1975) because the potentials set up by return currents can bias recordings made relative to a distant indifferent electrode in the body cavity. More importantly, the return current can alter the potential across the presynaptic terminals of the photoreceptors (Shaw, 1975) as it passes through the receptors on its way back to the retina (Fig. 24). Shaw (1975) demonstrated this effect by showing that when a photoreceptor was hyperpolarised relative to the body cavity, it was depolarised rela-

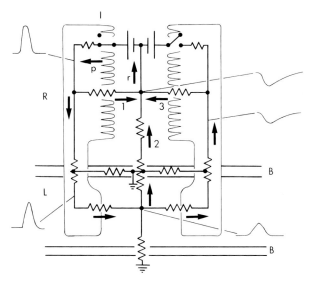

Fig. 24. The extra- and intracellular current flows induced in the retina *(R)* and lamina *(L)* of locust by stimulating receptors. The voltage responses to a light flash, recorded relative to earth, are shown alongside (after SHAW, 1975). Photocurrent *(p)* enters an active receptor, and induces an equal return current *(r)* in the surrounding extracellular space. The return current is provided by leakage from active receptors in either the retina, 1, or in the lamina. The lamina current either returns directly across the resistance barrier separating the two compartments, 2, or through the axon and cell body of a less strongly depolarised receptor, 3. The inversion of the response in the unstimulated receptor (RHS) results from there being an earth within the resistance barrier (SHAW, 1975). Note the light induced depolarisation of the lamina's extracellular space *(bottom right)*

tive to the retina's extracellular space, thus showing that return current was flowing up its axon (Fig. 24). Evidently strongly stimulated photoreceptors can inhibit the weak by driving current back up their lamina terminals but, to be potent, this effect requires a large differential in response (SHAW, 1975). The influence of this extracellular lateral inhibition on the smaller amplitude and more rapidly fluctuating potentials that constitute much of the receptor signal, still needs to be assessed. Nonetheless the extracellular potentials set up in the lamina must play an important role in setting the sensitivity of synapses in the lamina, and we will return to this in Sect. E.III.

Finally, by dye injecting large numbers of receptors in the worker bee retina, and measuring their spectral sensitivities, it was found that the colour types with broader spectral sensitivities had longer axon terminals in the lamina. This led to the proposal (MENZEL and BLAKERS, 1976) that positive electrical coupling in the retina results from a massive return current flow through axons. If this is so the pattern of retinal resistances in worker bee must differ from locust. Moreover, although apparently positive in the retina, the electrical coupling will really be inhibitory at the lamina synapses. Such uncertainties, and the fact that potentials recorded in the retina relative to an earth in the body cavity, need not represent, either the effects of transduction, or the presynaptic signal, emphasises the significance of extracellular currents.

9. Signal Transmission to the Lamina

Most of the available evidence suggests that the receptor potential is conducted passively, down the receptor axons, to its terminal in the lamina or the medulla. Direct recordings from photoreceptor axons (ZETTLER and JÄRVILEHTO, 1970, 1973; IOANNIDES and WALCOTT, 1971; SMOLA and GEMPERLEIN, 1972) show that the light induced signal is similar in shape to the receptor potential recorded in the retina, but is slightly smoothed in waveform and attenuated in amplitude (see also LAUGHLIN, 1974a). The intensity/response function recorded in the axons has a slightly depressed slope, and this may be due to the attenuation of high frequency components by passive transmission (IOANNIDES and WALCOTT, 1971). Because most insect photoreceptor axons are shorter than those of barnacle photoreceptors or of ocellar L-neurons, no specialised high resistance properties have been postulated for the membrane, although SHAW (1978b) points out that extracellular resistance barriers will help prevent attenuation.

Finally, it must be emphasised that the types of extensive biophysical measurement performed on barnacle photoreceptors, and locust ocellar L-neurons, have so far been precluded in insect retina, by the axons' small diameters (1–4 μm). The membrane of the axon terminal is certainly specialised because in fly (Fig. 26) and dragonfly the receptor terminals are postsynaptic to several interneurons (STRAUS-FELD, 1976a; ARMETT-KIBEL et al., 1977). There are also voltage sensitive channels in some species. Action potentials are recorded in the receptor soma of drone bees and probably originate in the axon (SHAW, 1969a), while light induced action potentials, which are severely attenuated and appear to originate at a distant site, are also seen in the axons of the dragonfly UV-PS cell (LAUGHLIN, 1974a). Given the regional specialisations of the receptor membrane seen in barnacle photoreceptors, it may be a dangerous oversimplification to think of the retinula cell's axon terminal as a simple closed cable.

10. Principles and Performance

The previous sections have shown how the retina's ability to present a neural image to the brain is constrained by a number of factors associated with the gathering and transduction of light. These include the well known optical limitations of angular sensitivity, interommatidial angle and photon catch (SNYDER, 1979), and the relatively unexplored parameters associated with transduction – namely non-linear summation, transducer noise, response speed and their modification through light and dark adaptation. The relationships between these quality factors, the structure of the retina and its measurement capabilities suggest that a compound eye is carefully organised in an endeavour to maximise its ability to present good neural images over a wide intensity range. Such matchings of structure to function are most important principles. They convert the description of structure and transfer functions into an appreciation of how the visual system works. Let us consider some proven and some possible examples. At the molecular level of membrane architecture, the dichroic rhodopsin molecules are often aligned within microvilli to ensure that the entire receptor absorbs the maximum number of photons with the minimum number of photopigment molecules (SHAW, 1969 b; SNYDER and LAUGHLIN, 1975). At the level of transduction, our discussions of intensity coding have suggested that voltage and conductance gain are carefully regulated to ensure that cells of different colour type operate at similar voltages within the same retina, despite receiving different mean quantum catches; that a quantum bump is produced whose amplitude is appropriate for the type of processing employed in the optic lobe; and that voltage gain is traded for response speed. At the organ level, light adaptation is a complex of interrelated processes involving the control of transducer gain, and the optical properties of receptors, cone cells and pigment cells. These are adjusted, in concert, over a wide intensity range to ensure that angular sensitivity, photon catch and range sensitivity provide a neural image with the best signal to noise ratio. Last and not least, developmental processes ensure that the spatial sampling characteristics and spectral sensitivity of the retina are regulated over the entire eye surface so that specific regions can be specialised for particular functions (e.g. blue sensitive dorsal retina for looking at the sky – rev. LAUGHLIN and McGINNESS, 1978; STAVENGA, 1979) and foveas (HORRIDGE, 1978 b; SHERK, 1977, 1978 b). Quite remarkably, these optical eye parameters can be varied throughout development to accommodate changes in eye size and visual habits (SHERK, 1978 a, c).

No matter how sensible they appear, many of these design principles are hypotheses, begging substantiation. How can we avoid fallacies of the type "Everything that is must be, because it is?" In as much as one can ever hope to achieve a definitive explanation of the design of a biological system, the solution to this tautology comes from relating the quality of the neural image to the capability of the entire visual system. We must correlate receptor transfer functions with visual thresholds to discover the limitations that the neural image places upon vision. If we find that factors such as increment sensitivity or temporal smearing curtail acuity then an interpretation of retinal organisation in terms of some design principles which minimise these constraints, is valid.

A few examples of correlations of receptor performance with visual behaviour can be given from the available data. These illustrate the types of questions that one can ask, and the utility of the answers one derives. The correlation of spatial acuity with the optical parameter, interommatidial angle, has been thoroughly investigated in muscoid flies. The smallest correctly resolved spatial frequency is set by receptor spacing, and narrower gratings appear to rotate in the wrong direction, due to aliasing (e.g. BUCHNER, 1976). Measured acceptance angles have not been correlated with contrast resolution in any species. The effective contrast transfer function of the entire visual system has been measured from the fall-off of contrast resolution with increased spatial frequency (e.g. GÖTZ, 1964; THORSON, 1966; WEHNER, 1975). For the locust *Schistocerca*, THORSON (1966) found that the fall-off in contrast resolution implied a receptor point spread function of half width 2–3°, and this agreed with acceptance angles measured electrophysiologically. Refinement of techniques led to a narrower physiological measure of acceptance angle 1.5° in *Locusta* (WILSON, 1975), which raises the possibility that the modulation transfer function of photoreceptors does not limit spatial acuity in the optomotor reflex. If this is so, the optomotor response does not test the full spatial acuity of the receptor mosaic, and highlights the problems associated with developing satisfactory behavioural tests to exploit the full capacity of the visual system, and give animals the motivation to use the full capacity. For this reason the study of the pursuit of prospective mates should continue to provide excellent assays for acuity (COLLETT and LAND, 1975; KIRSCHFELD and WENK, 1976).

The effects of transduction on resolution are poorly understood. In a pioneer correlative study, GLANTZ (1971) showed that the increment thresholds of higher order neurons in the crayfish optic tract were determined by the increment sensitivity of receptors over a wide intensity range. This emphasises the importance of maximising increment sensitivity in the face of non-linear summation. It is also apparent that small receptor signals generate behavioural responses. The minimum detectable contrast in fly optomotor responses is 0.005 for light adapted *Musca* (FERMI and REICHARDT, 1963). If one assumes that, as in *Calliphora*, the maximum value of photoreceptor contrast efficiency is 40% V_{max} per log unit and V_{max} is 60 mV (LAUGHLIN and HARDIE, 1978; HARDIE, 1979), then the corresponding threshold modulation in single receptor outputs is about 0.1 mV. This shows that as in barnacle photoreceptors (SHAW, 1972; Sect. D.VIII), insect retinula cells pass small signals across the first synapse and these are resolved at the highest level. As for the limitations imposed by transduction on temporal resolution, AUTRUM and STÖCKER (1952) showed that flies still resolved movements when individual receptor signals were modulating at 200 Hz and they correlated this with the flicker fusion frequency of the ERG. Their behavioural observations were confirmed by MCCANN and MACGINITIE (1965) who used extremely accurate stripe patterns containing negligible subharmonics, and these observations fit well with measurements of rapid turning and tracking during courtship behaviour (COLLETT and LAND, 1975). The actual blurring effects of motion, as outlined in Sect. E.II.6.c, have not been studied directly but the optomotor contrast threshold does increase rapidly with high rates of pattern flicker (e.g. MCCANN and MACGINITIE, 1965).

The inconclusive nature of these few examples drives home a major point. Although we can measure the transformations performed by the receptor mosaic with some precision, our grasp of receptor function is based upon commonsense interpretations of how a visual system should work, rather than knowledge of the receptors' roles in visual perception. The time is now ripe to correlate the receptor response properties and transfer functions, with behavioural thresholds, by recording directly the receptor mosaic's responses to threshold stimuli. These studies would help explain the forms of many threshold functions, and demonstrate the real limitations to vision that reside within receptors. Even in conditions where receptors alone are not restricting performance such correlations would peel off the receptor contribution to the overall transfer function of the visual system and so expose a different aspect to central performance.

III. The Lamina, a Neural Image Transformed

The lamina is the site of the first synaptic transformation of the receptors' neural image. Indeed the physiological analysis of lamina interneurons suggests that one of its prime functions is to maximise the transfer of object detail across the first synapse. It has proved possible to analyse this transfer rigorously because the lamina is a highly ordered neuropile, well suited to anatomical and physiological investigations at the cellular level. We will begin by looking at the neuroanatomy because this provides us with a wiring diagram which, through its unprecedented completeness and complexity, cries out for physiological analysis at the single cell level. We will then examine the physiological data to see how the retinal image is transformed, and how this transformation is related to the function of the arthropod compound eyes, and to general principles of vision.

1. Anatomy of the Lamina

When discussing the anatomy of the lamina, as it relates to the known physiology, one is usually discussing the lamina of *Musca*, and other muscoid flies, because it is in flies that the most comprehensive studies have been made. A limited amount of comparative data from other families of insects and Crustacea is included to emphasise that laminas show the same range of adaptation of structure to function as the retinas they serve.

a) Unit Structure

The lamina lies as a curved plate, beneath the retina, and is surrounded by a sheath of glial cells. In many cases, and in particular the apposition and neural superposition eyes of diurnal insects, the lamina is divided into a series of subunits, the lamina cartridges, and a patent sheath of epithelial glial cells can often be found, delineating each unit (fly, BOSCHEK, 1971; bee, RIBI, 1975, 1977; dragonfly, ARMETT-KIBEL et al., 1977). In any given eye region each cartridge contains an identical complement of neurons, and this redundancy greatly assists in the analysis of structure and function. The lamina consists of a restricted number of cell types, making a limited and regular set of connections. Consequently the same cell types are encountered repeatedly in one histological section or one electrode track. By comparison, some laminas show little or no evidence of a unit structure. In the firefly one can make out repeated groups of interneurons but there is no definite anatomical demarcation between groups (OHLY, 1975), while in cockroach lamina no unit structure is detectable (RIBI, 1977). In both cases the loss of cartridge structure is associated with an increased lateral spread of interneuron dendrites.

b) Retinotopic Projection of Photoreceptor Axons

All the projections that have been completely described, follow a pattern of great functional significance. The surface of the lamina is an ordered map of visual space, created by a projection of receptors with the same field of view to the same cartridge, or point on the lamina. Thus in the fused rhabdom apposition eyes of dragonfly, locust, the butterfly *Pieris* (HORRIDGE and MEINERTZHAGEN, 1970b; MEINERTZHAGEN, 1976), the crab *Scylla* (STOWE, 1977) and the small crustacean *Daphnia* (MACAGNO et al., 1973) all photoreceptors in the same ommatidium project to one lamina cartridge. This same pattern is seen in the superposition eyes of the skipper butterfly (MEINERTZHAGEN, 1976) and the male mayfly (WOLBURG-BUCHOLZ, 1977).

In the open rhabdom eyes of many muscoid flies, the spatial mapping of receptor signals onto the lamina requires a complicated pattern of projections. There are seven different rhabdomeres in each ommatidium, each looking in a different direction. Because the angle between rhabdomeres in one ommatidium equals the angle between adjacent ommatidia, there are seven rhabdomeres looking in the same direction, but situated in seven different ommatidia (STAVENGA, 1979). The projection of individual photoreceptor axons to the lamina ensures that all the receptors looking in the same direction project to one lamina cartridge, thus achieving a *neural superposition* of signals from one point in space (KIRSCHFELD, 1967; BRAITENBERG, 1967; TRUJILLO-CENÓZ and MELAMED, 1966). This strategy requires a complex pattern of receptor projections from any one ommatidium but the end result is worth it. Each neural cartridge in the lamina receives signals from rhabdomeres behind seven different lenses [or eight in the two equatorial facet rows where the two mirror symmetrical dorsal and ventral eye regions abutt – a fascinating complication (HORRIDGE and MEINERTZHAGEN, 1970a)]. Thus the photon count from each point in space is increased sevenfold (KIRSCHFELD, 1972), so achieving a substantial improvement in the photon signal:noise ratio. Consequently a neural superposition eye generally performs better than a standard apposition eye of the same dimensions (e.g. SNYDER et al., 1977b). The neural superposition eye is a beautiful example of the matching of structure to function in the nervous system. A highly desirable spatial transform is brought about through the directed growth of receptor axons. Any mistakes in the projection pattern will blur the neural superposition "image," just as lens aberrations blur an optical image, and it is not surprising that the neural wiring is extremely accurate (see Sect. E.III.1.d).

It is not certain that the fly uses the full potential of neural superposition, by summing receptor signals from all seven rhabdomeres looking in the same direction. The receptors with larger rhabdomeres, R 1–6, terminate in the lamina and sum onto large monopolar cells and T 1, the basket fibre (Fig. 26) but the two smaller receptors, R 7 and R 8, which make up the central rhabdomere, project to the medulla and have not been observed synapsing in the lamina.

The association of the two projection patterns with a difference in rhabdomere diameter has led to the notion of there being two receptor subsystems (e.g. KIRSCHFELD, 1972). The high sensitivity subsystem (HSS) is constituted through the lamina projection of R 1–6. The neural superposition of responses, and the larger rhabdomere diameter must give this system a photon catch that is many times greater than the corresponding R 7 and R 8 looking at the same point in space. On the other hand, R 7 and R 8, with their narrower rhabdomere should have higher angular sensitivity and they have been christened the HAS (high acuity subsystem). The central rhabdomeres' narrower acceptance angles have been confirmed by electrophysiological measurement (HARDIE, 1979). It has not proved possible to show that the two systems work independently, the HSS in dim conditions like rods, and the HAS under bright light, like cones. The change in spectral sensitivity of the optomotor response with light adaptation was initially ascribed to a changeover from HSS to HAS (ECKERT, 1971). It has since been found that *Drosophila* mutants, lacking the HAS system, show little impairment of optomotor response at high intensities (HEISENBERG and BUCHNER, 1977). Direct measurements of the sensitivities of R 1–6 and R 7 and R 8 emphasise just how tricky it can be to infer receptor properties from behavioural responses. The measured spectral sensitivities of R 7 and R 8 are incompatible with an either/or operation of the two subsystems: receptors R 1–6 are quite acute enough to respond strongly to the narrow stimulus patterns used at high intensities in ECKERT's experiments, and R 7 and R 8 produce large, albeit noisy, voltage responses at low intensities (HARDIE, 1979). Consequently the roles of the two pathways, which must differ in their sensitivities in the manner proposed by the two subsystem hypothesis, is as poorly defined as the medulla itself.

In other insects where receptor projections have been carefully examined there are usually six short fibres terminating in the lamina, and two or three long visual fibres projecting through the appropriate lamina cartridge, but continuing to the medulla (rev. MEINERTZHAGEN, 1976; and Chap. 1, this volume). In fly one of the long visual fibres, R 7, is both UV and weakly polarised light sensitive (e.g. HARDIE, 1979), and ingenious experiments, using stimuli directed to single rhabdomeres, indicated that the R 7/R 8 projection provided the substrate for a strong behavioural sensitivity to polarised light (KIRSCHFELD and LUTZ, 1974). In bee, one long visual fibre, the ninth cell, is the UV sensitive detector of polarised light, responsible for polarotaxis (MENZEL and SNYDER, 1974), while the other two are both UV sensitive (MENZEL and BLAKERS, 1976). Less conclusively, the long visual fibre identified in the dragonfly *Sympetrum* (ARMETT-KIBEL et al., 1977) is probably homologous to the UV and PS cell of *Hemicordulia* retina (LAUGHLIN and MCGINNESS, 1978). Thus a pattern could be emerging of a UV and polarisation sensitive pathway, direct from receptors to the medulla (WEHNER, 1976).

c) The Fly Lamina – a Highly Developed Wiring Diagram

A series of anatomical studies using silver and Golgi stains (CAJAL and SÁN-CHEZ, 1915; STRAUSFELD, 1971), electron microscopy (TRUJILLO-CENÓZ, 1965; TRUJILLO-CENÓZ and MELAMED, 1966; BOSCHEK, 1971; BURKHARDT and BRAITEN-BERG, 1976) and Golgi-EM (TRUJILLO-CENÓZ and MELAMED, 1970; CAMPOS-ORT-EGA and STRAUSFELD, 1973; STRAUSFELD and CAMPOS-ORTEGA, 1973 a, b) has given us an unprecedently detailed account of the fly lamina. Structurally, the lamina of *Musca* is one of the most completely described ganglia of any nervous system. Each cartridge is complicated, with 19 elements making regular and predictable contributions (STRAUSFELD, 1976 b). Eight are receptor axons, as discussed above, and five are the monopolar cells, L 1–5 (Fig. 25), with a distal cell body and a single axon projecting through the cartridge and across the chiasm to the medulla. The three spiny monopolars, L 1, L 2, and L 3 bear a dense brush of dendritic spines in the synaptic region of the lamina; L 1 and L 2 are almost indistinguishable in shape in the lamina but terminate at different levels in the medulla; L 4 and L 5 are smaller cells, with fewer spines and are termed smooth monopolars. The only lamina intrinsic cell, with dendrites entirely confined to the outer plexiform layer, is the amacrine cell (Fig. 25), which sends processes into at least 40 cartridges. The remaining cell types, the basket fibre, T 1, the centrifugals, ce and CE, and the tangential fibres, TAN 1 and TAN 2 (Fig. 25), are anatomically centrifugal because their cell bodies are located centrally, close to, or within the medulla. The five monopolar cells, the basket fibre and the two centrifugals are retinotopic elements projecting from each lamina cartridge to a single medulla cartridge, in the company of R 7 and R 8. L 4 also makes lateral connections with two adjoining cartridges. The amacrines and tangentials are extensive lateral elements and although their contributions to single cartridges are known, their distribution across the lamina has not been established.

The polarities and relative frequencies of lamina synaptic connections are shown in Fig. 26. This wiring diagram is taken from STRAUSFELD (1976 a, b) and STRAUSFELD and CAMPOS-ORTEGA (1977), and is based upon Golgi-EM studies. Until this work is complemented by extensive reconstructions from serial EM sec-

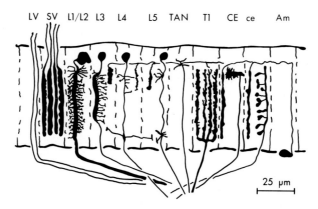

Fig. 25. The morphology of receptor axons and neural elements contributing to single lamina cartridges of the fly, *Musca*. For clarity the elements are distributed among several cartridges, two of the six short visual fibres have been omitted, and the pairs of cells, L 1 and L 2, and TAN 1 and TAN 2, are represented by the single elements, L 1/L 2, and TAN. *LV* = long visual fibres, R 7, 8; *SV* = short visual fibres from R 1–6; *L 1/L 2* and *L 3* = spiny monopolar cells; *L 4, L 5* = smooth monopolar cells; *TAN* = tangential fibre; *T 1* = basket fibre; *CE* and *ce* = centrifugal fibres; *Am* = lamina amacrine cell, note its spread into other cartridges. Drawing based upon the works of Strausfeld (1971, 1976 a)

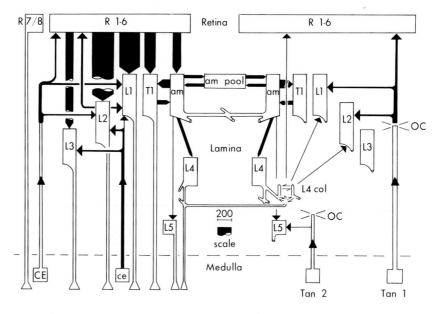

Fig. 26. The anatomical wiring diagram for lamina cartridges of the fly, *Musca*, showing the polarities and frequencies of synaptic contacts between neurons. *Intracartridge* pathways are shown in the left hand cartridge and *intercartridge* connections on the right. The width of *arrows* is proportional to the number of synapses reported by Strausfeld (1976 a, Tables 7.1 and 7.2) and the scale = 200 contacts. Connections are described in the text. *L 4 col* = collaterals from L 4 monopolar cells in adjacent cartridges; *OC* = tangential projections to other cartridges

tions, the list of connections cannot be regarded as exhaustive, and the synaptic frequencies can only be taken as a rough indicator of the strengths of pathways. Nonetheless the diagram is both impressive and revealing. The *intracartridge* connections are dominated by a massive throughput from the short visual fibres to the afferent interneurons, L 1, L 2, L 3, and T 1. In the upper lamina, each receptor forms many tetrads in which L 1, L 2, L 3 and an amacrine α-process are the four postsynaptic elements (BURKHARDT and BRAITENBERG, 1976). In the lower lamina the place of L 3 is taken by a glial element. A similar pattern of triadic connections and glial substitutions, have been found at dragonfly receptor → monopolar cell synapses (ARMETT-KIBEL et al. 1977). Some functional implications of dyads, triads, and tetrads are discussed in connection with the locust ocellus (Sect. C.II.4.c). The basket fibre, T 1, makes many separate contacts with receptor terminals and these are closely associated with synapses from the amacrine cell α-process (Fig. 26). Superimposed upon this dominant block of afferent synapses is a web of intracartridge feed-backs and lateral connections. The principal feed-back elements are the two centrifugals, ce and CE, but L 2 feeds back to the receptors and sideways to L 1. A similar feed-back and cross connection is made by one of the two large monopolar cells of the dragonfly's lamina cartridge (ARMETT-KIBEL et al., 1977). Note that, although L 1, L 2, L 3, and T 1 receive a substantial common input, the web of feed-backs and amacrine connections converts each of them into a unique parallel pathway.

The lateral or *intercartridge* connections are summarised on the right of Fig. 26, and most of these involve amacrine cells. Each cartridge contains α-processes from several amacrines, twining around the ascending basket fibre dendrites. The α-process is postsynaptic to receptor terminals and is both post- and presynaptic to the basket fibre. This could provide another powerful feed-forward interaction in a single cartridge, from receptors to basket fibres, via amacrines; and another feed-back from T 1 to amacrines (Fig. 26). In addition the amacrines could carry signals laterally. Every amacrine insinuates about 40 cartridges with at least one α-process, and amacrines covering the same areas form reciprocal synapses with each other. If one assumes that the lateral processes of amacrine cells sustain communication, and that the signals passed across amacrine-amacrine synapses are mutually supportive, then the amacrine system has the potential to pool receptor activity over many cartridges, and this lateral spread of signal would influence the responses of the basket fibre (STRAUSFELD and CAMPOS-ORTEGA, 1977).

The major lateral pathway powered by amacrines also involves the smooth monopolar cell L 4, which is the only fly monopolar cell to send processes to other cartridges. The axon of L 4 lies at the edge of the cartridge, and in the distal part of the cartridge it bears a small dendritic tree, receiving synaptic input from amacrine cells. At the proximal edge of the lamina, where its axon runs out towards the medulla, L 4 puts out three collaterals. One goes to the axis of its own cartridge, and the other two project along the x and y axes of the facet and cartridge mosaic, to the axes of two adjoining cartridges (Fig. 26). In each cartridge the three L 4 processes act as a unit, forming reciprocal synapses with each other, and synapsing onto the spiny monopolars, L 1, L 2, and the receptor axons R 1–6 (STRAUSFELD and CAMPOS-ORTEGA, 1973 b; STRAUSFELD, 1976 a). (Note the connection to receptors is not reported in STRAUSFELD, 1976 b or STRAUSFELD and CAMPOS-ORTEGA, 1977.)

Thus the input to L 4 might come from two lateral networks. The first is the amacrine pool and the second the L 4 collaterals. The collaterals then carry this lateral interaction to L 1, L 2, and receptor terminals. The significance of this two tier lateral network is unknown.

The remaining lateral pathways involve the two lamina tangential fibres. TAN 1 is strategically placed to modulate receptor input to the lamina, synapsing onto R1–6 axons at the top of the cartridge. It also contacts the spiny monopolars, L1–3, in this area. TAN 2 is presynaptic to L 5. This enigmatic smooth monopolar cell generates a retinotopic array of neurons, receiving two tiers of wide field input; one is afferent from the amacrines, and the other efferent, from TAN 1.

d) Diversity of Monopolar Cells

In the most general terms, the cell types of the laminas of compound eyes follow the pattern established in fly, and can be classified as monopolar cells, centrifugals, tangentials, amacrines, and long and short receptor axons (e.g. STRAUSFELD and BLEST, 1970). Only for the monopolar cells is the anatomy and physiology well enough understood to make a comparison between species worthwhile. In general, the Golgi studies find four or five monopolar cells in each species and these can be related to L 1–5 of muscoid flies. There are usually one or two large spiny monopolar cells, equivalent to L 1 and L 2 and in dragonfly (ARMETT-KIBEL et al., 1977), bee (RIBI, 1976), mayfly (WOLBURG-BUCHOLZ, 1977), and crayfish (NÄSSEL, 1977; NÄSSEL and WATERMAN, 1977) these cells run down the centre of the lamina cartridge and are postsynaptic to receptor axons. In the crab (STOWE et al., 1977), firefly (OHLY, 1975), in Lepidoptera (STRAUSFELD and BLEST, 1970), and in ants (WEHNER, 1976) similar spiny monopolar cells are found, but their position within the cartridge is not defined. Of the smaller monopolar cells, there is often a homologue of L 4, with a small proximal dendritic stump and proximal collaterals running to other cartridges [e.g. L 4 of bee (RIBI, 1977), M 5 in crayfish (NÄSSEL, 1977), and M 4 in firefly (OHLY, 1975)].

There are two major differences between the spiny monopolar cells of different species, which affect the organisation of the entire outer plexiform layer. These are the lateral spread of dendrites over a wide area of the lamina, corresponding to several cartridges, and the restriction of dendrites within one cartridge to a certain vertical level or layer of the lamina. A lateral spread, covering the inputs from more than ten ommatidia is seen in cockroach (RIBI, 1977), firefly (OHLY, 1975), and the privet hawk moth, in which a spread equivalent to one hundred ommatidia is described (STRAUSFELD and BLEST, 1970). In all cases these lateral projections of monopolar cell dendrites dissolve the cartridge structure. The occurrence of these wide field monopolar cells in nocturnal or crepuscular animals suggests that these interneurons are acting as spatial summation pools, and represent an adaptation for vision at low intensities (see Sect. E.II.4.a).

When the lamina is stratified, the divisions between layers are usually defined by the terminations of pairs of receptor axons. Some spiny monopolar cells restrict their dendrites to one or more layers, and this suggests that stratification is associated with the ordered segregation of receptors' outputs among interneurons, to generate colour or polarisation sensitive channels. Unfortunately no single study has produced a definitive correlation of receptor sensitivity characteristics with lamina connections but in bee, the stratification could divide blue and green receptor outputs among colour specific monopolar cells, while the UV receptors project to the medulla (MENZEL and BLAKERS, 1976; RIBI, 1977; rev. MENZEL, 1979). In crayfish, polarisation sensitivity may be segregated among two sets of stratified monopolar cells, each receiving inputs from receptors with the same polarisation sensitivity. Thus the two strata might generate two orthogonally sensitive channels (NÄSSEL and WATERMAN, 1977). The stratified laminas usually contain at least one spiny monopolar, equivalent to L 1 and/or L 2, which receives inputs from all the receptors terminating in one cartridge, e.g. dragonfly (ARMETT-KIBEL et al., 1977), bee (RIBI, 1977), crayfish (NÄSSEL and WATERMAN, 1977). In bee and dragonfly, intracellular recordings confirm that these cells are functioning as contrast coding channels, like L 1 and L 2 of fly (MENZEL, 1974; LAUGHLIN, 1976c; LAUGHLIN and HARDIE, 1978).

In conclusion, the limited data available to us shows the familiar pattern of a basic cellular organisation upon which is impressed a large number of structural variations, many of which can be related to different functional requirements. It is worth looking at this constancy and variability within the lamina in a little more detail, in the light of C.GOODMAN's findings from locust ocellus (C.GOODMAN, 1976; see also Chap. 3, this Handbook, Vol. VII/6C).

e) Constancy and Variability in the Lamina

An exhaustive study of ocellar interneurons suggests that the coexistence of constancy and variability is as much a characteristic of ganglia, as it is of any other structure capable of evolving. The lamina appears to conform to this principle. Although many studies of lamina structure have emphasised the precision with which a unit cartridge structure is replicated across the ganglion, there is little quantitative data on the accuracy with which cells and contacts are reproduced. This is partly because the complexity of wiring, and the large numbers of small cells, restrict the accuracy with which cell complement and connectivity can be analysed by simple methods. The two successful studies of constancy in the lamina have had to make laborious reconstructions of volumes of tract and neuropile, from thousands of sections. HORRIDGE and MEINERTZHAGEN (1970a) chose the neural superposition projection of fly photoreceptors as a suitable test pattern for studies of determinacy in the nervous system, because its complexity challenges developmental mechanisms. In the normal eye, all of the 650 axons traced from retina to lamina, projected to the correct cartridge, but errors were later encountered in eye regions where the ommatidial lattice was accidentally dislocated (MEINERTZHAGEN, 1972). MACAGNO et al. (1973) reconstructed the cyclopic retina and lamina of the small crustacean, *Daphnia*, principally because it contains just 286 cells, and because this organism is parthenogenetic, allowing one to compare isogenic individuals. Again, the comparison of many animals showed that a full and bilaterally symmetric complement of receptors and neurons was present, with the receptors all projecting to their correct cartridges and interneurons. Thus, both studies demonstrate that a complicated neuropile can be specified with a high degree of accuracy.

These painstaking analyses also detected small variations which did not disrupt the correct connectivity patterns. In the first projection of fly photoreceptors, there are axons entering the correct cartridge, but going to the wrong position within the ring of six terminals. In the *Daphnia* eye, although the receptors make correct connections to interneurons, each individual has an axon terminal of slightly different shape. This variation is similar to small differences in branching pattern observed in the locust ocellus and in insect motoneurons (see Sect. C.II.2). Nor are these the only sources of variability. Cartridges show small and consistent variations in cell size and shape across the lamina. In *Musca* the monopolar cell L4 has a thicker axon and more profuse proximal dendrites in the frontal eye region (Strausfeld and Campos-Ortega, 1973b), and the diameters of spiny monopolars also follow predictable gradients of size across the lamina, with L3 changing diameter independently of L1 and L2 (Braitenberg and Hauser-Holschuh, 1972). These differences suggest that certain aspects of cartridge structure can be modulated during development, to allow the lamina to match regional specialisations of the receptor mosaic. Some variability is also detected by comparing the connectivity patterns in related species. In *Musca*, both T1 and the amacrine cell, are postsynaptic to receptors R1–6 (Fig. 26) but in the fly *Lucilia* the amacrine is apparently presynaptic to receptors, and T1 is also predominantly presynaptic (Campos-Ortega and Strausfeld, 1973). This finding verifies an earlier and disputed finding from the same genus (Trujillo-Cenóz and Melamed, 1970).

The data from these few studies provides evidence for a continuous low level of variability that can be stabilised to generate evolutionary change. Does the lamina also provide the redundancy that facilitates change (see Sect. C.II.2)? In locust ocelli this redundancy is generated by duplications of single cells (C.Goodman, 1976), which allow for one member of a duplicate pair to sustain normal function while the other "experiments" with novel contacts. For the lamina, the evidence suggests that neuron duplications within single cartridges have played a minor role during its evolution. Despite a considerable structural diversity, the number of monopolar cells in each cartridge appears conservative, remaining at four or five. One cannot dismiss the possibility that duplications were used to acquire new connections, and the redundant duplicates then weeded out, but this hypothesis is made less attractive by the existence of two alternative sources of redundancy.

Closely related parallel pathways are one source of redundancy. For example, from the wiring diagram for *Musca* (Fig. 26) it is clear that L1, L2, and L3 receive a large element of common input from receptors, at tetrad synapses, and that their connectivity is similar to T1's. Consequently, any of these neurons could be drastically modified without necessarily reducing the amount of information crossing to the medulla. A second, and more important, source of redundancy is the repetition of cartridges. As we have seen, cartridges need not be slavishly reproduced across the lamina. In a situation where an animal can direct its gaze, a small area of the lamina can become specialised for a new function while neighbouring cartridges sustain the existing repertoire (providing that the function does not integrate over large numbers of cartridges). A similar redundancy also exists in the retina, where ommatidia are duplicated, and in the columnar structures of the medulla and lobula. This concept is probably applicable to many vertebrate eyes, where a columnar organisation is found in the cortex, and there are parallel pathways from the retina to the brain. Seen in this context, it is unfortunate that the regional specialisation of lamina cartridge structure has received little attention. Quantitative studies of variability among lamina cartridges, although technically demanding, could support the hypothesis that the redundancy found in arrays of sensory receptors and interneurons is an important catalyst for the remarkable adaptive radiation of visual systems. Given the increasing evidence for a columnar structure in the vertebrate cortex, this theory could find wider application.

2. Intracellular and Extracellular Potentials in the Lamina

a) Extracellular Potentials

A comprehensive series of experiments have measured extracellular resistance profiles and the distributions of dyes, radiotracers and electron dense markers to prove that the insect retina and lamina are separated from the haemolymph by a "blood-brain" or "blood-retina" barrier, and from each other by a barrier located just beneath the basement membrane, among pigmented glial cells. These barriers prevent the free diffusion of ions through the extracellular space and one must regard the retina and lamina as individual electrical and chemical compartments (SHAW, 1975, 1977, 1978 a).

In darkness the extracellular space of the lamina compartment is from 30 to 100 mV negative to both the haemolymph and the retina. Illumination of the receptors depolarises the lamina extracellular space by up to 50 mV (rev. LAUGHLIN, 1975 c). This lamina depolarisation is principally the result of photocurrent entering the lamina through receptor axons, and having to leave the lamina across resistance barriers (Fig. 24) (SHAW, 1975), consequently its intensity dependence and time course, is related to that of the receptors. An extracellular depolarisation might be a major inhibitory force because, by opposing the depolarisation of receptor terminals, it could curtail their transmitter release (LAUGHLIN, 1974 a; SHAW, 1975). To chart out this inhibitory influence we should describe the amplitude, time course, intensity dependence and spatial fields of the lamina depolarisation. Unfortunately this has not proved straightforward, because the extracellular compartment is a convoluted maze of clefts, narrower than the dendrites insinuating them, infiltrated by glia and occluded by intercellular junctions. It is not surprising that the interpretation of positive, light-induced potentials from the lamina is confused (LAUGHLIN, 1974 a). Recordings using large blunt electrodes report small depolarisations (LEUTSCHER-HAZELHOFF and KUIPER, 1964; HEISENBERG, 1971; cf. MOTE, 1970 a, b), perhaps because the blunt tips generate a cavity ringed by damaged cells, whose axons offer a spurious pathway from the lamina. The high resistance micropipettes used for intracellular recordings also produce a suspiciously broad spectrum of results and this could be due to the ease with which these electrodes confuse intra- and extracellular response. In fly lamina, MOTE (1970 a, b) recorded depolarisations of up to 50 mV, which resembled photoreceptor potentials, yet had a wider receptive field. In another study of fly lamina, SCHOLES (1969) mentioned wide field and smaller amplitude potentials, but confined his analysis to large potentials (ca. 50 mV), with narrow fields, and these probably corresponded to single photoreceptor axons. In dragonfly lamina a broad spectrum of depolarising responses was reported, with the obvious potentials from receptor axons at one extreme, and smoothed depolarising responses with wider receptive fields at the other (Figs. 27 and 29) (LAUGHLIN, 1974a). These latter responses were ascribed to the extracellular space, on the basis of their slower time constant and wider angular sensitivity. This contention is supported by the dye injection study of worker bee retina and lamina by MENZEL and BLAKERS (1976). They found slow potentials, with a narrow central part to their field and wide flank of lower sensitivity, similar to those reported in dragonfly (Fig. 29). They inferred an extracellular locus from the massive diffusion of dye (Procion Yellow) away from the injection site. To emphasise the difficulties encountered in monitoring these potentials, the recording described by MENZEL and BLAKERS (1976) slowly changed its sensitivity during the experiment. It began to acquire the characteristics of a UV photoreceptor axon, which was also partially stained by the dye injection. In summary, high resistance electrodes record a wide range of lamina responses, from receptor axons to extracellular potentials. Until improved techniques are developed for monitoring and marking the origins of extracellular potentials, we will have to guess at the receptive field characteristics of a very important influence in the lamina. The extracellular potentials undoubtedly bias intracellular recordings made in the lamina, relative to a distant earth (SHAW, 1978b) and this may explain why the dye injected axons of fly photoreceptors appear to have wider fields of view than their parent cell bodies (ZETTLER and WEILER, 1976).

b) Response of Lamina Interneurons

Of the ten or more types of lamina interneuron, only five have had their responses identified by intracellular recording and dye injection. The majority of cell markings have been made in the fly lamina, where the large monopolars, L1 and L2, and basket fibre, T1, the lamina amacrine cell, and the small monopolar cell, L4, have been intracellularly stained. The amacrine cell produces a noisy depolarisation on illumination (IOANNIDES, 1972) whereas L4 generates a train of action potentials, suggestive of ARNETT's (1972) "sustaining fibre" (HARDIE, 1978). In each case only one of these small cells was marked and the brief recording did not permit a characterisation of the cells receptive field and intensity/response function. T1 was also encountered once, but this was an excellent penetration, and the response was thoroughly investigated (JÄRVILEHTO and ZETTLER, 1973). The data accords with the lamina wiring diagram (Fig. 26). T1's hyperpolarising response is almost indistinguishable from L1 and L2 in waveform and latency, and the neuron has a narrow receptive field, indicative of inputs from receptors sharing the same field of view, and of lateral inhibition from amacrines, more powerful than that exerted on L1 and L2.

The two large spiny monopolar cells, L1 and L2, have been intracellularly stained in three genera of muscoid flies; *Calliphora* (AUTRUM et al., 1970; ZETTLER and JÄRVILEHTO, 1971; HARDIE, 1978), *Rutilia* (IOANNIDES, 1972), and *Phaenicia* (ARNETT, 1972). As far as we can tell at present, L1 and L2 have identical responses, as one might expect from their considerable shared input from receptors (Fig. 26). In darkness, the "resting" potential (measured relative to the extracellular space of the lamina) is small but a precise value is difficult to define. Reports

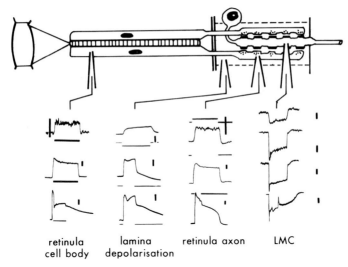

retinula   lamina   retinula axon   LMC
cell body   depolarisation

Fig. 27. Graded potentials recorded from the dragonfly lamina. Intracellular recordings from the retinula cell body, the retinula cell axon in the lamina, and the first order interneuron: the large monopolar cell, LMC. The lamina depolarisation is thought to be extracellular in origin. Responses to point sources of *approximately* equal intensities in each case, increasing from top to bottom. Note the smoothing of the extracellular response, and the amplification and transient nature of the LMC response. All stimuli are 500 ms in duration, range bars show 10 mV (LAUGHLIN, 1976b)

vary from $+20$ mV (ZETTLER and JÄRVILEHTO, 1971), through -5 mV (ZIMMERMAN, 1978) to -15 mV (LAUGHLIN and HARDIE, 1978). In all cases the resting membrane is really very active, even in darkness, displaying a consistent barrage of noise of up to 5 mV peak to peak amplitude. Illumination generates a large hyperpolarising response which is phasic at all but the lowest intensities, despite a tonic receptor input (Fig. 27). A brief, 10–20 ms, on transient, from 6 to 8 times larger than the corresponding receptor depolarisation, and of up to 30 mV saturated amplitude, is followed by a plateau phase of 0.5–1.0 s, during which time the hyperpolarising response decays to a steady level. When the light is extinguished, a depolarising off transient is generated (Figs. 27 and 28), and this is sometimes accompanied by a small and rapid spike-like depolarisation (ZETTLER and JÄRVILEHTO, 1971, 1973; LAUGHLIN and HARDIE, 1978). It is remarkable that the large ocellar neurons of insects show these same properties of a noisy resting membrane, amplified transient hyperpolarising response, and slow and fast depolarising off transients (Fig. 8).

The homologous large monopolar cells of dragonfly are similar to L 1 and L 2 in fly, although the hyperpolarising responses reach 50 mV in amplitude and represent an amplification of receptor input of $\times 14$ (LAUGHLIN, 1973). Essentially the same hyperpolarising response has been recorded from a large number of unidentified lamina units in locust (SHAW, 1968a), fly (SCHOLES, 1969; LAUGHLIN and HARDIE, 1978), dragonfly (LAUGHLIN, 1974b; LAUGHLIN and HARDIE, 1978), worker bee (MENZEL, 1974), and crab (ERBER and SANDEMAN, 1976). At the present time it is convenient to assign all these responses to a single physiological class of cells, the LMCs (large monopolar cells). This assumption is not as dangerous as

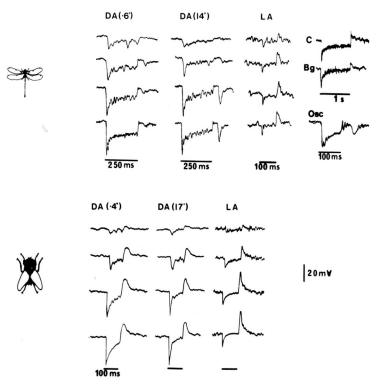

Fig. 28. The intracellular response waveforms of dragonfly and fly LMCs. Because of lateral inhibition the responses of dark adapted cells to a point source (DA 0.6° or 0.4°) decay less rapidly than the responses to wide angle stimuli (DA 14° or 17°). Light adaptation enhances both on and off transients *(LA)*. These responses are from a single cell in each animal. The effect of lateral inhibition in suppressing the sustained response is emphasised by comparing the prolonged response to a point source, centred in the visual field *(C)* with the response to a 14° background of the same luminous efficiency *(Bg)*. Some dragonfly LMC responses oscillate, e.g. *(Osc)* shows three superimposed responses. Stimulus durations are indicated below the responses and the range bar shows 20 mV for all recordings. From LAUGHLIN and HARDIE (1978)

it might first appear, for the following reasons. Extensive dye injection experiments show that of at least 24 hyperpolarising responses in the lamina all but one were from L1 or L2. The single exception was T1 (ZETTLER and JÄRVILEHTO, 1973; JÄRVILEHTO and ZETTLER, 1973). In addition all hyperpolarising units show the same responses to simple tests of waveform, sensitivity and receptive field. The one exception, MIMURA's unit (MIMURA, 1976), was easily distinguished by its enormous receptive field and UV sensitivity (see below). Thus, in this preliminary phase of investigation, the LMCs appear as a physiologically homogeneous class, which can be investigated more rapidly if we are freed from the necessity of marking and retrieving every recorded neuron. Ultimately we must return to marking experiments to see if there are significant differences between the parallel pathways, L1, L2, L3, and T1; but to make such an approach worthwhile we must first develop rapid and sensitive techniques for characterising small differences in receptive fields, response waveforms and intensity/response functions.

Additional pathways between the lamina and medulla of muscoid flies have been recorded from, but not identified anatomically. Two spiking units often occur in pairs with a regularity that suggests they are members of the retinotopic projections between lamina and medulla cartridges (ARNETT, 1972). Neither fibre shows a dark discharge. The ON-OFF fibre produces a transient response whenever a light spot is switched either on or off within its receptive field. Its field is elongated, with a horizontal half-width of 5.5° and a vertical of 4.4°. The ON-OFF fibre must receive an input from several cartridges. The other fibre, the sustaining unit is more complicated. The centre part of its receptive field corresponds to one cartridge and illumination of this region produces a sustained discharge. There are two antagonistic areas, each about the same size as the centre and on either side of it, along the horizontal axis. All three fields probably derive from adjacent cartridges along the z axis, but a definitive correlation of receptive fields with interommatidial angle and the acceptance function of each neuroommatidium, was not undertaken (ARNETT, 1972). The two antagonistic fields inhibit the sustaining discharge from the centre, and also generate transient off responses when a light is extinguished in either of their areas. The centre sustaining region is 1.3 log units more sensitive to a point source than the flanking off regions *and* the entire receptive field of the ON-OFF fibre. The fibres are part of the R 1–6 system, having no PS and the correct spectral sensitivity (McCANN and ARNETT, 1972) and they are probably centripetal because cutting through the first chiasm did not abolish their discharge (ARNETT, 1972). If one accepts this difficult lesion experiment and trusts both the anatomical wiring diagram (Fig. 26) and the conclusion that these fibres are retinotopic, then these units must be L 4 and L 5. All other fibres are either identified, centripetal, aperiodic or, in the case of L 3, so like L 1, L 2, and T 1 in their input that we can expect another hyperpolarising cell. This speculation agrees with HARDIE's single dye injection of L 4, but provides no ready anatomical explanation for the units' receptive fields, partly since L 4 does not project along the horizontal z axis. A resolution of this interesting possibility will depend upon a better correlation of the receptive fields with the ommatidial lattices and the acceptance angles, a correlation of thresholds with sensitivity among other members of the R 1–6 pathway through the lamina, and a further probing of the wiring diagram, perhaps guided by physiological interactions. This would provide a more complete account of the parallel pathways through each cartridge.

MIMURA (1974) has found additional spiking units in the first chiasm, with similar ON-OFF and centre-surround properties, but asymmetric receptive fields. In addition, he has characterised a hyperpolarising unit, identical in waveform, and sensitivity to point sources, with LMCs but with an enormous receptive field stretching over 50°, along each of three narrow arms. Between these arms are antagonistic depolarising areas which inhibit the light induced depolarisation. Because its hyperpolarising response is predominantly UV sensitive this input should come from the medulla, over a wide area of the medulla face, which makes TAN 1 and TAN 2 possible candidates.

3. The Neural Image Presented by the LMCs

In the lamina, the neural image in the photoreceptors is transformed into a neural image in the LMCs. This transformation is not so drastic as to render inappropriate the quality factors applied to the retinal neural image. It is still useful to view the LMC neural image as a fluctuating array of graded potentials, representing the distribution of intensity in space and time. Thus we will follow a line of argument similar to that applied to the receptors, looking at the spatial and intensity coding characteristics, noise levels and the temporal frequency responses of LMCs.

a) Spatial Coding Within the LMC Array

As expected from the orderly projections of axons from retina to lamina, each LMC has a narrow angular sensitivity function, similar to the receptor's but narrowed slightly by lateral inhibition (Fig. 29) (ZETTLER and JÄRVILEHTO, 1972). Lateral inhibition becomes more obvious when spots, bars or annuli of light are presented several degrees away from the axis, – the point of maximum sensitivity in

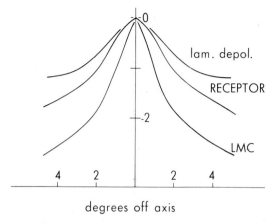

Fig. 29. Average angular sensitivity (in log units) for the lamina depolarisation, single photoreceptors (retinula cells), and the on transient of the LMC response. All data from dark-adapted dragonfly eye. The angular sensitivity of the single receptor represents the sensitivity of one ommatidium. The LMC angular sensitivity is compressed by lateral inhibition, while the extracellular lamina depolarisation has a wider field than one ommatidium (Laughlin, 1974b; 1976b)

the LMC's visual field. These off-axis stimuli elicit a small tonic depolarisation of the LMC (Laughlin, 1974b; Zettler and Weiler, 1976; Mimura, 1976), some of which may result from a passive pick up of the lamina extracellular response to light (Shaw, 1978b). Mimura (1976) finds that off-axis stimuli also decrease the sensitivity of the LMC to a test light on-axis, and that the inhibitory field is often asymmetrical about the axis. This asymmetry should be investigated in more detail because it could provide a useful functional difference between L1 and L2, producing a directionally selective response to moving stimuli. Although lateral inhibition affects the on transient response (Fig. 29), the angular sensitivity for small plateau responses (as measured 500 ms after stimulus onset) is much narrower, suggesting that lateral inhibition builds up over this longer time period (Laughlin, 1974b).

In summary, the spatial characteristics of the LMC neural image follow closely those of the receptor mosaic, with the same spacing or grain, and a similar narrow angular sensitivity at each point on the mosaic. The narrowing of the on transient field by lateral inhibition might give a slight emphasis to small angular displacements but this does not mean that the receptor mosaic's powers of resolution are improved upon. Information lost among the receptors cannot be retrieved. Lateral inhibition could improve the resolution of the entire visual system by helping to emphasise the small signals set up by fine detail, and making these signals more visible amid noise at higher levels, but the precise effects of lateral inhibition upon the spatial transfer properties of LMCs have yet to be established.

b) Intensity Coding by LMCs

As with photoreceptors, an outline of intensity coding characteristics can be obtained by plotting the $V/\log I$ curves (Fig. 30), derived from the responses to step intensity increments delivered in darkness, or increments and decrements superim-

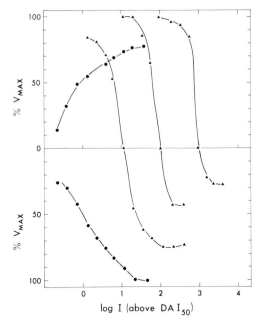

Fig. 30. Dark (●) and light adapted (▲) intensity/response functions for a fly LMC, plotted as $V/\log I$ curves. The absolute values of transient responses to step intensity changes, measured relative to the dark membrane potential, are plotted against the log of total intensity during the test stimulus. There is no standing background signal so that the zero intercepts of light adapted curves indicate the background intensities from which the sudden intensity increments or decrements were made. Intensity has been normalised relative to the intensity that produces a half maximal response in the dark adapted cell (DA $I_{50} = 1.3 \times 10^8$ quanta·cm^{-2}·s^{-1} from an axial point source of wavelength 484 nm). Voltage is expressed as a percentage of the maximum hyperpolarising response amplitude (mean $V_{max} = 30$ mV). In the dark adapted function the depolarising responses are from the off transient. From LAUGHLIN and HARDIE (1978) and HARDIE (1978)

posed upon maintained background levels of illumination (JÄRVILEHTO and ZETT-LER, 1971; LAUGHLIN, 1973; LAUGHLIN, 1975b). Unless stated otherwise, the data reviewed here comes from the most recent study on intensity coding (LAUGHLIN and HARDIE, 1978). This work gives a comprehensive description of receptor and LMC intensity/response functions over a 4 log unit range of background intensities, using wide angle adapting stimuli that represent natural conditions better than point sources, and it presents data from the retina and lamina of both fly and dragonfly. The responses and light adaptation properties of receptors and LMCs in these two animals are sufficiently similar for the results to be treated together.

In the dark-adapted LMC the amplification of receptor signal at the first synapse causes the LMC intensity/response function to rise more steeply than the receptor's, and compresses the dark-adapted dynamic range to about 2 log units of intensity (Fig. 30). This narrow range has led to the proposal that the rate of rise of LMC response amplitude, dV/dt, is a better metric of LMC signalling powers because, unlike the amplitude response, rate of rise does not easily saturate and increases over an intensity range of at least 6 log units. This argument suggests that LMCs are more efficient at coding the rate of change of intensity than intensity itself (JÄRVILEHTO and ZETTLER, 1971). It has since been found that highly effective light adaptation mechanisms prevent the saturation of the LMC amplitude response by high intensity backgrounds, thus nullifying any *a priori* argument for the coding of rate of change (LAUGHLIN, 1975b).

The light-adapted LMCs respond to changes in intensity, rather than absolute energy levels. After the application of a steady background intensity the membrane potential quickly returns to the dark level, when measured relative to the haemocoel, and small intensity increments and decrements produce large on and off responses according to a new light-adapted $V/\log I$ curve (Figs. 28 and 30). With no representation of background intensity, the light-adapted response amplitude can only code for intensity fluctuations relative to the background and it is in this sense that LMCs respond to change in intensity. This is not equivalent to responding to rate of change, it is more akin to coding contrast.

Both the shapes of the dark and light-adapted $V/\log I$ curves, and the spectral sensitivities of LMCs support this contrast coding hypothesis. The $V/\log I$ curves are approximately linear over much of their dynamic ranges, and this logarithmic relationship between intensity and response amounts to contrast coding (Sect. E.II.4.b). Moreover, amplification greatly increases the contrast efficiency of LMCs relative to the receptor input. Over the entire range of backgrounds investigated, the LMC contrast efficiency is consistently eight or ten times higher than the receptors' (Fig. 19a, cf. Fig. 30). As the receptor $V/\log I$ curves increase in slope with mean intensity (Fig. 19a), so do the LMC curves, with contrast efficiency rising from 70% V_{max}/log unit, when dark adapted, to over 250% V_{max}/log unit, when light adapted. Consequently the light adapted LMC is extremely sensitive to intensity fluctuations; a contrast of 0.1 produces a response of almost 10 mV. Note that the contrast efficiencies for on and off transients are the same: close to the background intensity (Fig. 30) so that small intensity increments and decrements are treated equally. As an inevitable consequence of this increased contrast efficiency, the LMC dynamic range about any one background decreases from about 2 log units, dark adapted, to about 1 log unit light adapted. For the light-adapted intensity/response function, as much as 80% of the response range is occupied by the responses to contrasts of less than 0.5 (Fig. 30).

The spectral sensitivities of fly and dragonfly LMCs are broad and are little changed by light adaptation (Fig. 31; LAUGHLIN and HARDIE, 1978). These cells respond well to wavelengths within the region of 300–600 nm, and show no trace of spectral opponency (LAUGHLIN, 1976c; ZETTLER and AUTRUM, 1975). Consequently the LMCs are a high sensitivity, non-chromatic pathway, integrating contrast signals over a wide spectrum of wavelengths, presumably to increase absolute sensitivity.

In summary, the LMCs of fly and dragonfly probably code contrast as response amplitude, with a higher sensitivity which results from signal amplification at the first synapse. This amplification expands a small voltage window of receptor output so that it fills the entire response range of the LMCs. Light adaptation mechanisms shift the window to keep it centred about the mean, so that the mean intensity level, or background, fails to generate a hyperpolarising response and, unlike the receptors, the range shift of LMC $V/\log I$ curves equals the change in background intensity (Fig. 32). In order to minimise the possibility of saturation by sud-

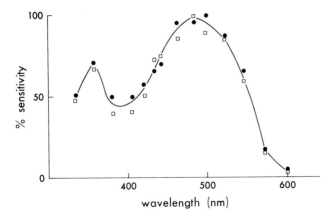

Fig. 31. The broad spectral sensitivity of a fly LMC is little changed during its transition from the dark-adapted (□) to light-adapted (●) state. Data for *Calliphora* from LAUGHLIN and HARDIE (1978) and HARDIE (1978)

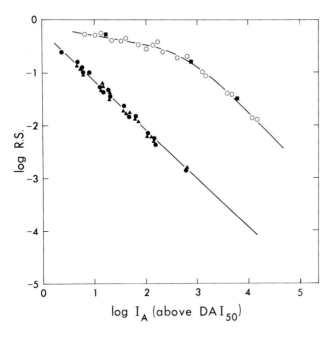

Fig. 32. The range shifts (R.S.) of photoreceptor and LMC V/log I curves plotted as a function of background intensity. ● = LMC on transient; ▲ = LMC off transient; ○ = photoreceptor range shift; ■ = photoreceptor range shift predicted from decay of response amplitude during light adaptation. Data from five LMCs and six photoreceptors from *Calliphora*. Background intensity is normalised relative to the DA I_{50}, as defined in Fig. 30. The LMC data has been fitted with a regression line of slope −0.98. From LAUGHLIN and HARDIE (1978) and HARDIE (1978)

den changes in mean intensity, LMC light adaptation mechanisms act extremely rapidly, producing a 2 log unit range shift, in either direction, in less than 0.5 s (Laughlin and Hardie, 1978). Thus the LMC's neural image is an inverted and amplified version of the smaller, contrast induced, fluctuations in potential across the receptor array.

c) Noise and Temporal Frequency Response

As we know little about the frequency responses of LMCs, and still less about noise levels, these two neural image quality factors can be considered together. In darkness the LMCs produce a constant level of noise (ca. 10% V_{max}) and with increasing levels of illumination, the noise first increases and then at higher intensities, falls again to around the dark level (Laughlin, 1973, and unpublished observations). This suggests that the intensity dependent noise in receptors (Fig. 20 a) is amplified and superimposed upon a constant noise source acting upon the LMCs. This constant noise could arise at synapses upon the receptor axon terminals, and the LMC membrane, and arguments presented in the next section suggest that the receptor→LMC synapse is always active, both in darkness and in light.

Is this constant barrage of noise a formidable obstacle to contrast signals? The noise certainly curtails the number of signal states the monopolar cell membrane can occupy (see Fig. 16), but it is deceptive to think of this noise in terms of voltage. Because of amplification this noise represents a 400 μV peak to peak amplitude signal in a receptor (Laughlin, 1973), and for a light-adapted fly LMC, with a contrast efficiency of 250% V_{max}/log unit, a noise level of 10% V_{max} is equivalent to a contrast of 0.05. As this latter value represents the peak to peak noise level, still smaller contrasts should be detectable in the outputs of single LMCs. Thus a high noise level is not necessarily a sign of a poor ability to resolve contrast, and arguments presented in the next section suggest that this high noise level arises from a strategy to increase the signal: noise ratio for the transmission of contrast signals across the first synapse.

Two studies compare the frequency responses of LMCs with receptors, under identical stimulus conditions, to derive a frequency response for voltage transfer across the first synapse (Järvilehto and Zettler, 1971, 1973; French and Järvilehto, 1978 b). Both find that the synaptic complex acts as a frequency dependent amplifier (Järvilehto and Zettler, 1971) boosting rapid fluctuations, and that transfer produces remarkably little change in phase, aside from the 180° shift brought about by signal inversion. These findings agree with the earlier observations, that the lamina components boosted the flicker fusion frequency of the ERG (Autrum, 1958), and are confirmed by a recent genetic dissection of lamina and retina ERG frequency responses in Drosophila (Wu and Wong, 1977), but some anomalies remain. Using conventional sinusoidally modulating stimuli Järvilehto and Zettler (1971, 1973) found that the synapse had a high gain, increasing from × 3 at 6 Hz, to × 8 at 100 Hz, and this agrees with the comparison of receptor and LMC response amplitudes to square wave stimuli (e.g. Laughlin and Hardie, 1978). Using a white noise technique, French and Järvilehto (1978 b) observed almost no gain (× 1 at 2 Hz and × 2 at 100 Hz). Their explanation, that gain is reduced by light adaptation, is not confirmed by the square wave studies, for gain remains high and constant over a wide background range (Laughlin and

HARDIE, 1978), and an alternative explanation must be sought. A second peculiarity is that both studies fail to find a massive attenuation of amplitude, and a large shift of phase at low frequencies. Both these effects might be expected from the transient response of LMCs, and their potent adaptation to new light levels. Perhaps, as FRENCH and JÄRVILEHTO suggest (1978 b), gain is reduced in step with the intensity modulation at low frequencies. Finally, FRENCH and JÄRVILEHTO (1978 b) found that lateral inhibition has no influence upon the frequency response. Inhibition may exhibit itself more clearly when the responses to frequencies of less than 2 Hz are tested.

In summary, although noise severely contaminates the voltage responses of LMCs, its effects are reduced by amplification at the first synapse, which renders small contrast signals more visible in the LMC neural image. Perhaps it is for this reason that the lamina selectively boosts the high temporal frequencies that are severely attenuated during transduction. In a moving retina this temporal boosting would also help save fine spatial detail from sinking below the noise level.

4. Mechanisms for Neural Image Transformation

The transfer of signals from photoreceptors to LMCs is dominated by three factors, inversion, amplification and the transient responses and range shifts indicative of powerful inhibitory mechanisms, antagonising the light-induced response. Although signal inversion is not of fundamental importance to intensity coding, signal amplification and transient responses are, because both these properties are found at the first synapse in the barnacle and insect ocelli (Sects. B.VIII; C.III.1) and the retina of lower vertebrates (Fig. 34), while transients are generated by self and lateral inhibition in the *Limulus* compound eye (Sect. D.IV). The large ocellar neurons of locust and the eccentric cells of *Limulus* eye are far more amenable to an exacting biophysical analysis of conductance mechanisms than insect monopolar cells (Sects. C.II.2; D.IV.3). Nonetheless, the insect lamina introduces some new and interesting hypotheses concerning optimal signal transfer at the visual system's first synapse. These ideas are generated from data on two factors, that are better understood in the insect lamina than in other visual systems, namely the wiring diagram and the extracellular field potentials.

Signal inversion and amplification is performed by the array of parallel chemical synapses made between each photoreceptor axon terminal and each LMC (LAUGHLIN, 1973). In fly (JÄRVILEHTO and ZETTLER, 1971), dragonfly (LAUGHLIN, 1973) and locust (SHAW, 1968 a, 1978 b) the synaptic delay is of the order of 1–2 ms; a value compatible with a monosynaptic pathway from receptors to LMCs. The LMC hyperpolarising response has a reversal potential that is 25–40 mV below dark resting potential and is associated with a conductance increase (SHAW, 1968 a; LAUGHLIN, 1974 c; ZIMMERMAN, 1978), suggesting that, as in locust ocellus (Sect. C.III.2), the response is generated by a conductance increase to potassium and/or chloride ions. Over a small amplitude range, where the non-linearities associated with self-shunting (Sect. E.II.3.b) at the postsynaptic membrane are presumed to be negligible, the postsynaptic response rises as an accelerating exponential function of the presynaptic voltage. This suggests that, in common with many other

chemical synapses, the transmitter release is an exponential function of presynaptic voltage. This exponential dependency boosts larger responses, and by
comparison with many other situations, the first synapse in the insect lamina is
highly sensitive, with a 0.8 mV input increment producing a tenfold postsynaptic
potential increase (Shaw, 1978 b). High sensitivity is associated with two related
factors, the large number of parallel synapses, and the convergence of several receptors onto a single LMC (Laughlin, 1973). With *each* fly LMC receiving over
400 synapses from receptors (Fig. 26), there must be a large population of synaptic
vesicles awaiting release from the receptor terminals and a small presynaptic signal
can produce a large transmitter dose. In this sense the action of many parallel synapses is equivalent to a single large synaptic site (Shaw, 1978 b).

Both receptor convergence and multiple parallel synapses (or large synapses)
have the additional advantage of improving signal : noise ratios (Laughlin, 1973).
If one considers uncorrelated noise within receptors sharing the same signal (e.g.
photon noise in the receptors entering one cartridge) the signal : noise ratio increases in proportion to the square root of the number of receptors (Smola and
Gemperlein, 1972; Laughlin, 1973). If one considers the shot noise associated
with the stochastic process of transmitter vesicle release, then the signal : noise ratio
for transfer across the synapse is proportional to the square root of the number
of identical synapses, or vesicles, involved (Laughlin, 1973). This is exactly
analogous to overcoming photon noise in an optical communication system by using more light. Thus parallel, or large, synapses increase the voltage gain at the first
synapse and improve the signal:noise ratio for synaptic transmission, particularly
when this latter parameter is expressed in terms of the smallest presynaptic input
detectable in the postsynaptic response. This may be why parallel synapses are also
found in the midget bipolar cells subserving single foveal cones (Laughlin,
1976 b).

The lamina extracellular field potential could also boost the sensitivity of the
first synapse. A chemical synapse, operating with exponential transmitter release
and suffering from self-shunting at the postsynaptic membrane achieves the
highest voltage gain in the mid-point of its operating range (Falk and Fatt, 1972).
It is possible that the standing negative potential of the lamina extracellular space
(Sect. E.III.2.a and Zimmerman, 1978) effectively depolarises the receptor terminals, keeping their synapses continuously active in the more sensitive mid-region
of their operating range. Note that the activity of the receptor→LMC synapse opposes the extracellular hyperpolarisation driving it, by inducing current to flow into the extracellular space, across the postsynaptic LMC membrane. The dark level
of activity of the synapse might be maintained at an equilibrium level, determined
by the current sinks generating the hyperpolarisation of the extracellular space.
There is some evidence to suggest that this hyperpolarisation is produced by current leaving the lamina extracellular space, via synapses on interneurons, and that
a part of this current is responsible for maintaining the LMC membrane potential
well above the equilibrium potential of the light-induced response, to ensure an adequate hyperpolarising response range (Zimmerman, 1978).

Such a synaptic equilibrium, mediated by field potentials, could be one of the
LMC light adaptation mechanisms responsible for producing a range shift far in
excess of the receptors' (Fig. 32) and suppressing the standing background signal.

Light adaptation must involve a shut down of the receptor→LMC hyperpolarising synapse because the plateau LMC response has approximately the same reversal potential as the on transient, and the decline in response from peak to plateau is associated with a fall in conductance (LAUGHLIN, 1974c; ZIMMERMAN, 1978). This shut down is not brought about by a desensitisation of the first synapse. The LMC contrast efficiency is consistently eight to ten times greater than the receptors', and this can only happen if the first synapse maintains its high voltage gain to transient stimuli. It follows that the synapse must be turned off by subtracting away the standing background signal from the presynaptic terminals (LAUGHLIN and HARD-IE, 1978). This is precisely the action expected of the light-induced depolarisation of the extracellular space (LAUGHLIN, 1974b; SHAW, 1975). To support this hypothesis, the light-induced depolarisation has the slower time constant required to produce transients (SHAW, 1978b) and, because it sums the receptor inputs from several cartridges, is capable of producing lateral inhibition. Note that stimuli subtending a broad angle are both more effective at generating large depolarising field potentials (SHAW, 1978b), and at producing a cut back in the LMC response to sustained stimuli (Fig. 28, C cf. Bg). To prove that the field potentials provide an elegantly simple and economical means for maintaining synapses in their optimum mid-range of operation, is a compelling challenge for future investigations of lamina function.

The depolarising bias of saturated on and off transient response amplitudes with increasing backgrounds (Fig. 30) correlates with the level of maintained receptor depolarisation, and hence the expected lamina field potential. It is proposed that the receptor-LMC synapse is not maintained at exactly the same level of activity over a wide range of backgrounds. Activity creeps up with increased mean intensity. This induces a standing hyperpolarisation in the LMCs which is offset by the subtraction of the lamina field potential at the LMCs postsynaptic membrane, so that there is, relative to the LMC terminals in the medulla, a complete annihilation of the background signal (LAUGHLIN and HARDIE, 1978).

Field effects are accompanied by synaptic interactions. The LMCs are part of a complex web of inter- and intracartridge feed-back and feed-forward circuits (Fig. 26), but the evidence for a significant shaping of the LMC waveform by these circuits is circumstantial. The rapid on transient is often accompanied by a damped oscillation at about 60 Hz (Fig. 28, Osc), and in aged preparations the oscillation can become unstable, and produces ringing of 20 mV amplitude (LAUGHLIN and HARDIE, 1978). Oscillations were also observed in the ERG of *Calliphora* (BURK-HARDT, 1954) and in lamina mutant ERGs from *Drosophila* (WU and WONG, 1977) where they have a similar frequency of 55 Hz. It is unlikely that rapid oscillations are produced by slow field potentials. In locust and dragonfly, the stimulation of single facets excites the receptors entering one cartridge, and under these conditions the on transient is still clearly visible (SHAW, 1978b; LAUGHLIN, unpublished observation). This proves an earlier inference (LAUGHLIN, 1974b), that the on transient is largely produced by intracartridge inhibition. The field potential within one cartridge is probably weak and the on transient could again result from synaptic interactions. The slow component of inhibition is much reduced during single facet stimulation, emphasising the importance of lateral inhibition, and there is plenty of scope (Fig. 26) for some of this being mediated synaptically (STRAUS-FELD and CAMPOS-ORTEGA, 1977). Synaptic interactions may also shape the off transient. This response increases in amplitude with hyperpolarisation of LMCs by current clamp (ZETTLER and JÄRVILEHTO, 1973; cf. ZIMMERMAN, 1978), and in locust ocellus this same finding indicated that a depolarising synaptic input generated the analogous slow off transient (WILSON, 1978b, see Sect. C.III.2). The fast spike-like potential riding on the leading edge of the off transient is not often seen in the lamina but is larger closer to the medulla (ZETTLER and JÄRVILEHTO, 1973; LAUGHLIN and HARDIE, 1978). This suggests that the spike is produced by excitable membrane at, or near, the LMCs central terminal – another remarkable similarity to ocellar L-neurons (WILSON, 1978b; see Sect. C.III.2). Could other slower components of the LMC response be generated at the medulla terminal, yet appear in lamina recordings? Graded potential neurons allow for two-way traffic and one might have to consider the lamina and medulla terminals as single integrating units, coupled by the axon. Given the complexity of the medulla cartridge this is indeed a daunting thought!

There is no doubt that the lamina end of the LMC is strongly coupled to the medulla terminal, although the ease with which signals pass in the opposite direction, from medulla to lamina, has not been directly examined. Definitive experiments, using precise electrode localisation techniques, show that the on transient amplitude decays by less than a half during its passage from lamina to medulla (ZETTLER and JÄRVILEHTO, 1973). For neurons of about 2–3 μm diameter, and up to 1,000 μm long, this is certainly good propagation, but the means by which it is achieved is disputed. ZETTLER and JÄRVILEHTO (1973) find voltage dependent conductances in the LMC axon, and suggest that these are part of an unspecified active propagation mechanism. They also measure the input resistance of the neuron by current clamp, and obtain a low value, indicative of a cable that is too leaky to support passive propagation over the required distance. WILSON (1978b) and SHAW (1978b) effectively counter their arguments. They point out that voltage dependent conductances occur in axons where signals propagate passively (e.g. barnacle, Sect. B.VI, and locust ocellus, Sect. C.III.2). These conductances may actually impede propagation (e.g. compare hyperpolarising signals with depolarising, in Fig. 2). They further suggest that the low values of LMC input resistance result from injected current flowing through active synaptic conductances in the lamina, and because these synapses produce the hyperpolarising response, their low impedance is not seen by the on transient propagating to the medulla. The issue of active vs. passive propagation will remain unresolved, until reliable biophysical measurements, of the type made in barnacle (Sect. B.VI; SHAW, 1972) or locust ocellus (WILSON, 1978b) are made in insect LMCs.

5. Principles for the Peripheral Processing of Contrast Signals

The retina and lamina of the compound eye share a set of common properties with the ocelli of barnacle and insects, *Limulus* lateral eye, and the outer plexiform layer and receptors of the vertebrate retina. These are a non-linear summation of intensity signals within receptors, as expressed by a sigmoidal $V/\log I$ curve, and the sensitive and transient responses of first order interneurons, symptomatic of an

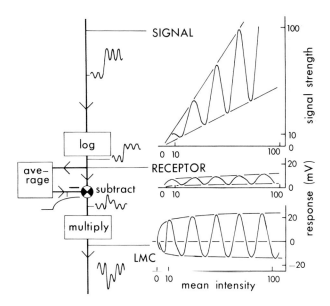

Fig. 33. The log transformation–subtraction–amplification strategy for light adaptation. Although the intensity range encompassed by a signal of contrast 0.5, expands with mean intensity, the responses of photoreceptors and LMCs are contained to an almost constant level by the operations shown in the block diagram. Further discussion in the text

amplification of receptor input and a delayed inhibition. In the insect compound eye there is sufficient data on intensity/response functions, measured in receptors and first order interneurons under identical conditions, to extract two general principles from these transient and non-linear effects. These are the *log transformation–subtraction–amplification* strategy and *high pass filtering*. These principles are interrelated and both help the peripheral visual system to code contrast efficiently over a wide range of intensities.

The log transformation–subtraction–multiplication strategy (LAUGHLIN and HARDIE, 1978) allows the eye to match the response range of neurons to the *expected* intensity range of contrast signals at any one of a number of mean intensities, as illustrated in Fig. 33. The upper graph depicts the problem associated with contrast coding. The absolute energy range encompassed by a contrast signal increases in proportion to mean intensity. The solution of this problem by fly photoreceptors and LMCs is shown in the lower two curves which plot their corresponding voltage response envelopes. These voltages were obtained by passing the contrast signal through measured intensity/response functions, and this empirical approach illustrates the inherent simplicity of the strategy, as outlined in the accompanying flow chart. The major task of adjusting sensitivity to mean intensity is performed by the receptors. Non-linear summation contains the expanding intensity envelope to almost constant dimensions, and this approximates to a logarithmic transformation (ZETTLER, 1969; and Sect. E.II.4.b). During synaptic transfer to LMCs, the standing background signal is subtracted away, and the fluctuating components carrying the contrast information amplified. Thus each retinal channel possesses this highly effective sensitivity control for handling changes in mean intensity.

All three processes have their own particular advantages. As discussed in Sect. E.II.4.b, the logarithmic transform helps objects to look alike at different intensities, by making the voltage responses of the neural image a function of contrast. Subtraction removes the redundant background signal from LMCs and allows for a fuller utilisation of their response range by contrast signals. A similar proposal has been made for retinal ganglion cells (Barlow and Levick, 1976). Amplification then protects these contrast signals from contamination by two sources of intrinsic noise. It reduces the equivalent contrast value of noise central to LMCs, and so helps in the central detection of small contrast signals. When amplification is achieved by recruiting large numbers of synaptic vesicles it also lessens the equivalent contrast of noise contamination at the receptor synapse (see Sect. E.III.4). By performing amplification and subtraction at an early stage the inevitable effects of intrinsic noise at synapses are minimised, and higher order neurons are provided with consistent signals, falling within defined amplitude limits.

Several arguments suggest that this simple adaptation strategy might match the receptor and LMC intensity/response functions to the statistical distribution of object detail (Laughlin and Hardie, 1978). The receptors' neural image encompasses all aspects of the information available to the optic lobe, and must be used for making comparisons between intensity levels in different retinal areas (e.g. dorsal light reactions). To do this, the receptors in different areas must operate with a similar sensitivity, and this requires that receptors have a broad dynamic range, capable of handling the extremes of highlight and shadow encountered in larger areas of object. As a consequence of a broader dynamic range, the voltage signals set up by contrasts within any one area are small, and susceptible to intrinsic noise. The LMCs filter the receptors' neural image to extract as much of this fine detail, as possible. Their instantaneous light-adapted dynamic range is approximately equal to the range of contrast, and the risk of signal clipping during changes in mean intensity level is minimised by the rapidity of light adaptation. Within the LMC voltage response range, the small contrast fluctuations are selectively amplified. Contrasts of less than 0.5 occupy over 80% of the voltage response and larger fluctuations are allotted progressively less and less (Fig. 30). If small signal fluctuations predominate, this is sound coding practice. Response range is allotted in proportion to signal probability, so that all signal levels within the LMC response range are fully utilised (Laughlin and Hardie, 1978). Small contrasts will predominate if reflectances are normally distributed. In addition, small fluctuations may carry most of the available contrast information because the high spatial and temporal frequencies are rich in detail, yet are attenuated by optical blurring and temporal smearing in the receptor mosaic. This would also explain why the first synapse boosts high temporal frequencies. As further support for a matching of neuronal input-output properties to the level of expected input, the fall in LMC contrast efficiency with intensity widens the dynamic range. Although this broadening is the simple consequence of operating the first synapse with a constant voltage gain, it conveniently accommodates the increased level of receptor noise, and allows the

LMCs to encompass signals over a wider retinal area, as might be required for spatial summation at lower intensities (LAUGHLIN and HARDIE, 1978).

The second principle, high pass filtering, has already been introduced in connection with *Limulus* lateral eye (Sects. D.IV and V) where self and lateral inhibition produce transient responses, giving spatial and temporal high pass filter properties to the eccentric cell array. In the insect compound eye the measurements of interneuron range shift during light adaptation enable one to see these high pass filter properties as a part of contrast coding. To adjust the intensity/response function of a contrast coding neuron to mean intensity one must take a measure of the mean input, and use this to drive the $V/\log I$ curve back and forth along the intensity axis (i.e. Figs. 30 and 32). If the mean is taken from the level of activity in a single channel, averaged over a certain time period, this amounts to self-inhibition. Similarly, if the mean is the ensemble average of receptor outputs over a larger retinal area, this amounts to lateral inhibition. Thus, the resulting high pass filter properties are necessary for an interneuronal mosaic to efficiently retrieve contrast detail from the receptor neural image, and accommodate this detail within a restricted range of voltage response states.

The most appropriate time span and retinal area over which to compute the mean is a question of some theoretical interest. If the time or area is too large then the probability of a change in mean intensity within this interval is increased, and the amplification of contrast signals must be reduced, to accommodate the larger *expected* intensity range. Conversely, if the time span or area is too small, inhibition attenuates higher frequencies and the light adaptation mechanisms start destroying the very signal they are designed to retrieve. The optimisation of contrast retrieval within these limits requires a complete description of the spatial and temporal distributions of intensity and the corresponding frequency responses of the receptor mosaic. As a preliminary suggestion, amplification and dynamic range should be related to the spatial and temporal characteristics of inhibition. The higher the amplification, the narrower the dynamic range and the more rapidly and locally must the mean signal be computed. Thus the interneurons most sensitive to contrast should show narrower inhibitory fields and faster adaptation than the neurons with broader dynamic range (e.g. LMCs cf. photoreceptors).

In conclusion, the data from the compound eyes of *Limulus*, fly and dragonfly, shows that two important principles of peripheral processing ensure that the response ranges within an interneuron array are matched to the appropriate levels of incoming intensity signal, in any one retinal area at any one time. A preliminary examination of the data also suggests that the parameters within the log transformation–subtraction–amplification strategy and the high pass filter principle, are carefully adjusted so that the intensity coding properties of receptors, and the voltage transfer properties at the first synapse, match the usual amplitude distributions of signals in space and time. This matching enables contrast detail to be transmitted with high efficiency from one neural image, the receptors', to another, the LMCs. This hypothesis can be tested by examining the responses of receptors and LMCs to natural stimuli, and by relating their responses to visual behaviour, in order to isolate the neural image quality factors limiting resolution (Sect. E.II.10). This approach could prove to be of some significance. The matching of receptor and interneuron input-output functions to the expected level of input could be as satisfying an adaptation of structure to function as the adjustment of receptor geometry to the properties of incoming light (SNYDER, 1979).

The proposal that these two strategies provide for the efficient peripheral processing of contrast signals is strengthened by the similarities between the response

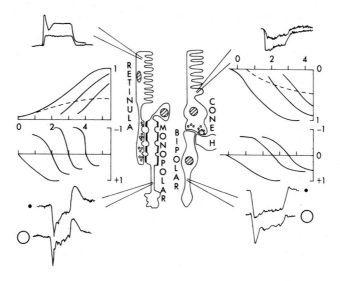

Fig. 34. The similarities between the responses and intensity/response functions of the receptors and first order interneurons of invertebrate and vertebrate retinas. Despite a difference in response polarity, the graded potentials of insect retinula cells and vertebrate cones both exhibit a broad dynamic range, a relatively small range shift with light adaptation, and a standing background signal (- - -). The analogous monopolar and bipolar cells also respond with graded potentials, but have a narrow dynamic range that is shifted in step with background intensity so that there is little representation of the standing background intensity level. Comparisons between the responses to a point source (●) and a broad stimulus (○) show that both interneurons are subject to lateral inhibition. Figure taken from Laughlin and Hardie (1978); vertebrate data from the mudpuppy *Necturus* is from Normann and Werblin (1974) and Werblin (1974)

characteristics of retinula cells and LMCs on the one hand, and vertebrate cones and bipolar cells on the other (Fig. 34). In both instances the receptors respond to light with graded potentials. Their intensity/response functions exhibit a broad dynamic range that is shifted by light adaptation, but always represents the background intensity. In first order interneurons, whether LMCs or bipolar cells, the intensity/response functions are steeper and exhibit a pronounced range shift with light adaptation, during which the background signal is removed. These characteristics are the hallmark of the log transformation–subtraction–amplification strategy. In addition, the interneuron responses are phasic, and adaptation is accelerated and increased by using broad field adapting stimuli, indicating spatial and temporal high pass filter properties which, incidentally, are more pronounced in retinal ganglion cells. As further support for a functional similarity, Werblin (1977) and Thibos and Werblin (1978) produce evidence that the voltage gain at the receptor → bipolar cell synapse is kept relatively constant, and bipolar range shift is brought about by a presynaptic subtraction of the standing light signal. Thus principles seen in invertebrate peripheral visual systems are of more general interest and applicability, a conclusion that is strengthened by the fuller comparison of vertebrate and invertebrate eyes, made in the next and final section.

F. Common Principles for Vertebrate and Invertebrate Visual Systems

A review of the cellular operations of receptors and first order interneurons in the ocelli of barnacles and insects, and the compound eyes of both *Limulus* and the more advanced insects and crustacea, produces a long list of similarities (Table 3). This table also gives the section in which the appropriate property is discussed, usually from a functional viewpoint. Now it is quite remarkable that many of these same properties are exhibited by the analogous photoreceptors and first order interneurons of vertebrate retinas, and examples are cited in the same table, with key references. In cases where the data is inconclusive I have interpreted it in terms of a similarity, because this often provides a functional interpretation worthy of discussion. These debatable cases are marked with a question mark. This list of similarities can be brought to life by taking a brief trip through the receptors and first order interneurons of a principled visual system.

We start with light entering the eye, and a set of optical principles reviewed by SNYDER (1979). Incoming light is directed by a dioptric system upon a matrix of directionally sensitive photoreceptors within which photopigment is densely packed to ensure maximum absorption. Being small and densely packed these receptors function as waveguides. The size of receptors and their angular spacing are matched to the optical quality factors of diffraction and photon noise.

The photoreceptor transducer has a gain sufficient to resolve single photons, and can approach the photon noise limit of resolution at low intensities. At higher light levels, intensity is signalled as the amplitude of a graded potential response. The relationship between intensity and voltage is inevitably non-linear, due to the saturation kinetics of the membrane responses, and this gives rise to a non-linear summation of response amplitudes so that the higher the intensity, the smaller the response per photon. The photoreceptor uses several light adaptation mechanisms to lower its sensitivity at higher intensities, so as to minimise the compressive effects of non-linear summation. The combination of non-linear summation and light adaptation produces an almost logarithmic transform of intensity. The mosaic of receptors, each representing intensity as voltage, generate a neural image of the object. In addition to the optical factors of receptor angular sensitivity and angular spacing, neural image quality is determined by the noise within receptors, and the smearing of moving objects, that results from the receptors' finite speed of response. The receptor signal is transmitted passively to the first synapse, and in this region one may encounter voltage sensitive calcium channels, responsible for boosting the synaptic response. The receptor neural image is often several overlapping sets of images, representing additional parameters such as the colour and the principal polarisation plane of light.

The graded potential in the receptor generates a graded response in the first order neuron by means of a chemical synapse (*Limulus* is an exception to this). These synapses often have a dyadic, triadic or tetradic structure, which could help increase the accuracy with which neural connections are made, and the flexibility with which they are employed. The chemical synapse releases transmitter as an ex-

Table 3. Similar properties of invertebrate and vertebrate peripheral visual systems

Property	Invertebrate example (section number)[a]	Vertebrate example	Reference
Transduction			
Single photon signals	C.III.1.b; D.III, E.II.3.a, 4.a	Toad rods	Baylor et al. (1979)
Non-linear summation of simultaneous single photon signals	B.IV; C.III.1.a; D.III; E.II.3	Turtle cones	Baylor and Fuortes (1970)
Sensitivity control for light adaptation	D.V.3; E.II.3	Gecko rods	Kleinschmidt and Dowling (1975)
Logarithmic transform	D.I; E.II.4.b	Gecko rods Mudpuppy cones	ibid. Normann and Werblin (1974)
Neural image generated within photoreceptor array	E.II.1	—	—
Neural image quality factors: temporal smearing and noise	E.II.5, 6	—	—
Electrical coupling of receptors	B.IV; D.III; E.II.8.a	Toad rods	Fain et al. (1976)
Synaptic Transfer			
Voltage sensitive channels at presynaptic site	B.VIII	Toad rods	Fain et al. (1977b)
Dyads, triads and tetrads	B.VIII; C.II.4.b; D.II; E.III.1.c	Widespread	rev. Stell (1972)
Exponential transmitter release	E.III.4	Salamander	Thibos and Werblin (1978)
Synapse poised in most sensitive mid-part of operating range	E.III.4?	General?	Falk and Fatt (1972)
Synapse active in darkness	E.III.4?	Skate rods	Ripps et al. (1976)
Large synapses or multiple small synapses	E.III.1, 4	Monkey midget bipolar cells	Boycott and Kolb (1973)
Transfer of small graded signals across first synapse	B.VII, VIII; C.III.1; E.III.3, 4	Dogfish bipolars Turtle retina	Ashmore and Falk (1976) Fain et al. (1977a)
Interneuron response			
Amplification of signal	C.III.1.b; E.III.3, 4	Dogfish	ibid.
Narrow dynamic range at any one mean intensity	C.III.1; E.III.3, 5	Mudpuppy bipolars Salamander bipolars	Werblin (1971, 1973) Thibos and Werblin (1978)
Rapid light adaptation shifts dynamic range to suit new mean intensity	E.III.3, 5	Salamander bipolars (rapid?)	ibid.
Subtractive inhibition at receptor's presynaptic terminal	E.III.4, 5	Salamander bipolars	Werblin (1977)

Table 3. (continued)

Property	Invertebrate example (section number)[a]	Vertebrate example	Reference
Inhibition mediated by extra-cellular field potentials	E.III.2.a, 4?	General at dyads triads etc.?	BYZOV et al. (1977)
Self and lateral inhibition produce temporal and spatial high pass filter properties	B.VIII; C.III.; D.IV, V.; E.III.5	Mudpuppy retina	WERBLIN (1972)
Parallel pathways via several arrays of interneurons	C.II, E.III.1	General, e.g. fish bipolars	STELL et al. (1977)
Structural			
Constancy of neuronal connections	C.II, E.III.1.e	—	—
Low level of variability	C.II, E.III.1.e	—	—
Redundancy as a catalyst for evolutionary change	C.II, E.III.1.a	—	—

[a]   B, barnacle ocellus; C, insect ocellus; D, *Limulus* lateral eye; E, compound eyes of insects and crustaceans

ponential function of presynaptic membrane potential, while postsynaptic conductance signals are subject to self-shunting. Consequently the synapse is at its most sensitive in the mid-region of its postsynaptic response range, and is actively maintained in this state at all levels of background illumination. This means that the synapse is continuously active in the dark. The receptor terminal also contains large numbers of presynaptic vesicles, either by making a few large synapses, or many smaller synapses. This again boosts the sensitivity of the synapse and ensures that a presynaptic signal is carried across the cleft by the release of many vesicles, so minimising the shot noise associated with synaptic transmission.

Because of the synapses' high sensitivity, large postsynaptic signals are generated by small presynaptic inputs. Amplification helps resolution by allowing small inputs to produce a neural response that is detectable against the backdrop of intrinsic noise, but a high gain also restricts the operating range of the first order neurons. To avoid saturation this range is adjusted neurally, with extreme rapidity, in response to changes of mean intensity within a small retinal area. This light adaptation is partially carried out by a subtraction of standing background signal from the receptor's presynaptic terminal, perhaps using extracellular field potentials. By continually adjusting its operating range to local changes in mean intensity, the first order interneuron has become a high pass filter, producing transient responses to spatially and temporally sustained stimuli. These filter properties result from the self and lateral inhibitory mechanisms that adjust the operating range. As a result of these properties the phasic first order interneuron is specialised to retrieve contrast information from the receptors, and present it within a second neural image. Other interneurons exist alongside it, and should provide alternative pathways for other types of information.

A close look at the structure of the principled visual system shows that it combines the constancy required for predictable and reliable function with the low level of variability required for evolutionary change. The redundancy that catalyses change is provided by neuronal duplication in small sets of specified cells, and by the duplication of unit structures in large arrays of neurons.

Although these principles of operation make good sense, and tend to minimise many of the constraints imposed upon the peripheral visual system by the materials from which it is constructed, some may doubt their validity. To counter this I suggest that the sharing of these properties by vertebrates and invertebrates confirms their importance. These animals see similar objects in the same environments, using neuronal building blocks which are essentially identical. One should expect the properties which coexist in different animals to derive from common solutions to common operational problems. If one is trying to resolve small signals transmitted across noisy synapses, or struggling with a non-linear receptor, does it matter that one has a backbone? The division between warm and cold blooded creatures might be more relevant. The isolation of common properties, as indicators of important functional principles is one attribute of the comparative approach to visual physiology. There is a second benefit. If one accepts that one is often studying the general principles of vision, then the opportunities offered by ocelli and insect compound eyes are the same opportunities offered by *Limulus*, the large retinal cells of lower vertebrates, and the accessible retinal ganglion cells of cats. They are preparations which allow one to ask fundamental questions about vision, and obtain unambiguous answers.

Acknowledgements. Special thanks to Ray Stone for tireless editorial assistance and for preparing the diagrams in Sects. C and E, and Pam Coote for typing most of the manuscript with unfailing accuracy. Joe Howard, Sam Rossel, and "Srini" Srinivasan contributed many useful comments to several drafts, while Sandy Smith prepared the figures for Sects. B and D.

References

Abramov, I.: Retinal mechanisms of colour vision. In: Handbook of sensory physiology, Vol. VII/2 (ed. M. G. F. Fuortes), pp. 567–608. Berlin-Heidelberg-New York: Springer 1972

Armett-Kibel, C., Meinertzhagen, I. A., Dowling, J. E.: Cellular and synaptic organisation in the lamina of the dragonfly *Sympetrum rubicundulum*. Proc. R. Soc. Lond. (Biol.) **196**, 385–413 (1977)

Arnett, D. W.: Spatial and temporal integration properties of units in first optic ganglion of dipterans. J. Neurophysiol. **35**, 429–444 (1972)

Ashmore, J. F., Falk, G.: Absolute sensitivity of rod bipolar cells in a dark-adapted retina. Nature **263**, 248–249 (1976)

Autrum, H.: Die Belichtungspotentiale und das Sehen der Insekten (Untersuchungen an *Calliphora* und *Dixippus*). Z. Vergl. Physiol. **32**, 176–227 (1950)

Autrum, H.: Electrophysiological analysis of the visual systems in insects. Exp. Cell Res. Suppl. **5**, 426–439 (1958)

Autrum, H., Kolb, G.: The dark adaptation in single visual cells of the compound eye of *Aeschna cyanea*. J. Comp. Physiol. **79**, 213–232 (1972)

Autrum, H., Metschl, N.: Die Arbeitsweise der Ocellen der Insekten. Z. Vergl. Physiol. **47**, 256–273 (1963)

Autrum, H., Stöcker, M.: Über optische Verschmelzungsfrequenzen und stroboskopisches Sehen bei Insekten. Biol. Zbl. **71**, 129–152 (1952)

Autrum, H., Zettler, F., Järvilehto, M.: Postsynaptic potentials from a single monopolar neuron of the ganglion opticum I of the blowfly *Calliphora*. Z. Vergl. Physiol. **70**, 414–424 (1970)

Autrum, H., Zwehl, V. von: Die spektrale Empfindlichkeit einzelner Sehzellen des Bienenauges. Z. Vergl. Physiol. **48**, 357–384 (1964)

Bader, C. R., Baumann, F., Bertrand, D.: Role of intracellular calcium and sodium in light adaptation in the retina of the honey bee drone (*Apis mellifera* L.). J. Gen. Physiol. **67**, 475–491 (1976)

Barlow, H. B.: Comment – three points about lateral inhibition. In: Sensory communication (ed. W. A. Rosenblith). Cambridge, Mass.: MIT Press 1961

Barlow, H. B.: The physical limits of visual discrimination. In: Photophysiology, Vol. II (ed. A. C. Giese). New York: Academic Press 1964

Barlow, H. B.: Retinal and central factors in human vision limited by noise. In: Vertebrate photoreception (eds. H. B. Barlow, P. Fatt). New York: Academic Press 1977

Barlow, H. B., Levick, W. R.: The mechanism of directionally selective units in the rabbit's retina. J. Physiol. (Lond.) **178**, 477–504 (1965)

Barlow, H. B., Levick, W. R.: Three factors limiting the reliable detection of light by retinal ganglion cells of the cat. J. Physiol. (Lond.) **200**, 1–24 (1969)

Barlow, H. B., Levick, W. R.: Threshold setting by the surround of cat retinal ganglion cells. J. Physiol. (Lond.) **259**, 737–757 (1976)

Barlow, R. B.: Inhibitory fields in the *Limulus* lateral eye. J. Gen. Physiol. **54**, 383–396 (1969)

Barlow, R. B., Bolanowski, S. J., Brachman, M. L.: Efferent optic nerve fibers mediate circadian rhythms in the *Limulus* eye. Science **197**, 86–89 (1977)

Barlow, R. B., Kaplan, E.: Properties of visual cells in the lateral eye of *Limulus in situ*. Intracellular recordings. J. Gen. Physiol. **69**, 203–220 (1977)

Barlow, R. B., Lange, G. D.: A nonlinearity in the inhibitory interactions in the *Limulus* eye. J. Gen. Physiol. **63**, 579–589 (1974)

Barlow, R. B., Quarles, D. A.: Mach bands in the lateral eye of *Limulus*. Comparison of theory and experiment. J. Gen. Physiol. **65**, 709–730 (1975)

Baumann, F.: Slow and spike potentials recorded from retinula cells of the honeybee drone in response to light. J. Gen. Physiol. **52**, 855–875 (1968)

Baumann, F.: Electrophysiological properties of the honey bee retina. In: The compound eye and vision of insects (ed. G. A. Horridge), pp. 53–74. Oxford: Oxford University Press 1975

Baylor, D. A., Fettiplace, R.: Kinetics of synaptic transfer from receptors to ganglion cell in turtle retina. J. Physiol. (Lond.) **271**, 425–448 (1977)

Baylor, D. A., Fuortes, M. G. F.: Electrical responses of single cones in the retina of the turtle. J. Physiol. (Lond.) **207**, 77–92 (1970)

Baylor, D. A., Lamb, T. D., Yau, K.-W.: Responses of retinal rods to single photons. J. Physiol. (Lond.) **288**, 613–634 (1979)

Beersma, D. G. M., Stavenga, D. G., Kuiper, J. W.: Organization of visual axes in the compound eye of the fly, *Musca domestica* L., and behavioural consequences. J. Comp. Physiol. **102**, 305–320 (1975)

Behrens, M. E.: Photomechanical changes in the ommatidium of the *Limulus* lateral eye during light and dark adaptation. J. Comp. Physiol. **89**, 45–57 (1974)

Behrens, M. E., Krebs, W.: The effect of light-dark adaptation on the ultrastructure of *Limulus* lateral eye retinular cells. J. Comp. Physiol. **107**, 77–96 (1976)

Békésy, G. von: Mach band type lateral inhibition in different sense organs. J. Gen. Physiol. **50**, 519–532 (1966)

Biederman-Thorson, M., Thorson, J.: Dynamics of excitation and inhibition in the light adapted *Limulus* eye *in situ*. J. Gen. Physiol. **58**, 1–19 (1971)

Blackwell, H. R.: Luminance difference thresholds. In: Handbook of sensory physiology, Vol. VII/4 (eds. D. Jameson, L. M. Hurvich), pp. 78–101. Berlin-Heidelberg-New York: Springer 1972

Blest, A. D.: The rapid synthesis and destruction of photoreceptor membrane by a dinopid spider: a daily cycle. Proc. R. Soc. Lond. (Biol.) **200**, 463–483 (1978)

Blest, A. D., Day, W. A.: The rhabdomere organization of some nocturnal Pisaurid spiders in light and darkness. Phil. Trans. R. Soc. Lond. **283**, 1–23 (1978)

Boschek, C. B.: On the fine structure of the peripheral retina and lamina ganglionaris of the fly, *Musca domestica*. Z. Zellforsch. **118**, 369–409 (1971)

Boycott, B. B.: Aspects of the comparative anatomy and physiology of the vertebrate retina. In: Essays on the nervous system; a festschrift for Professor J. Z. Young (eds. R. M. Bellairs, E. G. Gray). Oxford: Clarendon Press 1974

Boycott, B. B., Kolb, H.: The connections between bipolar cells and photoreceptors in the retina of the domestic cat. J. Comp. Neurol. **148**, 91–114 (1973)

Braitenberg, V.: Patterns of projection in visual system of the fly. I. Retina-lamina projections. Exp. Brain Res. **3**, 271–298 (1967)

Braitenberg, V., Hauser-Holschuh, H.: Patterns of projection in the visual system of the fly. II. Quantitative aspects of second order neurons in relation to models of movement detection. Exp. Brain Res. **16**, 184–209 (1972)

Brown, H. M., Hagiwara, S., Koike, H., Meech, R. M.: Membrane properties of a barnacle photoreceptor examined by the voltage clamp technique. J. Physiol. (Lond.) **208**, 385–413 (1970)

Brown, J. E., Blinks, J. R.: Changes in intracellular free calcium concentration during illumination of invertebrate photoreceptors. J. Gen. Physiol. **64**, 643–665 (1974)

Brown, J. E., Mote, M. I.: Ionic dependence of reversal potential of the light response in *Limulus* ventral photoreceptor. J. Gen. Physiol. **63**, 337–350 (1974)

Buchner, E.: Elementary movement detectors in an insect visual system. Biol. Cybernetics **24**, 85–101 (1976)

Bullock, T. H., Horridge, G. A.: Structure and function in the nervous systems of invertebrates. San Francisco: Freeman 1965

Burkhardt, D.: Rhythmische Erregungen in den optischen Zentren von *Calliphora erythrocephala*. Z. Vergl. Physiol. **36**, 595–630 (1954)

Burkhardt, W., Braitenberg, V.: Some peculiar synaptic complexes in the first visual ganglion of the fly, *Musca domestica*. Cell Tissue Res. **173**, 287–308 (1976)

Byzov, A. L., Golubtsov, K. V.: Model of the neuron-regulator of the effectiveness of synaptic transmission. Biophysics **23**, 119–126 (1978)

Byzov, A. L., Golubtsov, K. V., Trifonov, J. A.: The model of mechanism of feedback between horizontal cells and photoreceptors in vertebrate retina. In: Vertebrate photoreception (eds. H. B. Barlow, P. Fatt). London: Academic Press 1977

Cajal, S. R.: Observaciones sobre la estructura de los ocelos y vias nerviosas ocelares de algunos insectos. Trab. Lab. Invest. Biol. Univ. Madrid **16**, 109–139 (1918)

Cajal, S. R., Sánchez, D.: Contribución al conocimiento de los céntros nerviosos de los inséctos. Parte I, rétina y centros ópticos. Trab. Lab. Invest. Biol. Univ. Madrid **13**, 1–164 (1915)

Campenhausen, C. von: The ability of *Limulus* to see visual patterns. J. Exp. Biol. **46**, 557–570 (1967)

Campos-Ortega, J. A., Strausfeld, N. J.: Columns and layers in the second synaptic region of the fly's visual system: the case for two superimposed neural architectures. In: Information processing in the visual systems of arthropods (ed. R. Wehner). Berlin-Heidelberg-New York: Springer 1972

Campos-Ortega, J. A., Strausfeld, N. J.: Synaptic connection of intrinsic cells and basket arborizations in the external plexiform layer of the fly's eye. Brain Res. **59**, 119–136 (1973)

Chamberlain, S. C., Barlow, R. B.: Morphological correlates of efferent circadian activity and light adaptation in the *Limulus* lateral eye. Biol. Bull. **153**, 418–419 (1977)

Chappell, R. L., DeVoe, R. D.: Action spectra and chromatic mechanisms of cells in the median ocelli of dragonflies. J. Gen. Physiol. **65**, 339–419 (1975)

Chappell, R. L., Dowling, J. E.: Neural organisation of the median ocellus of the dragonfly. I. Intracellular electrical activity. J. Gen. Physiol. **60**, 121–147 (1972)

Collett, T., Land, M. F.: Visual control of flight behaviour in the hoverfly, *Syritta pipiens* L. J. Comp. Physiol. **99**, 1–66 (1975)

Compton, J. C.: Facts behind exposure determination. J. Biol. Photogr. Assoc. **46**, 159–166 (1978)

Cowan, W. M.: Neuronal death as a regulative mechanism in the control of cell number in the nervous system. In: Development and aging in the nervous system (eds. M. Rockstein, M. L. Sussman). New York: Academic Press 1973

DeVoe, R. D., Ockleford, E. M.: Intracellular responses from cells of the medulla of the fly. Biol. Cybernetics **23**, 13–24 (1976)

DeVries, H.: The quantum character of light and its bearing upon threshold of vision, the differential sensitivity and visual acuity of the eye. Physica **10**, 553–564 (1943)

Ditchburn, R. W.: Eye movements and visual perception. Oxford: Clarendon Press 1973

Dodge, F. A., Knight, B. W., Toyoda, J.: Voltage noise in *Limulus* cells. Science **160**, 88–90 (1968)

Dörrscheidt-Käfer, M.: Die Empfindlichkeit einzelner Photorezeptoren im Komplexauge von *Calliphora erythrocephala*. J. Comp. Physiol. **81**, 309–340 (1972)

Dowling, J. E.: Discrete potentials in the dark adapted eye of *Limulus*. Nature (Lond.) **217**, 28–31 (1968)

Dowling, J. E., Chappell, R. L.: Neural organisation of the median ocellus of the dragonfly. II. Synaptic structure. J. Gen. Physiol. **60**, 148–165 (1972)

Dvorak, D., Snyder, A. W.: The relationship between visual acuity and illumination in the fly *Lucilia sericata*. Z. Naturforsch. **33c**, 139–143 (1978)

Eckert, H.: Die spektrale Empfindlichkeit des Komplexauges von *Musca* (Bestimmung aus Messungen der optomotorischen Reaktion). Kybernetik **9**, 145–156 (1971)

Eckert, H., Bishop, L. G.: Nonlinear dynamic transfer characteristics of cells in the peripheral visual pathway of flies. Part I. The retinula cells. Biol. Cybernetics **17**, 1–6 (1975)

Eguchi, E., Waterman, T. H.: Freeze-etch and histochemical evidence for cycling in crayfish photoreceptor membranes. Cell Tissue Res. **169**, 419–434 (1976)

Erber, J., Sandeman, D. C.: The detection of real and apparent motion by the crab *Leptograpsus variegatus*. II. Electrophysiology. J. Comp. Physiol. **112**, 189 197 (1976)

Fahrenbach, W. H.: The micromorphology of some simple photoreceptors. Z. Zellforsch. **66**, 233–254 (1965)

Fahrenbach, W. H.: The visual system of the horseshoe crab *Limulus polyphemus*. Int. Rev. Cytol. **41**, 285–349 (1975)

Fain, G. L.: Quantum sensitivity of rods in the toad retina. Science **187**, 838–841 (1975)

Fain, G. L., Gold, G. H., Dowling, J. E.: Receptor coupling in the toad retina. Cold Spring Harb. Symp. Quant. Biol. **40**, 547–561 (1976)

Fain, G. L., Granda, A. M., Maxwell, J. H.: Voltage signal of photoreceptors at visual threshold. Nature (Lond.) **265**, 181–183 (1977a)

Fain, G. L., Quandt, F. N., Gerschenfeld, H. M.: Calcium-dependent regenerative responses in rods. Nature (Lond.) **269**, 707–710 (1977b)

Fales, D. E.: The light receptive organs of certain barnacles. Biol. Bull. **54**, 534–547 (1928)

Falk, G., Fatt, P.: Physical changes induced by light in the rod outer segment of vertebrates. In: Handbook of sensory physiology, Vol. VII/1 (ed. H. J. A. Dartnall), pp. 200–244. Berlin-Heidelberg-New York: Springer 1972

Fein, A., Charlton, J. S.: A quantitative comparison of the effects of intracellular calcium injection and light adaptation on the photoresponse of *Limulus* ventral photoreceptors. J. Gen. Physiol. **70**, 591–600 (1977)

Fermi, G., Reichardt, W.: Optomotorische Reaktionen der Fliege *Musca domestica*. Kybernetik **2**, 15–28 (1963)

Franceschini, N.: Sampling of the visual environment by the compound eye of the fly: fundamentals and applications. In: Photoreceptor Optics (eds. A. W. Snyder, R. Menzel), pp. 98–125. Berlin-Heidelberg-New York: Springer 1975

French, A. S.: Automated spectral analysis of neuro-physiological data using intermediate magnetic tape storage. Comput. Prog. Biomed. **3**, 45–57 (1973)

French, A. S., Järvilehto, M.: The dynamic behaviour of photoreceptor cells in the fly in response to random (white noise) stimulation at a range of temperatures. J. Physiol. (Lond.) **274**, 311–322 (1978a)

French, A. S., Järvilehto, M.: The transmission of information by first and second order neurons in the fly visual system. J. Comp. Physiol. **126**, 87–96 (1978b)

French, A. S., Snyder, A. W., Stavenga, D. G.: Image degradation by an irregular retinal mosaic. Biol. Cybernetics **27**, 229–233 (1977)

Frieden, B. R.: Image enhancement and restoration. In: Picture processing and digital processing (ed. T. S. Huang). Berlin-Heidelberg-New York: Springer 1975

Frisch, K. von: The dance language and orientation of bees. Cambridge, Mass.: Harvard University Press 1967

Fuortes, M. G. F.: Electrical activity of cells in the eye of *Limulus*. Am. J. Ophthalmol. **46**, 210–223 (1958)

Fuortes, M. G. F., Hodgkin, A. L.: Changes in the time scale and sensitivity in the ommatidia of *Limulus*. J. Physiol. (Lond.) **172**, 239–263 (1964)

Fuortes, M. G. F., O'Bryan, P. M.: Generator potentials in invertebrate photoreceptors. In: Handbook of sensory physiology, Vol. VII/2 (ed. M. G. F. Fuortes), pp. 279–320. Berlin-Heidelberg-New York: Springer 1972a

Fuortes, M. G. F., O'Bryan, P. M.: Responses to single photons. In: Handbook of sensory physiology, Vol. VII/2 (ed. M. G. F. Fuortes), pp. 321–338. Berlin-Heidelberg-New York: Springer 1972b

Fuortes, M. G. F., Yeandle, S.: Probability of occurrence of discrete potential waves in the eye of *Limulus*. J. Gen. Physiol. **47**, 443–463 (1964)

Gallego, A.: Comparative study of the horizontal cells in the vertebrate retina: mammals and birds. In: Neural principles in vision (eds. F. Zettler, R. Weiler), pp. 26–62. Berlin-Heidelberg-New York: Springer 1976

Gavel, L. von: Die „kritische Streifenbreite" als Maß der Sehschärfe bei *Drosophila melanogaster*. Z. Vergl. Physiol. **27**, 80–135 (1939)

Gemperlein, R., Smola, U.: Übertragungseigenschaften der Sehzelle der Schmeißfliege *Calliphora erythrocephala*. I. Abhängigkeit vom Ruhepotential. J. Comp. Physiol. **78**, 30–52 (1972a)

Gemperlein, R., Smola, U.: Übertragungseigenschaften der Sehzelle der Schmeißfliege *Calliphora erythrocephala*. 3. Verbesserung des Signal-Störungs-Verhältnisses durch präsynaptische Summation in der Lamina ganglionaris. J. Comp. Physiol. **79**, 393–409 (1972b)

Glantz, R. M.: Light adaptation in the photoreceptors of the crayfish, *Procambarus clarki*. Vision Res. **8**, 1407–1421 (1968)

Glantz, R. M.: Peripheral versus central adaptation in the crustacean visual system. J. Neurophysiol. **34**, 485–492 (1971)

Glantz, R. M.: Visual adaptation: a case of non-linear summation. Vision Res. **12**, 103–109 (1972)

Goldsmith, T. H., Bernard, G.: The visual system of insects. In: The physiology of insects, 2nd Ed., Vol. II (ed. M. Rockstein). New York: Academic Press 1973

Goodman, C. S.: Anatomy of locust ocellar interneurons: constancy and variability. J. Comp. Physiol. **95**, 185–201 (1974)

Goodman, C. S.: Anatomy of the ocellar interneurons of acridid grasshoppers. I. The large interneurons. Cell Tissue Res. **175**, 183–203 (1976)

Goodman, C. S.: Neuron duplications and deletions in locust clones and clutches. Science **197**, 1384–1386 (1977)

Goodman, C. S., Williams, J. L. D.: Anatomy of the ocellar interneurons of acridid grasshoppers. II. The small interneurons. Cell Tissue Res. **175**, 203–225 (1976)

Goodman, L. J.: The structure and function of the insect dorsal ocellus. Adv. Insect Physiol. **7**, 97–195 (1970)

Goodman, L. J.: The neural organisation and physiology of the insect dorsal ocellus. In: The compound eye and vision of insects (ed. G. A. Horridge), pp. 514–548. Oxford: Clarendon Press 1975

Götz, K. G.: Optomotorische Untersuchung des visuellen Systems einiger Augenmutanten der Fruchtfliege *Drosophila*. Kybernetik **2**, 77–92 (1964)

Götz, K. G.: Die optischen Übertragungseigenschaften der Komplexaugen von *Drosophila*. Kybernetik **2**, 215–221 (1965)

Gray, E. G., Pease, H. L.: On understanding the organisation of the retinal receptor synapses. Brain Res. **35**, 1–15 (1971)

Gur, M., Purple, R. L., Whitehead, R.: Ultrastructure within the lateral plexus of the *Limulus* eye. J. Gen. Physiol. **59**, 285–304 (1972)

Gwilliam, G. F.: The mechanism of the shadow reflex in Cirripedia. I. Electrical activity in the supraesophageal ganglion and ocellar nerve. Biol. Bull. **125**, 470–485 (1963)

Gwilliam, G. F.: The mechanism of the shadow reflex in Cirripedia. II. Photoreceptor cell response, second-order responses, and motor output. Biol. Bull. **129**, 244–256 (1965)

Gwilliam, G. F.: The mechanism of the shadow reflex in Cirripedia. III. Rhythmical patterned activity in central neurons and its modulation by shadows. Biol. Bull. **151**, 141–160 (1976)

Gwilliam, G. F., Bradbury, J. C.: Activity patterns in the isolated central nervous system of the barnacle and their relation to behaviour. Biol. Bull. **141**, 502–513 (1971)

Gwilliam, G. F., Millecchia, R. J.: Barnacle photoreceptors: their physiology and role in the control of behaviour. Prog. Neurobiol. **4**, 211–239 (1975)

Hagiwara, S.: Calcium spike. Adv. Biophys. **4**, 71–102 (1973)

Hamdorf, K.: The physiology of invertebrate visual pigments. In: Handbook of sensory physiology, Vol. VII/6 A (ed. H. Autrum), pp. 145–224. Berlin-Heidelberg-New York: Springer 1979

Hamdorf, K., Kaschef, A. H.: Der Sauerstoffverbrauch des Facettenauges von *Calliphora erythrocephala* in Abhängigkeit von der Temperatur und dem Ionenmilieu. Z. Vergl. Physiol. **48**, 251–265 (1964)

Hamdorf, K., Schwemer, J.: Photoregeneration and the adaptation process in insect photoreceptors. In: Photoreceptor optics (eds. A. W. Snyder, R. Menzel), pp. 363–389. Berlin-Heidelberg-New York: Springer 1975

Hanani, M., Shaw, C.: A potassium contribution to the response of the barnacle photoreceptor. J. Physiol. (Lond.) **270**, 151–163 (1977)

Hardie, R. C.: Peripheral visual function in the fly. Ph.D. Thesis. Australian National University, Canberra 1978

Hardie, R. C.: Electrophysiological analysis of fly retina. I. Comparative properties of R 1–6 and R 7 and 8. J. Comp. Physiol. **129**, 19–33 (1979)

Hartline, H. K.: Visual receptors and retinal interaction. Science **164**, 270–278 (1969)

Hartline, H. K., MacDonald, P. R.: Light and dark adaptation of single photoreceptor elements in the eye of *Limulus*. J. Cell. Comp. Physiol. **30**, 225–253 (1947)

Hartline, H. K., Ratliff, F.: Inhibitory interaction of receptor units in the eye of *Limulus*. J. Gen. Physiol. **40**, 357–376 (1957)

Hartline, H. K., Ratliff, F.: Spatial summation of inhibitory influences in the eye of *Limulus*, and the mutual interaction of receptor units. J. Gen. Physiol. **41**, 1049–1066 (1958)

Hartline, H. K., Ratliff, F.: Inhibitory interaction in the retina of *Limulus*. In: Handbook of sensory physiology, Vol. VII/2 (ed. M. G. F. Fuortes), pp. 381–448. Berlin-Heidelberg-New York: Springer 1972

Hartline, H. K., Wagner, H. G., MacNichol, E. F.: The peripheral origin of nervous activity in the visual system. Cold Spring Harb. Symp. Quant. Biol. **17**, 125–141 (1952)

Hartzell, H. C., Kuffler, S. W., Stickgold, R., Yoshikami, D.: Synaptic excitation and inhibition resulting from direct action of acetylcholine on two types of chemoreceptors on individual amphibian parasympathetic neurones. J. Physiol. (Lond.) **271**, 817–846 (1977)

Hassenstein, B.: Ommatidienraster und afferente Bewegungsintegration (Versuche an dem Rüsselkäfer *Chlorophanus viridis*). Z. Vergl. Physiol. **33**, 301–326 (1951)

Hausen, K.: Functional characterization and anatomical identification of motion sensitive neurons in the lobula plate of the blowfly *Calliphora erythrocephala*. Z. Naturforsch. **31 c**, 629–633 (1976)

Hecht, S., Shlaer, S., Pirenne, M.: Energy, quanta, and vision. J. Gen. Physiol. **25**, 819–840 (1942)

Heisenberg, M.: Separation of receptor and lamina potentials in the electroretinogram of normal and mutant *Drosophila*. J. Exp. Biol. **55**, 85–100 (1971)

Heisenberg, M., Buchner, E.: The role of retinula cell types in visual behaviour of *Drosophila melanogaster*. J. Comp. Physiol. **117**, 127–162 (1977)

Hochstein, S., Minke, B., Hillman, P.: Antagonistic components of the late receptor potential in the barnacle photoreceptor arising from different stages of the pigment process. J. Gen. Physiol. **62**, 105–128 (1973)

Hodgkin, A. L., Huxley, A. F.: A quantitative description of membrane current and its application to conduction and excitation in nerve. J. Physiol. (Lond.) **117**, 500–544 (1952)

Honegger, H.-W., Schürmann, F. W.: Cobalt sulphide staining of optic fibres in the brain of the cricket, *Gryllus campestris*. Cell Tissue Res. **159**, 213–225 (1975)

Horridge, G. A.: Optical mechanisms of clear zone eyes. In: The compound eye and vision of insects (ed. G. A. Horridge), pp. 255–298. Oxford: Clarendon Press 1975 a

Horridge, G. A.: Arthropod receptor optics. In: Photoreceptor optics (eds. A. W. Snyder, R. Menzel), pp. 459–478. Berlin-Heidelberg-New York: Springer 1975 b

Horridge, G. A.: The compound eye of insects. Sci. Am. **237**, 108–120 (1977)

Horridge, G. A.: A different kind of vision: the compound eye. In: Handbook of perception, Vol. 8 (eds. E. C. Carterette, M. P. Friedman). New York: Academic Press 1978 a

Horridge, G. A.: The separation of visual axes in apposition compound eyes. Phil. Trans. R. Soc. Lond. (Biol.) **285**, 1–59 (1978 b)

Horridge, G. A., Giddings, C., Stange, G.: The superposition eye of skipper butterfly. Proc. R. Soc. Lond. (Biol.) **182**, 457–495 (1972)

Horridge, G. A., Meinertzhagen, I. A.: The accuracy of the patterns of connexions of the first- and second-order neurons of the visual system of *Calliphora*. Proc. R. Soc. Lond. (Biol.) **175**, 69–82 (1970 a)

Horridge, G. A., Meinertzhagen, I. A.: The exact neural projection of the visual fields upon the first and second ganglia of the insect eye. Z. Vergl. Physiol. **66**, 369–378 (1970 b)

Horridge, G. A., Tsukahara, Y.: Distribution of bumps in the tail of the locust photoreceptor afterpotential. J. Exp. Biol. **73**, 1–14 (1978)

Hoyle, G.: Functioning of the insect ocellar nerve. J. Exp. Biol. **32**, 397–407 (1955)

Hubel, D. H., Wiesel, T. N.: Receptive fields, binocular interaction and functional architecture in the cat's visual cortex. J. Physiol. **160**, 106–154 (1962)

Hubel, D. H., Wiesel, T. N.: Functional architecture of macaque monkey visual cortex. Proc. R. Soc. Lond. (Biol.) **198**, 1–59 (1977)

Hudspeth, A. J., Poo, M. M., Stuart, A. E.: Passive signal propagation and membrane properties in median photoreceptors of the giant barnacle. J. Physiol. (Lond.) **272**, 25–43 (1977)

Hudspeth, A. J., Stuart, A. E.: Morphology and responses to light of the somata, axons, and terminal regions of individual photoreceptors of the giant barnacle. J. Physiol. (Lond.) **272**, 1–23 (1977)

Iles, J. F.: Structure and synaptic activation of the fast coxal depressor motoneuron of the cockroach, *Periplaneta americana*. J. Exp. Biol. **56**, 647–656 (1972)

Ioannides, A. C.: Light adaptation and signal transmission in the compound eye of the giant water bug *Lethocerus* (Belastomatidae: Hemiptera). Ph.D. Thesis. Australian National University, Canberra 1972

Ioannides, A. C., Horridge, G. A.: The organization of visual fields in the hemipteran acone eye. Proc. R. Soc. Lond. (Biol.) **190**, 373–391 (1975)

Ioannides, A. C., Walcott, B.: Graded illumination potentials from retinula cell axons in the bug *Lethocerus*. Z. Vergl. Physiol. **71**, 315–325 (1971)

Jacobson, M.: Developmental neurobiology. New York: Holt, Rinehart, and Winston 1970

Järvilehto, M., Zettler, F.: Micro-localisation of lamina-located visual cell activities in the compound eye of the blowfly *Calliphora*. Z. Vergl. Physiol. **69**, 134–138 (1970)

Järvilehto, M., Zettler, F.: Localized intracellular potentials from pre- and postsynaptic components in the external plexiform layer of an insect retina. Z. Vergl. Physiol. **75**, 422–440 (1971)

Järvilehto, M., Zettler, F.: Electrophysiological-histological studies on some functional properties of visual cells and second order neurons of an insect retina. Z. Zellforsch. **136**, 291–306 (1973)

Johnston, D., Wachtel, H.: Electrophysiological basis for the spatial dependence of the inhibitory coupling in the *Limulus* retina. J. Gen. Physiol. **67**, 1–25 (1976)

Kaplan, E., Barlow, R. B.: Properties of visual cells in the lateral eye of *Limulus in situ*. Extracellular recordings. J. Gen. Physiol. **66**, 303–326 (1975)

Kaplan, E., Barlow, R. B.: Energy, quanta and *Limulus* vision. Vision Res. **16**, 745–751 (1976)

Katz, B.: Nerve muscle and synapse. New York: McGraw-Hill 1966

Katz, B., Miledi, R.: The statistical nature of the acetylcholine potential and its molecular components. J. Physiol. (Lond.) **224**, 665–699 (1972)

Katz, M. J., Lasek, R. J.: Evolution of the nervous system: role of ontogenetic mechanisms in the evolution of matching populations. Proc. Natl. Acad. Sci. U.S.A. **75**, 1349–1352 (1978)

Kirschfeld, K.: Discrete and graded potentials in the compound eye of the fly *Musca*. In: The functional organisation of the compound eye (ed. C. G. Bernhard). Oxford: Pergamon Press 1966

Kirschfeld, K.: Die Projektion der optischen Umwelt auf das Raster der Rhabdomere im Komplexauge von *Musca*. Exp. Brain Res. **3**, 248–270 (1967)

Kirschfeld, K.: The visual system of *Musca:* studies on optics, structure, and function. In: Information processing in the visual systems of arthropods (ed. R. Wehner). Berlin-Heidelberg-New York: Springer 1972

Kirschfeld, K.: The resolution of lens and compound eyes. In: Neural principles in vision (eds. F. Zettler, R. Weiler), pp. 354–372. Berlin-Heidelberg-New York: Springer 1976

Kirschfeld, K., Feiler, R., Franceschini, N.: A photostable pigment within the rhabdomere of fly photoreceptors No. 7. J. Comp. Physiol. **125**, 275–284 (1978)

Kirschfeld, K., Franceschini, N.: Ein Mechanismus zur Steuerung des Lichtflusses in den Rhabdomeren des Komplexauges von *Musca*. Kybernetik **6**, 13–22 (1969)

Kirschfeld, K., Franceschini, N., Minke, B.: Evidence for a sensitising pigment in fly photoreceptors. Nature (Lond.) **269**, 386–390 (1977)

Kirschfeld, K., Lutz, B.: Lateral inhibition in the compound eye of the fly, *Musca*. Z. Naturforsch. **29 c**, 95–97 (1974)

Kirschfeld, K., Reichardt, W.: Die Verarbeitung stationärer optischer Nachrichten im Komplexauge von *Limulus*. Kybernetik **2**, 43–61 (1964)

Kirschfeld, K., Wenk, P.: The dorsal compound eye of Simuliid flies: An eye specialised for the detection of small, rapidly moving objects. Z. Naturforsch. **31 c**, 764–765 (1976)

Kleinschmidt, J., Dowling, J. E.: Intracellular recordings from gecko photoreceptors during light and dark adaptation. J. Gen. Physiol. **66**, 617–648 (1975)

Klingman, A., Chappell, R. L.: Feedback synaptic interaction in the dragonfly ocellar retina. J. Gen. Physiol. **71**, 157–175 (1978)

Knight, B. W., Toyoda, J., Dodge, F. A.: A quantitative description of the dynamics of excitation and inhibition in the eye of *Limulus*. J. Gen. Physiol. **56**, 421–437 (1970)

Koike, H., Brown, H. M., Hagiwara, S.: Hyperpolarization of a barnacle photoreceptor membrane following illumination. J. Gen. Physiol. **57**, 723–737 (1971)

Krebs, W., Helrich, C. S., Wulff, V. J.: The role of restricted extracellular compartments in vision. Vision Res. **15**, 767–770 (1975)

Krebs, W., Schaten, B.: The lateral photoreceptor of the barnacle, *Balanus eberneus*. Quantitative morphology and fine structure. Cell Tissue Res. **168**, 193–207 (1976)

Krischer, C. F.: On the mechanism of electric response of the photoreceptors of the barnacle and other animals. Z. Naturforsch. **27 c**, 409–413 (1971)

Kuffler, S. W., Nicholls, J. G.: From neuron to brain. Sunderland, Mass.: Sinauer 1976

Land, M. F.: Visually guided movements in invertebrates. In: Function and formation of neural systems (ed. G. S. Stent). Berlin: Dahlem Konferenzen 1977

Laughlin, S. B.: Neural integration in the first optic neuropile of dragonflies. I. Signal amplification in dark-adapted second order neurons. J. Comp. Physiol. **84**, 335–355 (1973)

Laughlin, S. B.: Neural integration in the first optic neuropile of dragonflies. II. Receptor signal interactions in the lamina. J. Comp. Physiol. **92**, 357–375 (1974 a)

Laughlin, S. B.: Neural integration in the first optic neuropile of dragonflies. III. The transfer of angular information. J. Comp. Physiol. **92**, 377–396 (1974 b)

Laughlin, S. B.: Resistance changes associated with the response of insect monopolar neurons. Z. Naturforsch. **29 c**, 449–450 (1974 c)

Laughlin, S. B.: Receptor function in the apposition eye. An electrophysiological approach. In: Photoreceptor optics (eds. A. W. Snyder, R. Menzel), pp. 479–498. Berlin-Heidelberg-New York: Springer 1975 a

Laughlin, S. B.: Receptor and interneuron light adaptation in the dragonfly visual system. Z. Naturforsch. **30 c**, 306–308 (1975 b)

Laughlin, S. B.: The function of the lamina ganglionaris. In: The compound eye and vision of insects (ed. G. A. Horridge), pp. 341–358. Oxford: Oxford University Press 1975 c

Laughlin, S. B.: The sensitivities of dragonfly photoreceptors and the voltage gain of transduction. J. Comp. Physiol. **111**, 221–247 (1976 a)

Laughlin, S. B.: Adaptation of the dragonfly retina for contrast detection and the elucidation of neural principles in the peripheral visual system. In: Neural principles in vision (eds. F. Zettler, R. Weiler), pp. 175–193. Berlin-Heidelberg-New York: Springer 1976 b

Laughlin, S. B.: Neural integration in the first optic neuropile of dragonflies. IV. Interneuron spectral sensitivity and contrast coding. J. Comp. Physiol. **112**, 199–211 (1976 c)

Laughlin, S. B., Hardie, R. C.: Common strategies for light adaptation in the peripheral visual systems of fly and dragonfly. J. Comp. Physiol. **128**, 319–340 (1978)

Laughlin, S. B., McGinness, S.: The structures of dorsal and ventral regions of a dragonfly retina. Cell Tissue Res. **188**, 427–447 (1978)

Leggett, L. M. W.: Some visual specialisations of a crustacean eye. Ph.D. Thesis. Australian National University, Canberra 1977

Leutscher-Hazelhoff, J. T.: Linear and non-linear performance of transducer and pupil in *Calliphora* retinula cells. J. Physiol. (Lond.) **246**, 333–350 (1975)

Leutscher-Hazelhoff, J. T., Kuiper, J. W.: Responses of the blowfly *(Calliphora erythrocephala)* to light flashes and to sinusoidally modulated light. Doc. Ophthalmol. **18**, 275–283 (1964)

Levi-Setti, R., Park, D. A., Winston, R.: The corneal cones of *Limulus* as optimised light concentrators. Nature (Lond.) **253**, 115–116 (1975)

Lillywhite, P. G.: Single photon signals and transduction in an insect eye. J. Comp. Physiol. **122**, 189–200 (1977)

Lillywhite, P. G.: Coupling between locust photoreceptors revealed by a study of quantum bumps. J. Comp. Physiol. **125**, 13–27 (1978a)

Lillywhite, P. G.: Signal and noise in the insect visual system. Ph.D. Thesis. Australian National University, Canberra 1978b

Lillywhite, P. G., Laughlin, S. B.: A neglected source of intrinsic noise in photoreceptors. Proc. Aust. Physiol. Pharmacol. Soc. **9**, 49P (1978)

Lillywhite, P. G., Laughlin, S. B.: Transducer noise in a photoreceptor. Nature (Lond.) **277**, 569–572 (1979)

Lipetz, L. E.: The relation of physiological and psychological aspects of sensory intensity. In: Handbook of sensory physiology, Vol. I (ed. W. R. Loewenstein), pp. 191–225. Berlin-Heidelberg-New York: Springer 1971

Lisman, J. E.: Effects of removing extracellular Ca^{2+} on excitation and adaptation in *Limulus* ventral photoreceptors. Biophys. J. **16**, 1331–1335 (1976)

Lisman, J. E., Brown, J. E.: The effects of intracellular Ca^{2+} on the light response and on light adaptation in *Limulus* ventral photoreceptors. In: The visual system: neurophysiology, biophysics, and their clinical applications (ed. G. B. Arden). New York: Plenum 1972

Lisman, J. E., Brown, J. E.: Light induced changes of sensitivity in *Limulus* ventral photoreceptors. J. Gen. Physiol. **66**, 473–488 (1975)

Listøl, K., Nja, A., Walløe, L.: Enhanced contrast arising from reflex inhibition in an array of stretch receptors. Biol. Cybernetics **24**, 75–83 (1976)

Loewenstein, W. R.: The generation of electrical activity in a nerve ending. Ann. N.Y. Acad. Sci. **81**, 367–387 (1958)

Macagno, E. R., Lopresti, V., Levinthal, C.: Structure and development of neuronal connections in isogenic organisms: variations and similarities in the optic system of *Daphnia magna*. Proc. Natl. Acad. Sci. U.S.A. **70**, 57–61 (1973)

McCann, G. D.: Nonlinear identification theory models for successive stages of visual nervous systems of flies. J. Neurophysiol. **27**, 869–895 (1974)

McCann, G. D., Arnett, D. W.: Spectral and polarisation sensitivity of the dipteran visual system. J. Gen. Physiol. **59**, 534–558 (1972)

McCann, G. D., MacGinitie, G. F.: Optomotor response studies of insect vision. Proc. R. Soc. Lond. (Biol.) **163**, 269–401 (1965)

Marmarelis, P. Z., Naka, K.-I.: Identification of multi-input biological systems. IEEE Trans. Biomed. Eng. **BME 21**, 88–101 (1974)

Martin, A. R.: A further study of the statistical composition of the end-plate potential. J. Physiol. (Lond.) **130**, 114–122 (1955)

Meinertzhagen, I. A.: Erroneous projection of retinula axons beneath a dislocation in the retinal equator of *Calliphora*. Brain Res. **41**, 39–49 (1972)

Meinertzhagen, I. A.: The organization of perpendicular fibre pathways in the insect optic lobe. Phil. Trans. R. Soc. Lond. **274**, 555–596 (1976)

Menzel, R.: Spectral sensitivity of monopolar cells in the bee lamina. J. Comp. Physiol. **93**, 337–346 (1974)

Menzel, R.: Spectral sensitivity and colour vision in invertebrates. In: Handbook of sensory physiology, Vol. VII/6A (ed. H. Autrum), pp. 503–580. Berlin-Heidelberg-New York: Springer 1979

Menzel, R., Blakers, M.: Colour receptors in the bee eye – morphology and spectral sensitivity. J. Comp. Physiol. **108**, 11–33 (1976)

Menzel, R., Snyder, A. W.: Polarised light detection in the bee, *Apis mellifera*. J. Comp. Physiol. **88**, 247–270 (1974)

Millecchia, R., Gwilliam, G. F.: Photoreception in a barnacle: electrophysiology of the shadow reflex pathway in *Balanus cariosus*. Science **177**, 438–441 (1972)

Miller, W. H., Cawthon, D. F.: Pigment granule movement in *Limulus* photoreceptors. Invest. Ophthalmol. **13**, 401–405 (1974)

Mimura, K.: Analysis of visual information in lamina neurones of the fly. J. Comp. Physiol. **88**, 335–372 (1974)

Mimura, K.: Some spatial properties in the first ganglion of the fly. J. Comp. Physiol. **105**, 65–82 (1976)

Mobbs, P.G.: Development of the locust ocellus. Nature (Lond.) **264**, 269–271 (1976)

Mote, M.I.: Focal recordings of responses evoked by light in the lamina ganglionaris of the fly *Sarcophaga bullata*. J. Exp. Zool. **175**, 149–158 (1970 a)

Mote, M.I.: Electrical correlates of neural superposition in the eye of the fly *Sarcophaga bullata*. J. Exp. Zool. **175**, 159–168 (1970 b)

Muller, K.J.: Photoreceptors in the crayfish compound eye: electrical interactions between cells as related to polarized-light sensitivity. J. Physiol. (Lond.) **232**, 573–596 (1973)

Mulloney, B., Selverston, A.: Antidromic action potentials fail to demonstrate known interactions between neurons. Science **177**, 69–72 (1972)

Munz, F.W., McFarland, W.N.: Evolutionary adaptations of fishes to the photic environment. In: Handbook of sensory physiology, Vol. VII/5 (ed. F. Crescitelli), pp. 193–274. Berlin-Heidelberg-New York: Springer 1977

Naka, K.-I., Kishida, K.: Retinal action potentials during dark and light adaptation. In: The functional organization of the compound eye (ed. C.G. Bernhard). Oxford: Pergamon Press 1966

Naka, K.-I., Rushton, W.A.H.: S-potentials from colour units in the retina of fish (Cyprinidae). J. Physiol. (Lond.) **185**, 536–555 (1966)

Nässel, D.R.: The organization of the lamina ganglionaris of the prawn, *Pandalus borealis* (Kroyer). Cell Tissue Res. **163**, 445–464 (1975)

Nässel, D.R.: The retina and retinal projection on the lamina ganglionaris of the crayfish *Pacifastacus leniusculus* (Dana). J. Comp. Neurol. **167**, 341–360 (1976)

Nässel, D.R.: Types and arrangements of neurons in the crayfish optic lamina. Cell Tissue Res. **179**, 45–75 (1977)

Nässel, D.R., Waterman, T.H.: Golgi EM evidence for visual information channelling in the crayfish lamina ganglionaris. Brain Res. **130**, 556–563 (1977)

Normann, R.A., Perlman, I.: Evaluating sensitivity changing mechanisms in light-adapted photoreceptors. Vision Res. **19**, 391–394 (1979)

Normann, R.A., Werblin, F.S.: Control of retinal sensitivity. I. Light and dark-adaptation of vertebrate rods and cones. J. Gen. Physiol. **63**, 37–61 (1974)

Ochs, A.L.: Is Fourier analysis performed by the visual system or by the visual investigator? J. Opt. Soc. Am. **69**, 95–98 (1979)

Ohly, K.P.: The neurons of the first synaptic regions of the optic neuropil of the firefly, *Phausis splendidula* L. (Coleoptera). Cell Tissue Res. **158**, 89–109 (1975)

Ohno, S.: Evolution by gene duplication. Berlin-Heidelberg-New York: Springer 1970

O'Shea, M., Rowell, C.H.F., Williams, J.L.D.: The anatomy of a locust visual interneuron; the descending contralateral movement detector. J. Exp. Biol. **60**, 1–12 (1974)

Ozawa, S., Hagiwara, S., Nicolaysen, K., Stuart, A.E.: Signal transmission from photoreceptors to ganglion cells in the visual system of the giant barnacle. Cold Spring Harb. Symp. Quant. Biol. **40**, 563–570 (1976)

Palay, S.L., Chan-Palay, V.: A guide to the synaptic analysis of neuropil. Cold Spring Harb. Symp. Quant. Biol. **40**, 1–16 (1976)

Palka, J.: Abnormal neural development in invertebrates. In: Function and formation of neural systems (ed. G.S. Stent). Berlin: Dahlem Konferenzen 1977

Patterson, J.A., Goodman, L.J.: Intracellular responses of receptor cells and second-order cells in the ocelli of the desert locust, *Schistocerca gregaria*. J. Comp. Physiol. **95**, 237–250 (1974)

Perrelet, A.: The fine structure of the retina of the honeybee drone. Z. Zellforsch. **108**, 530–562 (1970)

Pinter, R.B.: Frequency and time domain properties of retinula cells of the desert locust *(Schistocerca gregaria)* and the house cricket *(Acheta domesticus)*. J. Comp. Physiol. **77**, 383–397 (1972)

Pirenne, M.H.: Vision and the eye. London: Chapman and Hall 1967

Poggio, T., Reichardt, W.: Visual control of orientation behaviour in the fly. II. Towards the underlying neural interactions. Q. Rev. Biophys. **9**, 377–438 (1976)

Purple, R.L., Dodge, F.A.: Interaction of excitation and inhibition in the eccentric cell in the eye of *Limulus*. Cold Spr. Harb. Symp. Quant. Biol. **30**, 529–537 (1965)

Ratliff, F.: Mach bands: quantitative studies on neural networks in the retina. San Francisco: Holden-Day 1965

Ratliff, F., Hartline, H.K.: Studies on excitation and inhibition in the retina. A collection of papers from the laboratories of H. Keffer Hartline. London: Chapman and Hall 1974

Ratliff, F., Hartline, H. K., Miller, W. H.: Spatial and temporal aspects of retinal inhibitory interaction. J. Opt. Soc. Am. **53**, 110–120 (1963)

Ratliff, F., Knight, B. W., Dodge, F. A., Hartline, H. K.: Fourier analysis of dynamics of excitation and inhibition in the eye of *Limulus*: amplitude, phase, and distance. Vision Res. **14**, 1155–1168 (1974)

Ratliff, F., Knight, B. W., Graham, N.: On tuning and amplification by lateral inhibition. Proc. Natl. Acad. Sci. U.S.A. **62**, 733–740 (1969)

Reichardt, W.: Über das optische Auflösungsvermögen der Facettenaugen von *Limulus*. Kybernetik **1**, 57–69 (1961)

Reichardt, W.: Transduction of single-quantum effects. (Evidence from behavioural experiments on the fly). In: Processing of optical data by organisms and machines (ed. W. Reichardt). New York: Academic Press 1969

Reichardt, W.: The insect eye as a model for analysis of uptake, transduction, and processing of optical data in the nervous system. In: The neurosciences, second study programme (ed. F. O. Schmitt). New York: Rockefeller University Press 1970

Reichardt, W., Braitenberg, V., Weidel, G.: Auslösung von Elementarprozessen durch einzelne Lichtquanten im Fliegenauge. Kybernetik **5**, 148–170 (1968)

Reichardt, W., Poggio, T.: Visual control of orientation behaviour in the fly. Part I. A quantitative analysis. Q. Rev. Biophys. **9**, 311–375 (1976)

Ribi, W. A.: Neurons in the first synaptic region of the bee, *Apis mellifera*. Cell Tissue Res. **148**, 277–286 (1974)

Ribi, W. A.: The first optic ganglion of the bee. I. Correlation between visual cell types and their terminals in the lamina and the medulla. Cell Tissue Res. **155**, 103–111 (1975)

Ribi, W. A.: The first optic ganglion of the bee. II. Topographical relationships of the monopolar cells within and between cartridges. Cell Tissue Res. **171**, 359–373 (1976)

Ribi, W. A.: Fine structure of the first optic ganglion (lamina) of the cockroach, *Periplaneta americana*. Tissue Cell **9**, 57–72 (1977)

Ribi, W. A.: Gap junctions coupling photoreceptor axons in the first optic ganglion of the fly. Cell Tissue Res. **195**, 299–308 (1978)

Ripps, H., Shakib, M., MacDonald, E. D.: Peroxidase uptake by photoreceptor terminals of the skate retina. J. Cell Biol. **70**, 86–96 (1976)

Rodieck, R. W.: The vertebrate retina. Principles of structure and function. San Francisco: W. H. Freeman 1973

Rose, A.: The relative sensitivities of television pickup tubes, photographic film and the human eye. Proc. I.R.E. **30**, 293–300 (1942)

Rose, A.: Vision, human, and electronic. New York, London: Plenum Press 1972

Ross, W. N., Stuart, A. E.: Voltage sensitive calcium channels in the presynaptic terminals of a decrementally conducting photoreceptor. J. Physiol. (Lond.) **274**, 173–191 (1978)

Rossel, S.: Regional differences in photoreceptor performance in the eye of the praying mantis. J. Comp. Physiol. **131**, 95–112 (1979)

Rowell, C. H. F.: The orthopteran descending movement detector (DMD) neurones: a characterisation and review. Z. Vergl. Physiol. **73**, 167–194 (1971)

Rowell, C. H. F., O'Shea, M., Williams, J. L. D.: The neuronal basis of a sensory analyser, the acridid movement detector system. IV. The preference for small field stimuli. J. Exp. Biol. **68**, 157–185 (1977)

Ruck, P.: Electrophysiology of the insect dorsal ocellus. I. Origin of the components of the electroretinogram. J. Gen. Physiol. **44**, 605–627 (1961)

Saktor, B.: Energetics and respiratory metabolism of muscular contraction. In: The physiology of insecta. 1st Ed. (ed. M. Rockstein). New York: Academic Press 1965

Sandeman, D. C.: Regionalization in the eye of the crab *Leptograpsus variegatus:* eye movements evoked by a target moving in different parts of the visual field. J. Comp. Physiol. **123**, 299–306 (1978)

Scholes, J. H.: Discrete subthreshold potentials from the dimly lit insect eye. Nature (Lond.) **202**, 572–573 (1964)

Scholes, J. H.: Discontinuity of the excitation process in locust visual cells. Cold Spring Harb. Symp. Quant. Biol. **30**, 517–527 (1965)

Scholes, J. H.: The electrical responses of the retinal receptors and the lamina in the visual system of the fly *Musca*. Kybernetik **6**, 149–162 (1969)

Scholes, J.H., Reichardt, W.: The quantal content of optomotor stimuli and the electrical responses of receptors in the compound eye of the fly *Musca*. Kybernetik **6**, 74–80 (1969)

Schwartz, E.A.: Retinular and eccentric cell morphology in the neural plexus of *Limulus* lateral eye. J. Neurobiol. **2**, 129–133 (1971)

Shapley, R.: Effects of lateral inhibition on fluctuations of impulse rate. J. Gen. Physiol. **57**, 557–575 (1971)

Shaw, S.R.: Organization of the locust retina. Symp. Zool. Soc. Lond. **23**, 135–163 (1968a)

Shaw, S.R.: Polarized light perception and receptor interaction in arthropod compound eyes. Ph.D. Thesis. University of St. Andrews 1968b

Shaw, S.R.: Interreceptor coupling in ommatidia of drone honeybee and locust compound eyes. Vision Res. **9**, 999–1029 (1969a)

Shaw, S.R.: Sense-cell structure and interspecies comparisons of polarised light absorption in arthropod compound eyes. Vision Res. **9**, 1031–1040 (1969b)

Shaw, S.R.: Decremental conduction of the visual signal in the barnacle lateral eye. J. Physiol. (Lond.) **220**, 145–175 (1972)

Shaw, S.R.: Retinal resistance barriers and electrical lateral inhibition. Nature (Lond.) **255**, 480–483 (1975)

Shaw, S.R.: Restricted diffusion and extracellular space in the insect retina. J. Comp. Physiol. **113**, 257–282 (1977)

Shaw, S.R.: The extracellular space and blood-eye barrier in an insect retina: an ultrastructural study. Cell Tissue Res. **188**, 35–61 (1978a)

Shaw, S.R.: Signal transmission by graded slow potentials in the arthropod peripheral visual system. In: The neurosciences: 4th study programme (eds. F.O. Schmitt, F.G. Worden). Cambridge, Mass.: MIT Press 1978b

Sherk, T.E.: Development of the compound eyes of dragonflies (Odonata). I. Larval compound eyes. J. Exp. Zool. **201**, 391–416 (1977)

Sherk, T.E.: Development of the compound eyes of dragonflies (Odonata). II. Development of the larval compound eyes. J. Exp. Zool. **203**, 47–60 (1978a)

Sherk, T.E.: Development of the compound eyes of dragonflies (Odonata). III. Adult compound eyes. J. Exp. Zool. **203**, 61–80 (1978b)

Sherk, T.E.: Development of the compound eyes of dragonflies (Odonata). IV. Development of the adult compound eyes. J. Exp. Zool. **203**, 183–200 (1978c)

Simon, E.J., Lamb, T.D.: Electrical noise in turtle cones. In: Vertebrate photoreception (eds. H.B. Barlow, P. Fatt). New York: Academic Press 1977

Smith, T.G., Baumann, F.: The functional organisation within the ommatidium of the lateral eye of *Limulus*. In: Progress in brain research, Vol. 31 (eds. K. Akert, P.G. Waser). Amsterdam: Elsevier 1969

Smola, U.: Voltage noise in insect visual cells. In: Neural principles in vision (eds. F. Zettler, R. Weiler), pp. 194–213. Berlin-Heidelberg-New York: Springer 1976

Smola, U., Gemperlein, R.: Übertragungseigenschaften der Sehzelle der Schmeißfliege *Calliphora erythrocephala*. 2. Die Abhängigkeit vom Ableitort: Retina-Lamina ganglionaris. J. Comp. Physiol. **79**, 363–392 (1972)

Smola, U., Gemperlein, R.: Rezeptorrauschen und Informationskapazität der Sehzellen von *Calliphora erythrocephala* und *Periplaneta americana*. J. Comp. Physiol. **87**, 393–404 (1973)

Snodderly, D.M.: Processing of visual inputs by brain of *Limulus*. J. Neurophysiol. **34**, 588–611 (1971)

Snyder, A.W.: Acuity of compound eyes: physical limitations and design. J. Comp. Physiol. **116**, 161–182 (1977)

Snyder, A.W.: Physics of vision in compound eyes. In: Handbook of sensory physiology, Vol. VII/6A (ed. H. Autrum), pp. 225–314. Berlin-Heidelberg-New York: Springer 1979

Snyder, A.W., Laughlin, S.B.: Dichroism and absorption by photoreceptors. J. Comp. Physiol. **100**, 101–116 (1975)

Snyder, A.W., Laughlin, S.B., Stavenga, D.G.: Information capacity of eyes. Vision Res. **17**, 1163–1175 (1977a)

Snyder, A.W., Menzel, R., Laughlin, S.B.: Structure and function of the fused rhabdom. J. Comp. Physiol. **87**, 99–135 (1973)

Snyder, A.W., Stavenga, D.G., Laughlin, S.B.: Spatial information capacity of compound eyes. J. Comp. Physiol. **116**, 183–207 (1977b)

Srinivasan, M. V., Bernard, G. D.: The effect of motion on visual acuity of the compound eye: a theoretical analysis. Vision Res. **15**, 515–525 (1975)

Stavenga, D. G.: Pseudopupils of compound eyes. In: Handbook of sensory physiology, Vol. VII/6 A (ed. H. Autrum), pp. 357–440. Berlin-Heidelberg-New York: Springer 1979

Stell, W. K.: The morphological organisation of the vertebrate retina. In: Handbook of sensory physiology, Vol. VII/2 (ed. M. G. F. Fuortes), pp. 111–214. Berlin-Heidelberg-New York: Springer 1972

Stell, W. K., Ishida, A. T., Lightfoot, D. O.: Structural basis for on- and off-centre responses in retinal bipolar cells. Science **198**, 1269–1271 (1977)

Stevens, C. F.: A quantitative theory of neural interactions: theoretical and experimental investigations. Thesis. New York: Rockefeller Institute 1964

Stevens, C. F.: Study of membrane permeability changes by fluctuation analysis. Nature (Lond.) **270**, 391–396 (1977)

Stowe, S.: The retina lamina projection in the crab *Leptograpsus variegatus*. Cell Tissue Res. **185**, 515–525 (1977)

Stowe, S., Leggett, M.: Retina-lamina connectivity and polarization sensitivity in crustacea. Vision Res. **18**, 1087 (1978)

Stowe, S., Ribi, W. A., Sandeman, D. C.: The organization of the lamina ganglionaris of the crabs *Scylla serrata* and *Leptograpsus variegatus*. Cell Tissue Res. **178**, 517–532 (1977)

Strausfeld, N. J.: The organizations of the insect visual system (light microscopy). I. Projections and arrangements of neurons in the lamina ganglionaris of diptera. Z. Zellforsch. **121**, 377–441 (1971)

Strausfeld, N. J.: Atlas of an insect brain. Berlin-Heidelberg-New York: Springer 1976 a

Strausfeld, N. J.: Mosaic organizations, layers, and visual pathways in the insect brain. In: Neural principles in vision (eds. F. Zettler, R. Weiler), pp. 245–279. Berlin-Heidelberg-New York: Springer 1976 b

Strausfeld, N. J., Blest, A. D.: Golgi studies on insects. I. The optic lobes of Lepidoptera. Phil. Trans. R. Soc. Lond. (Biol.) **258**, 81–134 (1970)

Strausfeld, N. J., Campos-Ortega, J. A.: L 3, the 3 rd second order neuron of the 1 st visual ganglion in the "neural superposition" eye of *Musca domestica*. Z. Zellforsch. **139**, 397–403 (1973 a)

Strausfeld, N. J., Campos-Ortega, J. A.: The L 4 monopolar neurone: a substrate for lateral interaction in the visual system of the fly *Musca domestica*. Brain Res. **59**, 97–117 (1973 b)

Strausfeld, N. J., Campos-Ortega, J. A.: Vision in insects: pathways possibly underlying neural adaptation and lateral inhibition. Science **195**, 894–897 (1977)

Thibos, L. N., Werblin, F. S.: The response properties of the steady antagonistic surround in the mudpuppy retina. J. Physiol. (Lond.) **278**, 79–99 (1978)

Thorson, J.: Small-signal analysis of a visual reflex in the locust. I. Input parameters. Kybernetik **3**, 41–53 (1966)

Tisdale, A. D., Nakajima, Y.: Fine structure of synaptic vesicles in two types of nerve terminal in crayfish stretch receptor organs: Influence of fixation methods. J. Comp. Neurol. **165**, 369–386 (1976)

Toh, Y., Kuwabara, M.: Fine structure of the dorsal ocellus of the worker honeybee. J. Morphol. **143**, 285–305 (1974)

Toh, Y., Kuwabara, M.: Synaptic organisation of the fleshfly ocellus. J. Neurocytol. **4**, 271–287 (1975)

Tomita, T., Kikuchi, R., Tanaka, I.: Excitation and inhibition in lateral eye of horseshoe crab. In: Electrical activity of single cells. Tokyo: Igakushoin, Haga 1960

Trujillo-Cenóz, O.: Some aspects of the structural organisation of the intermediate retina of Dipterans. J. Ultrastruct. Res. **13**, 1–33 (1965)

Trujillo-Cenóz, O., Melamed, J.: Compound eye of dipterans: anatomical basis for integration – an electron microscope study. J. Ultrastruct. Res. **16**, 395–398 (1966)

Trujillo-Cenóz, O., Melamed, J.: Light and electronmicroscope study of one of the systems of centrifugal fibers found in the lamina of muscoid flies. Z. Zellforsch. **110**, 336–349 (1970)

Tsukahara, Y., Horridge, G. A.: Miniature potentials, light adaptation and after potentials in locust retinula cells. J. Exp. Biol. **68**, 137–149 (1977 a)

Tsukahara, Y., Horridge, G. A.: Interaction between two retinula cell types in the anterior eye of the dronefly, *Eristalis*. J. Comp. Physiol. **115**, 287–298 (1977 b)

Tyrer, N. M., Altman, J. S.: Motor and sensory flight neurons in a locust demonstrated using cobalt chloride. J. Comp. Neurol. **157**, 117–138 (1974)

Wachtel, H., Kandel, E.: Conversion of synaptic excitation to inhibition at a dual chemical synapse. J. Neurophysiol. **34**, 56–68 (1971)

Walcott, B.: Unit studies on light-adaptation in the retina of the crayfish, *Cherax destructor*. J. Comp. Physiol. **94**, 207–218 (1974)

Walcott, B.: Anatomical changes during light adaptation in insect compound eyes. In: The compound eye and vision of insects (ed. G. A. Horridge), pp. 20–36. Oxford: Oxford University Press 1975

Walls, G. L.: The vertebrate eye and its adaptive radiation. (Facsimile of 1942 ed.). New York: Hafner 1967

Wasserman, G. S., Kong, K.-L.: Temporal summation in a photoreceptor: dependence on response magnitude. Vision Res. **15**, 1297–1299 (1975)

Waterman, T. H.: Directional sensitivity of single ommatidia in the compound eye of *Limulus*. Proc. Natl. Acad. Sci. U.S.A. **40**, 252–257 (1954)

Wehner, R.: Pattern recognition. In: The compound eye and vision of insects (ed. G. A. Horridge), pp. 75–113. Oxford: Clarendon Press 1975

Wehner, R.: Structure and function of the peripheral visual pathway in Hymenopterans. In: Neural principles in vision (eds. F. Zettler, R. Weiler), pp. 280–333. Berlin-Heidelberg-New York: Springer 1976

Werblin, F. S.: Adaptation in a vertebrate retina: Intracellular recording in *Necturus*. J. Neurophysiol. **34**, 228–241 (1971)

Werblin, F. S.: Functional organisation of a vertebrate retina: sharpening up in space and intensity. Ann. N.Y. Acad. Sci. **193**, 75–85 (1972)

Werblin, F. S.: The control of sensitivity in the retina. Sci. Am. **228**, 70–79 (1973)

Werblin, F. S.: Control of retinal sensitivity II. Lateral interactions at the outer plexiform layer. J. Gen. Physiol. **63**, 62–87 (1974)

Werblin, F. S.: Regenerative hyperpolarisation in rods. J. Physiol. (Lond.) **244**, 53–81 (1975)

Werblin, F. S.: Synaptic interactions mediating bipolar response in the retina of the tiger salamander. In: Vertebrate photoreception (eds. H. B. Barlow, P. Fatt). New York: Academic Press 1977

Werblin, F. S., Dowling, J. E.: Organisation of the retina of the mudpuppy, *Necturus maculosa*. II. Intracellular recordings. J. Neurophysiol. **32**, 339–355 (1969)

Westheimer, G.: Optical properties of vertebrate eyes. In: Handbook of sensory physiology, Vol. VII/2 (ed. M. G. F. Fuortes), pp. 449–482. Berlin-Heidelberg-New York: Springer 1972 a

Westheimer, G.: Visual acuity and spatial modulation thresholds. In: Handbook of sensory physiology, Vol. VII/4 (eds. D. Jameson, L. M. Hurvich), pp. 170–187. Berlin-Heidelberg-New York: Springer 1972 b

White, R., Lord, E.: Diminution and enlargement of the mosquito rhabdom in light and darkness. J. Gen. Physiol. **65**, 583–598 (1975)

Whitehead, R., Purple, R. L.: Synaptic organisation in the neuropile of the lateral eye of *Limulus*. Vision Res. **10**, 129–133 (1970)

Wiggin, J. F.: Gamma correction in live color TV cameras. IEEE Trans. **BC-14**, 8–13 (1968)

Wilson, M.: Angular sensitivity of light and dark adapted locust retinula cells. J. Comp. Physiol. **97**, 323–328 (1975)

Wilson, M.: The functional organisation of the locust ocellus. J. Comp. Physiol. **124**, 297–316 (1978 a)

Wilson, M.: Generation of graded potential signals in the second order cells of locust ocellus. J. Comp. Physiol. **124**, 317–331 (1978 b)

Wilson, M.: The origin and properties of discrete hyperpolarising potentials in the second order cells of locust ocellus. J. Comp. Physiol. **128**, 347–358 (1978 c)

Wolburg-Bucholz, K.: The superposition eye of *Cloeon dipterum:* the organization of the lamina ganglionaris. Cell Tissue Res. **177**, 9–28 (1977)

Wu, C.-F., Pak, W. L.: Quantal basis of photoreceptor spectral sensitivity of *Drosophila melanogaster*. J. Gen. Physiol. **66**, 149–168 (1975)

Wu, C.-F., Pak, W. L.: Light-induced voltage noise in the photoreceptor of *Drosophila melanogaster*. J. Gen. Physiol. **71**, 249–268 (1978)

Wu, C.-F., Wong, F.: Frequency characteristics in the visual system of *Drosophila* – genetic dissection of electroretinogram components. J. Gen. Physiol. **69**, 705–724 (1977)

Wyszecki, G., Stiles, W. S.: Color Science. New York: Wiley 1967

Yeandle, S.: Evidence of quantized slow potentials in the eye of *Limulus*. Am. J. Ophthalmol. **46**, 82–87 (1958)

Zettler, F.: Die Abhängigkeit des Übertragungsverhaltens von Frequenz und Adaptationszustand, gemessen am einzelnen Lichtrezeptor von *Calliphora erythrocephala*. Z. Vergl. Physiol. **64**, 432–449 (1969)

Zettler, F., Autrum, H.: Chromatic properties of lateral inhibition in the eye of a fly. J. Comp. Physiol. **97**, 181–188 (1975)

Zettler, F., Järvilehto, M.: Histologische Lokalisation der Ableitelektrode, Belichtungspotentiale aus Retina und Lamina bei *Calliphora*. Z. Vergl. Physiol. **68**, 202–210 (1970)

Zettler, F., Järvilehto, M.: Decrement-free conduction of graded potentials along the axon of a monopolar neuron. Z. Vergl. Physiol. **75**, 402–421 (1971)

Zettler, F., Järvilehto, M.: Lateral inhibition in an insect eye. Z. Vergl. Physiol. **76**, 233–244 (1972)

Zettler, F., Järvilehto, M.: Active and passive axonal propagation of non-spike signals in the retina of *Calliphora*. J. Comp. Physiol. **85**, 89–104 (1973)

Zettler, F., Weiler, R.: Neural processing in the first optic neuropile of the compound eye of the fly. In: Neural principles in vision (eds. F. Zettler, R. Weiler), pp. 227–237. Berlin-Heidelberg-New York: Springer 1976

Zimmerman, R.P.: Field potential analysis and the physiology of second order neurons in the visual system of the fly. J. Comp. Physiol. **126**, 297–316 (1978)

Chapter 3

Polarization Sensitivity

Talbot H. Waterman, New Haven, Conn., USA

With 150 Figures and 1 Table

Contents

A. Introduction

Our virtual blindness to the polarization of light tends to block an appreciation of its widespread occurrence in nature. This blind spot has largely deprived us of potentially useful knowledge about the world around us. It has also kept us quite unaware, until rather recently (1948), that many other organisms do not share our deficiency. Instead, a large number of animals are significantly sensitive to at least some parameters of the polarization state.

The specific mechanisms involved, as well as their adaptive significance, are still rather imperfectly known. They are, however, increasingly lively areas of current research. This is not surprising in view of the inherent interest of the physiological problems involved, as well as their broad implications, for direction finding, visual contrast enhancement, and local station keeping. To introduce the background and present status of this topic, which is the purpose of this chapter, some definitions may first be in order.

I. Definitions

Terminology and symbols often present dilemmas which seem inevitable. Definitions dealing with the biological relevance of polarized light are no exception. Conflicts arise between convenient qualitative verbalizations and precise quantitative specification, as well as between customary usages, in several relevant disciplines and the various animal groups involved. This situation is not simplified by the hierarchy of levels from environmental optics to behavior with which the biologist must deal.

For the most general qualitative case, a rather noncommittal, yet expressive, term is needed. Polarization sensitivity has been used here for this purpose. By this I qualitatively mean the inherent capacity (i.e., the detector in the animal, not its surroundings) of an animal or its component sensory, neural, or effector elements, including behavior to respond differentially to optical polarization in its environment. This broad usage does not specify either the kind of response or the specific parameter of the polarization state which may be evoking it.

As reviewed previously (WATERMAN, 1974a, 1975c) for fully polarized light, these parameters would basically include the size, shape, orientation, and handedness of the polarization ellipse. But since natural polarized light is almost exclusively linearly, and only rarely elliptically, polarized, just two of these four dimensions, e-vector orientation (ϕ) and size or intensity (I) should fully define practically all biologically significant cases. However, natural polarized light usually is only partially polarized, therefore an additional parameter, degree of polarization (p), which is usually defined as the ratio of polarized to total intensities,

$$p = I_p/I_t \tag{1}$$

is required to characterize it.

These three parameters (i.e., ϕ, p, and I) would fully describe linearly polarized light from any particular point in visual space. A minimum requirement for inherent polarization sensitivity in an animal, therefore, is that either ϕ or p, or both, are to some effective degree distinguishable from I. In addition to instantaneously detecting polarization at a point, such discrimination might involve either spatial or temporal changes in ϕ and p, as well as polarization independent parameters [e.g., wavelength (λ) or I_t] as discussed below.

If polarization sensitivity were limited to discrimination between ϕ and I in linearly polarized light, it could more specifically be called e-vector sensitivity. However, only when the parameters of natural polarized light, which are in fact being utilized in a particular case, can be specified would the general use of such a restriction be justified.

In many laboratory situations where ϕ is the experimental variable, e-vector sensitivity is a quite appropriate general term. Even this, however, needs to be specifically restricted for quantitative use. Thus the e-vector sensitivity of a dichroic element in the eye would be defined by the ratio $A_{0°}/A_{90°}$, which is the absorption ratio in the planes of maximum and minimum absorbance respectively.

Physiological measurements of polarization sensitivity need to be expressed as ratios of the number of quanta required to evoke a given response with different degrees of polarization or with maximally and minimally effective e-vector direction. Such quantitative functions will be symbolized by S_p for unspecified polarization sensitivity and S_e for specific e-vector sensitivity. In practice, the validity of S_p and S_e at the photoreceptor cell level will depend on the "univariance" of the unit in question, meaning that its responses vary only with the rate of quantal absorption independent of wavelength or intracellular location (RODIECK, 1973, p. 263).

Note that other more specific, but qualitative, terms for certain aspects of polarization sensitivity may be convenient. Hence polarization detection is the key initial event in the photoreceptor which, for example, in rhabdomeric eyes depends on dichroism of the rhabdom membrane. At a higher level, polarization perception ordinarily implies processing of the relevant sensory input by the central nervous system.

Finally, polarization sensitivity in efferent systems is expressed by postural, locomotor, or other behavioral outputs evoked or modulated by the initial polarization detecting input. Polarotaxis, therefore, has been defined as a directed locomotor or turning response to the e-vector of linearly polarized light (WATERMAN, 1966a). Note that direction finding from natural polarized light in the sky or underwater is a polarized light compass or e-vector menotaxis.

Referring to this, without some reservation, as polarized light navigation (WATERMAN, 1958; WEHNER and BERNARD, 1976; VAN DER GLAS, 1977a) would seem undesirable in the broader context of the terminology which is well accepted in referring to various aspects of animal navigation, particularly in birds (EMLEN, 1975). Following GRIFFIN (1955, 1969) it seems important to maintain distinctions between pilotage (i.e., course finding by use of landmarks), direction finding (i.e., azimuth orientation independent of landmarks), and bicoordinate navigation (i.e., goal seeking from unknown territory; sometimes called "true navigation") or reverse displacement navigation (i.e., inertial navigation) (WATERMAN, 1972). So far in this hierarchy, nothing more complex than time-compensated direction finding has been demonstrated for the polarization sensitivity of animals in nature.

Because of the range of organisms and workers involved, it now seems important to choose one's words with care in referring to sensitivity, detection, perception, vision, and behavior in relation to polarized light. This will minimize unnecessary confusion and help optimize effective communication.

II. Background

Since VON FRISCH'S first work on behavioral polarization sensitivity in the honeybee (1948), there has been a sustained growth of interest in this field. In a 1961 review, 25 references were cited (WATERMAN, 1961a), including the pioneering, but negative, results of CROZIER and MANGELSDORF (1924). Five years later, cited publications (WATERMAN, 1966a) had grown to 89, even though the tabular summary for Biological Handbooks included only explicit positive results. A revision of the table in 1973 had 123 references classified under four headings: 1) polarotaxis (72 citations), 2) electrophysiology (27), 3) microspectrophotometry (9), and 4) miscellaneous (15) (WATERMAN, 1973).

On the basis of the working bibliography for the present review, which grows at an astonishing rate, an additional 100 or so citations would probably be needed to update the 1973 table. The annual increment, therefore, has been around 15% during the past 4 or 5 years rather than about 5% during the period 1966–1973. Thus the growth of this field shows two striking accelerations after the first reported positive responses to polarized light, which were in *Daphnia* and *Drosophila* (VERKHOVSKAYA, 1940).

First, VON FRISCH'S spectacular initial work (1948, 1949) induced a sudden interest, including my own persistent preoccupation with polarization sensitivity. This was maintained by a moderate and steadily increasing output over the succeeding 2 decades. During the 1970–1974 period, a second major spurt occurred and a comparable accelerated growth rate has continued into the present 5-year period. This impulsive speedup of polarization sensitivity research in the 1970s seems to have originated not so much from some single discovery or particular research group as from the cumulative growth resulting from effective application of several powerful experimental and theoretical techniques.

Nevertheless, it is clear that a few research centers have been primarily responsible for sustaining interest in polarization sensitivity. Munich, of course, has played a seminal role since VON FRISCH launched the field (1948); AUTRUM, who later succeeded VON FRISCH as Professor of Zoology, was among the first to apply electrophysiological techniques to the problem and hypothesize that individual retinular cells are the units of polarization sensitivity (AUTRUM and STUMPF, 1950); LINDAUER (Würzburg), JANDER (Kansas), and DAUMER (Munich) all did their doctoral research under VON FRISCH. LINDAUER, in turn, trained WEHNER (Zürich) and MENZEL (Berlin) in Frankfurt. Recent work stems principally from the Australian National University (ADRIAN HORRIDGE, SIMON LAUGHLIN, ALLAN SNYDER), Yale University (GARY BERNARD, TIMOTHY GOLDSMITH, TALBOT WATERMAN), and the

University of Zürich (RÜDIGER WEHNER) and the Max-Planck-Institut für Biologische Kybernetik at Tübingen (KUNO KIRSCHFELD).

With regard to the importance of new techniques in the polarization sensitivity field, electrophysiology, electron microscopy, microspectrophotometry, and sophisticated optical, as well as theoretical, analyses have all had a major favorable impact from the 1960s onward. Therefore, the 15–20 relevant publications (1972–1978) of ALLAN SNYDER, mainly coauthored with various colleagues, including several others mentioned above, have stimulated considerable interest by taking an analytical look at some potentially important theoretical optical details largely ignored previously. Currently, membrane biophysics and genetic manipulation of experimental material also are beginning to exert some effect.

In particular, the simultaneous application of two or more of these various approaches has proved effective in accelerating progress and increasing interest. In the author's experience, for example, the correlation of fine structural knowledge obtained in collaboration with EISUKE EGUCHI, with electrophysiological and other evidence for crustacean compound eye mechanisms, has been particularly stimulating. Similarly the coupling of SNYDER's sometimes brash theoretical optical approach to various collaborators' experimental data has no doubt proved considerably more effective than either might have been alone.

While such progress has surely been welcome, it has largely been restricted to only the sensory mechanisms or the most peripheral aspects of the corresponding afferent information processing. Unfortunately, comparably rigorous study of more central pathways and behavior remain largely for the future. Although WEHNER's work on *Cataglyphis* and WELLINGTON's observations on mosquito flight patterns are rare exceptions, the virtual lack of recent field experiments also leaves a conspicuous gap in our knowledge. Experiments in nature, of course, are needed not only to establish the adaptive utility of polarization sensitivity, but also to define the specific tasks required of the relevant detecting and processing mechanisms.

As a result, the role of polarization sensitivity in spatial orientation, visual contrast, pattern recognition, homing, and migration, including its overall adaptive significance, especially for aquatic animals, are not well understood. The rather elegant hypotheses of sensory mechanisms currently being elucidated or postulated, therefore, may seem a bit top heavy for the field's somewhat makeshift foundation!

III. Objectives

Since so much remains to be learned, we cannot yet sum up the subject of polarization sensitivity in anything like a definitive form. Despite a plethora of partial reviews published in recent years, a broad survey of current understanding is still much needed. This is a rather challenging task because of the potential scope and depth of the subject.

To begin with, polarization sensitivity is a visual capacity shared by a wide variety of animals. Crustaceans, insects, arachnids, cephalopod mollusks, and vertebrates, including man, are well documented (VON FRISCH, 1965, 1967; LANGER,

1966; WATERMAN, 1973, 1974a, 1975a). Furthermore, understanding polarization sensitivity requires knowledge at many hierarchical levels, ranging from the polarization of natural light to the biophysics of photoreceptor membranes and the mechanisms, as well as the consequences, of visually oriented behavior.

Ideally, one should be able to cover the topic by a systematic comparative survey of the functional relations at all levels, from photons and molecules to behavior and adaptive significance. Necessity, however, dictates a more practical approach. The patterns of polarized light in nature will first be summarized. The data in this field are probably less well known to biologists than they need to be. Indeed, until we understand more precisely how the animals concerned are using the environmental optical information, it is not even certain that the available information on atmospheric and submarine optics is adequate for explaining its biological applications.

The primary biological data will then be treated through a series of major examples in which our knowledge is mainly centered. In keeping with the general plan of this volume, I will deal mainly with polarization sensitivity in invertebrates, yet comparative references will also be made to vertebrates. Actually I have fairly recently reviewed polarization sensitivity specifically in the vertebrates (WATERMAN, 1975a) and subsequent progress has not been striking. The discussion and summary of this material finally will indicate how far we have come in understanding this field. They may also serve to guide further progress.

B. The Light Stimulus

Direct sunlight is not polarized, yet a substantial fraction of it becomes partially linearly polarized in the atmosphere and hydrosphere by primary scattering and differential reflection. Consequently, for light in nature,

$$I_t = I_p + I_u \tag{2}$$

and the degree of linear polarization p may be defined by Eq. (1) or as

$$(I_{max} - I_{min})/(I_{max} + I_{min}), \tag{3}$$

where I is light intensity and the subscripts are defined as: I_t = total, I_p = polarized, I_u = unpolarized, and the maximum and minimum values are photometrically measured with a rotatable polarizer.

No doubt moonlight, starlight, and bioluminescence may also undergo some polarization in nature (GEHRELS, 1974a), but in the absence of evidence for any biological significance, we need not consider them further here. Similarly, this review may be simplified for present purposes by restricting it to linear polarization. This is the only type known to be visually important. Furthermore, since elliptical components are of secondary or tertiary origin, natural polarization is predominantly linear. It occurs often to a high degree in the sky (ARAGO, 1811), underwater (WATERMAN, 1954a), and at surfaces and interfaces (MALUS, 1808; FRESNEL, 1816).

The following reviews summarize this field and provide extensive references (CHANDRASEKHAR, 1950; CHANDRASEKHAR and ELBERT, 1954; SEKERA, 1957; SHUR-CLIFF, 1962; FESENKOV, 1965; ROZENBERG, 1966; JERLOV, 1968, 1976; CLARKE and GRAINGER, 1971; LUNDGREN, 1971; WATERMAN, 1972, 1975b; KATTAWAR et al., 1973; COULSON, 1974; IVANOFF, 1974; TIMOFEEVA, 1974; TYLER, 1974; McCARTNEY, 1976).

I. Polarization by Scattering

The basic processes are those of radiative transfer in which solar photons are absorbed, scattered, refracted, and reflected. When these events quantitatively depend on the wavetrain's plane of vibration, polarization patterns will be produced. These are determined primarily by the rather simple geometry of the optically active element and its radiance input and output. Thus for RAYLEIGH scattering in either air or water, the polarization patterns are directly related to the angle (α) between the directional radiation and the line of sight (Figs. 1 and 2).

1. Rayleigh Model

Single scattering of monochromatic light by isotropic molecules, or other particles with diameters much smaller than λ, produces linear polarization with its e-vector orthogonal to the direction of the light flux. Consequently, in a spherical coordinate system with the scattering particle at the origin (O), light scattered in all directions will have its e-vector uniformly perpendicular to all meridians intersecting the propagation axis z (Fig. 2).

The intensity of the scattered light varies as λ^{-4} so that, for example, violet light at 400 nm is scattered 10.5 times more strongly than red at 720 nm. In general, the degree of polarization

$$p = p_{max} \sin^2 \alpha / (1 + \cos^2 \alpha) \qquad (4)$$

(Fig. 1). Consequently, p ranges from 0 (i.e., no polarization) in directions parallel to the light flux to 1 (i.e., complete polarization) in a plane perpendicular to the rays x, y (Fig. 2).

The ideal natural polarization pattern is established by a uniform ensemble of such particles scattering originally parallel light rays and observed from some point within the particle space. Consequently, the basic distribution shows strong bimodal radial symmetry. There are two unpolarized "neutral points" in the direction of the sun and antisun and an "equatorial" belt of complete and partial polarization centered at 90°. As shown by Eq. 4, the half bandwidth of this polarization band is 54.74°, where p has decreased to 0.5 p_{max} on either side of the coordinate system's equator.

Actually this very simple polarization pattern seems to be more complex to an earthbound observer because the distribution of p and ϕ then is usually referred

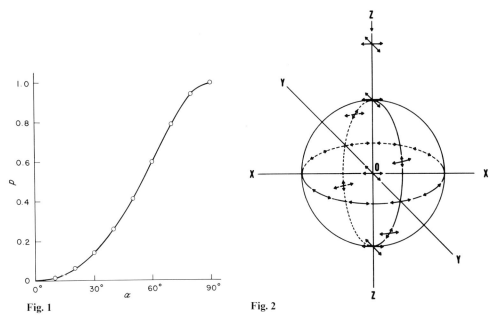

Fig. 1   **Fig. 2**

Fig. 1. Dependence of degree of polarization (p) of RAYLEIGH scattered light on the angle (α) between the line of sight and the propagation direction of an unpolarized collimated wavetrain like direct sunlight. (Eq. 4)

Fig. 2. E-vector direction (ϕ) of light scattered from an isotropic charged particle at 0 as projected on a concentric sphere. Unpolarized light is incident on 0 from above parallel to the z-axis, while the x, y plane ideally defines the directions of complete polarization indicated in Fig. 1 $(\alpha = \pi/2)$. If the upper end of the z-axis represents the solar point in the blue sky, the primary polarization pattern, relative to terrestrial axes, is determined by movement of the solar point through the sky (Figs. 3 and 7). (TYLER, 1974)

to terrestrial coordinates, most conveniently those determined by the horizontal plane and the gravitational vertical at the point of observation. If so, the direction of solar radiance (i.e., the z axis of Fig. 2) in the atmosphere and hydrosphere can be specified in the sky by a zenith angle θ_s for the sun's position, or underwater by the corresponding angle of refraction θ_r, and an azimuth angle γ_s between the intersection of the sun's vertical with the celestial horizon measured from a reference bearing of any other compass point.

The zenith angle θ_p and the azimuth angle γ_p of the point observed define the line of sight which forms an angle α (as in Fig. 1 and Eq. 4) with the solar flux direction. This stereogeometry establishes the following relationship (IVANOFF and WATERMAN, 1958a; TIMOFEEVA, 1974) between the "tilt" of the e-vector relative to the horizon for any radiance direction and line of sight.

$$\tan \phi = \frac{\tan \theta_s \cdot \sin|\gamma_s - \gamma_p|}{\sin \theta_p + \tan \theta_s \cdot \cos \theta_p \cdot \cos|\gamma_s - \gamma_p|} . \tag{5}$$

Obviously, in this equation, appropriate sign conventions must be observed for points right and left of the solar vertical and lines of sight above and below the horizontal. In general, $\phi = 0°$ for any point along the vertical great circle passing through the sun (i.e., $\gamma_s = \gamma_p$). When the sun is in the zenith (i.e., $\theta_s = 0°$), $\phi = 0°$ for all θ_p, γ_p. In horizontal lines of sight, ϕ_{max} occurs at $\pm 90°$ to the sun's azimuth.

2. Secondary Factors

Actually, such an ideal RAYLEIGH model for the hydrosphere and atmosphere must be modified in many ways to account for the real scattering of sunlight. The major influences are molecular anisotropy, higher order scattering, molecular absorption, scattering and absorption by aerosols and hydrosols, as well as effects due to reflected and diffusely scattered light. The outcome of all these is mainly to reduce p from 100% to some substantially smaller value and alter ϕ from RAYLEIGH model predictions; however, the details are complex and their analysis incomplete (ROZENBERG, 1966; MCCARTNEY, 1976).

For example, the sun's movement through the sky from dawn to dusk, of course, changes the patterns of p and ϕ *pari passu* (Figs. 147–149). Furthermore, since the sun's apparent path is strongly dependent on latitude and season, so is natural polarization (Figs. 3 and 4). These basic stereogeometric factors interact in complicated ways with the influence of the earth's albedo: the turbidity, as well as inhomogeneity, of the medium; and the optical path length

$$\tau = cr.\tag{6}$$

Here, r is the geometric path length and c is the total attenuation coefficient due to scattering and absorption. This coefficient is much greater in water than in air, but strongly influenced by λ in both media. Clearly, τ is a path standardized for the medium's attenuation properties. It may be important for both the directional radiance through the air or water, or both, as well as that in the line of sight.

Because of their intrinsic or analytic importance, many of these factors affecting polarization have been extensively studied by optical oceanographers, optical meteorologists, and astronomers interested in radiative transfer in planetary atmospheres (CHANDRASEKHAR, 1950; ROZENBERG, 1966; KONDRATYEV, 1969; GEHRELS, 1974a; JERLOV and STEEMANN NIELSEN, 1974; JERLOV, 1976; KATTAWAR and PLASS, 1976). Some are also undoubtedly of substantial biological importance. For obvious reasons, at least the main features of natural polarization patterns must be known to understand polarization sensitivity and its adaptive significance.

Consequently, the present review will take a primarily descriptive approach to the main features of natural polarization in addition to providing bibliographic access to analytical and theoretical aspects of the field, which may be zoologically relevant. Indeed, it is more than likely that certain features or correlates of natural polarization, so far overlooked or poorly known, will turn out to have a critical role in polarization sensitivity. Biologists themselves, therefore, may have to initiate their own optical studies that can be correlated with sensory and behavioral data (WATERMAN, 1954a; BRINES, 1978).

To illustrate, let me cite the nontrivial displacements of the "neutral" points, where $p = 0\%$ on the solar vertical, from their location at $\alpha = 0°$ predicted by RAY-

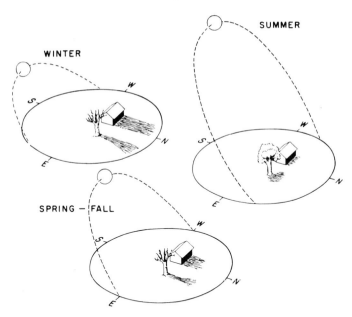

Fig. 3. Changes in the sun's path with the seasons, as observed in middle north latitudes. The basic pattern of scattered polarized light (p, ϕ) depends on the sun's position at any given moment, as shown in Figs. 1 and 2. (HASLER, 1966)

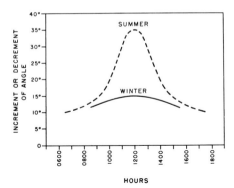

Fig. 4. Rates of change in the sun's bearing and, consequently, apparent celestial rotation of the polarization pattern, depend in general, on the latitude, time of day, and season. The hourly angular rates, as shown, are for the solstices at middle latitudes (compare Fig. 3). (HASLER, 1966)

LEIGH scattering (Fig. 1). In fact, it has long been known that such points above and below the solar and antisolar points do occur on the sun's vertical in the sky (Figs. 5 and 6). Their displacements may range from 15° to 35°, mainly depending on interactions between τ, λ, and θ_s. Similar neutral points (Fig. 6) have more recently been demonstrated underwater (TIMOFEEVA, 1974).

Actually, multiple scattering, in addition to displacing neutral points, distorts the sky distribution of ϕ (e.g., compare Figs. 4 and 5, Appendix B, SEKERA et al., 1955). This distortion is dramatic in the sun's vertical where ϕ is parallel to this

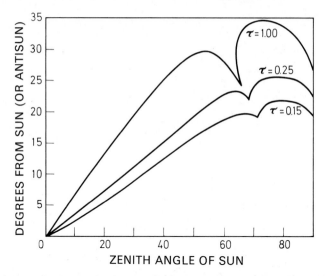

Fig. 5. Deviations of two neutral points (p=0% in the sun's vertical) in sky polarization (i.e., BREW-STER's point from the sun and the ARAGO point from the antisun) as a function of the sun's zenith angle at three different optical thicknesses (τ) of a RAYLEIGH atmosphere. (Simplified from COULSON, 1974). See Fig. 6 for locations on the celestial sphere

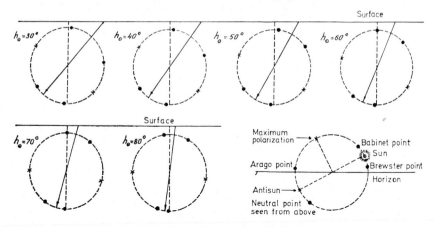

Fig. 6. Comparison of neutral points in the sky (lower right) with their analogs in an aqueous scattering medium at various refracted angles of directional irradiance between 30° and 80°. Neutral points are shown as filled circles; p_{max} locations by x's. (TIMOFEEVA, 1974)

celestial circle between the neutral points and the sun or antisun. This so-called "negative polarization", where the light intensity component in the scattering plane is greater than that perpendicular to it, may be quite extensive. For example, with $\theta_s = 46°$, such complementary ϕ might occur in the whole arc between zenith angles of 30° and 60° in the solar vertical.

No biological effects are known for these displaced neutral points and the in-tervening anomalous polarization, but no one seems to have looked for any. In fact, the value of p in these sky regions is less than 10%, or even less than 5%, so *e*-vector orientation may be academic; however, the neutral point displacements related to large θ_s may significantly expand the sky area, with p at or below biological threshold.

Natural polarization patterns in the atmosphere and hydrosphere are fundamentally similar in their origin through primary scattering of directional sunlight in the medium, yet there are obviously a number of differences between them which could be biologically significant.

3. Sky Polarization

For clear blue sky, p_{max} at best has been found to be 75%–85% when the sun is near the horizon and the point of observation near the zenith. The discrepancy between a measured 75% and an ideal RAYLEIGH expectation of 100% has been partitioned as follows: 6%, multiple scattering; 6%, molecular anisotropy, 5%, ground reflection; and 8%, influences of atmospheric aerosols (GEHRELS, 1974b).

As the sun drops below the horizon, p_{max} increases by perhaps 5%–10% for $\theta_s = 94°$–95° before again decreasing to the $\theta_s = 90°$ value when $\theta_s = 96°$–97°. Zenith p has dropped to about 0.5 p_{max} when $\theta_s = 102°$. The period of enhanced zenith polarization, around sunset and sunrise, corresponds approximately to civil twilight and will of course vary from a minimum of about 20 min twice a day on the earth's equator to something like 13 weeks around the annual dawn and dusk for the midnight sun at the poles.

As expected from simple theory, the location of p_{max} moves by about 90° (Fig. 7) during the day along the solar vertical preceding and following the sun, but secondary factors cause its magnitude and precise location to vary with θ_s. Thus, on a clear day with a p_{max} of 75%–80% at sunrise, its value at local noon was found to be about 60% (SEKERA et al., 1955). Thereafter, p_{max} increased again, but temporal asymmetry was also present, presumably due to changes in atmospheric optics during the day (Fig. 8). Measurements in a polluted smoggy atmosphere demonstrated much greater effects of θ_s on p_{max}. At 320 nm, for instance, p_{max} was 55% with $\theta_s = 93°$ and only 28% for $\theta_s = 36°$.

a) Depolarization by Haze and Clouds

Obviously, such effects become acute as haze or smog thickens to fog or clouds (Fig. 9). These reduce or entirely eliminate the polarization originating in the upper atmosphere. Although this is well known, the great spatial and temporal variability of atmospheric optics has made it hard to analyze. Suffice it to say here that with broken, but dense, cloud cover, the cloudy areas are partially or fully depolarized and the clear areas are polarized essentially as if the clouds were not there. Indeed, although the distribution of p is quite variable in different sky locations and at different times, the distribution of ϕ is quite stable for a given θ_s, γ_s and sometimes persistent even with apparently heavy overcast and precipitation (BRINES, 1978).

With certain types of cloud cover, various degrees of depolarization and altered patterns of radiance distribution can markedly affect the resulting polarization. Thus, if clouds are at high altitude, directional light beneath them will be sub-

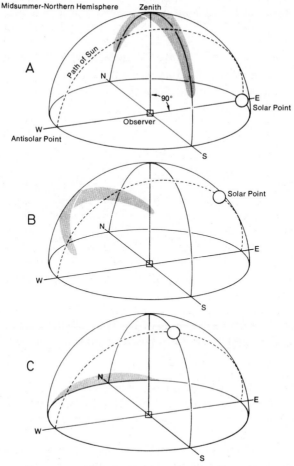

Fig. 7 A–C. Effect of sun's position in the sky on location and orientation of the band of maximum sky polarization apparent from a terrestrial observation point at sunrise **A**, midmorning **B**, and local noon **C**. (WELLINGTON, 1974c)

sequently polarized in the lower atmosphere to generate a substantial pattern. Note also that water droplets in clouds of several kinds have extinction coefficients about the same from 300 nm to 700 nm, or more (McCARTNEY, 1976). Consequently, despite some statements to the contrary in the insect literature, no selective transmission of violet or ultraviolet would be expected. The depolarizing effects of multiple scattering, or more properly multiple reflection, by such large particles also are quite insensitive to λ. Hence, λ selective effects on the polarization transmitted would not be expected either (but see VON FRISCH, 1965, p. 387).

b) Dependence on λ

Nevertheless, an important feature of p, and consequently p_{max}, is its strong dependence on wavelength (Fig. 10). Indeed, quite discrepant conclusions may be reached in comparing broad band with narrow monochromatic data for the blue

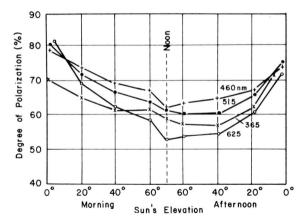

Fig. 8. Changes with time of day in p_{max} along the sun's vertical measured at four selected λ's. On this particular day, the early morning sky was the most strongly polarized, a condition which deteriorated steadily to an early afternoon minimum sustained through much of the afternoon. Note that decrease in p_{max} was greatest (36%) at 625 nm and least at 365 nm (19%), but, at all λ's measured, p_{min} was greater than 50%, well above the honeybee's or *Daphnia*'s polarotactic threshold for white light (10%–20%). (Redrawn from SEKERA et al., 1955). (Compare with Figs. 9 and 10)

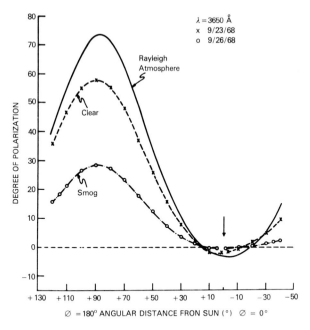

Fig. 9. Comparison of sky polarization at 365 nm measured along the sun's vertical under clear and smoggy conditions with corresponding values calculated for a RAYLEIGH atmosphere. At this near ultraviolet wavelength, p_{max} for the particular smog prevailing was reduced to half that for the clear atmosphere. Note the neutral points (where $p\% = 0$) on either side of the solar point (arrow). In the region between the sun and the neutral points, note that p is plotted as if it were "negative," a rather confusing convention (defined in the text) used where ϕ is parallel rather than perpendicular to the scattering plane. (COULSON, 1974)

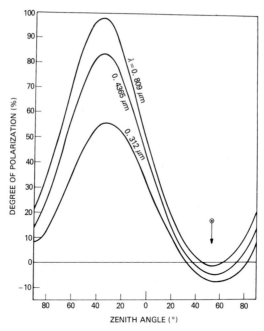

Fig. 10. Effect of λ on p at various zenith angles along the sun's vertical for a RAYLEIGH atmosphere. Note that p_{max} in the near ultraviolet is about half p_{max} at 809 nm. Also note that the location of the neutral points relative to the sun (arrow) is strongly affected by λ. See legend of Fig. 9 for explanation of "negative" p. (COULSON, 1974)

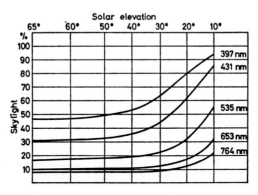

Fig. 11. Influence of solar elevation on the relative contribution of skylight to global radiation shown for selected λ's. (JERLOV, 1968)

or red (SEKERA, 1957), but when rapid monochromatic measurements are made photoelectrically under sufficiently stable optical conditions, reasonably consistent results have been obtained. At the risk of oversimplification, some λ dependent effects of possible biological relevance may be cited.

   With very clear sky in lines of sight neither too close to the sun nor too far from the zenith, p_{max} (Fig. 8) has been reported at about 460 nm (SEKERA et al., 1955), even though polarization calculated for an ideal RAYLEIGH atmosphere is greater at longer wavelengths (Fig. 10). This value of 460 nm is a significantly longer wave-length than λ_{max} for the diffusely scattered blue sky light which is near 410 nm. Di-rect radiant flux from the sun has its peak *power* at 476 nm (Fig. 12). At sea level, when the sun is reasonably near the zenith and the sky quite clear, it has a λ_{max} about 500 nm (KONDRATYEV, 1969), but its spectral distribution is fairly flat from 480 to 570 nm. With increased atmospheric turbidity and greater solar zenith angles approaching 90°, marked shifts toward longer wavelengths usually develop (Fig. 8).

Note that despite its far greater radiant intensity compared with the diffuse sky-light (about $6.6 \times 10^5 \times$), the sun's disc subtends only 0.543° (or $7.1 \times 10^{-6} \times$ of the whole sky). Consequently, the fraction of global radiation contributed by the sky is not trivial and is strongly dependent on both solar zenith angle and wave-length (Fig. 11). Thus, at near ultraviolet wavelengths (397 nm), skylight con-tributes 93% to the total when $\theta_s = 80°$, but only 48% when $\theta_s = 25°$. The corre-sponding values are much less for 764 nm; 21% for $\theta_s = 80°$, and only 9% at $\theta_s = 25°$.

Of course, during twilight, the sky provides the full irradiance reaching that particular geographic area. During this period also, the relative amounts of blue or red, or both, wavelengths in the clear sky increase with a corresponding loss in the yellow–green (McFARLAND and MUNZ, 1975). This spectral characteristic of twilight may be critical in determining the λ_{max} of certain fish visual pigments (MUNZ and McFARLAND, 1973, 1977), but its influence on polarization sensitivity is not known, yet could be significant (see below).

c) Importance of Intensity Units

Before turning from the relation of λ to sky polarization, an important caveat should be made. This depends on the nature of photoreception. Most meteorolog-ical optical data are presented in physical units deliberately independent of biolog-ical systems which may be affected. Thus, irradiance is usually measured in power units of watts per square meter and, in much of this review, such units are quoted or implied. Yet, the visual or photosynthetic effect of irradiance, because it de-pends on photochemical change, is strongly dependent on spectral distribution and on the quantum nature of light.

Consequently, the biologically relevant units are quanta per s per unit area per unit wavelength (i.e., dN per dλ) or frequency band (i.e., dN per dv) (GOVARDOV-SKII, 1972)[1]. Because of the shape of the visual pigment absorbance spectra, the frequency unit plot seems the better of these two for comparing spectral irradiance with sensitivities of visual systems (DARTNALL, 1975). While irradiance spectra can be transposed from one to another of these systems of units by simple arithmetic (see DARTNALL, 1975), the graph of power (e.g., watts) per square meter per λ for the environmental irradiance unit is very different from that for quanta per second per square meter per v (Fig. 12).

For example, the λ_{max} in the dE per dλ units is in the blue at 476 nm for sunlight outside the atmosphere, whereas the λ_{max} for the dN per dv units is at about 1,500 nm in the infrared! At the earth's surface, this quantum frequency solar ir-

[1] For a discussion of comparable relations, with regard to photosynthetic action spectra and effi-ciency, see BJÖRN, 1976

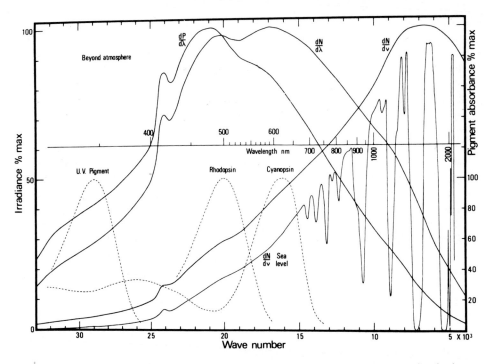

Fig. 12. Dependence of normalized solar spectral irradiance curves on measurement unit selection. Three plots, reaching maxima of 100%, are for the same data beyond the earth's atmosphere drawn respectively as watts per unit λ ($dP/d\lambda$), quanta per s per unit λ ($dN/d\lambda$) and quanta per s per unit frequency (dN/dv). Atmospheric absorption produces the sharp fluctuations in the sea level curve for dN/dv. Since vision depends on the rate of quantal absorption, either of the two types of quantal plots may be used for vision and photosynthesis, depending mainly on convenience. For comparison, DARTNALL nomograms are shown (dotted curves) for a rhodopsin, cyanopsin, and an insect ultraviolet pigment ($\lambda_{max} = 345$ nm). (DARTNALL, 1975)

radiance curve is basically of the same form, but starting at about 700 nm, increasingly strong absorption bands punctuate the red and infrared. Note that the insect visual pigment, shown with a peak in the ultraviolet at 345 nm, lies in a region where dN per dv of direct sunlight is relatively minute (Fig. 12).

However, natural polarization will be more related to the spectral distribution of the sky than to that of direct sunlight. Indeed, the λ for sky p_{max} observed by SEKERA et al. (1955) at 460 nm is very close to the peak of the measured dN per $d\lambda$ curves for clear sky reported by MCFARLAND and MUNZ (1975). If these sky curves were replotted for dN per dv, their peaks would be shifted to longer wavelengths, probably to about 550 nm for sky 30° above the horizon and 120° from the sun. This peak seems rather remote for correlation with the "sensitivity" of an ultraviolet receptor like the proposed polarized light receptor R 9 in the honeybee ($\lambda_{max} = 340$ nm).

However, the ultraviolet receptor of the ventral eye region of the dragonfly *Hemicordulia* (C.I.6.b.γ.) has significantly greater transducer gain than the other retinular cell color types (LAUGHLIN, 1976a); this was postulated to be an adaptation to the low level of daylight mentioned above. The location of this receptor, however, would seemingly prevent it from having any correlation with direct viewing of the sky.

d) Sky Summary

From the above brief review, the potential richness of the celestial panorama for a photoreceptive system with appropriate polarization sensitivity is obvious. When p or ϕ is perceived either separately or together over the sky, they would establish a characteristic pattern dependent primarily on the sun's position and RAYLEIGH scattering (Figs. 147–149). Secondarily, it would be modulated or distorted by many other factors mentioned above. In terms of visual subtent, the polarization pattern would greatly predominate over the "tiny" sun. When the latter is covered by a cloud, behind an obstacle like a mountain or immediately below the horizon, the polarization, the radiance distribution, or the sky's color pattern would be the only visible celestial directional cues. In our virtual e-vector blindness, it is hard to imagine what kind of visual surroundings natural polarization establishes for the many animals that perceive it well. As discussed elsewhere, this is particularly acute where animals can choose unambiguous compass directions from inherently ambiguous e-vector orientation.

4. Underwater Polarization

The natural polarization pattern in the hydrosphere differs in a number of important ways from that in the atmosphere (WATERMAN, 1954 a). To begin with, it occupies a full sphere rather than a hemisphere. Theoretically, one might expect that FRESNEL reflection of solar irradiance at the air–water interface and in situ RAYLEIGH and MIE scattering of directional sun's rays would together establish the underwater polarization.

Yet, nearly all of it depends on scattering so that ϕ in all lines of sight is approximately perpendicular to the apparent direction of the light in the water. No gross effect on underwater polarized light has yet been found attributable to selective reflection and refraction at surface incidence. The water surface does, however, have other important influences.

a) Effects of Air–Water Interface

First, of course, refraction changes the direction of the light entering the water so that

$$\sin \theta_r = {}^3\!/_4 \sin \theta_s \qquad (7)$$

(Fig. 13). This alters ϕ since its orientation relative to the horizontal is θ_r (WATERMAN and WESTELL, 1956). To an underwater observer then, ϕ is $0°$ in lines of sight in the bearings of the sun or antisun and maximal at about $90°$ to those directions. Maximal tilt, however, because of refraction, does not exceed the critical angle of about $48.6°$, even when the sun is on the horizon.

Near the surface, as is well known, the whole aerial hemisphere can be seen underwater as distorted and reduced by surface refraction to a cone angle of about

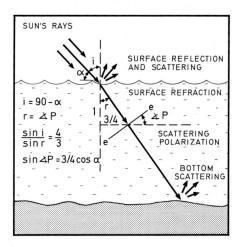

Fig. 13. Basic mechanism of underwater polarization of refracted sun's rays by RAYLEIGH scattering. Observed in a horizontal line of sight, the *e*-vector reaches maximum tilt towards the sun about 90° to the sun's bearing, where $\phi = <P = \frac{3}{4} \cdot \cos \alpha$, where α in this figure is the sun's altitude. External surface reflection and scattering have little detected effect on underwater polarization, but bottom scattering and secondary or higher order scattering by the medium reduce *p*. (WATERMAN and WESTELL, 1956)

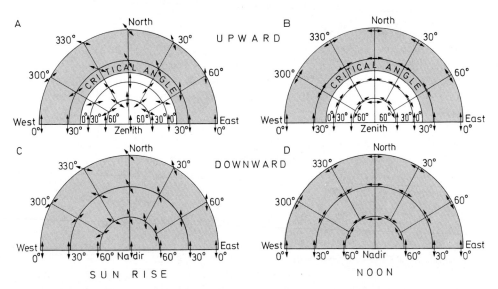

Fig. 14 A–D. Underwater polarization pattern as observed from a point 2–3 m below a calm surface with 0 cloud cover. Note that the whole underwater field of view is partially linearly polarized. The half circles represent solid angle quadrants upward (**A** and **B**) and downward (**C** and **D**) at sunrise (**A** and **C**) and noon (**B** and **D**). Double headed arrows indicate *e*-vector tilt relative to the horizon at the coordinate intersection in question. Elevation and depression of the lines of sight (drawn as half circles) are labeled on the horizontal diameter relative to the horizon (0°). Radii are bearings of the lines of sight. Note that in the upper hemisphere at shallow depths the underwater horizontal direction (0°) is accompanied by an apparent terrestrial horizon (also labeled 0°) at the critical angle near 48.6°. (WATERMAN, 1954a)

97.2° (Fig. 14). As a result, with clear skies, nearly 25% of the underwater polarization at shallow depths is due primarily to polarization of the blue sky; the other three quarters originate in the water itself. With increasing depth, the sky's contribution is rapidly attenuated (SMITH, 1974). As this happens, polarized light, arising within the water itself, becomes the exclusive source of polarization within the critical angle as well as elsewhere.

Second, natural water surfaces are seldom completely calm. Hence, the geometric simplicity of the basic polarized light pattern is overlaid with transient influences of the wave pattern on light refraction. This expands the sun's image underwater into a large glitter pattern, but has less dramatic effect on the apparent sky polarization because of the latter's greater angular extent. However, ripples and waves do cause underwater e-vectors to oscillate about a mean angle ϕ, with an amplitude and frequency dependent on surface movement. At shallow depths, such polarized light variations may be conspicuously present, but they have not been studied carefully.

b) Effects of the Medium

Beyond the interface, water as a medium has a profound effect because scattering and absorption of light in the hydrosphere are several orders of magnitude greater than in the atmosphere. Thus, the total attenuation coefficient (i.e., c) of a RAYLEIGH atmosphere is 1.1×10^{-5} m^{-1} at 550 nm (ELTERMAN, 1970). In contrast, c for pure water at 550 nm is 6.9×10^{-2} m^{-1} (JERLOV, 1976).

Accordingly, c for H$_2$O is about $6.3 \times 10^3 \times$ that of air. Obviously, this greatly reduces penetration of sunlight into the medium with all its well known consequences for photosynthesis (STEEMANN NIELSEN, 1974) and vision (WATERMAN, 1972, 1974b; DARTNALL, 1975). Thus, the meteorologic range in the ideal RAYLEIGH atmosphere is about 336 km, whereas a visibility range, calculated from the differences in c, would be a mere 54 m for distilled water.

This agrees with the horizontal sighting range estimated by DUNTLEY's (1963) rule of thumb $4/c$ (one attenuation length $= 1/c$) for a large dark object against a light background but it is less than that calculated from a more generous allowance of attenuation lengths ($6/c = 87$ m) (DUNTLEY, 1974). Indeed, if six attenuation lengths are computed for pure water at 475 nm instead of 550 nm, they give nearly double the estimated blue–green range, or 167 m. In any case, such estimates show that visual pilotage underwater is not much use for animals which venture more than 100–200 m away from shore or bottom even in ideally clear water.

α) *Interaction of Absorption and Scattering.* With regard to underwater polarized light, it is important to note that attenuation is the relative radiant flux lost in the medium both by absorption and by scattering. Hence, $c = a + b$, where a and b are the total absorption and scattering coefficients respectively. The complex relations between these inherent properties of the natural water masses seem almost paradoxical. Attenuance in pure water, and also in pure seawater, therefore, is largely due to absorbance. Yet, it is the primary scattering of directional radiance that establishes natural polarization. Nevertheless, multiple scattering by hydrosols in turbid water is well known usually to decrease p and the theoretical maximum degree of polarization is approximated only in the clearest water with highly directional irradiance.

For such pure water, the angular distribution of scattered radiant intensity, defined as the volume scattering function $\beta(\theta)$ (JERLOV, 1976), is nearly symmetrical about a minimum at 90° to the radiance direction (θ_r taken as 0°). Hence, the least light is scattered in the direction of maximum p (Eq. 4). Most natural waters, however, show much stronger forward scattering than pure water and the scattering minimum, as well as the direction of p_{max}, may be displaced backwards to angles as great as 100°–120° (i.e., differing from the RAYLEIGH model by as much as 30°) (KULLENBERG, 1974; TIMOFEEVA, 1974).

In general, for natural waters and turbid media in the laboratory, when the irradiance is vertical (i.e., with zenith sun), the angular distribution of p is symmetrical in various azimuthal planes. However, in the more general case of oblique illumination (i.e., sun not in zenith), the two lobes of these distributions are apparently asymmetrical, except in the plane normal to the sun's bearing (IVANOFF, 1974; TIMOFEEVA, 1974).

β) p_{max} *in Natural Waters*. In natural water, $\beta(\theta)$ depends in a complex way on the concentration, size, refractive index, and shape of the suspended particles. Although p and $\beta(\theta)$ are generally independent parameters, in vitro measurements have shown that $p_{90°}$ in sea water samples shows a roughly inverse log linear relationship to $\beta(\theta)$ (IVANOFF, 1974). Actually, large particles typically decrease p, yet small particles ($d < 6\,\mu m$) may significantly increase it. Although some p_{max}'s greater than 80% have been reported (i.e., the theoretical p_{max} for pure water = 83.5%), p_{max} underwater seems usually to be not more than about 60%, even under highly favorable optical conditions (WATERMAN and WESTELL, 1956; IVANOFF and WATERMAN, 1958a; WATERMAN, 1958; TIMOFEEVA, 1962). Measurements in the Pacific south of Costa Rica showed that p_{max} at 520 nm ranged from 52% at the surface to 40% at 50 m on a clear day with $\theta_s = 5°–15°$ (LUNDGREN, 1971). With overcast skies at a nearby station, p at the surface was reduced to 32%, while at 50 m, it was the same as on the clear day. Near Sardinia, p_{max} at 1 m for $\lambda = 460$ nm was 64%, but at 190 m it was about 43% with $\theta_s = 14°–30°$ (LUNDGREN, cited by JERLOV, 1976) (Fig. 19).

γ) *Dependence on* λ. Polarization is related to the spectral distribution of the irradiance for several reasons. To begin with, for pure seawater, the volume scattering function at 90° ($\beta_{90°}$) varies approximately the same as $\lambda^{-4.32}$ (MOREL, 1974). Consequently, its value at 450 nm is about 34% of that at 350 nm and, at 550 nm, only 43% of that at 450 nm. As a result, the shorter wavelengths lose their directionality, and hence degree of polarization, more quickly than longer. On the other hand, clear seawater is most transparent around 470 nm so that longer wavelengths are absorbed more rapidly (Fig. 15). In deep clear water, red light would be the most collimated and, therefore, most strongly polarized. Yet the downwelling daylight would contain little or no red photons because of absorption.

On the other hand, the deep water would have roughly monochromatic downwelling irradiance, with a λ_{max} near 465 nm. This would therefore comprise nearly all of the polarized light, even though it lies at the minimum of the λ–p curve. In fact, in situ measurements have shown that p is minimum in horizontal lines of sight at λ's near that for maximum transmission and increases slightly at longer and shorter λ's (IVANOFF and WATERMAN, (1958a).

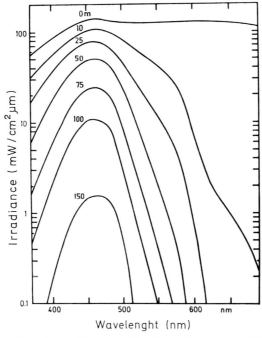

Fig. 15. Effect of depth on downwelling spectral irradiance (measured as $dP/d\lambda$) in very clear oceanic water. By 150 m, the broad surface spectrum of sunlight has been filtered by the medium to a narrow wavelength band peaking at 465 nm. (LUNDGREN and HØJERSLEV, 1971). Compare with Figs. 12 (for the sky) and 16 (for the influence of plotting the data in units of quanta per unit frequency)

The somewhat lesser polarization at shorter λ's indicates that the $\lambda^{-4.32}$ rule for scattering in pure seawater was not evident here, probably due to increased absorption below about 465 nm. The λ-sensitivity of scattering by nonabsorptive particles is generally stated not to be large in the visible range, but it may be significant when scattering angles are 90° or greater and dependent on the diameter of the suspended elements.

In inshore marine locations and many freshwater sites, colored substances dissolved in the medium frequently are present (HUTCHINSON, 1957; JERLOV, 1968). These will affect a (λ) and alter the spectral distribution of underwater light accordingly.

c) Importance of Intensity Units

As already mentioned above with relation to sky polarization, the most critical comparison between spectral sensitivity of a photoreceptor and the underwater spectral irradiance would seem to be in terms of photons per frequency interval rather than the usual oceanographic optics units of radiant power per wavelength interval (DARTNALL, 1975). While such a change in units makes a rather spectacular difference in the curve for direct solar irradiance, the effect of such a transposition is much less striking underwater, particularly when $z > 10$ m (Fig. 16).

Another important item in evaluating the importance of the λ_{max} of the irradiance, including the polarization, in relation to the λ_{max} of visual elements re-

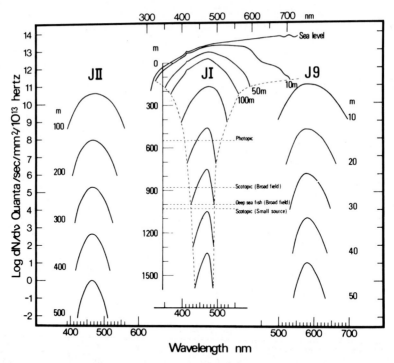

Fig. 16. Measured as log dN/dv downwelling irradiance curves for sunlight at various depths are fairly similar to the power per unit λ plots in Fig. 15 for very clear oceanic water (J I). Broken lines indicate limits of vision. J II was less clear oceanic water than J I, while J 9 was a much less transparent coastal water. (DARTNALL, 1975)

sponding to it is the density of the photosensitive pigment in the receptor organelles. Both in fish (O'DAY and FERNANDEZ, 1976) and algae (RAMUS et al., 1977), pigment density may be great enough in dim light to broaden the action spectrum in such a way as to uncouple its apparent and previously widely accepted dependence on λ_{max} of the downwelling light.

d) Effect of Depth

At any given point underwater, p and ϕ depend on the radiance distribution of the light impinging on that location. Near the surface, the reflected sun's rays and skylight make major distinct contributions to the downwelling light (SMITH, 1974). Consequently, the radiance distribution at $z = 1$–2 m gives strong evidence of this within the critical angle (i.e., θ_c) (Fig. 17).

The sun's refracted image (i.e., $\theta_r = 21.5°$ in the case reported by SMITH) draws out the radiance distribution in a long conical peak and the marked intensity drop caused by the "disappearance" of the sky at the critical angle produce sharp knees on either side. By $z = 5$ m, the sun's effect is still strong, but the intensity decreases at θ_c are reduced and asymmetrical. At 20 m, the effect of the sky is detectable but minor; the direct sun's influence is still considerable. By 53 m, however, both have

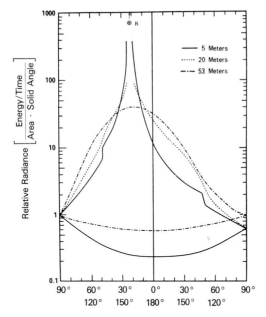

Fig. 17. Radiance distribution for downwelling and upwelling light measured in various lines of sight at three different depths (Gulf of California). Upward curve at 20 m is almost the same as at 5 m. Sky clear, $\theta_r = 21°30'$ (indicated by R), sea moderate. Photometer bandwidth 60 nm with λ_{max} about coincident with the water's maximum transmittance. (SMITH, 1974)

disappeared and downwelling irradiance has a smooth eggshape asymmetrical about the vertical with its maximum approximately at θ_r.

If a were zero in natural waters and b large, this smooth radiance distribution present at moderate z would become spherical when the optical path length, including depth (i.e., z), becomes great. Light scattered from such nondirectional irradiance of course would be unpolarized. On the other hand, if some absorption occurs, as it indeed does in water, residual directionality will remain even with high turbidity. Consequently, some polarized light will persist underwater as deep as surface light penetrates.

$\alpha)$ *Asymptotic Depth.* However, the interaction between absorption and scattering gradually reduces ϕ from its maximum subsurface value determined by $^4/_3 \sin \theta_s$ to $0°$ at the so-called asymptotic depth z_a (WATERMAN, 1954a, 1955). The radiance distribution there becomes a prolate ellipsoid symmetrical about the vertical because the path length followed by downward scattered light is shorter than that of the obliquely transmitted component. Hence, the vertical downwelling light gradually comes to predominate, regardless of θ_s and the state of the sky and water surface. TYLER (1963) has argued that at z_a and deeper $p = \varepsilon^2$, where ε is the eccentricity of the ellipsoid.

Below z_a, the angular distributions of p and ϕ remain constant. Like the radiance, the polarization in this region depends only on the optical properties of the medium. As far as any daylight penetrates, they are independent of z and of the angular distribution of the radiance incident at the water surface. A precise

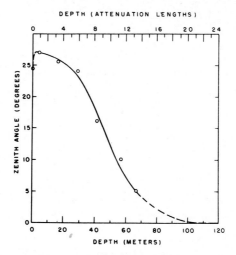

Fig. 18. Effect of depth on direction of maximum in the radiance distribution for downwelling light. As shown in Fig. 13, the ordinate (labeled zenith angle) has the same values as ϕ observed at 90° to the sun's bearing. Measured in Lake Pendoreille, Oregon, with a filter having its λ_{max} at 480 nm. θ_s was 33.4°; θ_r 24.4°. Measurements were made only to 66.1 m, but extrapolation indicates z_a was between 16 and 20 attenuation lengths. (DUNTLEY, 1963)

analytical solution derived from a complete STOKES formulation has been recently achieved (KATTAWAR and PLASS, 1976). Tabular and graphic data have been presented as a function of single scattering albedo for the RAYLEIGH phase matrix, as well as two meteorological cases (i.e., cloud, haze). While asymptotic p_{max} is at 90° (i.e., horizontal) for RAYLEIGH scattering, phase matrices for nonideal media yield p_{max} nadir angles of less than 90° (KULLENBERG, 1974 and TIMOFEEVA, 1974, cited above).

In the sea, both measurement (Fig. 18) and theory (ZANEVELD, 1974; HØJERSLEV and ZANEVELD, 1977) indicate that the near asymptotic radiance distribution, and hence the asymptotic p and ϕ, are approached at depths involving perhaps 15–20 attenuation lengths (WHITNEY, 1941; TYLER, 1960; BEARDSLEY, 1966; TIMOFEEVA, 1974; PREISENDORFER, 1976, Vol. I, pp. 50–53, Vol. III, pp. 19–24). Note that at such a z_a, downward irradiance, which decreases exponentially, is less than 10^{-6} of its surface value.

The actual depths involved vary strongly with the inherent optical properties of the medium and, λ (JERLOV, 1968). Thus, when c and b are large, symmetry will be reached in moderate depths, with small coefficients z_a occurs at several hundred meters. With regard to λ, for example in the Sargasso Sea, with $\theta_s = 40°$, near asymptotic distributions were measured for 375 nm at $z = 150$ m, but for 475 nm, the corresponding z was 400 m (JERLOV, 1968).

More generally, the asymptotic depth will be a function of $1/b$, but the number of photons present to be polarized by scattering is a function of $1/a$ (λ). As the asymptotic depth is approached, p and ϕ vary less and less in azimuth or the sun's position. Hence, biological use of natural polarized light for a sun compass would be impossible when $z \geq z_a$. Yet, its potential effectiveness as a visually mediated ho-

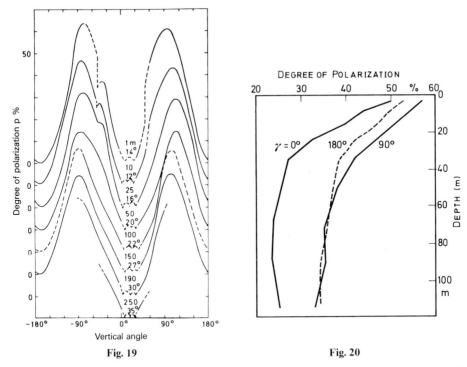

Fig. 19. Effect of depth on *p* measured at vertical angles between the zenith (0°) and nadir (180°) off Sardinia. As shown, θ_s ranged from 14° to 35° during the measurements. Peaks of polarization lobes show that p_{max} near 90° to θ_r was 64% at a depth of 1 m and about 43% at 190 m. (LUNDGREN cited by JERLOV, 1976)

Fig. 20. Effect of depth on *p* at 500 nm measured off Bermuda in three horizontal lines of sight: $\gamma = 0°$ sun's bearing, $\gamma = 90°$ perpendicular to sun's bearing, and $\gamma = 180°$ antisun's bearing. (Redrawn from IVANOV and WATERMAN by JERLOV, 1976)

rizon or vertical indicator, as well as input for a reflex position stabilizer, would persist throughout this part of the photic zone.

Clear evidence was obtained photographically that the sun's position still affects ϕ at 200 m in relatively clear water near Barbados (WATERMAN, 1955), but quantitative polarization measurements are practically nonexistent in deep water (max. 115 m, IVANOFF and WATERMAN, 1958a; 100 m, TIMOFEEVA, 1962; 50 m, LUNDGREN, 1971). However, LUNDGREN (cited by JERLOV, 1976) has more recently made some measurements to 250 m off Sardinia (Fig. 19). Extrapolation and theoretical calculations have suggested p_{max} at asymptotic depths to be 13%–38% (TYLER, 1963; BEARDSLEY, 1966), which overlaps with p_{max}'s observed above this level ranging from 30% to 60%–67% (Fig. 20).

β) Biological Implications. *Daphnia*, the only aquatic animal for which *p* threshold has been studied, was shown to have a polarotaxis threshold with *p* of 10%–20% (WATERMAN and JANDER cited by WATERMAN, 1966a and discussed below). On the basis of this one case, polarization sensitive animals should be able to detect both p and ϕ throughout the photic zone in natural waters. In surface layers and down to some level above z_a, ϕ could be used to determine the sun's azimuth (Fig. 18).

Near and below z_a, the polarization pattern could still provide visual information useful for the animal's spatial orientation and its changes, as suggested by WATERMAN (1958) and recently by LEGGETT (1976). Under conditions where no landmarks are visible and the radiance distribution may not have enough contrast to evoke an effective dorsal light reflex, such an aid to stabilizing position and locomotion may be quite important (RINGELBERG et al., 1975). Of course, most organisms will use statocysts for such purposes, but these are widely supplemented by visual reflexes (SCHÖNE, 1975).

e) Effect of Twilight

One further point should be made about underwater polarization. This relates to the quite different but largely unknown conditions which occur at twilight. With the sun below the horizon, the first order polarization pattern, due to quasi-RAYLEIGH scattering of the refracted sun's rays, obviously will disappear. All the radiance entering the sea will be from the sky and, if the latter is clear, will be strongly polarized in a band centered on the vertical circle normal to the sun's bearing (Fig. 7). As mentioned above (B.I.3.b.), spectral irradiance from the sky also shifts considerably at twilight.

Thus, around sunrise or sunset, there are sharp changes in the directionality and spectrum of the downwelling light. At the same time, polarization of the irradiance at the surface is altered accordingly. It has been known for a long time that quite offbeat polarization patterns occur underwater at such times of the day (WATERMAN, 1954a). However, no measurements have been published on exactly how they affect p and ϕ. Twilight underwater appears to be important in the orientation and behavior of at least fishes (GROOT, 1965; MUNZ and MCFARLAND, 1973, 1977; MCFARLAND and MUNZ, 1975). Both the hydrological optics and the relevant biology need further study.

II. Polarization by Reflection

Dielectric interfaces in nature will give rise to partially polarized light by differential reflection and refraction. For example, unpolarized light entering a smooth water surface from the atmosphere will be polarized to an extent dependent on the angle of incidence and the ratio of refractive indices of the two media. Theoretically,

$$p = \frac{R_\perp - R_{||}}{R_\perp + R_{||}}, \tag{8}$$

where the R's are intensity reflection coefficients for the components of the externally incident light vibrating perpendicular and parallel respectively to the

plane of incidence (CLARKE and GRAINGER, 1971). These coefficients are related to
the refractive index ratio and light directions as follows:

$$R_\perp = \frac{\sin^2(\theta_i - \theta_r)}{\sin^2(\theta_i + \theta_r)}, \tag{9}$$

$$R_\parallel = \frac{\tan^2(\theta_i - \theta_r)}{\tan^2(\theta_i + \theta_r)}. \tag{10}$$

Of course, by Snell's law:

$$\frac{\sin \theta_i}{\sin \theta_r} = \frac{n_{H_2O}}{n_{air}} = 1.33. \tag{11}$$

Actually, when $\theta_i = 0$, reflection is about 2%. As θ_i increases, overall reflection
increases monotonically slowly out to 65°–75°, then it rapidly approaches total reflection at grazing angles to the surface. In contrast, p, which is also 0% when $\theta_i = 0$,
increases to 100% when arctan $\theta_i = 1.33$ (hence BREWSTER's angle is 53° where about
7.6% of the incident light is reflected), but then decreases again to 0% when $\theta_i = 90°$.
Note that these simple geometrical optical relations hold for unpolarized collimated light incident on uncontaminated and smooth, relative to λ, water surfaces.

1. Natural Air–Water Interfaces

a) External Reflection

In fact, none of these restrictions is ordinarily met in the field. Even laboratory
measurements of water surface reflections (Fig. 21) show considerable variations
of p as a function of nadir angle θ_n from the basic FRESNEL predictions (CHEN and
RAO, 1968). If, in addition, the incident light is polarized, the p vs. θ_n curves vary
markedly with ϕ_i. In nature, where the skylight is partially polarized and more diffuse than the unpolarized strongly directional sunlight, reflection and refraction of
both these components will affect the resulting patterns of p and ϕ.

These relations have not been carefully studied but some qualitative information is available (HULBURT, 1934; WATERMAN, 1954a). More recently, I have recorded reflected p's on water surface imaging strongly polarized areas of the sky
at large values of θ_i. Under such conditions, reflected ϕ around sunrise or sunset
was commonly observed to be as great as 90° in azimuths normal to the sun, which
is quite different from the $\phi = 0°$ expected from FRESNEL reflection of unpolarized
incident light. The latter condition could be observed in the same line of sight at
the same θ_s, but only when the sky region reflected was heavily overcast. Indeed,
it was sometimes possible in lines of sight perpendicular to the sun's bearing near
the horizon to observe almost any ϕ between 0 and 90°, depending on the θ of the
observer's line of sight (unpublished).

Since natural water surfaces are not mirror smooth, further complications are
introduced by waves and ripples. In general, rough surfaces do not show FRESNEL
reflection, but instead sometimes yield diffuse LAMBERT reflection or more com-

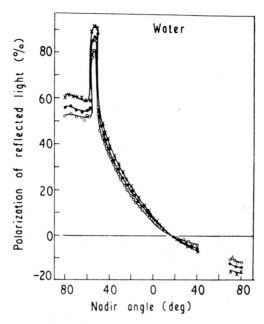

Fig. 21. Polarization *(p)* of light reflected in the principal plane from a smooth water surface in the laboratory. Three wavelengths were used: open circles 398 nm; filled circles 500 nm; and *x*'s, 605 nm. (CHEN and RAO, 1968)

monly tilted *e*-vectors in the reflected light which are inclined towards the direction of incidence (WATERMAN, 1954a). Again, these effects have not been carefully studied in the field, but biologists wishing to determine the relation between visual polarization sensitivity and reflected light need to consider them. For example, there may be some significant effect due to directions and spatial frequency components of surface waves (COX, 1974).

b) Internal Reflection

For an underwater observer, internal reflection also has polarizing effects. This may need to be considered in addition to the transmission of sky polarization and the in situ pattern reviewed above. Thus, 2% of the upwelling underwater light in lines of sight towards the zenith is reflected downward and this percentage increases slowly out to about 30°–35°, then rapidly to 100% at the critical angle (i.e., θ_c). Beyond that, reflection is complete out to $\theta'_i = 90°$.

As with external reflection, p in internal reflection is 0% when $\theta'_i = 0°$, rises to a maximum (i.e., 100%) at an intermediate angle (i.e., $\theta'_i = 37°$), and then falls to 0% again at θ_c and beyond. Because of strong attenuation, these phenomena have significant influences only near the surface, but upwelling irradiance available for internal reflection is not more than 6% of the downwelling irradiance (JERLOV, 1968). Hence, the contribution of internal reflection to the polarization pattern in the field has not been recognized within θ_c.

However, just beyond θ_c, a considerable amount of the internally reflected light is elliptically polarized due to surface reflection of the linearly polarized rays scat-

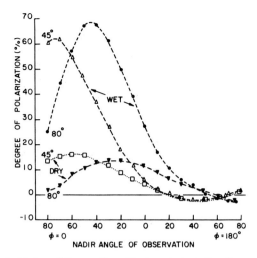

Fig. 22. Polarization *(p)* of light at 520 nm reflected in the principal plane from wet and dry soil at two angles of incidence. Laboratory measurements. (COULSON, 1974)

tered in the water (WATERMAN, 1954a; IVANOFF and WATERMAN, 1958b). This circumscribed case is an exception to the general rule cited above that primary components of naturally polarized light are linearly polarized. Even so, its biological significance is dubious, particularly since we know nothing so far about polarization sensitivity to elliptically polarized light.

2. Terrestrial Surface Reflection

Although intuitively less familiar than water reflection, terrestrial surfaces like soil, rocks, and vegetation also give rise to substantial polarization in the light they reflect (COULSON, 1968, 1974). Depending on a number of factors, p_{max}'s as great as 30%–40% may be reflected by black loam or grass, for instance. If soil is wet, p_{max}'s of 60%–70% (Fig. 22), comparable to those underwater or in the sky, have been reported.

In general, there is an inverse relationship between reflectance and polarizance. Thus, light sand reflects lower p's than dark soil or rocks. Neutral point locations, analogous to those in the atmosphere and hydrosphere, are also dependent here on the reflecting medium (CHEN and RAO, 1968). Complex changes in p are again introduced if the incident light is polarized and soil and desert sand, at least, show considerable dispersion, with p being inversely related to λ.

3. Biological Implications

Interface polarization has been thought to be of possible biological significance to animals with polarization sensitivity for three reasons. As with Polaroid sunglasses, a properly oriented polarizer in an aerial visual system could first reduce glare

from reflection (SCHNEIDER and LANGER, 1969; BOHN and TÄUBER, 1971; TRU-
JILLO-CENÓZ and BERNARD, 1972) and, second, increase underwater visibility in
certain air–water lines of sight. Third, the use of water surface polarization as a horizon indicator for dragonflies recently has been suggested (LAUGHLIN, 1976a;
C.I.6.b.δ). Note that the natural polarization patterns actually are considerably
more complex than usually assumed. Furthermore, no direct evidence is yet available to support any of these three interesting hypotheses.

C. Responses and Mechanisms

The distribution of polarization sensitivity in the animal kingdom is, no doubt,
rather imperfectly known. As cited in the introduction, it has been demonstrated
to occur in well over 100 species in three major phyla of higher metazoans. Among
these cases, the photoreceptors concerned are variously compound eyes, camera
eyes, "simple" ocellus-like eyes, and even extraocular light sensitive elements (e.g.,
pineal of lower vertebrates).

However, most of our knowledge of this area is typified by a few species which
have been more than casually studied. Thus, much of the available information on
polarization sensitivity is provided by six invertebrate types discovered between
1940 and 1961 to possess this sensory capability. Five of these are arthropods having compound eyes, while the sixth is a cephalopod mollusk having camera eyes.

All of them have their photoreceptor membranes organized as rhabdoms. The
polarization sensitivity of these six cases in fact depends on the organization of the
photoreceptor membrane into innumerable regularly ordered microvilli (Figs. 23–
27). Presumably this is also true in those four cases where simple eyes of arthropods
have been shown to mediate polarization sensitivity, but these will be discussed
separately below (C.II.).

The notion that dichroism of the visual pigment is the most likely basis of e-
vector detection in insects was put forward by DE VRIES et al. (1953) and STOCK-
HAMMER (1956, 1959). It was seconded by a number of others and appropriately
correlated with the microvillus nature of rhabdoms in general (GOLDSMITH and
PHILPOTT, 1957; JANDER and WATERMAN, 1960; MOODY and PARRISS, 1961; GOLD-
SMITH, 1962). Later, the hypothesis that polarization sensitivity input comprises
two or more differently oriented dichroic channels, dependent on the specific
microvillus pattern in the rhabdom, was proposed for various specific cases (for
the octopus, MOODY and PARRISS, 1961; for the bee, GOLDSMITH, 1962; for decapod
crustaceans, WATERMAN, 1966b).

Rhabdoms are composite organelles made up of rhabdomeres each contributed
by the individual photoreceptive cells (e.g., in arthropods most often 7–9 in number) clustered around the axial photon absorbing structure so formed. The numerous microvilli of each rhabdomere project from the lateral surface of the retinular
cell soma. Ordinarily, they are all aligned with great regularity perpendicular to the
direction of incident light. With important exceptions, all microvilli from a given

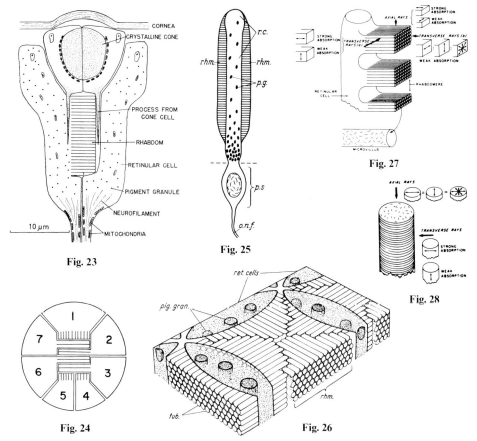

Fig. 23

Fig. 24

Fig. 25

Fig. 26

Fig. 27

Fig. 28

Figs. 23 and 24. Ommatidium of *Daphnia* compound eye. (WATERMAN, 1966b). **Fig. 23**. Axial longitudinal diagram to show fused unbanded rhabdom. Microvilli from only one rhabdomere from retinular cell at left (comparable to R6 or R7 in Fig. 24) can be seen in this section. In decapods and most insects, microvilli extend only part way across the rhabdom (Figs. 30, 35, and 36). **Fig. 24**. Diagrammatic cross section at midrhabdom level. Note two orthogonal microvillus directions, despite several other differences from a typical decapod crustacean rhabdom pattern

Figs. 25 and 26. Rhabdom structure in *Octopus; o.n.f.*, optic nerve fiber; *p.g.* (pig. gran.), pigment granules; *p.s.*, proximal segment; *r.c.* (ret.cells), retinular cells; *rhm*, rhabdomere; *tub*, microvilli. (MOODY and PARRISS, 1961). **Fig. 25.** Photoreceptor cell showing, diagrammatically, two rhabdomeres on opposite lateral surfaces. Relations of cells and rhabdomeres to fused rhabdom shown in Fig. 26. **Fig. 26.** Retinal mosaic schematically showing that four rhabdomeres comprise a fused rhabdom. Each retinular cell contributes two sets of parallel microvilli to adjacent rhabdoms, as shown. Stereodiagram has its broad surfaces normal to the incident light and, hence, to the rhabdom axis

Figs. 27 and 28. Comparison of crustacean and vertebrate photoreceptive membrane fine structure (GOLDSMITH and BERNARD, 1974). **Fig. 27.** Diagram of part of toothed rhabdomere in a decapod crustacean (e.g., crayfish) showing how one rhabdomere contributes to the overall rhabdom. The gaps between its microvillus layers are filled with orthogonal microvilli from an adjacent retinular cell in the same ommatidium. Subsidiary diagrams show that rays perpendicular to the microvilli, whether axial or transverse (a), are preferentially absorbed if their *e*-vector is parallel to the long axis of the microvilli and if the visual pigment chromophores are oriented in the photoreceptor membrane, as shown by the single microvillus drawn below. Absorption of transverse rays (b) parallel to the microvillus axis would be independent of their *e*-vector direction. **Fig. 28.** Part of vertebrate rod outer segment, shown diagrammatically. Subsidiary figures indicate that if the chromophores of visual pigment are randomly oriented in the plane of the membrane disks, absorption is isotropic for axial light rays and dichroic for transverse rays, with major absorption normal to the rod axis

receptor cell are parallel, but those from different rhabdomeres in a rhabdom have two or more radial directions relative to the optic axis. Obviously, this establishes a photoreceptor membrane geometry quite different from that of typical vertebrate rod and cone outer segments (Figs. 28 and 142).

In a given rhabdom-bearing species, the resulting retinal mosaic typically demonstrates an astonishing regularity of cellular and rhabdomere geometry closely correlated with polarization sensitivity, among other things. However, the collaborative pattern of these structures varies widely in different arthropods (Fig. 10 in WATERMAN, 1975 b) and mollusks.

In the present context, this rhabdom variety can be subsumed under a few basic fine structural and functional types. Most important in such a classification are the lateral and longitudinal relations of the components. Both optical and electrical coupling or independence are of prime importance at the retinal level in supporting or dissipating the dichroism inherent in individual rhabdomeres. Obviously, their geometry and fine structure do not provide direct evidence for these functional relations, but do show whether or not certain necessary conditions are met.

With regard to their lateral organization, rhabdoms of arthropods can structurally be either open or fused (Figs. 29–33). Longitudinally, rhabdomeres may be tiered in either case. In fact, one or more rhabdomeres in optical sequence are widespread, if not universal, in insect and crustacean compound eyes. Tiering indeed occurs in vertebrate retinas, but only in quite specialized cases (FINERAN and NICOL, 1976, 1978; LOCKET, 1977; MILLER and SNYDER, 1977).

Open rhabdoms have rhabdomeres which are isolated parallel rod-like units well separated from each other by extracellular medium of lower refractive index (Fig. 29). These are typical of the higher flies (e.g., Diptera Brachycera) where they have been extensively studied (KIRSCHFELD and SNYDER, 1975) and in perhaps half of the 300,000 species of Coleoptera (HORRIDGE and GIDDINGS, 1971; WACHMANN, 1977). They also occur in Collembola (PAULUS, 1972), Dermaptera (ECKERT, 1968), Hemiptera (e.g., LÜDTKE, 1953; RENSING and BOGENSCHÜTZ, 1966; BURTON and STOCKHAMMER, 1969; SCHNEIDER and LANGER, 1969; IOANNIDES and HORRIDGE, 1975), and in the isopod *Ligia* (EDWARD, 1969; EGUCHI [cited by WATERMAN, 1975 b]). At least in flies like *Musca* and *Calliphora*, each rhabdomere of this type has a different field of view (Fig. 29) (AUTRUM and WIEDEMANN, 1962; FRANCESCHINI, 1975).

Fused rhabdoms, which occur widely in arthropods (Figs. 23, 24, 30, and 34) and cephalopods (Fig. 26), have their constituent rhabdomeres in close longitudinal contact. The resulting structure in crustaceans and insects may range from a long thin cylinder occupying a major fraction of total ommatidial length, typical of EXNER's apposition compound eyes (Figs. 31 and 63), to short thick ellipsoids occupying only a minor basal fraction of the ommatidium's total length, typical of EXNER's superposition compound eyes (Figs. 32 and 63). Rhabdomeres in a fused rhabdom are generally assumed (Fig. 30) to share the same field of view (HORRIDGE and MEINERTZHAGEN, 1970 a; but see BERNARD, 1975).

Typically, the microvilli of fused rhabdoms extend only partway across the rhabdom diameter (Figs. 26, 30 b, 35 and 36). Hence, they are contiguous with those of adjacent rhabdomeres only at their closed tips. However, in the spider *Agelena*, microvilli of apposed retinular cells were described as reaching all the way

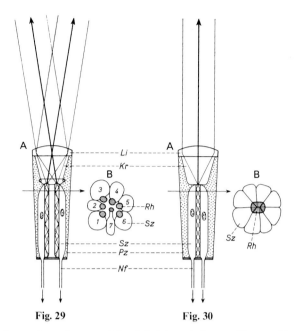

Fig. 29   **Fig. 30**

Figs. 29 and 30. Comparison of open and fused rhabdoms in insects. *Kr*, crystalline cone; *Li*, corneal lens; *Nf*, primary axons; *Rh*, rhabdom; *Sz*, retinular cell. (KIRSCHFELD, 1971). **Fig. 29.** Open rhabdom in dipteran ommatidium. **A** Longitudinal axial diagram showing two separate rhabdomeres borne on the axial lateral surfaces of R 2 and R 5. Ray tracings indicate different fields of view of the rhabdomeres and their individual light trapping (guiding) action. **B** Transverse diagram at level shown by arrow. Seven separate rhabdomeres are obvious and an eighth is tiered in optical series below that of R 7. **Fig. 30.** Fused rhabdom in ommatidium of apposition type eye. **A** Longitudinal axial diagram. **B** Cross section diagrammed at level shown by arrow. Note that eight constituent rhabdomeres are found axially in longitudinal contact forming a single columnar structure oblong in cross section. Ray tracings indicate that all rhabdomeres share the same field of view and act together as a single light guide

across the rhabdom (SCHRÖER, 1974). Hence, they must interdigitate those of their opposite cell and be in longitudinal contiguity with the latter's microvilli.

This kind of overlapping relationship was not found in another spider [i.e., *Lycosa* (MELAMED and TRUJILLO-CENÓZ, 1966)], but a possibly similar dovetailing of parallel microvilli from apposing retinular cells forming a rhabdom is cited below for dipteran dorsal ocelli (C.II.2.a.β). While it is not known that such interdigitated microvilli affect polarization sensitivity, another pattern of rhabdomere overlapping, known as banding, has been repeatedly correlated with *e*-vector discrimination (Figs. 34–37).

Banded fused rhabdoms are typical of mysid, stomatopod, and decapod crustaceans (EGUCHI and WATERMAN, 1966; WATERMAN, 1977). One instance has been reported in an isopod (i.e., Crustacea Peracarida) (NILSSON and ELOFSSON, 1977). They also occur sporadically in insects [i.e., some Thysanura, Coleoptera (MEYER-ROCHOW, 1972; FRANTSEVICH et al., 1977); Lepidoptera (HESSE, 1901; MEYER-ROCHOW, 1971; PAULUS, 1975; KOLB, 1977); Diptera (WADA, 1974a); and Neuroptera (SCHNEIDER and LANGER, 1975)]. The microvilli of individual rhabdomeres are periodic in their longitudinal distribution (Fig. 27) so that typically

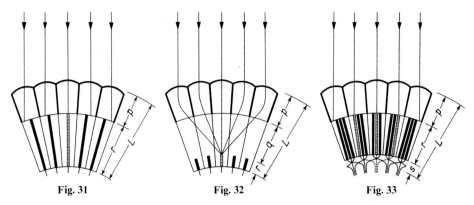

Figs. 31–33. Diagrammatic structure of three basic compound eye types. *L*, ommatidial length, *p*, dioptric length; *g*, "clear zone" length; *r*, rhabdom length; *s*, primary fiber crossover zone. (Kirschfeld, 1967). **Fig. 31.** Classic apposition eye with long thin fused rod-like rhabdom (*r*) extending from the distal dioptric system (*p*) to the basement membrane. Rays show axial light stimulating the ommatidium parallel to the incoming light, but not those out of line. **Fig. 32.** Classic superposition type eye (e.g., the firefly *Lampyris*) with short rhabdoms separated from the distal dioptric system by a considerable optically open "clear space." In such a system, parallel light is concentrated on a single rhabdom (as suggested by the ray paths shown) thereby substantially increasing an ommatidium's effective aperture. **Fig. 33.** Neural superposition eye as exemplified by dipterans. Three rhabdomeres of the open rhabdom appear and ray paths shown indicate parallel rays stimulate different rhabdomeres in three adjacent ommatidia with slightly different axial alignments (see also Figs. 101 and 104). Optically, this type is essentially apposition, but neural superposition below the basement membrane summates input from rhabdomeres located in adjacent ommatidia, yet looking at the same point in space. Like optical superposition, neural superposition in effect increases sensitivity of the eye, in this case, by significantly augmenting the signal to noise ratio of the system

two groups of different cells contribute alternate orthogonal layers of microvilli to the overall banded structure (Figs. 34–37).

From an optical point of view, the three main arthropod rhabdom types (i.e., open, unbanded fused, banded fused) should have quite different functional properties. These have been extensively analyzed by Allan Snyder and his colleagues (Snyder, 1973, 1974, 1975 a, b, 1977; Snyder and Menzel, 1975; Snyder et al., 1977; McIntyre and Snyder, 1978). Such properties include some which are highly important for polarization sensitivity. Consequently, these are reviewed in detail below.

Still another fused rhabdom type occurs in cephalopod retinas (Zonana, 1961; Yamamoto et al., 1965). This differs basically from the arthropod pattern in having fewer, typically only four, rhabdomeres and in the occurrence of two rhabdomeres with parallel microvilli on opposite lateral faces of each photoreceptor cell. Typically in cephalopod retinas, each primary visual axon then can be activated by two different parallel sets of microvilli, each set belonging to a different rhabdom. The consequences of such sharing have not been analyzed in detail either theoretically or experimentally.

No vertebrates have been thoroughly studied for polarization sensitivity, although a wide range of species from fish to man have been explored to some extent (Waterman, 1975a). Normally, the fine structural geometry of their photorecep-

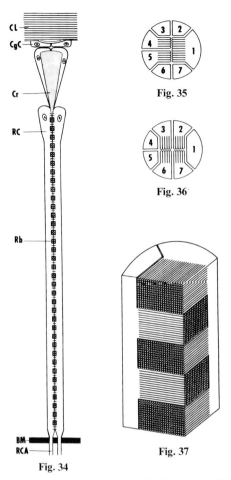

Fig. 35

Fig. 36

Fig. 37

Fig. 34

Figs. 34–37. Ommatidium of the crab *Callinectes* with a highly developed banded fused rhabdom. Over-all compound eye is of apposition type (Fig. 31) (EGUCHI and WATERMAN, 1966). **Fig. 34.** Longitudinal axial section. Although only a few are drawn, there are actually 450 bands of microvilli along this very thin (5 μm) elongate (400 μm) rhabdom. R 8 is not shown in this schematic. *BM*, basement membrane; *CgC*, corneagenous cells; *CL*, corneal lens; *Cr*, crystalline cone; *Rb*, rhabdom; *RC*, retinular cell; *RCA*, primary axon. **Fig. 35.** Diagrammatic cross section of ommatidium showing cells of origin of three rhabdomeres with horizontal microvilli. This kind of band alternates with one having orthogonal microvillus organization (Fig. 36). **Fig. 36.** Diagrammatic cross section of ommatidium showing cells of origin of four rhabdomeres with vertical microvilli. Compare with Fig. 35. **Fig. 37.** Stereodiagram indicating basic microvillus structure of one quarter of the rhabdom. Compare with Figs. 27, 35, and 36 for further details

tive membranes differs sharply from that of the rhabdom-bearing arthropods and cephalopods (EAKIN, 1972); hence, their general mechanism of ocular polarization sensitivity must differ accordingly (WATERMAN, 1975c). However, there is now elegant fine structural evidence that a few teleosts (i.e., *Anchoa* and some related anchovies) may have a special polarization sensitive receptor system (FINERAN and NICOL, 1976, 1978). As discussed below, this implies that there are two orthogonal dichroic cone receptor types.

I. Arthropod Compound Eyes

Rhodopsin in situ in the rhabdom has been shown directly by microspectro-photometry to act as a dichroic analyzer (HAGINS and LIEBMAN, 1963; LANGER, 1965; LANGER and THORELL, 1966; WATERMAN et al., 1969). The highly ordered parallel arrangement of microvilli in arthropod rhabdomeres, combined with a more or less restricted dipole moment of their visual pigment molecules, establishes the inherent polarization sensitivity as suggested by GOLDSMITH and PHILPOTT (1957).

If the chromophore orientation in arthropods were like that of vertebrate rod or cone outer segments (Fig. 28), rhabdom dichroism would be at a low level (i.e., <2). Microspectrophotometry has often yielded ratios smaller or not much greater than this; yet, polarization sensitivity measured electrophysiologically in retinular cells has often given substantially higher ratios yielding maximum S_p's of 9–12 (SHAW, 1966, 1969b; WATERMAN and FERNÁNDEZ, 1970; BUTLER and HORRIDGE, 1973; MOTE, 1974; GOLDSMITH, 1975).

Despite considerable research, there is yet no case for which a reasonably complete analysis can be presented all the way from visual pigment photochemistry and rhabdom dichroism through sensory input processing to polarotactic behavior. The sort of partial explanations currently possible for arthropod compound eyes are illustrated by the two crustacean and three insect types reviewed below.

1. *Daphnia* and Other Cladocerans

The first positive report of an animal's response to linear polarization was VERKHOVSKAYA's finding (1940) that *Daphnia* presented with a two light phototactic choice behaved as if linearly polarized light had 2–3 times the brightness of unpolarized light of the same photometric intensity. She obtained similar results with *Drosophila* adults. In *Locusta*, photokinetic velocity was reported to be 23% greater in polarized than unpolarized light (CASSIER, 1960). This kind of polarization sensitivity has not been studied much further, but it is suggested by AUTRUM and STUMPF's data on *Apis* and *Calliphora* (1950), indicating 16%–36% greater electro-retinogram (ERG) amplitudes with polarized, compared with unpolarized, stimuli of the same photometric intensity. If the organism responds to polarized light by orienting the major axis of an anisotropic photoreceptor parallel to the *e*-vector of the plane polarized stimulus, this stronger excitation should then occur.

Such differential intensity effects, however, have not generally been found in subsequent work. However, rates of O_2 consumption in *Daphnia pulex* are reported higher when adapted to polarized light than to an unpolarized light of the same photometric intensity (BUIKEMA, 1972). Since metabolic rate was also found to increase with higher light intensity, these results suggest that the polarized light looks brighter to the *Daphnia*. Other effects of polarized light on metabolism and growth have been reported, but their physiological implications are not yet clear (BUIKEMA, 1975).

a) Oriented Behavior

Further research on polarization sensitivity in *Daphnia* was not published for more than a decade after VERKHOVSKAYA's paper until BAYLOR and SMITH (1953)

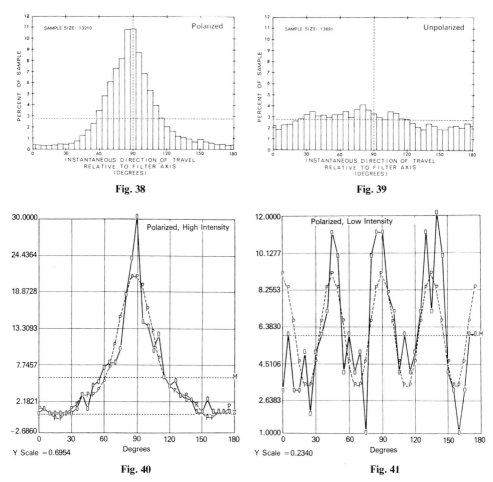

Fig. 38

Fig. 39

Fig. 40

Fig. 41

Figs. 38–41. Polarotactic orientation in *Daphnia* swimming in a vertical beam of light. **Fig. 38.** Orientation with light linearly polarized; *e*-vector at 0° (180°). Course distribution in 5° groups for over 13,000 measurements. Compare with Fig. 39 (R.S.WILSON and T.H.WATERMAN, original). **Fig. 39.** Control behavior with the overhead beam unpolarized. Here, 0° is a geographical azimuth reference. (R.S. WILSON and T.H. WATERMAN, original). Compare with Fig. 38. **Fig. 40.** Earlier data obtained with high light intensities showing single peak responses in 180° similar to that in Fig. 38. The observed points are plotted as o's connected by continuous lines. The result of a periodic regression curve fitting appears as P's and broken lines. *E*-vector at 0° (180°). Compare with Fig. 41. (WATERMAN, 1963). **Fig. 41.** Effect of decreasing *I* by two log units on polarotaxis of the same *Daphnia* and protocol as in Fig. 40. Here, there was a four peaked response to the *e*-vector at 0° (180°), with maxima at 0°, 45°, 90°, and 135°. Such multiple peaked polarotaxis is found in many groups. Symbols and plot as in Fig. 40. (WATERMAN, 1963)

and ECKERT (1953) independently discovered its strong orientation in a vertical beam of linearly polarized light. Soon after, HARRIS and WOLFE (1955) confirmed this. Polarotaxis under the conditions tested was at 90° to the *e*-vector (Figs. 38–40). Similar responses were reported by BAYLOR and SMITH (1953) for eight additional cladoceran genera, among other freshwater plankton, without quantitative data.

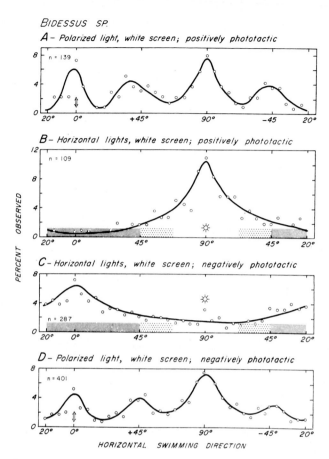

Fig. 42 A–D. Direct experimental evidence that polarotaxis and phototaxis are independent in the aquatic beetle *Bidessus*. Reversing the animal's phototactic sign from positive **B** to negative **C**, as expected, shifted the preferential orientation in relation to horizontal lights (at 90° and 270°) and intermediate dark sectors without significantly affecting the four peaked polarotaxis in a vertical linearly polarized beam with its *e*-vector at 0° **A** and **D**. (JANDER and WATERMAN, 1960)

α) *Question of Artifacts.* During the late 1950s, BAYLOR and some others became convinced that differential scattering or differential reflection–refraction, either in the surround or the cornea or lens, was the basis of the apparent polarization sensitivity in *Daphnia* and even the bee (BAYLOR and KENNEDY, 1958; BAYLOR and SMITH, 1958; KALMUS, 1958; DEVRIES and KUIPER, 1958; SMITH and BAYLOR, 1960; BAYLOR and SMITH, 1961).

Naturally, such claims focused attention on the threat of intensity artifacts in research on polarization sensitivity. However, careful control of differential scattering and reflection, as well as appropriate experimental design, showed that polarotaxis in *Daphnia* is indeed distinct from phototaxis. Yet, the two may often be synergistic. Thus, to pursue earlier experiments on the marine mysid *Mysidium* (BAINBRIDGE and WATERMAN, 1957, 1958), an extensive study was made with *Daphnia* on the correlation of responses to differential light scattering by the medium and those to *e*-vector orientation per se (WATERMAN, 1960). The results strongly implied, but did not directly prove, that polarotaxis in *Daphnia*, as well as in the less strongly orienting *Mysidium*, is based on distinct sensory mechanisms.

Proof that such a distinction is real for *Daphnia*, as well as some other arthropods (Fig. 42), was soon forthcoming from experiments demonstrating the effect of reversal of the animal's phototactic sign. This did not alter its preferred polarotactic direction (i.e., usually 90° to the *e*-vector) despite the reversed response expected if the scattered light intensity pattern was determining the observed orientation (JANDER and WATERMAN, 1960). Similar results were obtained with the hemipteran *Corixa* (RENSING and BOGENSCHÜTZ, 1966).

During the *Daphnia* experiments, both low light intensities or low contrast between the level of horizontal illumination and the vertically downward beam of polarized light were found to induce orientation at four different angles (Fig. 41) to the *e*-vector (i.e., 0°, 45°, 90°, 135°) rather than the one (i.e., 90°) previously observed with high intensities or high contrast, or both. Steady oblique orientation (i.e., 45°, 135°) is not uncommon in polarotactic responses [WATERMAN, 1973, and discussion below for various crustaceans, insects (Fig. 42) and cephalopods]. It has not been reported for phototaxis, but can occur in interactions of geotaxis and phototaxis (JANDER, 1963a). Thus, these behavioral data proved that an intrinsic polarization sensitivity is present among others in *Daphnia*.

Somewhat later, BAYLOR conceded rather obliquely that an intraocular dichroic model, as proposed for insects by AUTRUM (quoted by VON FRISCH, 1950), by WATERMAN (1951), by DE VRIES et al. (1953), and by STOCKHAMMER (1956, 1959), must be invoked to explain *Daphnia*'s *e*-vector responses. Neither an extraocular nor an intraocular reflection–refraction mechanism can account for the crucial data (BAYLOR and HAZEN, 1962; HAZEN and BAYLOR, 1962). However, direct evidence for intraocular dichroism in *Daphnia* has yet to be obtained. Available information on rhabdom fine structure is given below.

β) Effect of p on Polarotaxis. During the early 1960s, *Daphnia*'s polarotaxis was studied further in the author's laboratory, but the results were never published in detail. The first study was done in collaboration with Dr. RUDOLF JANDER and addressed the problem of how much polarization is required in a partially polarized stimulus for *Daphnia* to orient to the *e*-vector. This should settle the question whether or not the natural *p* in its environment (B.II.) is adequate to induce polarotaxis. Several extensive series of experiments were done to test this with *Daphnia* swimming in vertical or horizontal beams of light, with *p* ranging from 0 to 100%.

Two different methods were used to produce partial polarization for the experiments. One comprised a set of multiple glass plates tilted at appropriate angles in the stimulus beam; the other mixed together various amounts of polarized and unpolarized light with a beam splitter. With such partially polarized stimuli, two kinds of oriented response were quantified. In one of them, spontaneous orientation to the *e*-vector was recorded in a vertical beam (Fig. 43).

In the other, the interaction between the gravity reflex and polarotaxis was determined with a horizontal beam polarized at 45° to the vertical and varied in *p* from 0° to 100% (Fig. 44). The actual measurement was the displacement of the

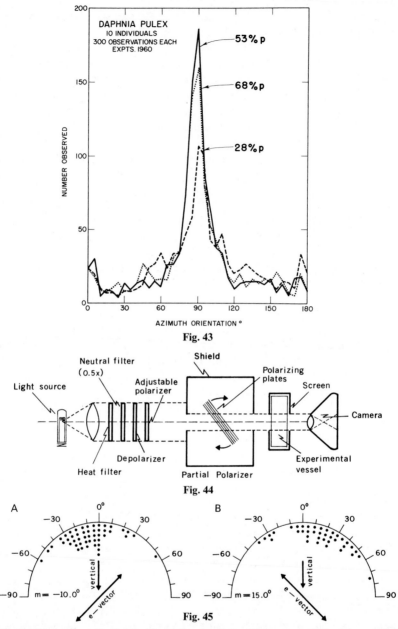

Fig. 43

Fig. 44

Fig. 45

Figs. 43–45. Effects of p on *Daphnia*'s polarization sensitivity. (WATERMAN and JANDER, unpublished).
Fig. 43. Polarotaxis observed as spontaneous swimming azimuths in a vertical beam of partially polarized light. Note that strong preference for 90° swimming directions was still present at $p=28\%$. Although not plotted here it persisted at 20%, but became more diffuse and significantly weaker at 10%.
Fig. 44. Experimental setup used to measure angular displacements of the dorsoventral axis evoked by a horizontal linearly polarized light beam of variable p, with its ϕ at 45°. Here, the orienting effect of polarized light is estimated by opposing the torque, due to gravity, to an opposing one, due to e-vector direction. **Fig. 45.** Tilt measurements of angles between longitudinal axis of the animal's body and the vertical, obtained using the setup in Fig. 44, with $p=100\%$ and $\phi=\pm45°$. In **A**, the mean vector was $-10°$; in **B** it was $+15°$

dorso-ventral axis of the *Daphnia* from the vertical induced by various p's in the oblique polarization (Fig. 45). Comparative experiments were made with animals responding to a natural blue sky overhead which was 40%–50% linearly polarized (Fig. 46).

In the laboratory, significant polarization sensitivity was found at eight different p's ranging from 10% to 100%. Similar results were obtained with both methods of producing the partially polarized light and with both measures of polarotactic response. Estimated from the log mean sum of squares, the directional uncertainty of the polarotaxis is high at 10% p, but decreases sharply at 20%, and remains essentially constant at higher p's to 100%. Thus, the variances are such that the apparent differences between the three intermediate p's of Fig. 42 are not significant.

Thus, beginning with p between 10% and 20%, significant orientation appears and is maintained at all higher levels of polarization. Note that in the honeybee also, a p of 10%–15% is about the threshold for good polarotaxis (VON FRISCH, 1965). For *Daphnia*, it is interesting to note that at asymptotic depths in clear water p_{max} ranges from 13% to 38% and even in milky media at great optical depths (i.e., $\tau = 55$) p_{max} is about 10% (TIMOFEEVA, 1974). A p_{max} around 30%, which should evoke strong polarotaxis, is probably common in sunlit natural waters.

γ) Orientation to the Clear Sky. In clear blue sky, p_{max} is usually greater than underwater, as it was in the *Daphnia* field studies we did to complement the laboratory experiments. Under an overhead sky 40%–50% linearly polarized, the animals were set out in small shallow experimental cylinders so that sky irradiance was a major component of their visual field. When both sun and clear sky were visible to the *Daphnia*, their azimuth distribution showed highly significant orientation with a peak in the sun's bearing (i.e., solar elevation angle 56°) and two other maxima of 45° right and left of the solar peak (Fig. 46 A).

Using periodic regression (WATERMAN, 1963), the first harmonic (i.e., period 360°) is found to account for 53.5% of the total variance, while the second (i.e., 180°) and fourth (i.e., 45°) harmonics are next in order of significant components of the distribution. While these experiments do not discriminate between the contributions of the sun itself and the sky polarization in evoking the strong 0° peak, the two peaks near 45° and 315° are almost certainly responses to the polarization pattern of the sky.

With the sun lower in the sky, *Daphnia* could be screened so that they could see the overhead sky, but not the sun directly. Another screen was used to prevent asymmetrical illumination of the tall white cylinder surrounding the experimental vessel. *Daphnia*'s orientation under this second field condition (Fig. 46 B) was basically like that with both the sun and blue sky visible (Fig. 46 A). However, the differential responses were weaker and the 0° peak less prominent than when the sun was in view. Regression analysis shows that the first harmonic has the highest semiamplitude to mean ratio followed in order by the eighth and the fourth.

The decrease in the apparent polarotactic preference for 45° and 315° when the sun is not visible is not explained, but is perhaps similar to the deterioration of field polarotaxis found in the halfbeak fish *Zenarchopterus* when a small cloud covered only the sun (WATERMAN and FORWARD, 1972). Comparable behavior was observed in the field for insects (WELLINGTON, 1974a). Tested as a control, a waxpaper depolarizer covering the experimental vessel in the field was found to disori-

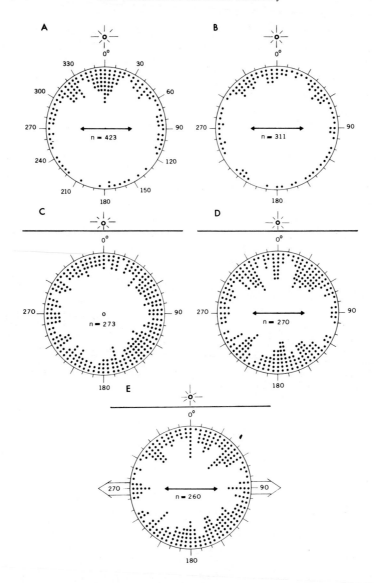

Fig. 46 A–E. Azimuth orientation of *Daphnia* outdoors under clear blue sky and sun. (Waterman and Jander, unpublished). **A** Sun's zenith angle 34°. Both sun (0°) and sky polarization (45° and 315°) peaks were present, but overall distribution was biased towards the sun. **B** Sun's zenith angle 70°–72° and sun not visible to animals. Significant orientation occurred similar to, but weaker than, **A**. **C** Same condition as **B**, but with depolarizer placed overhead. On basis of χ^2 tests, no significant orientation was found. **D** Same condition as **B**, except black cylindrical screen used as surround for experimental vessel, rather than white cylinder used in **A, B** and **C**. Note oblique orientation stronger and 360° symmetry better than in **B**. **E** Same conditions as **D**, but with imposed 100% linear polarization overhead with *e*-vector parallel to that in zenith sky. Orientation less certain than under open sky, only reaches $p < 0.05$ for χ^2 if data are folded over within 180° to increase counts of the angular groups

ent the *Daphnia* (Fig. 46 C). Hence, significant responses obtained in the two previous series of experiments were, in fact, due to the natural overhead illumination and not to some other visual stimulus or modality.

When the cylindrical screen around the experimental vessel was black instead of white, the 0°, 45°, and 315° orientation to the blue sky alone was stronger. In addition, the 180° symmetry of the distribution was distinctly improved (Fig. 46 D). Thus, even with a black surround, the oblique orientation to the polarization plane was significant in the field, whereas we had found in the laboratory that only 90° peaks occurred with this background at high light intensities (JANDER and WATERMAN, 1960).

δ) *Effect of λ on Polarotaxis.* A second study of *Daphnia* polarotaxis was done with Dr. KARL DAUMER in the early 1960s on the dependence of polarization sensitivity on λ. This was briefly reported in the BERNHARD Symposium on Compound Eyes (WATERMAN, 1966 b), but never published in detail. Our interest in this was sharpened by VON FRISCH's finding that polarotaxis in the honeybee was wavelength dependent and that, in fact, ultraviolet wavelengths (i.e., 330–400 nm) alone are apparently adequate for *e*-vector implemented orientation (VON FRISCH, 1954, 1965). Reports of ultraviolet sensitivity in crustaceans are rare (GOLDSMITH and FERNÁNDEZ, 1968; WALD and SELDIN, 1968), but it had been more than once attributed to *Daphnia* (VIAUD, 1938; HEBERDEY, 1949; ROBERT et al., 1958).

Polarotaxis in *Daphnia magna*, responding to a vertical beam of linear polarized light, was measured photographically with flashes at far red wavelengths which did not affect the animal's behavior. The number of quanta required to evoke equal degrees of polarotactic orientation were determined at 20 nm intervals between 320 and 600 nm (Fig. 47). Significant polarotaxis occurred from 360 to 580 nm, with the most effective wavelength being not in the ultraviolet, but at 440 nm. In addition, a shoulder was present on the action spectrum at 520 nm.

Thus, *Daphnia* differs from the bee, as reported by VON FRISCH, by orienting well to polarized light at wavelengths longer than 500 nm. In the crab *Rhithropanopeus*, polarotaxis of the stage II zoea was reported maximal near 500 nm, with a rise in the response curve in the violet suggesting another peak at shorter wavelengths which were not actually tested (VIA and FORWARD, 1975). Polarotaxis in the cladoceran does occur in the near ultraviolet (i.e., 360–400 nm), but not as strongly as in the blue violet. The spectral region between 400–450 nm is the one in which *Daphnia* shows a preponderance of horizontal swimming compared with vertical hop and sink movements typical at longer monochromatic wavelengths (SMITH and BAYLOR, 1953; STEARNS, 1975). Previous work had shown *Daphnia* to be positively phototactic to long λ's and negative to short (VON FRISCH and KUPELWIESER, 1913; HEBERDEY, 1936).

Both the natural importance of *Daphnia*'s polarotactic responses, as well as their correlation with wavelength discrimination and the so-called color dances, remain to be studied adequately. Nothing is yet known about how the underlying basitaxis to polarized light is transformed into a biological goal in the form of a menotaxis. Presumably, the relationship between the two is similar to that between phototactic basitaxis and phototactic menotaxis. Field experiments are much needed, as well as more detailed structural and functional studies in the laboratory.

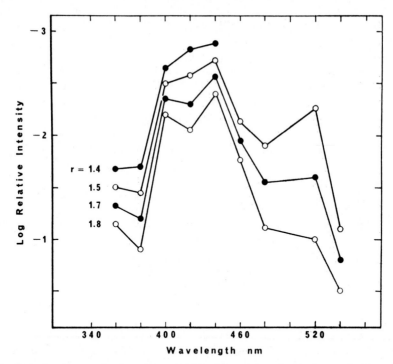

Fig. 47. Action spectrum for the polarotaxis of *Daphnia magna* swimming in a vertical beam of linearly polarized light. Narrow band interference filters transmitting equal numbers of quanta were used every 20 nm from 320 nm to 600 nm. Significant polarotactic responses 90° to the *e*-vector were found between 360 nm and 580 nm, but suitable data for equal degrees of orientation *(r)* were available only as plotted. These equal response curves are essentially parallel, whether or not the polarotaxis was relatively strong (*r* = 1.8) or weak (*r* = 1.4). (DAUMER and WATERMAN, unpublished; figure from WATERMAN, 1966 b)

Our measurements showing the interaction of polarotactic orientation and gravity orientation certainly are congruent with the idea, cited below, that natural polarized light may provide an important reference for spatial position under circumstances where landmarks and other directional cues are weak or absent. Almost certainly, complex polarotactic and phototactic behavior patterns, like those cited for *Daphnia*, are ubiquitous not only in freshwater but also marine plankton (BAYLOR and SMITH, 1957; WATERMAN, 1958; FORWARD, 1975). Hence, their careful study is of more than parochial interest and importance.

b) Compound Eye Organization

It is unfortunate that *Daphnia*, which exhibits one of the strongest and most persistent polarotaxes known is so small that the underlying sensory and integrative physiology have not yet proved feasible for proper study. Nevertheless, some of the relevant sensory fine structure and neurology have been explored. Four distinct photoreceptive sites have been attributed to *Daphnia*.

Most obvious is the cyclopean compound eye (BULLOCK and HORRIDGE, 1965, pp. 1168 ff; YOUNG, 1974 for reviews). Also conspicuous is a much smaller naupliar eye (i.e., ocellus) (Fig. 48). Then, the so-called frontal organ comprises several pairs of neurosensory cells located in the head region (Fig. 49) and connected to the protocerebrum (ELOFSSON, 1966). As these cells may bear rhabdomere-like microvilli, at least in some crustaceans, they have been assumed to be photoreceptive in such cases. Finally, selective irradiation of parts of the body remote from the head evokes reflex responses attributed to a generalized "dermoptic" sense (VIAUD, 1938; ROBERT et al., 1958).

The last is believed to be responsible for the typical ultraviolet avoidance reaction of *Daphnia*, although whether or not this is in fact independent of both the compound eyes and ocelli has been controversial (SCHULZ, 1928; BAYLOR and SMITH, 1957). Indeed, despite considerable interest in *Daphnia*'s light responses, little critical work has been done on their extraocular light perception. Thus, using fiber optic stimulation (i.e., 0.3 mm spot), YOUNG (1974) could not confirm the ROBERT et al. (1958) report that extraocular stimulation could affect compound eye movement reflexes. Yet, YOUNG does accept the notion of a low sensitivity extraocular ultraviolet receptive system. Even the specific contribution of the naupliar eye is uncertain.

In *Daphnia magna*, this organ comprises only ten inverse rhabdom-bearing receptor cells enclosed in four pigment cups directed respectively up, down, right, and left. The down looking ocellar unit has four receptor cells; the other three have two each (KLOTSCHE, 1913). The naupliar eye of daphnids is much smaller than the compound eye; however, the relative size and conspicuousness of the naupliar eye varies considerably even within the genus *Daphnia* (BROOKS, 1959).

In cladocerans, more generally, there sometimes appears to be a reciprocal relation between the relative sizes of these two visual organs. Thus, *Polyphemus* and *Leptodora* have elaborate compound eyes, but the naupliar eye is absent or vestigial, while the chydorid *Monospilus* has only a well developed naupliar eye. Yet, the chydorid *Dadaya* has both compound and naupliar eyes which are unusually large.

α) *Cyclopean Pattern.* The *Daphnia* compound eye (Figs. 48–51) has only 22 ommatidia, with their optic axes separated by nearest neighbor angles of about 40°. Nevertheless, it represents the median fusion, both ontogenetically and phylogenetically, of the paired lateral eyes into a roughly spherical organ. With its crystalline cones protruding from a dark pigment mass it looks like an irregular mulberry. Overlapping broad receptive fields, with a half width of 30°, have been estimated from optical measurement (YOUNG and DOWNING, 1976). Comparison shows that except for *Polyphemus* (which has about 160 ommatidia) and *Leptodora* (which has 300 or more ommatidia) cladoceran compound eyes, including those of *Daphnia*, are substantially reduced from eyes of other more generalized branchiopods (e. g.,*Artemia*).

β) *Ommatidial Components.* Despite a number of electron microscopic studies, critical details of both the retina and the visual pathways through the optic ganglia are still unknown. For polarization sensitivity, the pattern and structure of the rhabdomeres and their dichroism, as well as any optical or electrical coupling between retinular cells, obviously are critical but still inadequately known. Actually, EGUCHI and I started a fine structural study of the retina in the mid 1960s but, be-

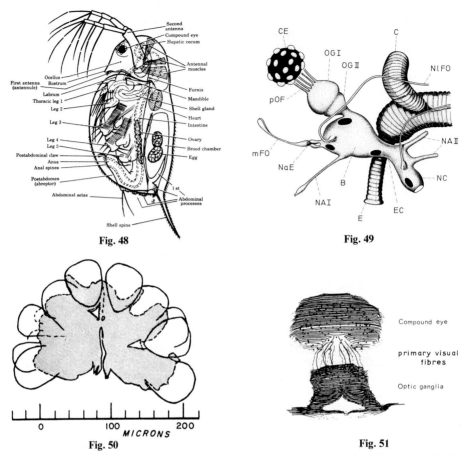

Figs. 48–51. *Daphnia* and its fused median compound eye. **Fig. 48.** Lateral view of adult female *D. similis*; head plus carapace length 2–3 mm. Locations of compound and naupliar eyes are shown. (Brooks, 1959). **Fig. 49.** Internal anatomy of *Daphnia* head showing, in lateral view, relation of compound eye, naupliar eye, and frontal organs to the brain and digestive tract. Dark ovals in CNS are four different clusters of neurosecretory cells. Orientation similar to Fig. 48. *B*, brain; *C*, caecum; *EC*, circumesophageal commissure; *CE*, compound eye; *E*, esophagus; *mFO*, median frontal organ; *NAI*, *NAII*, first, second antennal nerves; *NaE*, nauplius eye; *NC*, nerve cord; *NlFO*, nerve to lateral frontal organ; *OGI, OGII*, first, second optic ganglion; *pOF*, primary optic fibers (redrawn from Sterba, 1957). **Fig. 50.** Frontal section through cyclopic compound eye, suggesting relation of ommatidial lenses to ocular mass of screening pigment. (Baylor and Hazen, 1962). **Fig. 51.** Computer reconstruction of compound eye and optic ganglia in frontal view. Dark spots locate cell nuclei of retinular cells in the eye and of interneurons in the lamina ganglionaris (first optic ganglion). Lines in optic nerve area represent 22 strands, each comprising eight primary axons from an ommatidium (compare Fig. 49 optic nerve). (Macagno et al., 1973)

cause the topic seemed to have been preempted by Röhlich and Törö (1965), we completed only an exploratory beginning (Waterman, 1966b).

   The basic structure of the *Daphnia* ommatidium is reasonably well known from both light and electron microscopic studies (Figs. 23 and 24). Beneath a spheroidal crystalline cone, which focuses images well behind the rhabdom (Young and Downing, 1976), lies an axial rhabdom without the longitudinal banding typical of decapods, mysids, and stomatopods. But, like these malacostracans, *Daphnia* has its constituent microvilli aligned in two orthogonal directions, in this case parallel to the sides of the rectangular cross-section of the rhabdom. Its typical cross sectional dimensions (i.e., $9.5 \times 5.5 \ \mu m$), which is much larger than λ for visible light, suggest that waveguide like properties are not important (YOUNG and DOWNING, 1976).

In our electron micrographs only seven retinular cells (Fig. 24) and their rhabdomeres were located (WATERMAN, 1966b). In fact, all eight rhabdomeres present do not appear in any given cross section (MACAGNO et al., 1973). Usually four of the seven we saw had their microvilli perpendicular to the longer transverse axis of the rhabdom (Fig. 24). The microvilli of the remaining retinular cells were significantly shorter and parallel to this longer axis of the rhabdom cross section. Note that these rhabdoms are special in two ways: (1) the microvilli of the four central rhabdomeres extend all the way across the rhabdom instead of only halfway, as in typical fused rhabdoms in general, and (2) these four units interdigitate their layers of microvilli transversely in an axially successive layered pattern.

Actually, it has been clear for a long time that each ommatidium gives rise to a bundle of eight afferent axons (Fig. 51). Yet, we did not identify R8 and its rhabdomere, while RÖHLICH and TÖRÖ (1965) were ambiguous about their occurrence and location. However, they were subsequently reported to be localized in the proximal half of the retinula, where they replace, presumably in a tiered optical sequence, one of the other distal retinular cells and its rhabdomere (MACAGNO et al., 1973).

On the basis of current knowledge, each ommatidium thus could have two orthogonal dichroic input channels. No fine structural evidence for junctions suggestive of electrical coupling between retinular cells has been reported in adult *Daphnia* compound eyes, but transient gap junctions between first and second order neurons, as well as between neurons and glia, occur during optic tract development (LOPRESTI et al., 1974).

In the eye as a whole, a distal group of five contiguous ommatidia have their rectangular rhabdom axes closely parallel (MACAGNO et al., 1973) and aligned with the sagittal and transverse planes of the animal (YOUNG and DOWNING, 1976). In fact, previous study had indicated that all rhabdoms in the eye have the long edge of their rectangular cross section parallel to the sagittal plane (RÖHLICH and TÖRÖ, 1965).

In the cladoceran *Leptodora*, which shows a strong polarotaxis (a major peak at $90°$ to the *e*-vector), the fused compound eyes have about 300 ommatidia. The rhabdoms again have two orthogonal microvillus directions and, at least in local regions of the retina, show closely parallel alignment in the ommatidia and, hence, in their presumptive dichroic absorption maxima (WOLKEN and GALLIK, 1965). Indeed, it is not known whether or not polarization sensitivity in *Daphnia* is mediated by particular ommatidia or is possible with all of them; nor is it known whether or not all or only certain specific retinular cells in each retinula are important in polarization sensitivity.

γ) Eye Movements. In *Daphnia*, the compound eye is suspended in the hemocoele in such a way that it can rotate freely in three planes. A sort of hydraulic ball and socket mechanism permits this free rotation to occur through an annular suspensory membrane loosely attaching the eye to the hypodermis (KLOTSCHE,

1913; DOWNING, 1974). The extent of these angular movements, which are behaviorally important, are 160° in the sagittal plane and 50°–60° in the coronal and transverse planes (DOWNING, 1974). Three pairs of fine muscles execute these fixation movements, as well as the characteristic 3°–4° continuous tremor of the eye (FROST, 1975).

In visual orientation, the compound eye of *Daphnia* is usually rotated by its muscles to achieve a specific relation to directional light stimulus patterns (JANDER, 1965, 1975). This is a prelude to subsequent body orientation responses which execute a sort of dorsal light reflex (MITTELSTAEDT, 1961). In this way, the body is aligned with the eye which had previously directed itself relative to the radiance distribution. Thus, three median pairs and two dorsolateral pairs of ommatidia participate in contrast orientation (RINGELBERG et al., 1975). Note, however, that phototaxis can be positive, negative, or transverse, depending on the "set" of the animal (JANDER, 1965).

Now violet and ultraviolet light are only effective in evoking eye orientation when they fall on the dorsal ommatidia, whereas responses to yellow–green wavelengths depend on illumination of lateral ommatidia (YOUNG, 1974). This seems consistent with the λ_{max} for polarotaxis being at 440 nm as cited above. The shoulder found at 520 nm presumably would result from the contribution of yellow–green sensitive lateral ommatidia. The interaction between these orienting effects of radiance distribution, wavelength specific visual channeling, and polarotaxis obviously needs more effective coherent study in these cladocerans. It will be particularly interesting to consider eye geometry, retinular dichroism, and the four basitactic directions typical of polarized light orientation (i.e., 0°, 45°, 90°, 135°).

In another briefly reported experiment, results were obtained when an effort was made to evoke optomotor nystagmus in *Daphnia* with vertical moving stripes alternately polarized in different planes (FROST, 1975). However, we know (see below) that such responses in crabs and insects are critically dependent on the angular relation between the specific *e*-vector direction of the stimulus pattern and the orientation of the dichroic receptor mechanism. Consequently, lack of optomotor response to polarized stripes reported for *Daphnia* is critical only if such correlation is tested.

δ) *Ganglionic Connections.* We do, of course, have some data on the basic organization of the visual information processing system in *Daphnia*. Thus, the input from the 176 retinular cells of the eye runs with no exchanges or crossovers in 22 bundles of eight axons from their ommatidia of origin to the lamina ganglionaris, the outer of two optic ganglia (Fig. 51). There, the bundles of retinular cell axons from a given ommatidium each become associated with four monopolar cells which run to the medulla, the second more proximal ganglion (MACAGNO and LEVINTHAL, 1975). Six of the receptor neurons terminate synaptically on the laminar monopolars, while two run straight through the lamina with little or no synaptic contact and terminate in the medulla.

c) *Summary for* Daphnia

Current understanding of *Daphnia* polarization sensitivity may be summarized as follows. Their strong *e*-vector response and continuous swimming pattern have provided some of the best data on polarotaxis. Depending on stimulus conditions, basic *e*-vector orientation may be symmetrical in 180° (i.e., two peaks in a circle) or in 45° (i.e., eight peaks in a circle). Even though natural polarized light in their environment is well above their threshold for orientation, few field data are available. There is no information on the adaptive significance of their polarization sensitivity nor any evidence for its menotactic application to possible course steering.

Fine structural evidence suggests two orthogonal dichroic polarizer channels are present in their aberrant reduced eye. Constant muscular jitter of the eye might establish a shifting retinal image, but acceptance angles of the ommatidia seem too large to make its significance obvious. Perhaps, however, the resulting apparent *e*-vector oscillation is important in polarization sensitivity (discussed below). The problem of processing both polarization and λ information in the retina and visual afferents is probably similar in *Daphnia* and the higher crustaceans, but our present state of knowledge makes such a conclusion rather speculative.

While the compound eye is generally assumed to be the intermediary for polarization sensitivity, the possible contributions of the nauplial eye, the frontal organs, and the dermoptic sense are not really known.

2. *Procambarus* and Other Decapod Crustaceans

Except for a preliminary and not adequately controlled experiment on the hermit crab *Eupagurus* (KERZ, 1950), behavioral polarization sensitivity was not demonstrated in decapod crustaceans until the early 1960 s (*Podophthalmus*, WATERMAN, 1961 b; *Uca*, ALTEVOGT, 1963; *Ocypode*, DAUMER et al., 1963; *Goniopsis*, SCHÖNE, 1963). Relatively little quantitative work of this sort has been done recently. In contrast, electrophysiology, microspectrophotometry, and electron microscopy have been extensively applied to other levels of the problem, especially in various crayfish like *Procambarus*.

a) Oriented Behavior

Relevant behavioral studies in this major group of crustaceans have so far been limited to brachyuran crabs (Figs. 52–54). Especially, certain semiterrestrial crabs (e.g., *Ocypode*, *Grapsus*) have a highly developed visual sense which contributes strongly to their alert and lively behavior. Like other shore living animals, such crustaceans typically demonstrate strong long range orientation dependent on celestial clues (i.e., sun and sky polarization) and landmarks (HERRNKIND, 1972). Polarization sensitivity has been studied in several types of responses, both in the field and laboratory.

α) *Laboratory Orientation.* Thus, in the long eyestalked swimming crab *Podophthalmus*, spontaneous azimuth alignment of the longitudinal body axis in a vertical beam of linearly polarized light shows, in the laboratory, a systematic preference for four directions relative to the *e*-vector (WATERMAN, 1961 b). As in the case of *Daphnia* (Fig. 41), under certain conditions cited above, these are at 0°, 45°, 90°, and 135° to the polarization direction. Similar preferences demonstrated (Fig. 53), both by body orientation and direction of walking, occur in the Pacific ghost crab *Ocypode ceratophthalma* (DAUMER et al., 1963).

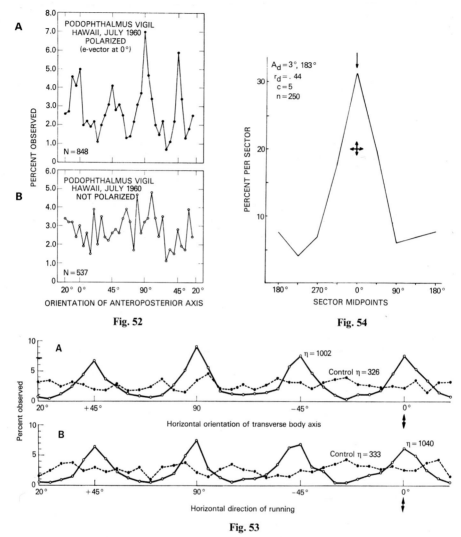

Fig. 52

Fig. 54

Fig. 53

Figs. 52–54. Laboratory demonstration of polarotaxis in various crabs. **Fig. 52. A** Spontaneous four peaked polarotaxis of the portunid crab *Podophthalmus* in a vertical beam of linearly polarized light (*e*-vector at 0°). **B** Control experiment for Fig. 52 A; vertical beam not polarized. No evidence present for four preferential directions found with polarization. (WATERMAN, 1961 b). **Fig. 53.** Effect of *e*-vector on the ghost crab *Ocypode*, measured from the horizontal orientation of the transverse body axis **A** and the horizontal direction of running **B**. Both show spontaneous preference for 0°, ±45°, and 90° directions relative to the *e*-vector (open circles connected by continuous lines). In neither case was significant preferential orientation present in an unpolarized vertical beam (filled circles and broken lines in the two graphs). Comparable 45° multiple peaks were obtained in the field with the *Ocypode* responding to sky polarization. In other species, "simple" menotaxis *(Uca)* (Fig. 54) and time compensated menotaxis *(Goniopsis)* have also been found, as detailed in the text. (DAUMER et al., 1963). **Fig. 54.** Polarotactic orientation of fiddler crabs *(Uca)* in the laboratory. Directions of walking were primarily perpendicular to a simulated shoreline cued by overhead polarization, with *e*-vector either perpendicular or parallel to its direction. Preferential orientation shown here for individuals reared in this setup and more than two months old was absent in younger specimens reared under the same conditions. (HERRNKIND, 1972)

The oblique orientation is a special feature of the four basic orientation directions of polarotaxis and has been found in a wide range of animals with habits and eye structure as different as *Daphnia*, the copepod *Diaptomus* (UMMINGER, 1969), the amphipod *Hyallela* (JANDER and WATERMAN, 1960), brachyuran crabs, hymenopteran insects (JACOBS-JESSEN, 1959; JANDER, 1963a; VAN DER GLAS, 1975), beetles (BIRUKOW, 1953, 1954; JANDER and WATERMAN, 1960), the hemipteran *Corixa* (RENSING and BOGENSCHÜTZ, 1966), a water mite *Arrenurus* (JANDER and WATERMAN, 1960), and the cephalopods *Euprymna* (a sepiolid) and *Sepioteuthis* (a squid) (JANDER et al., 1963). Further discussion of basitaxis and its relation to ambiguity in polarization sensitivity is given in Sects. C.I.3.a. and D.

To prove that the apparent polarotaxis of *Ocypode* was a specific response to the *e*-vector and not just a secondary one to light intensity patterns effected by the polarization, the following control was carried out (DAUMER et al., 1963). A strong fixed intensity pattern was set up with black and white quadrants horizontally surrounding the experimental area. When each crab introduced into the vessel ran across its center, the *e*-vector of the overhead illumination was rotated through a large angle. The number of crabs turning with the *e*-vector was significantly greater than the number turning against the *e*-vector plus those not turning at all.

Hence, the crab's polarization sensitivity mechanism is independent of its means of intensity discrimination. Another set of experiments on *Ocypode* (DAUMER et al., 1963) showed that polarized and unpolarized stimuli of identical photometric intensities have the same phototactic effect on the crab, unlike the early report cited above for *Daphnia*. In contrast, light induced eyestalk deviations in the Atlantic ghost crab *Ocypode quadrata* were reported to indicate that the brightness of polarized light with vertical *e*-vector was 3 times as great as with horizontal polarization (SCHÖNE and SCHÖNE, 1961). On the other hand, eye movements to stimulus displacement were found in *Carcinus* not to be dependent on *e*-vector orientation at wavelengths in the green, but became so for blue or red stimuli (HORRIDGE, 1967).

Laboratory experiments on the mangrove crab *Goniopsis* showed that an overhead *e*-vector could be used for choosing an azimuth direction which demonstrated 24-h compensation for the overhead polarization changes expected to result from the sun's movement through the sky (SCHÖNE, 1963). This confirms polarization sensitivity as an astromenotaxis comparable to that first demonstrated directly for the sun by VON FRISCH (1950) for bees and by KRAMER (1950) for starlings. The orientation direction which mangrove crabs chose by this means was perpendicular to their native shoreline.

Larval stages of a xanthid crab *Rhithropanopeus* were found to have a complex ontogeny of polarotaxis (VIA and FORWARD, 1975). Stages I and IV did not orient to *e*-vector direction, but both stages II and III did. However, polarotaxis in stage II was at 90° to the plane of polarization in a vertical beam, whereas stage III was oriented parallel to the plane. Polarotaxis and phototaxis were shown to be different phenomena. Interestingly, the former disappeared during dark adaptation of stage II zoeas, whereas their phototactic reactions became stronger. As mentioned above, λ_{max} for polarotaxis was about 500 nm, but tests were not run at short enough λ's to ensure that there was not a violet or near ultraviolet peak.

β) Field Orientation. In addition to the laboratory experiments summarized above, *Ocypode ceratophthalma* was also found, on exposure to the natural blue sky, to show four peaked polarotaxis (i.e., 0°, 45°, 90°, 135°) at times when the zenith sky was polarized, even if *p* was weak (DAUMER et al., 1963). Training experiments in which the crabs learned to run to and from their burrows in the sand demonstrated that menotactic course steering was also possible using only the polarization pattern of the blue sky. Thus, the same polarized stimulus which evokes basitaxis in azimuth directions determined by *e*-vector direction can, with other clues or another behavioral "set," or both, give rise to a menotaxis in azimuth directions relevant to the animal's "needs."

Comparable laboratory and field studies of polarotaxis and astromenotaxis have been carried out on several species of the fiddler crab *Uca*, which is also shore living. After earlier unsuccessful attempts to demonstrate polarotaxis, ALTEVOGT (1963) induced directional preferences in *Uca tangeri* using an overhead polarizing filter. Juveniles below a certain size failed to respond, but individuals of carapace widths ≥ 7 mm responded to changes in *e*-vector directions. Field and laboratory studies on this species from northwest Africa and southern Spain were continued for several years by ALTEVOGT and his associates (ALTEVOGT and VON HAGEN, 1964; ALTEVOGT, 1965; KORTE, 1965, 1966).

Near orientation (i.e., short range), as required for rapid retreat to a nearby burrow opening, was shown to be kinesthetically mediated and independent of vision. In contrast, far orientation (i.e., long range) by these crabs is a visually guided menotaxis potentially involving three mechanisms. One of these is the use of landmarks, which is not considered further here. The other two require only a view of the clear sunny sky.

Certain individuals using only the sky showed spontaneous azimuth preferences. Others could be trained to select particular compass directions. Either the sun or polarized areas of the blue sky could be used independently for such celestial direction finding. When both were obscured, neither spontaneous nor learned directional preferences were evident.

Similar results were obtained with North American species of *Uca* (HERRNKIND, 1968, 1972). In addition, polarotaxis in a learned direction was obtained in a simulated shore line habitat under a linear polarizer (Fig. 54). It was concluded that a time compensated celestial menotaxis, dependent both on the sun's position and the sky's polarization pattern, is an important orienting clue for adults of these beach crabs.

Examination of the capacity to orient as a function of developmental stage showed that juveniles until they were several months old did not orient to celestial cues or *e*-vector direction. Thus, *Uca* was apparently different from *Ocypode* whose juveniles, including postmegalopa stages, showed strong polarotaxis both on the beach and in the laboratory (JANDER et al., 1963). Results of studies on polarotaxis in zoeal *Rhithropanopeus* (VIA and FORWARD, 1975) just cited were still different. Some larval stages responded to polarized light and others did not. Clearly, these must be complex interactions between maturation of the sensory and neural mechanism involved and the adaptive behavioral requirements of various species as emphasized by HERRNKIND (1972).

γ) Optomotor Responses. Some interesting, but unresolved, problems were raised by KORTE (1965, 1966) when various visual parameters, including polarization sensitivity, were studied in *Uca tangeri* using optomotor techniques. An overhead rotating polarized sector disk was found to evoke optomotor responses, while a similar black and white disk was ineffective. He concluded from this that distal ommatidia in the fiddler crab eye are specialized for polarization sensitivity and virtually lack intensity or movement discrimination; however, these experimental results are in conflict with others which indicate that *Uca pugnax* is sensitive to a rotating black and white pattern presented to the distal ommatidia (CLARK, 1935).

Furthermore, any implication of KORTE's results that lateral ommatidia of decapod compound eyes cannot discriminate *e*-vector orientation is unwarranted. Fresh experiments, preferably along the lines of those done on *Musca* by REICHARDT and his colleagues (for review, REICHARDT and POGGIO, 1976), are clearly needed in this area. Actually, we attempted long ago to study optomotor responses evoked by polarized light in the mangrove crab *Goniopsis* (BARBER and WATERMAN, 1954, unpublished).

Vertical stripes of polaroid film mounted without gaps on the inside of a rotating drum had their optic axes alternately at 90° to one another. The crab's response was tested under experimental conditions, which we had proved to be highly effective for optomotor stimulation with corresponding black and white stripes. No convincing eyestalk nystagmus or turning–walking responses were obtained with the polarized stripe pattern.

We concluded from this negative result that optomotor experiments were not as good a technique as we had hoped for studying polarization sensitivity in crustaceans. Indeed, VON FRISCH et al. (1960) even argued that optomotor responses to polarization patterns would not be expected in the bee eye, according to the eight channel model of the retinular analyzer. In our case, we did not entertain the related conclusion for *Goniopsis* that the lateral ommatidia lack polarization sensitivity. In fact, there is a plausible explanation for our negative result, even though such optomotor responses still need to be restudied for direct evidence.

The explanation rests on the fact that in order to avoid intensity artifacts from polarized stripes oriented in different directions on a concave cylindrical surface, we had "ingeniously" oriented our alternate stripes at 45° and 135° to the vertical. Now we know that, at least in a number of crustaceans, this would be the least likely pair of orthogonal *e*-vector directions to be discriminated. Details will become clear below, but suffice it to say here that this depends on the fact that the two dichroic analyzers, apparently responsible for polarization sensitivity in each ommatidium, are oriented vertically and horizontally in the central retina.

Clearly, the input from these two channels would be the same for both 45° or 135° *e*-vectors. Support for this explanatory hypothesis comes from much more recent optomotor tests done on the crab *Carcinus* (KIRSCHFELD, 1973a), which confirm that, in this species also, stripes with alternating *e*-vectors at 45° and 135° have no optomotor effect.

However, an important discovery by KIRSCHFELD was that if the stripes are polarized successively at 0° and 90° relative to the vertical, clear optomotor responses appear in the green crabs, a stimulus condition we did not check in *Goniopsis* for the reason cited. Therefore, optomotor responses can be evoked by polarization patterns, but the response may be specifically dependent on particular e-vector directions.

These are not necessarily the same in different arthropods. Thus, dipterans, as well as the honeybee, with the frontal eye region illuminated under similar circumstances respond positively to 45° and 135° polarized stripes, but not to 0° and 90° (KIRSCHFELD and REICHARDT, 1970; KIRSCHFELD, 1973a, b). Note that DE VRIES and KUIPER (1958) had already reported no optomotor response in *Apis* to polarized stripes with e-vectors alternately oriented at 0° and 90°. Their failure to obtain a response was parallel to ours in *Goniopsis*, even though they drew different conclusions from it. In *Carcinus* and dipterans, white, orange, and blue wavelengths are effective, but in the bee only blue and ultraviolet evoke this response (KIRSCHFELD, 1973b). Clearly, these different aspects of optomotor polarization sensitivity reflect underlying features of the receptive channels and visual information processing involved (discussed below).

b) Problem of Sensitivity and Discrimination

Soon after hearing about VON FRISCH's bee polarotaxis, we began trying to learn something about the channeling and information processing responsible for the underlying sensory capability. Thus, single units of the classic *Limulus* compound eye preparation (HARTLINE and GRAHAM, 1932) were found to be e-vector sensitive (WATERMAN, 1950), but this was dependent on oblique light entry into individual ommatidia (WATERMAN, 1954b). Differential responses to e-vector direction were absent when stimulus incidence was parallel, or nearly so, to the unit's optic axis.

Hence, the e-vector discrimination depended, in this case, on an external reflection–refraction mechanism and was not intrinsic to the eye. Furthermore, we showed that the spikes ordinarily recorded in the *Limulus* optic nerve are spikes in eccentric cell axons. These are second order axons apparently activated transsynaptically by any of 8–20 retinular cells present in a given ommatidium, which typically converge on a single eccentric cell (WATERMAN and WIERSMA, 1954).

These studies showed that the aberrant *Limulus* compound eye was not the correct one in which to study polarization sensitivity, despite HARTLINE's demonstration of its basic importance in the general study of visual physiology. As a result, WIERSMA and I turned to the optic tract of decapod crustaceans in 1955 when we recorded single unit activity especially in *Goniopsis*, *Grapsus*, and *Panulirus* eyestalks. Recently, I reviewed the results of this collaboration (WATERMAN, 1977) so I need not do so in detail here.

Our results, while otherwise productive, were negative with regard to significant polarization sensitivity at the optic nerve level (WATERMAN and WIERSMA, 1963; WATERMAN et al., 1964). In contrast, high S_e's have been repeatedly demonstrated by intracellular recordings of retinular cells in a variety of decapods (SHAW, 1969b; WATERMAN and FERNÁNDEZ, 1970; MOTE, 1974; LEGGETT, 1976, 1978). As discussed below, it remained for later experiments to demonstrate that a rotating e-vector seems to be required to evoke differential responses at the optic nerve level.

c) Compound Eye Organization

Meanwhile, it seemed prudent, in trying to discover the mechanism of polarization sensitivity, to retreat from higher order neurons to the primary level in the retina. Incentive for such an approach came directly from new information on the functional organization of decapod crustacean compound eyes (Figs. 55–58). This knowledge suggested a rather simple model for the mechanism of polarization sensitivity. The relevant details in decapods have become well known, beginning with the pioneer electron microscopic studies of EGUCHI (1964, 1965) and RUTHERFORD and HORRIDGE (1965).

These confirmed the fact, already well described by PARKER (1890, 1891, 1895) and some other light microscopists, that the rhabdom in various decapods is made of about 10 to 400 layers comprising orthogonal "fibrous" units in alternate bands contributed mainly by the seven regular retinular cells in each ommatidium (Figs. 34–37, and 64). Even the toothed pattern of rhabdomeres (Fig. 27), comprising such a fused rhabdom, was clearly and correctly described by PARKER for the crayfish.

α) *Importance of Fine Structure.* Beginning in the mid-1960s, electron microscopy revived interest in these details and added much new information. One basic contribution was the fact that the fine striations barely visible in the best light microscopy are, in fact, microvilli which protrude axially from the retinular cells. This had been demonstrated for insects and *Limulus* about 10 years before (GOLDSMITH and PHILPOTT, 1957; MILLER, 1957; WOLKEN et al., 1957; FERNÁNDEZ-MORAN, 1958). As discussed above, this elaborate membrane system contains the visual pigment rhodopsin and is, in fact, the site of the dichroism basic to arthropod and cephalopod polarization sensitivity.

Between the publication of part of EGUCHI's thesis in 1965 and 1971, quite a few interesting aspects of how decapods are able to perceive polarized light were illuminated. Testing the obvious implications of the fine structural organization of the retinula selective adaptation of the ERG showed that there are, in fact, only two orthogonal *e*-vector discriminating channels (Fig. 62, below) in the land crab *Cardisoma*'s retina (WATERMAN and HORCH, 1966). Similarly, intracellular recording in the green crab *Carcinus* showed that two types of polarization sensitive cells are present in a given area of the retina; their maximum *e*-vector responses are also orthogonal (SHAW, 1966). In subsidiary experiments (WATERMAN and HORCH, 1966), the lobster *Homarus* and the crayfish *Orconectes* gave the same responses as *Cardisoma*. In this land crab, the polarization sensitivity peaks coincided with the directions of the two sets of rhabdom microvilli. This certainly reinforced the notion that polarization sensitivity receptor channels are directly correlated with selective transverse alignment of rhabdom microvilli perpendicular to the ommatidial optic axis.

Fine structural changes induced by selective adaptation confirmed this in the spider crab *Libinia* (Figs. 59 and 60) and showed that maximum absorption in rhabdomeres occurred parallel to the long axis of their microvilli (EGUCHI and WATERMAN, 1968). This had been predicted in the octopus (MOODY and PARRISS, 1961) and later demonstrated optically (MOODY, 1964). In dipterans electrophysiological (GIULIO, 1963), as well as microspectrophotometric (LANGER, 1965; LAN-

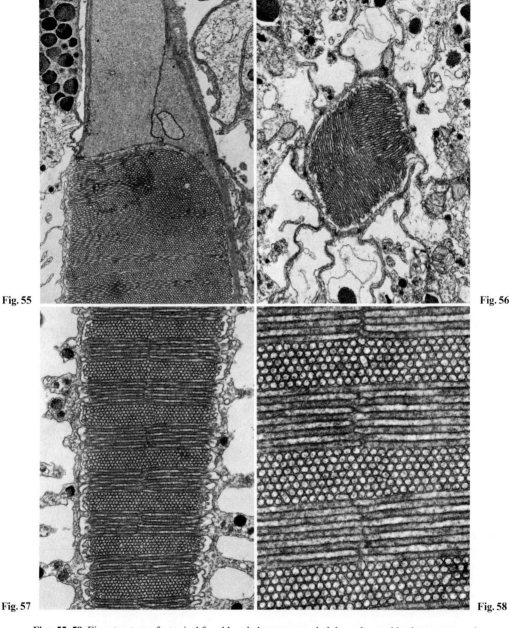

Fig. 55

Fig. 56

Fig. 57

Fig. 58

Figs. 55–58. Fine structure of a typical fused banded crustacean rhabdom observed in the stomatopod *Gonodactylus bredeni*. Essentially similar organization has been found in other stomatopods, mysids, and decapods with apposition type compound eyes. (EGUCHI and WATERMAN, original). **Fig. 55.** Axial section showing the proximal end of the dioptric crystalline cone where it meets the distal end of the rhabdom. In the latter, two orthogonal sets of microvilli arise from the distal R 8, as in the rock crab *Grapsus*. **Fig. 56.** Cross section of the distal rhabdom showing its rhombic shape at this level. Two approximately perpendicular microvillus directions are apparent in this slightly oblique section. Radial cell membranes anchored close to the rhabdom by desmosomes show eleven sectors around the axis;

GER and THORELL, 1966), evidence had also shown its occurrence in insects. In subsequent decapod studies correlating fine structure, electrophysiology, and microspectrophotometry, the dichroic components of rhabdomeres in a number of species were found to have this same orientation of maximum absorption. It is, in fact, the general rule not only in decapod crustaceans, but also in insects and cephalopods. Only two particular rhabdomeres are known (i.e., R 7 in dipterans [KIRSCHFELD, 1969] and R 8 in the hemipteran *Lethocerus* (IOANNIDES and HORRIDGE, 1975]), which are exceptions. Their aberrant principal axis occurs normal to the microvillus long axis (discussed below).

β) Role of Rhodopsin. Direct measurements of dichroism, using microspectrophotometry of transverse light beams through the isolated crayfish rhabdom [*Orconectes* (WATERMAN et al., 1969), *Procambarus* (WATERMAN and FERNÁNDEZ, 1970)], further demonstrated that the major absorption axis is parallel to the microvilli, and added the further point that the spectral distribution of the dichroism is the same as the absorption spectrum of rhodopsin in the microvilli (Fig. 61). This substantiated the hypothesis proposed by DE VRIES et al. (1953), which was seconded by STOCKHAMMER (1956, 1959) and a number of others (JANDER and WATERMAN, 1960; LANGER, 1966), that the visual pigment in typical rhabdom bearing eyes serves both as a photon absorber and an intrinsic dichroic polarizer[2].

Visualization of the rhodopsin in decapod photoreceptor membranes has recently become possible through the application of freeze–fracture techniques (EGUCHI and WATERMAN, 1976; FERNÁNDEZ and NICKEL, 1976). The fracture face of the protoplasmic leaflet (PF) of split microvillus membrane in the crayfish *Procambarus* is richly particulate with conspicuous 80–90 Å spheroids having center-to-center spacing of about 120 Å. Note that intramembranous particles of similar size and location have also been observed in rhabdom microvilli of insects (SEITZ, 1970; PERRELET et al., 1972; HARRIS et al., 1977) and a snail (EAKIN and BRANDENBURGER, 1970).

Several lines of evidence favor the identification of these components with molecules of photopigment, probably in small aggregates. Now, if their dichromophores lie randomly distributed approximately in the plane of the receptor membrane, as in the vertebrate outer segments, a single microvillus should be dichroic,

---

[2] Note that λ_{max} for S_e in these decapods determined by microspectrophotometry is near 530 nm, far from the ultraviolet, even though both violet and yellow sensitive retinular cells, recorded intracellularly, yielded high polarization sensitivities (WATERMAN and FERNÁNDEZ, 1970)

◀ seven from R 1–R 7, plus four lobes of R 8. **Fig. 57.** Axial section showing more proximal part of the regular rhabdom comprising rhabdomeres of R 1, R 4, and R 5 with horizontal microvilli (relative to the animal's body axes) and R 2, R 3, R 6, and R 7 with vertical. As typical of crabs, extensive perirhabdomal vacuoles surround the photoreceptor organelle (also prominent in Fig. 56). These are traversed by cytoplasmic strands connecting the rhabdom with the rest of its parent retinular cell. **Fig. 58.** Magnified view of rhabdom axis showing highly regular orthogonal pattern of microvilli in alternate bands. Closed ends of microvilli, which extend only half way across each layer, are shown in those bands cut parallel to the microvillus axis, the plane of maximum absorption by this dichroic structure (Figs. 59 and 60). Note that microvilli in each half band come from opposite retinular cells with toothed rhabdomeres (compare Fig. 27)

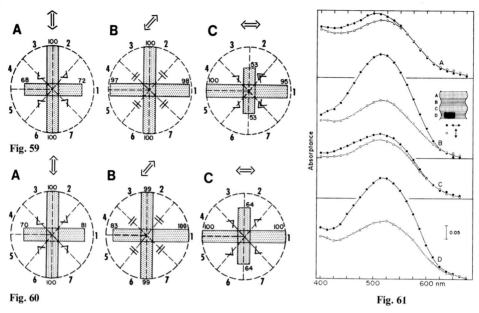

Fig. 59

Fig. 60

Fig. 61

Figs. 59–61. Evidence in a typical decapod crustacean rhabdom for two orthogonal dichroic channels with their major absorption axes parallel to their microvilli. **Figs. 59 and 60.** Fine structural effects of selective light adaptation (6 h) with linear polarized light (*e*-vector horizontal, 45°, and vertical, as indicated) in the spider crab *Libinia*. Numbers of two types of cytoplasmic organelles per unit cross section of retinular cell were compared for the horizontal (R 1, R 4, and R 5) and vertical (R 2, R 3, R 6, and R 7) channels under these three conditions. Previous experiments showed that both multivesicular bodies and pinocytotic vesicles increased substantially in light. Standardized counts for the two channels are shown by the vertical and horizontal bar lengths. Statistical differences indicated between channels: $=$ same as; $>$ greater than 5% level; $>>$ greater than 1% level. (EGUCHI and WATERMAN, 1968). **Fig. 59.** Distribution of multivesicular bodies in the perirhabdomal cytoplasm shows that vertically polarized light is selectively absorbed by R 2, R 3, R 6, and R 7 with vertical microvilli; horizontal *e*-vector differentially light adapted R 1, R 4, and R 5 with horizontal microvilli, whereas 45° *e*-vector affected both channels equally. **Fig. 60.** Counts of pinocytotic vesicles near the rhabdom yielded similar evidence to that of Fig. 59 that the major absorption axis of dichroic rhabdomeres is parallel to their microvillus axis. **Fig. 61.** Microspectrophotometric evidence that rhabdomeres in the crayfish *(Orconectes)* eye show a dichroic ratio of about 2.0 at their λ_{max} of 525 nm to transverse illumination confined within a single rhabdom band with major absorption parallel to their microvilli. In addition to confirming the fine structural results on *Libinia* (Figs. 59 and 60), these data demonstrate that rhodopsin is the molecular basis of rhabdomere dichroism; its molecules must, therefore, have some restrictions in their chromophore orientation in the photoreceptor membrane. (WATERMAN et al., 1969)

with a ratio just less than 2, with the major absorption axis parallel to the long axis of the microvillus (MOODY and PARRISS, 1961; WATERMAN et al., 1969).

γ) Dichroism and Polarization Sensitivity. In a perfect array of parallel straight microvilli, the overall dichroism should also approach this value. Actually, the original microspectrophotometric measurements of this parameter in *Procambarus* (WATERMAN et al., 1969) and *Libinia* (HAYS and GOLDSMITH, 1969) rhabdomeres were consistent with such a model (Fig. 61). However, *e*-vector sensitivity ratios (i.e., S_e's) measured electrophysiologically, are often sharply in excess of 2 (maximum values 9–12) in a number of decapods [e.g., *Astacus, Procambarus, Carcinus, Callinectes* (SHAW, 1969b; WATERMAN and FERNÁNDEZ, 1970; MOTE, 1974)].

If, as is generally assumed, the high sensitivity ratios are to be accounted for strictly in terms of rhodopsin dichroic ratios, preferential dichromophore alignment favoring the microvillus longitudinal axis would be required (e.g., KIRSCHFELD, 1969; SHAW, 1969b). Thus, microvillus photoreceptor membranes must be different in this regard from vertebrate outer segment disks (Fig. 28). In addition, there is considerable discrepancy between the earlier microspectrophotometry measurements and electrophysiological estimates of polarization sensitivity (GOLDSMITH, 1975; WATERMAN, 1975c). While this anomaly has not been completely explained, the general approach followed assumes that microspectrophotometric dichroic ratios of around 2 are substantially lower than the real in situ values.

Evidence has been obtained from microspectrophotometry of isolated crayfish rhabdoms that Brownian rotational and translational motion of rhodopsin molecules is significantly less than in vertebrate rod outer segments (GOLDSMITH and WEHNER, 1977). Also, photoinduced dichroism in crayfish photoreceptor membranes in the presence of formaldehyde has been interpreted as a measure of the normal dichromophore distribution.

The data are consistent with a model in which the absorption vectors are uniformly distributed between $\pm 50°$, relative to the microvillus long axis and at an inclination of about 20° to the membrane surface (GOLDSMITH and WEHNER, 1977). The predominantly axial dichromophore orientation has been attributed to thermodynamic constraints on these membranes arising from their cylindrical form and its 700 Å diameter (LAUGHLIN et al., 1975; SNYDER and LAUGHLIN, 1975).

In addition, photoreceptor membranes more viscous than those of vertebrate rod outer segments could account for the observed reduction or absence of translational and rotational Brownian movement of the rhodopsin in the membrane (GOLDSMITH, 1975; GOLDSMITH and WEHNER, 1977). While microspectrophotometric dichroic ratios between three and four have quite often been measured in decapods (GOLDSMITH, 1975), these are still too small, by a factor of two or three, to account for the maximum polarization ratios of 10–12 electrophysiologically measured in crabs and crayfish (SHAW, 1969b; WATERMAN and FERNÁNDEZ, 1970). Clearly interesting problems of photoreceptor membrane molecular structure and transduction–excitation mechanisms remain to be solved here.

δ) *Other Factors in Sensitivity.* Note that although microvillus dichroism is obviously an initial requirement for polarization sensitivity, a wide range of other factors at a variety of levels may modify or even eliminate its differential effects. Indeed, SNYDER has argued repeatedly that the dichroism of rhabdoms is, in general, a secondary byproduct of other more essential visual adaptations (SNYDER et al., 1973; SNYDER, 1975a; SNYDER and LAUGHLIN, 1975). For present purposes, however, it is primary because the whole system for sensing, encoding, and processing polarized light parameters depends on it. Thus, we need to review the subsequent fate of the initial dichroic selectivity of the photoreceptor membrane.

To begin with, the effective dichroism Δ_e of a rhabdomere theoretically depends not only on the dichroism (Δ) of the regularly ordered microvilli, but also on their absorbance (γ) and the length (l) of the light path through them (SNYDER, 1975 b; SNYDER and LAUGHLIN, 1975; McINTYRE and SNYDER, 1978), so that:

$$\varDelta_e = \frac{1 - e^{-\gamma l}}{1 - e^{-\gamma l / \varDelta}}. \qquad (12)$$

Here, it is assumed that if all photons are absorbed, the light power input is one. Also in this equation, the γ is specifically taken as the absorption parallel to the microvillus axes. Clearly, very long or very absorbent rhabdomeres have polarization sensitivities approaching unity (i.e., no e-vector discrimination). Thus, for a given absorption coefficient and dichroic ratio, long rhabdomeres would have a low polarization sensitivity and low absolute sensitivity. GRIBAKIN (1975) has argued that the optimum length for units in an open rhabdoms is between 50 and 100 μm. Rhabdomeres in many fused rhabdoms are considerably longer nonetheless.

Thus, in decapods, the length of the rhabdom has been found to be between 150 and 450 μm (EGUCHI and WATERMAN, 1966; NÄSSEL and WATERMAN, unpublished). Self-absorption could be quite substantial [3] in such a case; hence, a decrease in polarization sensitivity and a corresponding increase in band width of the absorption spectrum would be expected. Thus, in an unfused rhabdomere 250 μm long, a dichroic absorptance ratio of 10 would theoretically be decreased, by this factor, to an absorbance ratio of 4.11 (GOLDSMITH and BERNARD, 1974). However, the typical layering of decapod rhabdoms ideally should eliminate such losses in discrimination. Even in a very long banded rhabdom, the absorbance ratio could equal the dichroic ratio (SHAW, 1969 b; SNYDER, 1973; GRIBAKIN, 1975).

This effect would be optimal if 1) the microvillus directions are symmetrical (e.g., orthogonal), 2) the absorption is equal in the channels, and 3) the wavelength sensitivity is equally distributed between them (SNYDER, 1973). Consequently, a banded rhabdom would seem to be organized for both maximum absolute sensitivity and maximum polarization sensitivity. Unequivocal experimental evidence for this remains to be demonstrated.

ε) *Retinular Cell Eight.* Another complicating factor, which is widespread if not universal in decapod as well as some mysid and stomatopod retinulas, is the presence of a distal eighth retinular cell (R 8) in addition to the seven regular retinular cells (R 1–R 7). The rhabdomere of R 8 optically precedes the main rhabdom comprising rhabdomeres R 1–R 7 (Fig. 62). At least the nucleus and axon of R 8 have been known since the time of late nineteenth century light microscopists [e.g., G.H. PARKER (1891, p. 113)]. Only recently, however, has knowledge of its detailed structure drawn attention to its probable visual importance (Table 1 in WATERMAN, 1977).

The electron microscopic demonstration that R 8 in decapods, indeed, has a rhabdomere (KUNZE and BOSCHEK, 1968, for *Ocypode*) was foreshadowed by earlier findings of a similar R 8 in mysids (MAYRAT, 1962; EGUCHI and WATERMAN,

---

[3] In the lobster *Homarus*, total axial absorbance for a 240 μm rhabdom has been estimated to be 80% (BRUNO et al., 1977)

1966, 1973). The caridean *Pandalus* has eight axons from each ommatidium, although the rest of R 8 has not been identified (Nässel, 1976 b) but, in the common *Palaemonetes*, a four-lobed R 8 with rhabdomere is present (Eguchi and Waterman, unpublished).

Now 10 or more additional genera of decapods have been shown to have a four-lobed cross retinular cell with an axial rhabdomere and a proximal axon arising from one of its lobes which also contains the nucleus. In the crayfishes *Pacifastacus* (Nässel, 1976 a) and *Procambarus* (Eguchi and Waterman, unpublished), the R 8 rhabdomere is not banded and has microvilli oriented in the horizontal plane and, thus, parallel to those of cells R 1, R 4, and R 5 of the regular rhabdom. In *Grapsus* (Eguchi and Waterman, 1973), *Cardisoma* (Eguchi and Waterman, unpublished), and *Panulirus* (Meyer-Rochow, 1975), the R 8 rhabdomere is banded with the microvilli in alternate bands being orthogonal. Thus, a single four-lobed cross retinular cell gives rise to two discretely oriented sets of microvilli (Fig. 63).

Since spiny lobsters and crayfish are both macruran decapods, the comparative fine structure of R 8 in other members of this reptantian group containing 600–700 species should be a matter of considerable interest. In the Anomura, we have encountered typical brachyuran type R 8 cells in the galatheid crab *Petrolisthes* and the hermit crab *Pagurus* (Eguchi and Waterman, unpublished). In several genera of stomatopods, which are hoplocaridans rather than eucaridans like decapods and euphausiids, not only are the regular rhabdoms banded in typical decapod fashion, but R 8 is present and of the brachyuran type (Eguchi and Waterman, unpublished).

Thus, in *Squilla empusa* and *Gonodactylus bredeni* distal, four-lobed R 8's have been observed with two layered sets of microvilli in their rhabdomeres. Curiously, *Squilla mantis* has been reported to lack such an R 8 (Schönenberger, 1977). Instead, a minute basal cell with no rhabdomere was identified as R 8; a kind of proximal retinal cell not previously noted in stomatopods or decapods. Obviously, this exception needs further study; however, among five species of mysids from as many different genera, a distal R 8 was found to be present in three and absent in two (Hallberg, 1977). So uniformity of fine structural details is not necessarily the rule, even within limited taxonomic groups.

The functional significance of R 8 has not yet been demonstrated; however, from our general knowledge of polarization sensitivity in the regular rhabdom, the following predictions may be made. Where the same cell has two apparently balanced sets of orthogonal microvilli (*Panulirus* and *Grapsus*), the dichroism inherent in each would cancel out at least optically. Whether or not the dynamic properties of such a system in practice reduce the polarization sensitivity of R 8 to 1 (i.e., no discrimination) remains to be shown. On the other hand, R 8 in the crayfish should have polarization sensitivity with its maximum response to horizontal *e*-vector.

ζ) *Interactions of R 8 and R 1–R 7 (Fig. 64).* Now, in addition to any direct contribution to photon absorption and excitation, these R 8's have another possible contribution resulting from their action as filters for the light which reaches the regular rhabdom with which they are in optical series. Such filtering could be of importance both with regard to polarization sensitivity and wavelength discrimination.

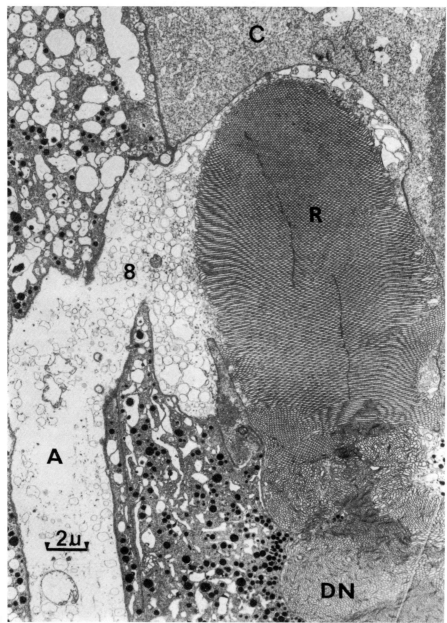

Fig. 62

Figs. 62–64. Comparison between the distally located R 8 and R 1–R 7 in crayfish and crab. In both types, its rhabdomere optically precedes the regular, more proximal, fusiform or cylindrical banded rhabdom constituted by rhabdomeres of R 1–R 7. For occurrence of R 8 so far documented, see Table 1 in WATERMAN (1977). **Fig. 62.** Axial section of *Procambarus* ommatidium showing the short (5% of total rhabdom length) nonbanded rhabdomere *(R)* of R 8, located between the proximal end of the crystalline cone *(C)* and the banded distal neck region *(DN)* of the regular rhabdom (rhabdomeres of R 1–R 7). All microvilli in R 8 are horizontal in orientation and, therefore, parallel to those of R 1, R 4, and R 5. The section also shows origin *(8)* of the R 8 axon *(A)* from one of four lobes of this cell; this runs proximally outside the regular retinular cells and their axons to its terminus in the medulla externa (Fig. 67) without synapsing in the lamina ganglionaris, as do R 1–R 7. Typically, R 8 cytoplasm lacks granules of screening pigment usual in R 1–R 7 (EGUCHI and WATERMAN, original). **Fig. 63.** Diagram

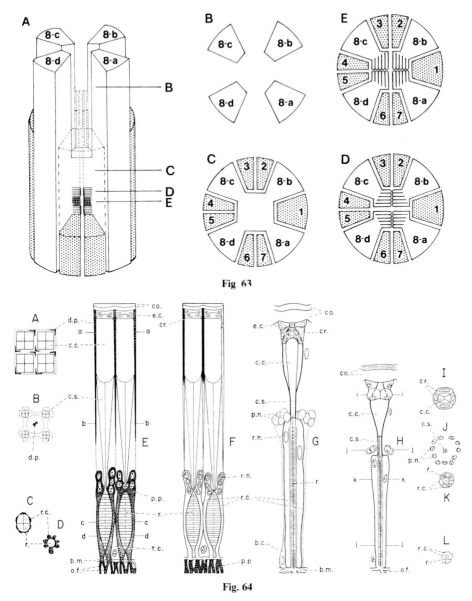

Fig. 63

Fig. 64

of R 8 in the rock crab *Grapsus*. Here R 8 is longer (20% of total rhabdom length) and banded in two sets of orthogonal microvilli originating from the four lobes (**A–D**) of this one cell. As in crayfish, one of these lobes gives rise to the cell's axon. Most distally, the rhabdom comprises only R 8; in an intermediate zone, R 1–R 8 all contribute to the microvillus bands, then, proximally, the whole regular rhabdom is formed by rhabdomeres of R 1–R 7. **A**. Stereodiagram of distal part of rhabdom. **B–E** Cross sections at the levels marked in A showing cellular organization and microvillus pattern. For further details, see original report (EGUCHI and WATERMAN, 1973). **Fig. 64.** Comparison of decapod crustacean ommatidia in the crayfish *Astacus* (**A–F**) and the crab *Macropodia* (**G–L**). The levels of the cross sections are indicated on the axial diagrams (**E** and **H**) (e.g., **A** is at level a–a). Note that **E** and **F** compare a light adapted and dark adapted ommatidium while **G** and **H** compare a fresh ommatidium with one fixed in alcoholic Bouin's. *b.c.*, basal cell; *h.m.*, basement membrane; *c.c.*, crystalline cone; *co*, cornea; *cr*, crystalline cone cell; *c.s.*, crystalline cone stalk; *d.p.*, distal pigment; *e.c.*, corneagenous cells; *o.f.*, primary axons; *p.p.*, proximal pigment; *p.n.*, pigment cell nuclei; *r*, rhabdom; *r.c.*, retinular cell; *r.n.*, retinular cell nucleus; *t.c.*, tapetal cell. (WATERMAN, 1961 a)

The polarization sensitivity of the underlying cell would theoretically be changed in the presence of a polarizing filter (i.e., the distal rhabdomere) preceding it with microvilli orthogonal to the proximal unit by a multiplicative factor $\exp \gamma l \left(1 - \frac{1}{\Delta}\right)$ (SNYDER, 1973, 1975a, and GRIBAKIN, 1975; MCINTYRE and SNYDER, 1978). In a hypothetical example, the modest dichroism (1.57) of the proximal unit was enhanced by this mechanism to an effective polarization sensitivity of 9.0 (GRIBAKIN, 1975). With the filter dichroism parallel to that of the underlying cell, the effective polarization sensitivity was calculated to be 3.6.

Note, however, that the strongest optical Δ reported for a rhabdomeric eye is a ratio of 6 for the squid *Loligo* (HAGINS and LIEBMAN, 1963). If this as yet unconfirmed value is typical, it is achieved without benefit of the banding and filtering which have been hypothesized to be important for polarization sensitivity in arthropod retinulas.

In *Procambarus* (EGUCHI and WATERMAN, unpublished), R 8 contributes only about 5% (i.e., about 50 μm) of the total rhabdom length and in *Grapsus* about 20% (i.e., about the same absolute length, 50 μm). Actually, as the above formula makes clear, the length of the filtering unit is one of three important parameters controlling its polarization sensitivity enhancing effect. A further distinction between crayfish and crab R 8 rhabdoms is their microvillus pattern cited above.

Consequently, if R 8 has the filtering action postulated above, it should enhance the polarization sensitivity of R 2, R 3, R 6, and R 7, which have their microvilli vertically oriented. At the same time, it should decrease polarization sensitivity of the horizontal regular retinular cells. Note, however, that such effects would probably be λ sensitive. Hence, the λ_{max} of R 8, which is not yet known, would determine which of the regular retinular cells could be affected and to what extent (EGUCHI et al., 1973).

In contrast, two orthogonal microvillus sets are present in the crabs *Grapsus* (EGUCHI and WATERMAN, 1973), *Callinectes*, *Carcinus*, and *Ocypode* (NÄSSEL and WATERMAN, unpublished) and the spiny lobster *Panulirus* (MEYER-ROCHOW, 1975). Note that in our preparations of *Ocypode* and other Brachyura, the R 8 rhabdomeres appear to have the two regular alternating sets of orthogonal microvilli, as previously described for *Grapsus* (EGUCHI and WATERMAN, 1973), in contrast to the irregular pattern of microvilli reported in R 8 for *Ocypode* (KUNZE and BOSCHEK, 1968).

Although these two directional rhabdomeres of R 8 should not optically show polarization sensitivity if the two sets of microvilli are equivalent in both spectral sensitivity and dichroism, the possibility of R 8 producing a weak *e*-vector sensitivity with orthogonal peaks has been suggested recently (STOWE et al., 1977). This was based on the intracellular evidence for such a response observed occasionally in both *Carcinus* and *Astacus* (SHAW, 1969b). However, the single direction of R 8 microvilli in crayfish make this correlation with the green crab questionable.

On the other hand, the brachyuran type R 8 might be involved in providing an independent isotropic channel to allow instantaneous *e*-vector perception, if that in fact exists, when coupled with two anisotropic channels in the regular rhabdom. Such an analyzer for plane polarized light is known to be feasible from the relation between the STOKES parameters (WATERMAN, 1975c, p. 340–341) and, as reviewed

below, it has been suggested as a possible model for the worker bee analyzer (BER-
NARD and WEHNER, 1977). Note, however, that for a three-channel system of this
kind, the difference between ϕ_1 and ϕ_2 cannot be 90° or 0°.

d) Afferent Channeling

Recall, however, that R 8 does give rise to an afferent axon which terminates
synaptically not in the lamina ganglionaris, as do R 1–R 7, but instead in the next
optic ganglion (i.e., medulla externa) (Figs. 65 and 66). Hence, some special function is implied. For instance, R 8 in dipterans and R 9 in the honeybee, which are
generally thought to mediate polarization sensitivity (as discussed below), also do
not terminate in the most distal optic ganglion, but in the next more central
ganglion. Quite apart from relevance to polarization sensitivity, R 8 in decapods
may be related to extreme scotopic sensitivity or λ discrimination (EGUCHI and
WATERMAN, 1973; WATERMAN, 1977)[4]. Obviously, appropriate experiments are
much needed here.

Beyond the initial detection of polarized light by dichroic rhabdomeric components of decapod eyes, the processing of the sensory input obviously involves,
first, the induction of receptor potentials in the retinular cell membrane and, then,
their transmission centrally. An important issue in view of the models discussed
above is whether or not individual rhabdomeres, despite their elaborate interdigi-
tation, are independently excitable and whether or not each retinular cell can respond as a distinct unit.

The alternative would presumably involve some kind of junctions between
rhabdomeres or retinular cells, which could give rise to electrical coupling. Excitatory coupling, which would dissipate polarization sensitivity between units with
different e-vector orientations, has been reported to occur in certain insect retinulas
and in Limulus, but apparently not in decapods (SHAW, 1969 a), although it has not
been widely tested. Inhibitory coupling, which would selectively sharpen discrimination between units, has been proposed for the crayfish (MULLER, 1973), but not
confirmed (MOTE, 1974).

From the receptor potentials in isolated or coupled retinular cells, sensory excitation is transmitted proximally to the optic ganglia, which are four in decapods
(Fig. 65), as reviewed by ELOFSSON and DAHL (1970). There is no evidence here for
spike trains either in the photoreceptor cells or their axons; hence, transmission
presumably is electrotonic, at least as far as the receptor terminal synapses[5]. For
R 1–R 7 in the crayfish, the latter occur on three types of monopolar secondary
neurons M 2–M 4 in the lamina ganglionaris, while the R 8 axon passes through it
without terminating and synapses in the medulla externa, the next more proximal
ganglion (NÄSSEL, 1976a, 1977). Similar relations have also been found in the
caridean shrimp Pandalus (NÄSSEL, 1976 b).

---

[4] Failure to find microspectrophotometric evidence for violet receptors in the regular rhabdom of
crayfish (R 1–R 7) (hypothesized by EGUCHI et al., 1973) raises the question of whether or not R 8, in
fact, may be the short wavelength receptor (GOLDSMITH, 1978). However, the absorbance of its rhabdomere and the specific location of marked violet receptors need to be determined

[5] In insects, the secondary neurons were reported to respond with a hyperpolarizing potential, also
unaccompanied by spiking (JÄRVILEHTO and MORING, 1974; LAUGHLIN, 1976a)

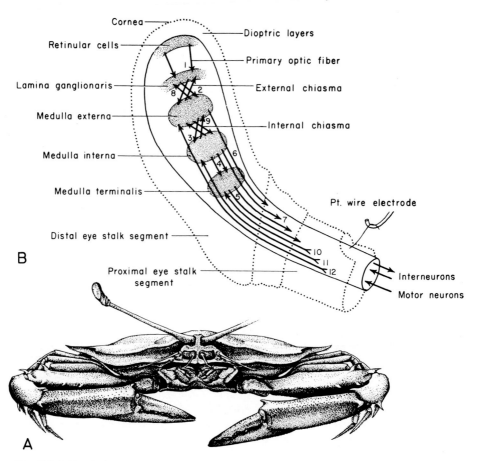

Fig. 65 A, B. Despite its extraordinarily long eyestalks, the swimming crab *Podophthalmus* **A** has its typical decapod visual processing system located close to the primary photoreceptive layer **B**. Only afferent primary fibers (1) occur between retina and lamina ganglionaris, but efferent interneurons (8–12) occur at many other levels, in addition to a variety of afferent interneurons (2–7). No attempt has been made to indicate horizontal interneurons well known to occur at various levels. (WATERMAN et al., 1964)

Presumptive evidence for polarization sensitivity occurs in the terminal patterns of R 1–R 7 in *Pacifastacus* (NÄSSEL and WATERMAN, 1977). Golgi-electron microscopic studies demonstrate that four of the regular retinular cells terminate on M 3 and the other three on M 4 (Fig. 66). It remains to be shown whether or not the grouping of retinular cell terminals corresponds with the two orthogonal microvillus sets [i.e., R 2, R 3, R 6, and R 7 vertical and R 1, R 4, and R 5 horizontal, as proposed in an earlier model (WATERMAN, 1966b)].

All of R 1–R 7 form another set of synaptic terminals with M 2 and, since all of the retinular cell terminals in the lamina ganglionaris appear to be triadic, there is one unidentified postsynaptic profile in each terminal on all three monopolar cells (Fig. 67). There is yet no clear suggestion how the wavelength discriminating information is handled at this level (NOSAKI, 1969; WATERMAN and FERNÁNDEZ, 1970).

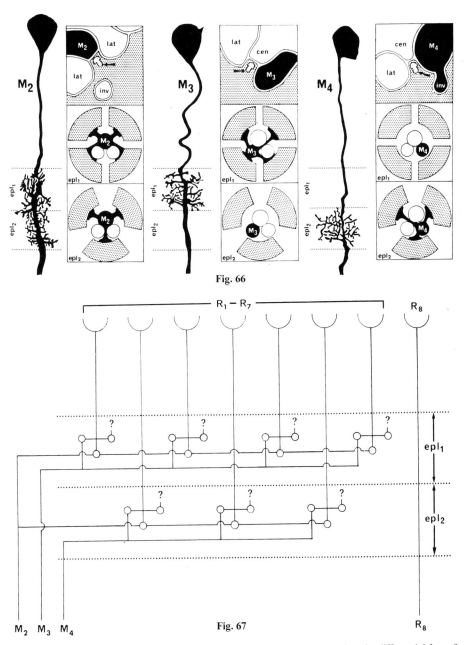

Fig. 66

Fig. 67

Figs. 66 and 67. Connectivity of crayfish retinular cells, possibly demonstrating the differential fate of the horizontal and vertical *e*-vector sensitive channels identified in the retina (NÄSSEL and WATERMAN, 1977). **Fig. 66.** Golgi-EM preparations demonstrate that R 1–R 7 make synaptic contact in neuroommatidia (cartridges) of the lamina ganglionaris with three types of monopolar interneurons. All seven synapse with M 2; only four of them synapse with M 3 in epl₁; the remaining three synapse with M 4 in epl₂. **Fig. 67.** Diagram summarizing these connections (Fig. 66) for one retinula. Since all terminals seem to be triadic (two lateral and one central), there is one unidentified connection for each R 1–R 7.

Note the quite different relations of R 8 which terminates in the next proximal optic ganglion

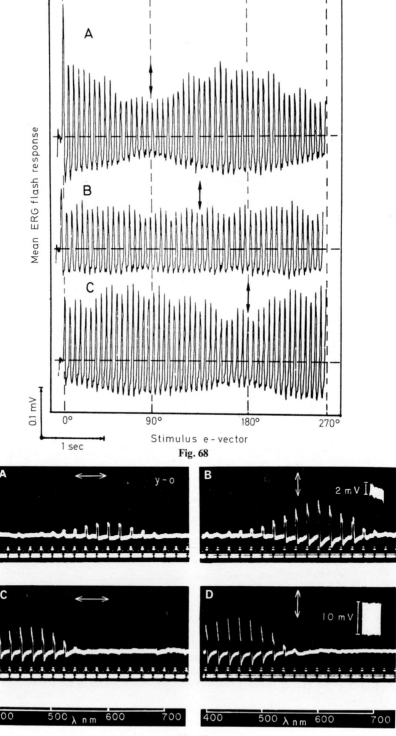

Fig. 68

Fig. 69

e) Electrophysiology

As mentioned above, electrophysiological evidence for post retinal polarization sensitivity was sought in the mid 1950s, and later, by WIERSMA and me (reviewed in WATERMAN, 1977). Recording from the optic nerve of *Panulirus, Grapsus, Podophthalmus*, and other decapods, no convincing evidence of *e*-vector discrimination was found, even though this research demonstrated a wide range of other types of visual interneurons (YORK and WIERSMA, 1975), as well as the prevalence of afferent signals in the optic nerve, including those from the contralateral eye (WIERSMA et al., 1964; BUSH et al., 1964). It remained for YAMAGUCHI (1967) to discover in *Procambarus* that differential responses could be regularly obtained in higher order fibers if the stimulus *e*-vector was rotating at some minimum angular velocity or faster.

These experiments proved that the differential response did not result from reflection–refraction artifacts by showing that polarization sensitivity was not dependent on the angle of stimulus incidence onto the cornea. Also, rotating the eye correspondingly displaced the angular locations of maximum and minimum responses to a fixed stimulus *e*-vector.

α) *Optic Nerve Spikes.* Sustaining fibers in the optic nerve (i.e., those having large visual fields) respond with maximum spike frequency at 0° and 90°, relative to the vertical and minimum rates at 45° and 135°. The interneuron response, therefore, has twice the angular frequency of the response in the photoreceptors themselves, as cited above, but the peaks correspond with the directions of the two orthogonal receptor channels demonstrated on several levels. Indeed, selective adaptation proved that the sustaining fibers in question do transmit input from both polarization sensitive receptor channels.

Thus, adapting the eye to vertical *e*-vector selectively suppressed the interneuron response peaks for *e*-vectors at 0° and 180°. Similarly, horizontal receptor adaptation suppressed the peaks at 90° and 270°. In both cases, the other orthogonal set of peaks was unaffected or not much suppressed by the selective adapting stimulus. With 45° or 135° adaptation, no selective suppression of the four peaks in sustaining fibers occurred.

Here, the behavior of the receptor components was closely similar to that demonstrated at the ERG level (Fig. 68) in *Cardisoma* (WATERMAN and HORCH, 1966) and directly at the retinular cell level (Fig. 69) in *Procambarus* (WATERMAN and FERNÁNDEZ, 1970). In contrast to most insect data, both violet and yellow retinular

---

◄ **Figs. 68 and 69.** Electrical evidence confirming the occurrence of two, and only two, *e*-vector sensitive channels in decapod crustacean eyes. **Fig. 68.** Selective adaptation of the ERG in the giant land crab *Cardisoma* demonstrates specific vertical and horizontal dichroic systems. Polarized test flashes showed that, with a horizontally polarized adapting light (double arrow at 90°), response amplitude was minimum in that direction and maximum vertically **A**. Relations were reversed with the adapting light vertical (180°) **C**. No significant amplitude modulation occurred with the adapting light at 45° (equidistant from both channels) **B** (WATERMAN and HORCH, 1966). **Fig. 69.** Intracellular recordings of retinular cell responses to equal quantum flashes of vertical and horizontal polarized light scanned at 20 nm intervals from 400 nm to 740 nm with a flash rate of 30 per min. Receptor units of quite different λ_{max} (440 and 590 nm) were confirmed and both shown to have good polarization sensitivity with either horizontal or vertical preferential responses. (WATERMAN and FERNÁNDEZ, 1970)

cells of the crayfish have substantial S_e's, with the mean greater for the more numerous longer wavelength units (WATERMAN and FERNÁNDEZ, 1970).

Note that the absorption of plane polarized light by the dichroic rhabdomeres in the two orthogonal sets present should roughly follow $\sin^2\theta$ and $\cos^2\theta$ functions. If so, as discussed in relation to R 8, their optical sum would obviously be isotropic; yet, if there is a power function or logarithmic relation between stimulus intensity and receptor potentials, as well as higher level responses, the physiological sum would not be.

Actually, the experimental results directly prove that the physiological addition of these two input channels is clearly polarization sensitive, with maxima both perpendicular and parallel to the stimulus e-vector. We know that the axons recorded have large receptive fields, but we do not yet know, beyond the receptor terminal connectivities reviewed above for the lamina ganglionaris how selective or inclusive their input is with regard to R 1–R 8.

An additional important point was reported by YAMAGUCHI (1967); namely, that dimming fibers in the crayfish optic nerve, which increase their firing rate in response to reduction in light intensity (YORK and WIERSMA, 1975), also show polarization sensitivity, but the peaks (i.e., 45°, 135°) and valleys (i.e., 0°, 90°) of their spike frequencies are shifted 45° compared to the sustaining fibers. No polarization sensitivity, to either stationary or rotating e-vectors, was found in on–off or movement fibers of the optic nerve. Since those findings were presented in Japanese, in a brief abstract only, their interest and potential significance have not yet been widely appreciated.

A fuller account, cited as in preparation in YAMAGUCHI et al. (1976), has not yet been published, but closely similar results have been reported in some detail for the stomatopod *Oratosquilla* (YAMAGUCHI et al., 1976) and in an independent experimental study on the Indo-West Pacific portunid crab *Scylla* (LEGGETT, 1976, 1978).

It is perhaps surprising that *Oratosquilla*, which is quite distinct from a decapod in much of its general morphology (WATERMAN and CHACE, 1960), should not differ significantly from *Procambarus* in the polarization sensitivity of its optic nerve fibers so far studied (YAMAGUCHI, personal communication). The close fine structural similarity of R 8 in some members of the two groups has already been reviewed above. In this stomatopod, only the sustaining fibers have been studied, so that the striking phase shift in the dimming fibers of decapods remains to be found in this suborder.

Interestingly enough, the vertical and horizontal polarization sensitivity channels do not appear to be functionally symmetrical. In both *Procambarus* and *Oratosquilla*, the spike response to vertical e-vector and the selective adaptation to this plane of polarization appeared to be stronger than the horizontal. However, current experiments (YAMAGUCHI and WATERMAN, unpublished) suggest that this asymmetry shifts from one channel to the other with the direction of e-vector rotation.

β) *Medulla Externa Responses*. The results in *Scylla* (LEGGETT, 1976) were obtained by extracellular recording in the crab's medulla externa and, hence, considerably more peripheral in the visual system from those reported by YAMAGUCHI in the optic nerve (Fig. 65 B for locations). Two types of unit were found in the crab; one was somewhat similar to the sustaining fibers in *Procambarus* and *Oratosquilla*. It responded to a rotating *e*-vector with a $\cos^2\theta$ function with peaks at $0°$ and $90°$, but only for one direction of rotation. In the opposite direction, a substantial decrease in spike rate was reported when *e*-vector rotation began, but no frequency modulation occurred with ongoing $d\phi/dt$. This kind of unit is perhaps reminiscent of the evidence that pigeons can discriminate rotating from nonrotating *e*-vector (KREITHEN and KEETON, 1974). However, further experiments (discussed below) have shown that pigeons can also specifically learn to discriminate stationary *e*-vector directions of an overhead light (DELIUS et al., 1976).

The second type of *Scylla* polarization sensitive medullary unit responded only with a ϕ insensitive increased firing rate in both directions of rotation. It showed neither discrimination of the sign of $d\phi/dt$ nor of ϕ itself, since no response frequency modulation resulted from $d\phi/dt$. In contrast, sustaining fibers in crayfish and stomatopods have not yet been found specifically sensitive to direction of rotation nor steadily responsive to a rotating *e*-vector independent of ϕ (YAMAGUCHI et al., 1976).

Clearly, discovery of several types of polarization sensitive elements in the visual interneurons of decapods and stomatopods is encouraging since we have long known that the corresponding behavior and retinal detecting mechanism are present. It is not yet clear, however, whether or not the elements now known are a fair sample of those actually determining polarization sensitivity at the behavioral level. Probably, the information most desirable in new experiments would be specific outputs of M 2–M 4 in lamina ganglionaris and the signal brought directly to medulla externa by R 8. In view of the demonstrated need for a rotating *e*-vector to evoke differential responses in optic nerve axons, recall that many animals, including arthropods, respond behaviorally only to detected changes in stimulus parameters; when the latter are stable, there is no orientation response (e.g., REICHARDT and POGGIO, 1976).

From an anthropomorphic point of view, the sorting out of λ and polarized light inputs would seem to be an important function of the processing system. Yet, we so far have no clue how or even whether or not it is, in fact, done. Previous experiments have shown that both the violet and yellow receptor channels also appear to be added together in the spike responses of crayfish higher order sustaining fibers (TREVIÑO and LARIMER, 1970; WOODCOCK and GOLDSMITH, 1970). However, the likelihood that the primary interneuronal channels have not yet been effectively sampled is not negligible in view of the rather rough and ready recording techniques which have been used and the compact complexity of the decapod optic tract (Fig. 65).

γ) Correlation with Orientation. While the electrophysiological results obtained so far seem quite incomplete, they do offer a number of suggestive correlations with data of other kinds. For example, *e*-vector sensitive spike frequency maxima in crayfish optic nerve fibers provide response peaks which coincide with basitactic behavioral responses (i.e., at $0°$, $45°$, $90°$, and $135°$ to the plane of polarization of a vertical light beam) in a variety of decapods and other animals (cited above). Clearly, such underlying multiple reference directions derived from a polarization pattern need to be replaced by an unambiguous menotactic compass direction for use in most biological applications.

Now, the mechanism of deriving a menotaxis from a basitaxis could be similar for polarotaxis to that required for course steering in a phototaxis, or even geotaxis. At least under certain laboratory conditions, two or four ambiguities may appear in geotactic and phototactic responses. The inherent ambiguity in 180° of plane polarized light doubles the problem for this submodality so that there can be eight preferred directions basically indicated by the detector analyzer system. Very little is known about this situation, although it has been widely discussed at the receptor level with regard to the necessary number of polarization sensitive input channels (e.g., MOODY and PARRIS, 1961; WATERMAN, 1966c, d, 1974a, 1975c; KIRSCHFELD, 1972; BERNARD and WEHNER, 1977; VAN DER GLAS, 1977; see discussion below).

Another interesting point emerges from the YAMAGUCHI and LEGGETT findings; namely, does the sensory stimulation specifically evoked by a moving e-vector play a role in the spatial stability of the animal concerned? LEGGETT (1976) does suggest (following LAUGHLIN, 1976b) that compensatory reflex orientation might be triggered by apparent e-vector rotation resulting from angular displacement of the animal. Particularly in a flying or swimming animal, its surround is typically between 50% and 100% occupied by a natural polarization pattern which is itself perfectly stable on a short time scale (Sect. B above).

Hence, it could provide good visual information on positional displacement under conditions when the habitat is otherwise devoid of appropriate orientation clues. We know that gravity is widely used by decapod crustaceans for such an orientation cue (SCHÖNE, 1975), but we also know that it is typically backed up by at least one visually dependent system. For the case in question, this could be mediated by the rotation detecting polarization sensitivity system[6]. Both the sensory and behavioral aspects of this hypothesis need further study. Since many normal functions depend on a maintained stable relation between the animal's coordinate system and that of its environment, this situation could be an important control mechanism.

f) Summaty for Decapods

Our current understanding of polarization sensitivity in crayfish and other decapods can be summarized as follows. Intraocular dichroic analyzers are present in the rhabdoms of their compound eyes. Both light sensitivity and dichroism of the photoreceptor membrane are dependent on the visual pigment rhodopsin. Despite the wide adaptive radiation of this, by far the largest, order of Crustacea [i.e., decapods comprise about one-third of the ca. 26,000 total species in the class (WATERMAN and CHACE, 1960)], the detailed structure of the compound eye seems remarkably uniform.

Thus, the banded rhabdom with orthogonal microvilli in two alternating sets arising from three and four regular retinular cells, respectively, is almost universal in those decapods studied, whether or not their compound eyes are apposition or

---

[6] Our *Daphnia* experiments (cited above), demonstrating behavioral interactions between gravity responses and polarotaxis to horizontal beams of polarized light, provide a highly relevant example

superposition. As far as known, the rhabdomal microvilli are all orthogonal to the optic axis of their ommatidium and all those in a single rhabdomere are nearly always parallel to one another; the *Panulirus* proximal rhabdom is a marked exception (EGUCHI and WATERMAN, 1966). Also, the alignment of these two microvillus directions, as well as the corresponding directions of maximum light absorption, is consistently just parallel to the vertical and horizontal axes of the animal's body in its normal attitude in space. The apparently universal R 8 in each retinula has microvilli either just parallel to the horizontal set in the regular rhabdom (e.g., the crayfish) or both perpendicular and parallel to it (e.g., crabs and the spiny lobster).

Overall, at least the central area of the eye provides a two channel polarization sensitive input to its polarimeter. Although the detailed processing mechanism is not yet known, this input, perhaps aided by other nonpolarization sensitive–specific inputs, permits both basitactic and menotactic orientation to be derived from the polarization plane of the light stimulus. The specific roles of R 8 and the comparative mechanism of processing both polarization and other visual parameters, especially color, remain important desiderata.

3. *Apis* and Other Bees (Apidae)

Bees, like ants (Sect. C.I.4. below), are capable of visually mediated vector orientation in which the location of their nest or sources of food are determined and remembered in a polar coordinate system characterized basically by range and azimuth (JANDER, 1963b). While landmarks may contribute importantly to such visual orientation, the celestial cues provided by sky polarization and the sun directly are crucial. Because of this and VON FRISCH's fundamental experiments and analysis, the honeybee has been and continues to be the central type in the study of polarization sensitivity. There is evidence, however, that basically similar sensory and behavioral responses also are present in a number of other kinds of bees (JACOBS-JESSEN, 1959; WELLINGTON, 1974a).

a) Oriented Behavior

α) *Original Field Discovery by* VON FRISCH *(Figs. 70–72)*. To begin with, this insect provides one of the few cases where the adaptive importance of its polarization sensitivity has been clear from the very beginning (VON FRISCH, 1948, 1949; reviews, 1965, pp. 384–443, 1967, 1974). Also, as one of the biologically most studied organisms, *Apis* provides an unusually sophisticated level of knowledge to use in understanding its polarization sensitivity. Despite this, surprising new discoveries have been made in the last few years (e.g., the importance of R 9 in polarization sensitivity and the elaborate longitudinal twistings of R 1–R 8 in most of the retina). Indeed, much remains to be learned about the perception of polarized light and the way in which its natural patterns are put to adaptive use.

In his rather incredible initial experiments, VON FRISCH showed that a $10°–15°$ spot of blue sky sufficed to permit a dancing worker bee to indicate correctly the azimuth of its feeding place. This was proved in an observation hive with a horizontal comb surface screened off from all view of the environment except for the small patch of sky, initially north, visible through a length of stove pipe. If clouds

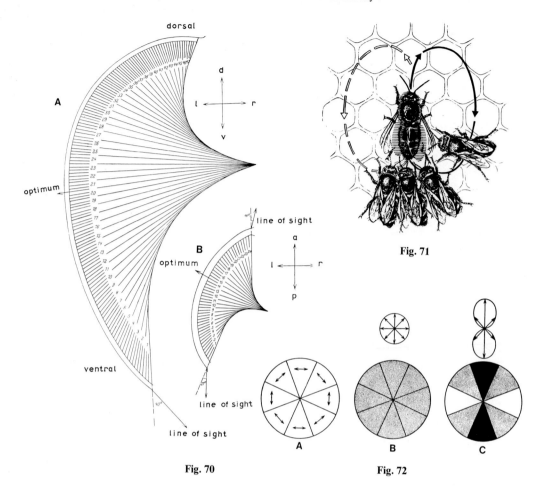

Fig. 70

Fig. 71

Fig. 72

Figs. 70–72. Classic components of polarization sensitivity in the honeybee worker. **Fig. 70.** Basic pattern of the compound eye showing idealized ommatidial pattern in vertical transverse **A** and horizontal longitudinal **B** sections of the left eye through the region of minimum separation of optic axes (indicated by arrows labeled "optimum" 10° down from horizontal, 60° forward of lateral). Orientation of sections shown by crosses. The 5,500 ommatidia are arranged in hexagonal packing on a convex elliptical surface with markedly astigmatic cornea and divergence angles. As shown, ommatidial axes, perpendicular to·the corneal surface in the central retina, deviate markedly from that orientation anteriorly, posteriorly, and particularly ventrally, with the resultant line of sight divergences shown. In the proximal areas, the boundary of every third ommatidium is projected, and numbered. In **A**, each ommatidium shown belongs to one of the 145 horizontal rows (z-rows) present in the long dorsoventral axis (BAUMGÄRTNER, 1928). **Fig. 71.** Most *Apis* behavioral data on polarization sensitivity involves the classic waggle dance performed on either a vertical or horizontal comb surface. The direction indicated is determined by the relation between a natural or imposed *e*-vector pattern and the direction of the food source being communicated to other workers (VON FRISCH, 1965). **Fig. 72.** Early model of *e*-vector sensitivity proposed for the bee ommatidium. Each of the eight regular retinular cells was hypothesized to be dichroic with its major absorptance tangential **A**. Such an assemblage obviously would respond unselectively to unpolarized light **B** and selectively (parallel to the *e*-vector) in partially linearly polarized light (e.g., blue sky) **C** (AUTRUM and STUMPF, 1950). This Sternfolie model was repeatedly used by VON FRISCH also (1950 and later)

passed over the sky area in question, the bees' orientation was lost and regained pari passu. If the visible sky patch was selected close to the sun where p approaches 0%, the oriented response also disappeared. Disoriented or misoriented dances resulted when the pipe aperture was covered.

In addition, displacement with a mirror of the sky area actually visible through the pipe correspondingly shifted the direction-indicating phase of the dance. Hence, the vectorial information was not inherent in the apparent location of the sky seen. In fact, the critical parameter of blue sky light proved to be its plane of polarization. Thus, placing a polarizer over the horizontal comb demonstrated that when its major transverse axis was parallel to the natural sky polarization in that line of sight, normal orientation was maintained. Yet, systematic displacements of the bees' directional behavior were evoked by certain orientations of the imposed e-vector (VON FRISCH, 1949).

β) *Challenges to* VON FRISCH's *Conclusions.* While one might expect to file these brilliant results with a comment that "the rest is history," such is not the case. As mentioned above, there was considerable argument in the late 1950s (KALMUS, 1958; DE VRIES and KUIPER, 1958; SMITH and BAYLOR, 1960) that VON FRISCH's supposed polarization sensitivity was merely a response to light intensity patterns external to the animal and dependent on differential refraction and reflection. Indeed, there always is a danger that such artifacts may fool the experimenter, but VON FRISCH presented a detailed rebuttal of the relevance of such arguments (VON FRISCH et al., 1960; VON FRISCH, 1965, p. 416 ff.). Much subsequent work has supported the reality of a true polarization sensitivity in the honeybee.

In addition, protracted challenges, largely by WENNER and his collaborators (WENNER, 1971), to the underlying experimental method VON FRISCH employed to study bees' visual orientation stirred up a lot of controversy. This, for a time, seemed to threaten the whole dance language hypothesis of bee communication. By implication, it cast something of a shadow on the significance of polarization sensitivity in the bee. Like the polarization "artifact" problem cited above, this basic criticism of methodology stimulated a beneficial, more critical quantitative, approach to experiments in the field, but left essentially intact the important basic discoveries (GOULD, 1976). It also made clear that, as in the realm of polarization sensitivity, so in the partly overlapping one of bee communication, much remains to be done.

An inherent handicap in studying e-vector orientation in the honeybee is the difficulty or impossibility of observing the actual course flown. Its readily observed behavior in the hive has of course been crucial, as has the arrival of marked individuals at feeding places, but the flight behavior between these end points has generally not been accessible to experimental analysis. In this regard, the desert ant *Cataglyphis* (discussed below) has proved to be an important species where this desideratum can be directly studied.

Beyond his initial discoveries, VON FRISCH contributed considerably more, both in further field experiments and modeling possible mechanisms of polarization sensitivity in the bee compound eye. For instance, he remarks (1965, p. 397) that periodic oscillations observed around the flight direction in bees orienting by sky polarized light could be necessary for their polarized light analysis. Detailed references to the original reports, quoted without further credits, are in VON FRISCH (1965).

γ) *Transposition to Geotaxis.* Another point of interest is related to the fact that normally dancing bees indicate the direction of a food source while performing on a vertical comb surface in a dark hive. The sun's bearing is transposed to a vertical $0°$ reference relative to which the goal direction is danced. No visual cue is required during such a normal dance. When bees dance on a horizontal comb, however, visual directional information is required for oriented dances, usually the sun or some polarized sky.

When performing on a vertical comb in the dark hive, minor errors occur in the angular transposition. These vary with time of day and have turned out to be relevant to the bee's sensitivity to the earth's magnetic field (LINDAUER and MARTIN, 1968). Similar small mistakes appear if the bee is dancing vertically in an open hive from which it can see only a uniformly cloud covered sky. However, when some blue sky appears between clouds, large errors (i.e., to $40°$) are made in the transposed angle.

Historically, this was another early indication of the bee's capacity to use blue sky for orientation. The explanation of such errors lies in their being a compromise angle between the sun's bearing, detected on the outward flight from the hive, and the supposed sun's bearing, estimated from the sky polarization. The latter is detected by the same dorsally directed ommatidia, but they look at a quite different area of sky when the bee is dancing on a vertical surface than when it is flying back to the hive. The interaction between the two orienting modes has been shown to be complex and depend on some, as yet, unidentified effect of the polarization pattern (EDRICH, 1977).

δ) *Problem of Deducing Sun's Bearing.* Using an octagonal analyzer comprising eight Polaroid triangles with their major absorption axes tangential to the assemblage (Fig. 72), VON FRISCH (1950) could correlate the bee dance directions with the currently observable sky polarization patterns. Most striking, perhaps, was the report that when there were, in fact, two areas visible in the sky with the same e-vector orientation, two ambiguous azimuths were danced; however, BRINES (1978) has recently obtained different results. Actually, since VON FRISCH's main research was done, the broader problem has been recognized that the sun's bearing, which the bee must know for its dance orientation, cannot be determined solely from the e-vector orientation at a given point in the sky (e.g., KIRSCHFELD et al., 1975; VAN DER GLAS, 1978).

Other information is therefore necessary if the bee dance is to be oriented at the required angle to the sun's azimuth when only a small patch of blue sky is available. For instance, if the animal knows the sun's altitude at that time, the observed e-vector orientation at a given θ_p would yield the sun's azimuth unambiguously only in a limiting case. In general, two alternative azimuths would be possible. Discrimination between these additional cues would still be needed. Obviously, further research is needed to learn how the bees actually do this.

ε) *Sky Area Required.* Field experiments by VON FRISCH and LINDAUER (1954), with the sun hidden by a nearby mountain ridge, confirmed the bees' ability to learn directions to a feeding place from the overhead polarization. In this case, of course, a very large area of sky was visible to the bees. First while flying in the shadow of the ridge they were trained to go to one of a set of four feeding sites set out at 90° angles from the hive. Then on the next day in another, but unfamiliar location with a flat terrain and at a different time of day, 9 of 11 bees which succesfully located a feeding place chose the one in the same compass direction from the transposed hive as the learned direction.

In a replication with a second hive of bees trained in the original mountain shadowed place and subsequently tested in still another unfamiliar location, 9 of 16 bees, which went to the four orthogonal feeding places, chose the trained direction. Note that although the n's are small, the observed behavior indicates that changes in sky polarization pattern can be reckoned with by the bee, just as can changes in the sun's position during the day (VON FRISCH, 1950). Therefore, VON FRISCH and LINDAUER (1954) concluded that bees are capable of using time compensated sky polarization as a compass.

Experiments using a screen and mirror to transpose the apparent position of the sun showed that large areas of sky had to be visible to the bee for its polarization to compete effectively with the sun itself when both were seen. Moreover, the relative orienting importance of sun and sky varied with time of day. Thus, the polarized light had a stronger influence in the early morning and late afternoon when the sun's orienting effect was maximum nearest the zenith.

These results of VON FRISCH are consistent with the important observations of WELLINGTON (1974a) that mosquitoes and other insects show conspicuous long ranging polarotaxis in the field only when the zenith angle of the sun is greater than 30°. This he interprets as evidence that strong zenith polarization is required for the sky dependent but direct sun independent oriented behavior in question.

Note that although large clear sky areas were required in the mirror and screen experiments for strong e-vector orientation, the early data had proved (VON FRISCH, 1948, 1949) that only a 10°–15° patch of blue sky was enough to orient waggle dances. This order of magnitude has been confirmed more recently by experiments showing this to be approximately the minimal field necessary for oriented dances to sky light, at 90° to the sun where $p = 30\%$–40% and $\lambda_{max} = 460$ nm. This 10°–15° stimulus was estimated to illuminate 25–50 ommatidia in the dorsal part of the retina (ZOLOTOV and FRANTSEVICH, 1973). For nearly perfect orientation, a 60°–80° area subtending 150–200 units was determined experimentally to be necessary. As in VON FRISCH's data where a threshold of $p = 11\%$ $\pm 4\%$ was found, $p = 15\%$ or more was quite adequate to induce good responses in this later research. Only minor improvement in oriented behavior resulted using $p > 15\%$, as also reported earlier by VON FRISCH.

The result of dividing an effective area of sky into four subthreshold areas and separating them to various degrees was also tested (ZOLOTOV and FRANTSEVICH, 1973). The data suggested that the effective summating area for this kind of polarization sensitivity was about 200 ommatidia. However, much smaller minimum effective stimulus angles were reported for an artificial light source in the zenith with $p = 100\%$ (EDRICH and VON HELVERSEN, 1976).

ζ) *Comparison with Laboratory Data.* In the latter experiments, dancing bees, illuminated on a horizontal comb by a controlled overhead light, were found in high intensity white light to orient well to very restricted stimuli (i.e., 0.5° in diameter) significantly smaller than the acceptance angle of one ommatidium (i.e., half

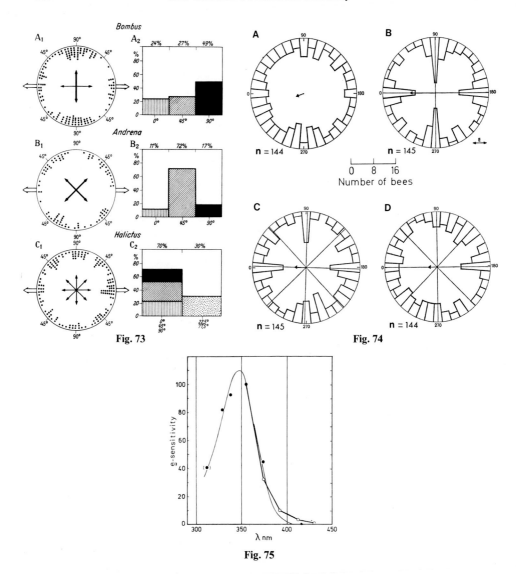

Fig. 73

Fig. 74

Fig. 75

Figs. 73–75. Polarotaxis in bees. **Fig. 73.** Spontaneous walking direction of three genera of bees in a vertical beam of linearly polarized light with the *e*-vector direction indicated by the open arrows outside the circles. Each data point in A 1, B 1, and C 1 indicates the orientation of an experimental animal. Percentage distribution in major angular groups plotted in A 2, B 2, and C 2. Under prevailing laboratory conditions, the basitactic preference of *Bombus* was normal to the *e*-vector, *Andrena's* was ±45° oblique to the *e*-vector and *Halictus'* was 0°, ±45°, and 90° relative to *e* (Jacobs-Jessen, 1959). **Fig. 74.** Multiple peaked walking responses obtained with *Apis* workers, also in a vertical beam of linearly polarized light of various spectral compositions. Observations in 10° angular groups are plotted radially within circles, with the full radius scaled to 18 data points. *E*-vector at 0°–180°. **A** Control in unpolarized white light (incandescent bulb). **B** Same, but linearly polarized. Appropriate statistics for such a circular distribution (Batschelet, 1965) show that four parallel and perpendicular peaks are highly significant (p < 0.0001). **C** Polarized blue–green light (broad band filters plus cutoff used). **D** Purple light. Both **C** and **D** evoked oblique (±45°), as well as parallel and perpendicular basitaxes. For **C**, p < 0.005; for **D**, p < 0.05. The author concludes that such polarotaxes would not occur if polarization sensitivity

width 3.2°). It was estimated that such a small patch would illuminate 3–7 contiguous ommatidia in the dorsal part of the compound eye, but no explanation was given for the marked difference between this minimum angle and ones estimated earlier from field data.

Combining the normal head position of a dancing bee with antidromic illumination, these dorsal ommatidia were found to be specifically located in a retinal area with a normal R 1–R 8 + R 9 retinular pattern, rather than the special R 1–R 9 configuration which occurs in an adjacent, more dorsal, area (WEHNER et al., 1975). It had previously been shown by VON FRISCH (1965, p. 418) that the lateral and ventral parts of the bee's eye were not essential for dance orientation to the blue sky, but that a dorsal sector certainly was.

While appropriate laboratory experiments have rarely been done, the honeybee and other Apidae, under certain conditions, clearly show multiple peak orientation to the e-vector like many other polarization sensitive animals. Apparently species' specific patterns (Fig. 73) were reported for several bee genera (JACOBS-JESSEN, 1959), but such behavior may be altered by experimental circumstances (JANDER, 1963 a). More recently, VAN DER GLAS (1975) has found different basitactic patterns in walking Apis workers dependent on wavelength of the overhead polarized light (Fig. 74). In Daphnia polarotaxis, both light intensity and its angular distribution have comparable effects, as cited above (Sect. C.I.1.).

η) *Dependence on* λ. Obviously, the minimum number of ommatidia required for polarization sensitivity in the bee dances is an important diagnostic cue for determining the perceptive mechanism involved. The mechanism's wavelength specificity is another such clue on which data have also been accumulating. First, VON FRISCH (reviewed in 1965) found that only near ultraviolet or blue light was required for polarization sensitive orientation and that longer λ's are not used. Later, an action spectrum (Fig. 75) was obtained for polarized light oriented bee dances (VON HELVERSEN and EDRICH, 1974); this was possible since the degree of orientation was found to be strongly dependent on intensity of the polarized light. The resulting sensitivity data peaked sharply at 355 nm and fell to nearly 0 at 430 nm (Fig. 75). Field evidence for the ant *Cataglyphis* indicates that the λ_{max} of its sky orientation peaks below 410 nm, but a full sensitivity curve is not yet available (DUELLI and WEHNER, 1973). Recall, in contrast, that the polarization sensitivity curve for *Daphnia* had its maximum at 440 nm, as mentioned above.

ϑ) VAN DER GLAS *Experiments*. Recently VAN DER GLAS (1975, 1976, 1977 a, 1978) has carried out extensive experiments on the bee in an effort to improve our

---

◄ is dependent only on the R 9 ultraviolet photoreceptor channel (VAN DER GLAS, 1975). **Fig. 75.** Wavelength dependence of polarization sensitivity obtained with worker bees dancing in the laboratory under imposed overhead polarization subtending a 17° conical angle. Scatter in danced directions was used to estimate S_e from orientation at various wavelengths and intensities. The strong peak in S_e near 350 nm surely confirms the crucial role of ultraviolet in polarization sensitivity, but the authors argue it does not necessarily eliminate the possibility of other retinal cells than R 9 from contributing to this visual modality. Filled and open circles represent the behavioral data points with the maximum estimated S_e at 355 nm scaled at 100. The smooth curve peaking at slightly shorter wavelengths is the DARTNALL nomogram for a visual pigment with λ_{max} at 347 nm. (VON HELVERSEN and EDRICH, 1974)

understanding of the polarization sensitivity mechanism by analyzing the parameters of skylight which are perceived. Both spontaneous orientation of walking bees in an arena and dancing bees in the hive have been studied. His initial hypothesis was that in the worker bee, due to the distribution of polarization sensitivity and λ_{max} among the various retinular cells (discussed below), the sky polarization pattern is, in fact, perceived as a color pattern. Note that this does not imply that normal sky color patterns are responsible for observed "polarotaxis." Actually, there is evidence that this is not the case (van der Glas, 1977 b), even though it is also clear that sky areas can be discriminated by color (Brines, 1978).

If van der Glas' color hypothesis is valid, the color plate used by Menzel (1975 a) to dramatize the pattern of sky polarization, by assigning different colors to different e-vector orientations, would be more than a pedagogic demonstration, although the spectral variety perceivable by the bee would presumably be smaller than that used in this example. Actually, green, blue, and ultraviolet receptors are present in the bee retina but, as already pointed out above, green wavelengths and longer are ineffectual in evoking responses to polarized light initiated by the compound eye.

In one set of van der Glas' (1975) experiments, workers were released into the center of a transparent covered arena in which their directions of walking to the periphery were recorded as a function of the color and polarization of an overhead light. The most striking feature of the resulting orientation patterns was their dependence on λ (Fig. 74). The stimulating effectiveness of each stimulus condition was calculated from the transmission of the broad band and cutoff color filters used and the spectral sensitivities of the three receptor types reported to be present (Autrum and von Zwehl, 1964). Thus, with "yellow" polarized light, highly significant orientation peaks (i.e., $p < 0.01\%$) occurred at 3° and 183° (i.e., essentially parallel to the stimulus e-vector).

With unfiltered polarized light from the incandescent overhead source, four peaks were present (i.e., $p < 0.01\%$) that were perpendicular, as well as parallel, to the e-vector. This confirmed Jacob-Jessen's (1959) and Jander's (1963 a) interesting earlier observations. With "blue–green" and "purple" polarized light stimuli, eight peak responses were obtained; the additional ones oriented at 45° and 135° to the e-vector.

The different orientation patterns, found by van der Glas under various wavelength conditions, obviously cannot be dependent solely on a single channel retinular input. The postulated λ related mechanism might improve polarization sensitivity because other research on bees (Daumer, 1956) has shown that a 5% difference in the amount of ultraviolet mixed with white light is detectable by them, whereas brightness differences alone have thresholds of 10%–15% or more.

In a second set of experiments, van der Glas (1976) tested his color hypothesis on bees dancing on a horizontal comb under a tent-like cover with a 27° or 36° view of the zenith sky at its apex. The sun's zenith distance ranged from 39° to 74° in the various experiments. Note, however, that zenith sky appears to have distinct stimulating effects (Brines, 1978). As in von Frisch's data and the walking bees, most dances observed by van der Glas were disoriented in orange light. The same broad band and cutoff filters were used here as in the walking experiments. Significant ($p < 0.01\%$) polarotaxis occurred with yellow and blue–green filters, but the accuracy of orientation was considerably less than in controls having no color filters.

Similar results were obtained with neutral filters which lowered the excitation of all three receptor types. The latter results suggest that, in the color filter experiments, receptors strongly stimulated by longer wavelengths are masking R 9 responses evoked by some ultraviolet passing the yellow and blue–green filters. Other evidence for such masking has been found by BRINES (1978). In all these test series, including controls, two peaked orientation distributions were found by VAN DER GLAS, with the preferred directions at 180° to each other. This was attributed to the ambiguity of the zenith color pattern hypothesized to be the orientation clue.

Polarizers in diagonal quadrants were oriented in two configurations so that corresponding sky sectors were transmitted or extinguished, respectively, depending on whether or not they were centered in the sun's vertical or along the perpendicular great circle through the zenith. In the former, blue light was predominantly effective in orienting the dances, whereas ultraviolet was predominant in the perpendicular band. Overhead color sector patterns, alternating areas of blue–green and purple filters, showed that orientation, similar to that normal with sky polarization, could be evoked with unpolarized color patterns.

Light through the blue–green filter was believed to be an effective stimulus for blue receptors of the bee eye, but not for the ultraviolet ones. The purple filter was thought to affect both blue and ultraviolet receptors. However, with these crude sector patterns, dances were often unstable. Later experiments done with gradual, rather than abrupt transition between two color areas at short wavelengths (i.e., ultraviolet, bee purple), evoked nearly normal dances (VAN DER GLAS, 1977b, 1978).

Similar effects of half shade screening of the visual field were demonstrated both to the normal sky polarization pattern and the two-color simulation (VAN DER GLAS, 1976). In both cases, better orientation was observed when the edge of the half shade was perpendicular to the sun's vertical than when it was parallel to it. Thus, segments towards the sun and antisun are more important than the perpendicular ones between them. This apparently is consistent with BRINES' conclusion (1978) that orientation is best with horizontal e-vector. These experiments, like the ones on walking, were interpreted by VAN DER GLAS to indicate that blue wavelengths evoke significant polarization sensitivity. However, it is considerably weaker than that induced by ultraviolet.

1) Conclusions. These experimental data indicate that bee polarized light perception involves a color discrimination mechanism, rather than one unique for polarization sensitivity or one based on intensity discrimination. It remains to be seen how this explanation will fare when confronted with seeming contradictions from other experimental approaches. For instance, it would be difficult to account for the polarotactic effectiveness, cited above, of a 0.5° patch of polarized light much smaller than the acceptance angle for one ommatidium (EDRICH and VON HELVERSEN, 1976) if the orientation of a color pattern must be discriminated by a receptor mosaic. This apparent discrepancy is considered in VAN DER GLAS' thesis (1978, p. 65). A somewhat different and, probably, more general hypothesis for celestial menotaxis (also proposed by VAN DER GLAS, 1978, p. 45) is reviewed in Sect. D, below.

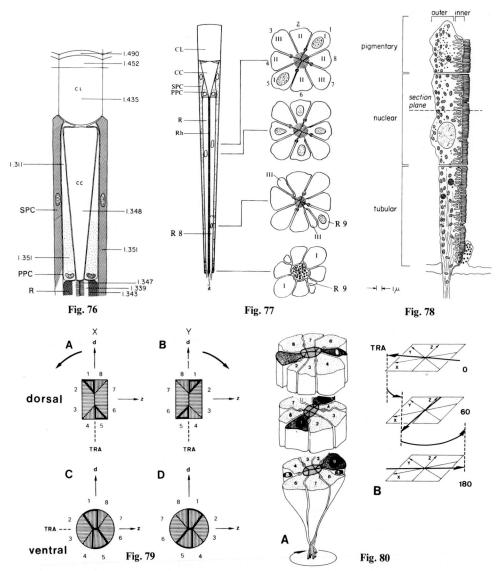

Figs. 76–80. Structure of the honeybee worker's ommatidium. *CC*, crystalline cone; *CL*, corneal lens; *PPC*, principal pigment cell; *R*, retinular cell; *Rh*, rhabdom; *SPC*, secondary pigment cell; *TRA*, transverse ommatidial axis. **Fig. 76.** Dioptric components, including measurements of refractive indices, of different regions of the cornea *(CL)*, crystalline cone *(CC)*, primary pigment cells *(PPC)*, secondary *(long)* pigment cells *(LPC)*, and various parts of the retinular cell *(R)*. (VARELA and WIITANEN, 1970). **Fig. 77.** Axial and selected transverse sections. The former (after PHILLIPS, 1905) shows the proximal location of R 9, while the latter indicate the author's terminology of the four (I–IV) diagonal pairs of regular retinular cells seen at different levels in a rhabdom shown as nontwisted. But see other terminology in Figs. 79 and 80, as well as the text (GRIBAKIN, 1975). **Fig. 78.** Axial view of single regular retinular cell showing relation of its lateral rhabdomere to other cell components. Note that the cell is only about 5 μm thick, but 200–300 μm long from CC tip to the basement membrane. As shown, the rhabdomere terminates and the retinular cell narrows to penetrate this layer as a primary optic axon. (VARELA and PORTER, 1969). **Fig. 79.** *X* and *Y* type rhabdoms from the worker bee retina. Upper row **A** and **B** from

b) Compound Eye Organization

To understand these behavioral results, the structure of the worker bee's eye and its probable mechanism of detecting and processing polarized light information must be reviewed. There are about 5,500 constituent ommatidia in the eye organized in a convex receptor surface and elliptical in outline. Along the major axis, the radius of curvature is about twice that along the minor axis, so the field of view (about $190° \times 145°$) is strongly astigmatic (Fig. 70). The facets are regularly arranged in a hexagonal packing pattern, with about 146 along the major axis and only 46 along the minor. At the point of least divergence along the former, the interommatidial angles are about $1°20'$ and, along the latter, about twice as great at $2°40'$ (DEL PORTILLO, 1936).

Each ommatidium, which is of the apposition type in the sense that its elongate rod-shaped rhabdom begins directly proximal to the crystalline cone, contains nine photoreceptor cells in its retinula (Figs. 76–80); however, most of the older standard descriptions cited eight, which is the number visible in any given cross section of most retinulas. On the basis of such an eight part receptor group in each ommatidium, VON FRISCH (1950) following the suggestion of AUTRUM, mentioned above, at first hypothesized that every retinula provided eight individual polarization sensitivity input channels, each with its maximum sensitivity axis perpendicular to the radial axis of the cell (Fig. 72).

As was demonstrated by his Polaroid "star sheet," such a model traversed by linear polarized light obviously would yield an intensity pattern symmetrical both around the pair of diagonal octants containing the *e*-vector (i.e., minimum transmission) and those perpendicular to it (i.e., maximum transmission) (Fig. 72). The other four pairs of octants would transmit at intermediate levels.

α) *Fine Structure.* Actually, when the microvillus pattern became known in the bee rhabdom (GOLDSMITH, 1962), R 1–R 8 were found to have only two orthogonal microvillus directions arranged in quadrants, each comprising two adjacent rhabdomeres with parallel microvilli (Fig. 77). Hence, a polarized light analyzer, based on their orientation and consequent dichroism, would presumably have two orthogonal channels, each with four synergistic cells (GOLDSMITH, 1962). This, of course, differs from the Sternfolie model. However, present evidence, as discussed below, suggests that the dichroism of R 1–R 8 has little, if any, direct effect on polarization sensitivity.

◀ dorsal half of eye, lower row **C** and **D** from ventral half. Note that the transverse axis *(TRA)*, defined by the plane in which microvilli of R 3 and R 7 (dorsal half) or R 1 and R 5 (ventral half) meet, coincides with the *z*-axis (horizontal rows) of the ommatidial pattern. This coincidence occurs at the distal tip of the rhabdom, but the axis will rotate proximal to that point with retinular twist, anticlockwise Type *X* (**A** and **C**); clockwise Type *Y* (**B** and **D**) indicated by the curved arrows (Fig. 80). *d* is dorsal. Retinular cell numbers correspond to those used in the text and have been revised by WEHNER to unify the terminology for bees and ants. **Fig. 80.** Diagram of single dorsal ommatidium (*X* type) in a worker bee eye. **A** Transverse section shows retinular pattern at three depths relative to the distal rhabdom tip, indicated in μm at the right. **B** Corresponding axial orientation demonstrates that TRA (arrow dorsal in orientation at 0 μm) has rotated 90° anticlockwise by 60 μm and 180° by 180 μm. The fixed axes (*x*, *y*, and *z*) of the ommatidial coordinates are shown for reference. More extensive bee data and a comparison with rhabdom twist in an ant are plotted in Fig. 81. (WEHNER, 1976 b)

Instead, R 9 (Fig. 77), previously known, at least as a nucleus, but largely ignored as "occasional" or "insignificant" (VON FRISCH, 1965, p. 433), has recently become a sharp focus of attention in this regard (PERRELET, 1970; GRUNDLER, 1971; GRIBAKIN, 1972, 1975; MENZEL and SNYDER, 1974; SKRZIPEK and SKRZIPEK, 1974; WEHNER et al., 1975). Actually, on theoretical grounds, SNYDER (1973) predicted that R 9 in the worker bee eye should have a lower absolute sensitivity than R 1–R 8, but a higher polarization sensitivity. Electrical recordings confirmed this (MENZEL and SNYDER, 1974) and, as discussed below, R 9 is currently believed to be the main, if not the sole, site of polarization sensitivity.

Structurally, the bee rhabdom as a whole (Fig. 78) is a fused unbanded cylindrical unit with its rhabdomeres continuous (i.e., not toothed as in decapods), and held in close contact by longitudinal desmosomes. It is only about 4 µm in diameter but 300 µm, or more in length (MENZEL and SNYDER, 1974). In general, the precise retinular cell and rhabdomere pattern differs between dorsal and ventral halves of the retina (GRUNDLER, 1974). Also, ommatidia of two mirror image patterns occur in each half (X and Y types described below), while a small marginal area of the dorsal half contains still another cell and rhabdomere arrangement. In addition, two types of R 9, one short and the other long, are present in different areas of the retina.

Note that, unfortunately, terminology and numbering of components in the bee retinula and optic cartridges are not, by any means, uniform (Figs. 77, 79, 80 and 82). Also, they have not been consistent with those used for ants. In an effort to standardize this for the hymenopteran retinula, WEHNER (1976 b, Table 1) has revised his bee cell numbers to match the pattern used for ants (MENZEL and SNYDER, 1974; MENZEL and BLAKERS, 1976), which we follow here in the text. Obviously, care is required in coping with the evolving terminology, as well as the inherently complex system itself!

β) Regular (Short R9) Ommatidia. Rhabdoms of retinulas with short R 9's comprise 99% of the worker bee's retina. They are characterized by having only eight rhabdomeres at all levels (Figs. 77, 79, and 80). In the distal 65%–75% of the retinula, these are contributed by R 1–R 8. The microvilli of R 1, R 4, R 5, and R 8 are predominantly vertical at the distal tip of the rhabdom, with R 1, R 5, and R 4, R 8 forming diagonal pairs of the same orientation or regrouped as R 1, R 8, and R 4, R 5 forming opposite vertical quadrants.

Similarly, the microvilli of R 2, R 3, R 6, and R 7 are approximately horizontal [i.e., parallel to the z-axis of the facet pattern and the horizontal axis of the bee's eye (WEHNER et al., 1975)]. Diagonal pairs and opposite quadrants with horizontal microvilli are roughly symmetrical with the vertical set. Note that although their orthogonal relation is maintained throughout the length of the rhabdom, the orientation of microvilli relative to body or eye axes changes continuously due to twisting.

In the proximal 25%–35% of the retinula, to which R 9 is restricted, it replaces either R 1 or R 5 in such a way that the distal end of the R 9 rhabdomere abuts on the proximal end of the R 1 or R 5 rhabdomere; at this juncture, their respective microvilli are parallel (Fig. 80). This detail could be important in determining the effect of filtering on polarization sensitivity of R 9 in optical series with R 1 or R 5

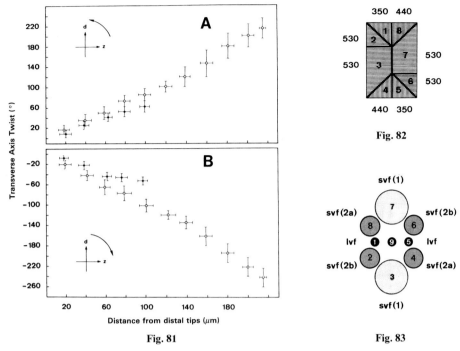

Fig. 81

Fig. 82

Fig. 83

Figs. 81–83. Further structural correlates of the worker bee ommatidium from dorsal half of compound eye. **Fig. 81.** Comparison of rhabdom twisting in X-type **A** and Y-type **B** units in *Apis* (open circles with $\pm$S.E. indicated) and in the ant *Myrmecia* (filled circles $\pm$S.E., data from MENZEL and BLAKERS, 1975). The horizontal *(z)* and dorsoventral *(d)* axes of the eye and the respective directions of twisting in the two types are also indicated. Note that transverse axis orientation *(TRA)* standardized at $0°$ (Figs. 79 and 80) is plotted on the ordinate. For samples of retinal orientation of retinular axes, see Figs. 84 and 85. (WEHNER, 1976b). **Figs. 82 and 83.** Correlation between retinular cell types and primary visual axons in a pseudocartridge of the lamina. (WEHNER, 1976b). **Fig. 82.** Rhabdom of an X-type ommatidium from the dorsal retina (distal cross section) identifying the pairs of diagonal cells with the same λ_{max} and microvillus directions. R 1–R 8 apparently lose most of their inherent dichroism because of the extensive twisting (Figs. 80 and 81), but the short R 9 (occurs proximally only) retains it (Figs. 86 and 87). **Fig. 83.** Nine primary axons from an ommatidium diagramed at the laminar cartridge level. R 2–R 4 and R 6–R 8 (short visual fibers, *svf*) terminate in the lamina, whereas R 1, R 5, and R 9 (long visual fibers, *lvf*) run through it to terminate in the medulla. All three long fibers have their λ_{max} in the ultraviolet but only R 9 has been found to have a high S_e (Fig. 87)

(SNYDER, 1973; GRIBAKIN, 1975). The idea that R 9 is the only effective polarization sensitive unit in the ommatidium was proposed by MENZEL and SNYDER (1974) and supported with some interesting experimental evidence.

At the level where it is displaced by R 9, R 1 or R 5 gives rise to its axon, which can be identified outside each retinula in proximal transverse sections. Ultimately, this axon joins those of R 5 or R 1 and R 9 (Fig. 83) as one of the three long visual axons which differ from the other six in terminating in the medulla externa (RIBI, 1975; SOMMER and WEHNER, 1975). This is reminiscent of the decapod crustacean pattern discussed above. There, R 8 terminates in the medulla terminalis, whereas R 1–R 7 terminate in the lamina ganglionaris, as do R 2–R 4 and R 6–R 8, in the worker bee's short R 9 ommatidia. Such distinctive receptor terminals for the long

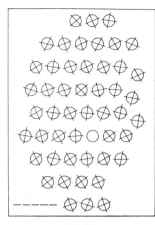

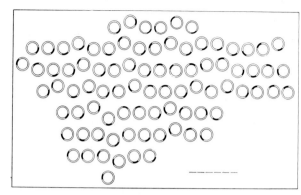

Fig. 84   Fig. 85

Figs. 84 and 85. Mapping of retinula orientation in z rows in central areas of the *Apis* retina (SKRZIPEK and SKRZIPEK, 1973). **Fig. 84.** Orientation of the rhabdom transverse axis (and the direction normal to it) (Fig. 79). **Fig. 85.** Location of R 9 shown by the dark sector of each annulus. Note that these short (40 μm) polarization sensitive ultraviolet receptors replace either R 1 or R 5 in a given retinula, as can be seen by comparing this map with Figs. 79 and 84. Data on R 9 microvillus orientation has also been mapped by MENZEL and SNYDER (1974)

visual cells of the bee obviously imply that they serve a particular function. As will become clear below, this is almost certainly correlated with the bees' polarization sensitivity and its ultraviolet perception.

It remains to describe the dramatic twisting of the rhabdom characteristic of all retinulas with short R 9's (GRUNDLER, 1974). All of them rotate either clockwise or anticlockwise (Fig. 81) at a rate of about 1° per μm (WEHNER et al., 1975). As a result, the long axes of microvilli in full length rhabdomeres rotate through about 180°, evenly distributed along their length; the shorter R 9 rhabdomere twists about 40°. Obviously, such marked departures from uniformly parallel microvilli for a given rhabdomere would be expected to decrease or, if extensive enough, completely cancel any effective dichroism in the rhabdomere of the corresponding retinular cell (McINTYRE and SNYDER, 1978). If, as is generally believed, these short R 9's mediate the animal's polarization sensitivity, how can they manage to do so?

Before trying to answer that one, however, a further aspect of the rhabdom twisting should be considered, namely that clockwise and anticlockwise rotation (WEHNER, 1976 b) occur with about equal frequency and in a random distribution in the dorsal retina, where it has been studied (WEHNER et al., 1975). Coupled with the direction of rhabdom twisting are the two mirror image patterns in which the retinular cells are assembled in the corresponding retinular types. In addition, the precise alignment of retinular cells in the retina shows considerable variation, as well as the two basic locations mentioned, for R 9 units (Figs. 84 and 85).

Thus, in the left eye of a worker bee, rhabdoms with an anticlockwise twist (i.e., Type X) have a cell pattern that reads clockwise as 1, 8, 7, 6, 5, 4, 3, and 2, but those with a clockwise twist (i.e., Type Y) have the clockwise sequence of cells 1, 2, 3, 4, 5, 6, 7, and 8 (GRUNDLER, 1974; MENZEL and SNYDER, 1974; SOMMER and

WEHNER, 1975; WEHNER et al., 1975). Obviously, such elaborate stereometry could have profound implications for the bee's polarization sensitivity. To explore these, we must examine the data on the polarization sensitivity of *Apis* worker's retinular cells and its possible correlation with oriented behavior (Sect. c. below).

γ) *Special (Long R9) Dorsal Ommatidia.* Long R9's occur only in about 60 ommatidia (i.e., about 1% of the retina) localized in the first four to five most dorsal *z*-rows of ommatidia (SCHINZ, 1975). In this special area, the fused rhabdomeres and their nine parent cells extend all the way from the crystalline cone tip to the basement membrane. Instead of the two orthogonal transverse microvillus directions present in the short R9 retinulas, there are apparently three or more. Furthermore, these special rhabdoms (i.e., *d*-type of WEHNER et al., 1975) are not twisted like those of most of the retina (GRUNDLER, 1974).

Hence, the microvilli of each rhabdomere are all parallel to one another, which should of itself provide strong *e*-vector discrimination. However, there is evidence that the polarization sensitivity expressed in the bee dance orientation is not limited to this very small marginal area. Indeed, it is centered in a different retinal region adjacent to it (EDRICH and VON HELVERSEN, 1976). Marginal retinulas with special structure are also known in eyes of many species of dipterans (WADA, 1974a; see below), but again their possible relations to orientation and polarization sensitivity are not known.

c) Retinal Receptor Types

Since the classic recordings of AUTRUM and VON ZWEHL (1964), three receptor types (i.e., green, blue, and ultraviolet) have generally been reported for the worker bee. Recent measurements of their λ_{max}'s yielded 540 nm, 440 nm, and 350 nm respectively (MENZEL and BLAKERS, 1976). To appreciate their possible correlation with the polarization sensitivity-related fine structural detail above, we need to know their location in the retina and their connections with secondary and higher order neurons.

The precise distribution of color receptor types has, until recently (GRIBAKIN, 1969, 1972), been somewhat uncertain. It was rather generally accepted, however, that all three were present in each retinula and diagonally opposite elements were of the same polarization sensitivity, as well as color type. Now, it seems there are two pairs of green receptors (i.e., R2, R6 and R3, R7), one pair of blue (i.e., R4, R8), and one pair of ultraviolet (i.e., R1, R5) units in the dorsal retina (reviewed by WEHNER, 1976b). The odd R9, which proximally pairs with R1 or R5, is a third ultraviolet receptor. In the ventral retina, blue receptors are absent (GRIBAKIN, 1969).

Why polarization sensitivity in the bee is so strongly coupled to receptors with a λ_{max} at 340 nm remains to be explained. We have already noted above that, on a power scale, blue sky polarization peaks at about 460 nm, far from the ultraviolet and certainly quite remote from 340 nm. Furthermore, if the alternative units of dN/dv are used, the blue sky λ_{max} shifts over to about 550 nm, much further still from R9's λ_{max}. To explain this apparent dilemma, we need to know considerably more about the relevant details of natural polarization (Sects. B.I.3 and D) and how they are used for polarization sensitivity.

d) Factors Controlling S_p

Despite the seminal role of worker bees for research on polarization sensitivity, no intracellular measurements of their retinular cell responses to e-vector orientation were published until recently (MENZEL and SNYDER, 1974). Surprisingly, these demonstrated that most of the photoreceptor cells recorded had little or no polarization sensitivity, which is consistent with, but not necessarily an explanation of the failure of e-vector rotation to affect the ERG amplitude (AUTRUM and STUMPF, 1950). Low polarization sensitivity (av.1.3) had previously been found intracellularly in the bee drone (SHAW, 1969 a). Such low sensitivity is quite different from the polarization sensitivity of the crayfish and other decapods cited above, where all or nearly all retinular cells tested typically gave high sensitivity ratios. In the worker bee, 70 green cells yielded an average polarization sensitivity of less than 1.2 (Fig. 86); the maximum encountered was 2.4 (MENZEL and SNYDER, 1974). Blue cells were rarely recorded, but the only one cited had a polarization sensitivity of 1.27.

Two types of ultraviolet units were encountered. Of 13 tested, 10 had low polarization sensitivity, coupled with considerable secondary sensitivity at $\lambda > 450$ nm. These were identified indirectly as long ultraviolet units R 1 or R 5. The other three (Fig. 87) found had a high polarization sensitivity (av.5, max.9). They were impaled near the basement membrane and their λ_{max} was about 350 nm, with sensitivity at $\lambda > 450$ nm down to 1%. Hence, they were taken to be R 9 units. On the basis of these data, the short ultraviolet receptor R 9 emerges as the e-vector discriminating cell type in the worker bee and has been widely accepted as such. This is quite a switch from its earlier neglect and the notion that the two orthogonal dichroic channels of R 2–R 4 and R 6–R 8 were basic to polarization sensitivity.

An immediate question is how to account for the low polarization sensitivity of R 2–R 4 and R 6–R 8 and the high polarization sensitivity of R 9. Optical analysis of a long fused symmetrical rhabdom suggests that it should combine high absolute sensitivity with strong polarization sensitivity, as well as good λ discrimination (SHAW, 1969 a; SNYDER et al., 1973). Initially, one might expect that the long length of such a photoreceptor organelle would reduce both polarization sensitivity and λ discrimination through self-absorption. Thus, in a hypothetically isolated simple rhabdomere 250 μm in length and having 1% absorption per μm, an inherent dichroic ratio $\Delta = 10$ would be reduced by self-absorption to an absorbance ratio of about 4 (GOLDSMITH and BERNARD, 1974, p.253). A higher concentration of visual pigment would augment the reduction.

SHAW (1969 b) and SNYDER (1973; SNYDER et al., 1973), however, have argued that, in a fused rhabdom, the dielectric waveguide optics could partly or fully eliminate such effects of self-filtering. Hence, both high absolute sensitivity and high polarization sensitivity would be present together. This is possible because of optical coupling in which light power incident on one rhabdomere is shared in a sort of lateral filtering by all other units of the whole rhabdom.

Clearly, such interactions, including their effect on polarization sensitivity, should be dependent on the arrangement of spectral sensitivities and pattern of microvillus orientation of the constituent retinular cells (SNYDER, 1973). If certain conditions of symmetry are met, even very long rhabdomeres can have polarization

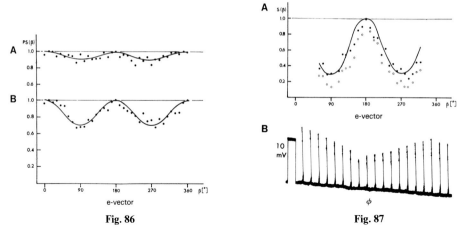

Fig. 86   **Fig. 87**

Figs. 86 and 87. *E*-vector sensitivity (S_e) of worker bee retinular cells calculated from intracellular recordings at ϕ intervals of 10° and wavelengths near λ_{max} Polarization sensitivities as a function of ϕ (abscissa) were obtained from an appropriate response–intensity function. The curves represent calculated average functions. (MENZEL and SNYDER, 1974). **Fig. 86.** Polarization sensitivity of green receptors ($\lambda_{max} = 530$ nm), the most numerous encountered. **A** Most cells ($n = 70$) had $S_e = 1.0$–1.2; these have a relatively high secondary peak in the ultraviolet. **B** Green cells with less ultraviolet sensitivity show higher $S_e = 1.2$–2.4 (with 2.4 being the maximum observed). Still a third group, not plotted, show greater mean S_e and a lower ultraviolet peak. Only one blue receptor was recorded and had an S_e of 1.27. **Fig. 87.** Polarization sensitivity of ultraviolet receptors. One group of 10 ultraviolet cells had considerable ($> 5\%$) sensitivity to $\lambda > 450$ nm, but low $S_e = 1.2$–1.6. **A** Three ultraviolet cells (judged on indirect evidence to be R 9) with negligible (10^{-2}) sensitivity to $\lambda > 450$ nm yielded high $S_e = 5$ mean, 9 max. Open circles show the data for the most sensitive unit, filled circles and the curve are averages and calculated function for all three recorded cases. Plot as in Fig. 86. **B** Sample intracellular record from an ultraviolet unit tested at successive 10° intervals of ϕ after > 30 min dark adaptation

sensitivity $= \varDelta$ in a fused rhabdom. However, we do not at present know for sure whether or not the absence of appropriate color symmetry of bee retinular cells R 2–R 4 and R 6–R 8 is a factor in their observed low polarization sensitivity (SNYDER, 1973) or whether that is fully accounted for by their rhabdom twisting (WEHNER et al., 1975).

While optical coupling should sharpen discrimination by fused rhabdom components, electrical coupling between these receptor cells would reduce or eliminate it. There is indirect evidence that this could be a major factor in the low polarization sensitivity of R 2–R 4 and R 6–R 8 (MENZEL and SNYDER, 1974; MENZEL and BLAKERS, 1976). Direct evidence for electrical coupling between retinular cells believed to be from the same ommatidium was found in honeybee drones using a double barrelled electrode (SHAW, 1969 a). Coupling was used to explain the observed low polarization sensitivity.

Positive electrical coupling is evidently involved in the secondary λ-sensitivities of the majority of receptor cells recorded in worker bees. Typically, such cells have, in addition to their own major λ_{max}, a minor peak coincident with the λ_{max} of another receptor type. On the other hand, evidence was also found for negative electrical coupling, perhaps counterbalancing such a "positive" effect (MENZEL and BLAKERS, 1976).

If these opposed influences can account for maintenance of effectively pure color inputs, perhaps they also might do so for polarization sensitivity channels, provided, of course, that twisting has not eliminated all polarization sensitivity except for short R 9. It should be recalled that neural sharpening has been evoked in explaining good acuity in visual systems which are optically inadequate (REICHARDT, 1965). However, as cited above (C.I.2.d), an effect of this sort to account for high S_p in crayfish has been proposed, but not confirmed.

Finally, however, there is rhabdom twisting to account for the low polarization sensitivity of R 2–R 4 and R 6–R 8 (MENZEL and SNYDER, 1974; SNYDER and McINTYRE, 1975; WEHNER et al., 1975; McINTYRE and SNYDER, 1978), but here we run into the apparent quandary that R 9 also twists about 40° between its upper and lower ends at the same rate as the other retinular cells[6]. To predict the optical results of this, the rhabdom's birefringence, as well as its dichroism must be considered in a model (WEHNER et al., 1975).

In a straight rhabdom with unidirectional microvilli, these functions are independent, but in a twisted rhabdom, they are not. Assuming birefringence in the bee rhabdom to be very low, WEHNER et al. (1975) calculated that polarization sensitivity in the long twisted ultraviolet retinular cells (i.e., R 1 and R 5) is unity (i.e., no discrimination) but, for the short ultraviolet cell (R 9), it is substantial (e.g., 4.2 if $\Delta = 5$; 7.1 for $\Delta = 10$) despite the rhabdom twist.

e) Models of ϕ Discriminating Mechanism

α) *Three Channel Instantaneous Model.* If R 9 is the one and only polarization sensitive receptor in a bee ommatidium, a single retinula obviously cannot provide instantaneous *e*-vector discrimination. As we have seen, three independent channels are needed for this task. Consequently, this function requires cooperation between two or more ommatidia in the bee (or ant: MENZEL and SNYDER, 1974; MENZEL and BLAKERS, 1975). Since R 9 cells in neighboring ommatidia in the dorsal half of the bee eye (Figs. 84 and 85) have two different orientations and, hence, presumably different ϕ_{max}s, their collaboration with an independent polarization insensitive unit would provide the theoretical minimum requirements for the system.

According to WEHNER et al. (1975), the planes of maximum sensitivity (ϕ_{max}) of the X and Y type rhabdoms differ by 36° if their birefringence is assumed to be low. On that basis, a minimal detector for stationary *e*-vector orientation could require 1) two differently oriented R 9's of opposite twist type from neighboring ommatidia to provide two differential polarization sensitive inputs (more than two of these would be redundant) and 2) at least one long ultraviolet cell to act as an independent third channel without polarization sensitivity (WEHNER et al., 1975). If all three have the same λ_{max}, then ϕ and I could be independently discriminated, provided the ϕ_{max}'s differ by some angle other than 90° or 0°. Actually, VAN DER GLAS (1977a) argued that such a three-channel model is unlikely for the bee, but no direct evidence is available either way.

---

[6] Despite this generality (WEHNER et al., 1975), other preliminary evidence suggests that the proximal rhabdom in the bee does not in fact twist; hence, the R 9 rhabdomere itself may not be twisted (MENZEL, personal communication)

Note that this question of e-vector detecting mechanism is essentially a sensory physiological and information processing problem. Yet, it is, of course, intimately related to the visual input being utilized and the adaptive use of the information obtained. Consequently, it has been tempting to accept rather glib assumptions about these input–output functions of the polarization sensitivity black box, even though they are inadequately known or understood. For instance, we do not know with certainty that the bee, or any other polarization sensitive animal, uses an instantaneous e-vector sensor in its sky orientation[7].

In most orienting responses of animals, especially arthropods, they behave as if they are bringing the stimulus pattern into some particular alignment with their body axes (JANDER, 1963a; WATERMAN, 1966d; MITTELSTAEDT, 1972; SCHÖNE, 1975; REICHARDT and POGGIO, 1976; EDRICH, 1977). Such a straightforward direction matching approach, however, will not work when successive turn-and-look sampling is used, as in *Cataglyphis* (WEHNER, 1975), although it is consistent with VAN DER GLAS' ϕ-symmetry model discussed below. Actually, little is known about how the worker bee can dance quite accurately at a given azimuth angle relative to the sun using only some area of clear blue sky as a reference. These problems are reviewed further in Sects. B and D. However, two recent theoretical papers, which are more directly related to modeling retinal mechanisms, will be considered.

β) *Four-Channel Consecutive Model.* The correlation between ideal RAYLEIGH sky polarization pattern and possible models for polarization sensitivity in the worker bee compound eye has been considered in some detail by VAN DER GLAS (1977a) and is discussed further in Sect. D. Of various possible generalized e-vector detecting systems, he rejects the one just discussed, as well as that proposed by MENZEL and BLAKERS (1975). Both seemed unlikely to him because of certain behavioral experiments done with polarization patterns (VON FRISCH, 1965). Instead, VAN DER GLAS proposed a consecutive model in which four polarization sensitive channels, two in each eye, successively evaluate a sky region either during the circling rotation of the dance or oscillation in flight.

For such a model, the consequences of various orientations of the maximum e-vector sensitivity planes of the two types of short R 9's were explored by VAN DER GLAS, assuming that the ratio of their responses is the critical input parameter. A variety of "optimal" solutions were obtained, depending on different ranges and restrictions assumed for relevant factors. These included an important constraint imposed by the fact that the dorsoventral axis of the head, and, therefore, the ommatidial coordinate system, is tilted posteriorly more than $40°$ in the flying bee compared with a walking bee.

Considering all this, the "best" solution to the basic optical geometry problem was that ϕ_{max} of the two types of short R 9 rhabdomeres should be oriented at $31°$ and $105°$ respectively, and anticlockwise from the z-axis. The angular distance between them would then be $74°$. This is twice the separation angle calculated for their optical model by WEHNER et al. (1975), but VAN DER GLAS (1977a) believes this could easily be accounted for if the assumed effective birefringence were

---

[7] The absence of strong frequency dependence of worker bee orientation to a fixed zenith e-vector, in which p was sinusoidally oscillated from 0 to 1.0 at frequencies between 0.1 and 50 Hz, was used to support the instantaneous alternative (VON HELVERSEN and EDRICH, 1977, preprint)

0.8×10^{-3}, rather than nearer zero. The resulting estimates of oblique orientations for ϕ_{max} could be consistent with the fact that bees show optomotor responses to alternate oblique angles of e-vector orientation in vertical polarized stripes, but not a pattern with e-vector directions at $0°$ and $90°$ (KIRSCHFELD, 1973 b).

γ) *Color Vision Model.* In an independent, more general but related, paper, BERNARD and WEHNER (1977) have developed a comparison between trichromatic color vision and "polarization vision" based on the three independent dimensions of partially linearly polarized light: 1) total intensity I_t, 2) e-vector orientation ϕ, and 3) degree of polarization p. The corresponding characteristics of a color stimulus are I_t, dominant wavelength λ, and purity.

If ϕ is to be unambiguously identified, regardless of the values of I_t and p, KIRSCHFELD (1972) has made clear that three independent receptor units are required for instantaneous recognition (i.e., without relative rotation of the stimulus and the detector). In optical polarimetry, intensity measurements are routinely made at three, or more, orientations of one measuring polarizer typically at angles $45°$ or $60°$ apart (SHURCLIFF, 1962; CLARKE and GRAINGER, 1971, p. 135). If three such dimensions need to be simultaneous, a minimal biological polarimeter would require three differently oriented e-vector sensors (the case KIRSCHFELD has emphasized). It could be sequential with fewer. Actually, as clearly pointed out by SHURCLIFF (1962) and discussed in detail above, one of these three receptors need not have polarization sensitivity. The response output R of a unit polarization sensitivity receptor may be formulated as follows (BERNARD and WEHNER, 1977):

$$R = 1 + \frac{p(S_p - 1)}{(S_p + 1)} \cos(2\phi - 2\phi_{max}), \tag{13}$$

where polarization sensitivity (i.e., S_p) is R_{max}/R_{min} when $p = 100\%$.

If there is only one polarization sensitivity channel with a response like the above, intensity cannot be discriminated from contributions due to ϕ if the channel is fixed. Even if it is rotated, however, there would always be a pair of angles, except at I_{max} and I_{min}, that would give the same R. As pointed out by MOODY and PARRISS (1961), such a detector could not discriminate the usual geometric quadrants I from IV and II from III. This does not seem consistent with KIRSCHFELD's (1972) statement that a single polarization sensitivity channel, if rotated, could be adequate for menotaxis. MOODY and PARRISS (1961) also clearly appreciated that a fixed two-channel analyzer would confuse angles in various quadrants like the rotating single polarizer.

Whereas most of the earlier work has ignored the quantitative influence of p, BERNARD and WEHNER's (1977) model allows them to explore its theoretical consequences in detail. For example, their plot of p and ϕ for a two-channel polarimeter demonstrates that, in general, there will be two "neutral" ϕ's, $90°$ apart, which yield the same output in both channels, regardless of p. Discrimination of ϕ is generally better near those angles and becomes poor at angles far from both. JANDER (1963 a, b) had suggested some time ago that basitactic orientation angles for polarotaxis might be directly derived from these neutral angles.

Specifically, for the orthogonal case, the neutral angles are at $\pm 45°$ and the worst angular discrimination estimated from the pattern of confusion loci would occur at and near ϕ_{max1} and ϕ_{max2}, except in the limiting case where $p = 1.0$ when those angles are unambiguous. Difference in S_{p1} vs S_{p2} or $|\phi_{max1} - \phi_{max2}|$ introduce asymmetries into the confusion loci. Interestingly, for a two-channel analyzer, overall best ϕ discrimination occurs when there is a 90° difference between their ϕ_{max}'s. However, for their polarization vision model, BERNARD and WEHNER (1977) assumed that the first order interneurons in the system comprise three polarization opponent cells, like those of the primate color system (DE VALOIS, 1973).

Yet, we should remember that a rigorously defined trichromatic color vision, like the well documented case for worker bees and man, has rarely been proved in other animals, despite an enormous amount of research (reviewed by AUTRUM and THOMAS, 1973). On the other hand, evidence for some sort of color discrimination is widespread in many invertebrates and vertebrates. While this requires two or more differentially sensitive receptor cell types, it does not follow that the number and response characteristics of the latter prove some sort of color vision (DE VALOIS, 1973). In fact, it has been argued that preoccupation with just various receptor types actually blocked progress in understanding vertebrate λ-discrimination for some time.

Discrimination depends on effective input comparisons that isolate, at some level, the important stimulus parameters. In addition, we know that the rather astonishing perceptual data, which support the retinex theory of human color vision, are far more complex and subtle than any simple peripheral model of three primary color receptors might imply (McCANN et al., 1977). Obviously, in comparing polarization sensitivity with color vision, we also need to keep these matters in mind.

f) Conclusion for Bees

It is striking that we remain so ignorant about key aspects of the honeybee's polarization sensitivity. Neither the information processing mechanism nor the stimulus input necessary for polarized sky orientation are adequately known. Consequently, both field work, effectively coupling measured sky polarization patterns with oriented behavior, and a continued search for the polarization discriminators among interneurons of the *Apis* visual system are much needed. It would be particularly interesting, in both approaches, to confirm or refute the hypotheses that polarization is perceived as a color pattern and the natural polarized light compass depends on matching symmetry of the sky pattern, as received in both eyes. Perhaps imaging is more important than discrimination in polarization sensitivity.

4. *Lasius* and Other Ants (Formicidae)

Since bees and ants are both hymenopterans, they might well have been discussed together, as were a wide variety of decapod crustaceans above. Indeed, WEHNER has recently synthesized the data on the peripheral visual system of bees and ants together (1976 b); however, the relevant information on the honeybee seemed so important, complex, and voluminous that here it has been dealt with alone. Now, ant polarization sensitivity will be reviewed.

a) Oriented Behavior

The recognition that ants can use polarized light in the sky for orientation came soon after the discovery of this complex vector orientation in the bee. Quite a number of species have been shown to have such a sky polaromenotaxis: *Lasius niger* (SCHIFFERER cited by VON FRISCH, 1950; JANDER, 1957), *Myrmica laevinodis* (VOWLES, 1950), *Formica fusca, F. rufa, Myrmica ruginodis, Tapinoma erraticum, Tetramorium caespitum* (JANDER, 1957), and *Cataglyphis bicolor* (WEHNER and DUELLI, 1971). Actually, SANTSCHI (1911, 1923), in some well cited experiments on *Cataglyphis* and *Monomorium salamanus*, showed that they could use the sun as a compass. Even at twilight without the sun, foragers were shown to orient accurately using only a view of overhead sky, the terrain and sky near the horizon were not needed. He suggested that this behavior was a kind of celestial orientation in which the stars, not visible to human eyes under the prevailing conditions, or the moon were seen by the ants and used as the steering clue (i.e., a sky compass), but von FRISCH (1949) proposed that sky polarization was a more likely basis for this twilight compass.

α) *Experiments with* Formica. With a different species e., *Formica rufa*, mirror experiments showed that the full moon can, in fact, be used in a photomenotaxis (JANDER, 1957). In addition, menotaxis was found with an artificial light source. Actually, *Cataglyphis* also can employ the moon for orientation according to WEHNER and DUELLI (1971), but only for a positive or negative tropotaxis, not a compass response. No evidence was obtained in this more recent work that *Cataglyphis* is able to use stars as SANTSCHI proposed. Its twilight compass generally is, in fact, sky polarized light, as reviewed below. Meanwhile, JANDER's thesis research (1957), carried out under VON FRISCH's direction, was devoted to visual orientation in *Formica rufa* and made substantial contributions, among other things, to this species' responses to sky polarization.

Thus, *Formica rufa* were trained to find their nest in a given compass direction (e.g., 245° from the sun's bearing). When a large circular Polaroid filter was placed over the experimental arena with its *e*-vector oriented parallel to that in the zenith sky (i.e., 90°–270° to the sun's bearing), the mean homing direction was unaffected (Fig. 88 A). However, with the imposed *e*-vector rotated 50° clockwise or anticlockwise relative to the sky, compromise running directions resulted which were displaced 23°–25° towards the polarizer's principal axis (Fig. 88 B). Such orienting effects of sky polarization are apparently quite general since qualitatively similar experimental results were obtained with both formicine and myrmicine ant species, as cited above.

JANDER was also able to show, with artificial light sources replacing the sun, that the memory trace in *Formica* for *e*-vector orientation is coupled to that for a direct light compass reaction. When one of these changes, so does the other. In contrast, orientation to landmarks can change independently of polarized light orientation and orientation to a light source; hence, JANDER concluded that these classes of orientation mechanism are not coupled and appear to be independent. Indeed, when sun and sky were completely clouded over, the ants oriented exclusively to landmarks (e.g., trees, buildings).

β) Experiments on Myrmica. Similar conclusions had been reached on the basis of stimulus substitution experiments in *Myrmica* (Figs. 89 and 90), whose orientation in the laboratory to gravity, directional light, and polarization was analyzed (VOWLES, 1950, 1954 a, b). From these data, it was postulated that all three types of sensory input converged on a common steering (i.e., taxis) component different from that mediating landmark orientation. According to JANDER's model (1957), the integrated output of each of these convergent sensory pathways would feed into a common orientation center in the nervous system which, in turn, would relay its convoluted information to the coordination center for locomotion.

It is interesting that ambiguities attributed to the nature of *Myrmica*'s gravity sensing (e.g., angles related as $\theta_1 = 360° - \theta_2$ were not distinguished) and phototactic mechanisms (e.g., angles related as $\theta_1 = 180° - \theta_2$ were confused) were apparent in the stimulus transfer experiments. Although VOWLES did not suggest it, extending this simple model of ambiguity to polarized light is tempting. Since the latter is a 2θ function, analogy would mean that $\theta_1 = 90° - \theta_2$ would be indistinguishable, which was later discussed as a general problem of polarotaxis by MOODY and PARRISS (1961). In general, these orientational ambiguities, basic to the simple sensory components, do not usually appear in normal field behavior except under special conditions (e.g., the twilight 180° polarotactic confusion of *Cataglyphis*).

Unlike the negative results reported for *Lasius* (BRUN, 1914), *Formica* was found to be capable of compensating its menotaxis for the sun's movement through the sky (JANDER, 1957). This had recently been discovered independently for bees (VON FRISCH, 1950) and starlings (KRAMER, 1950). JANDER did not comment on the possible tie-in of sky polarization with, in this case, the sun itself. However, a time compensated polaromenotaxis was demonstrated in another ant (DUELLI, 1972, 1973; WEHNER, 1972), as it had been for the bee (VON FRISCH and LINDAUER, 1954). Such an outcome could be consistent with the proposal that phototactic and polarotactic inputs both converge on a single taxis center in the nervous system.

γ) Experiments on Cataglyphis. Field experiments on directional training in the North African Middle Eastern desert ant *Cataglyphis* have substantially expanded our understanding of the behavioral aspects of ant polarization sensitivity (WEHNER, 1968, 1972, 1976 a). Its vector orientation is predominantly visual. Like the bee, it can learn to expect food at a given range and bearing from the nest. To a degree not possible in bees, however, the ant's hunting forays can be followed completely over extended distances. In the process, various polarizers, depolarizers, color filters, and other devices can be placed over them without disturbing their outward and return courses over the natural terrain. Despite changes in direction on the outward course, *Cataglyphis* at any moment can take a direct course back to its nest using visual celestial cues whenever the degree of sky polarization is above a certain minimum threshold and the pattern (Figs. 147–149) has only one axis of symmetry (DUELLI, 1972). In a single foray, the ant can learn the correct celestial reference directions and remember them for several days (Fig. 91).

Orientation was not less at twilight, although it was bimodal when the sun was below the horizon (WEHNER and DUELLI, 1971). Figure 147 shows the pattern for ϕ in the sky about that time. Shading the sun during the day, or even displacing

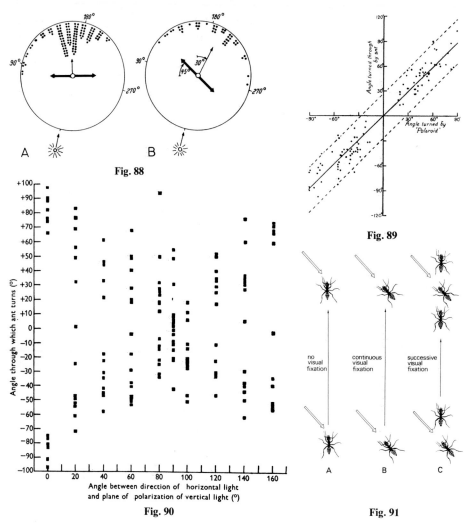

Fig. 88

Fig. 89

Fig. 90

Fig. 91

Figs. 88–91. Polarotaxis in ants. **Figs. 88 A.** *Formica* trained in the field to orient normal to an imposed overhead *e*-vector (heavy double headed arrows) ran in a mean direction indicated by the single headed vertical arrow. **B** Rotation of the *e*-vector clockwise through 45° resulted in a shift of the mean orientation by 30°±5° in the same direction. As diagramed, the sun was visible through the polarizer at 0°. Each point represents one run by an ant. The mean direction shown in **B** was apparently a compromise between the direction learned from the sun in **A** (*e*-vector not changed in **A**) and that derived from the *e*-vector which had changed in **B**. Similar experiments show that *Formica*, as well as other ant genera cited in the text, could learn azimuth directions from blue sky polarization (JANDER, 1957). **Fig. 89.** Directional responses made in the laboratory by walking *Myrmica* when the orientation of an overhead *e*-vector was rotated through various angles. Points show individual runs ($n = 105$). The straight oblique line is the calculated regression line of the response on the stimulus change (these angles are not significantly different). The broken lines indicate the 95% confidence interval $\pm 27°$ from the regression line. (VOWLES, 1950). **Fig. 90.** Turning angles shown by "escaping" *Myrmica* running on a horizontal surface in the laboratory when a directional unpolarized horizontal light beam (to which the ant orients photomenotactically) is replaced by a vertical linearly polarized beam (to which it orients polarotactically). Responses are plotted as functions of the angular difference between horizontal beam direction and vertical beam *e*-vector. Note that the course change induced by stimulus substitution is minimum

its apparent azimuth with a mirror, did not ordinarily decrease the precision of the ants' orientation to the sky (DUELLI and WEHNER, 1973). Nevertheless, the sun's bearing, but not its elevation, could be used to maintain course direction if the sky polarization pattern was disrupted optically. Courses with the sun compass were less accurate than with sky polarization alone. Apparently, the sun is relatively more important than sky polarization in bees and myrmecine ants, but has a subordinate effect in formicine ants like *Cataglyphis* and *Formica*, for which the polarization predominates.

Interestingly enough, WELLINGTON (1955) had maintained earlier that, for a wide range of larval and adult insects, travel across open spaces was steered with reference to sky polarization, whether or not the sun was visible. Much of this data was derived from many different kinds of caterpillars crawling on the ground. In their case, of course, the polarotaxis must be mediated by lateral ocelli (Sect. C.II.2.b.).

δ) *Factors Affecting* S_p. Interestingly, orientation by both the sun and sky polarization was not possible if all $\lambda < 410$ nm were removed with a low cutoff filter. However, normal orientation resumed when a $\lambda > 390$ nm cutoff filter was substituted. Therefore, λ's between 390 and 410 nm were adequate for accurate direction finding. Only the ultraviolet receptors, not the green, were concluded to be involved in orientation to sky polarized light (DUELLI and WEHNER, 1973). Comparable results have been reported for the beetle *Geotrupes* and *Cataglyphis* walking under the sky screened by various broad band filters (FRANTSEVICH et al., 1977). Good polarotactic orientation was reduced from about 90% to near 30% in both species when ultraviolet was screened out.

Not only is such orientation limited in *Cataglyphis* to violet and near ultraviolet λ's, but different parts of its retina vary in their importance for the sky polarotaxis (WEILER and HUBER, 1972; DUELLI, 1975; WEHNER, 1975). In fact, a restricted retinal area centered dorsomedially (i.e., 51° above the horizon and 45° out from the sagittal plane) is mainly responsible for such orientation (Figs. 92–96). Simultaneous binocular polarization sensitivity is not involved and e-vector discrimination can take place monocularly. It is not known whether or not the special area functions as it does because of receptor or connectivity specialization[8].

Restriction of the ant's view of the sky indicates (Figs. 94 and 95) that all parts of the sky appear to be effective for orientation, yet directional accuracy depends

---

[8] As cited above, polarotaxis in *Apis* workers depends on a dorsal retinal area, but not on the ventral part of the eye. Similar results were also reported for the hemipteran *Corixa* (RENSING and BOGENSCHÜTZ, 1966)

◄ when this angular difference is 90°, which in nature is the difference between the sun's bearing and zenith e-vector orientation. Note also the symmetrical ambiguities of most of these substitution responses. (VOWLES, 1954a). **Fig. 91.** Possible mechanisms of course steering by ants using celestial information as a compass from a given sky region (direction indicated by arrows). **A** Stimulus localized on corresponding retinal area dependent on standard posture (no fixation). **B** Body (head, eyes) turned so that stimulus is continuously localized on some specific retinal area (continuous fixation). **C** Body (head, eyes) turned periodically to localize stimulus on specific receptor area (successive fixation, a mechanism reviewed for insects and stomatopods by HORRIDGE, 1977). Orientation of *Cataglyphis* by sky polarization employs intermittent directional data acquisition **C** (WEHNER, unpublished, 1978)

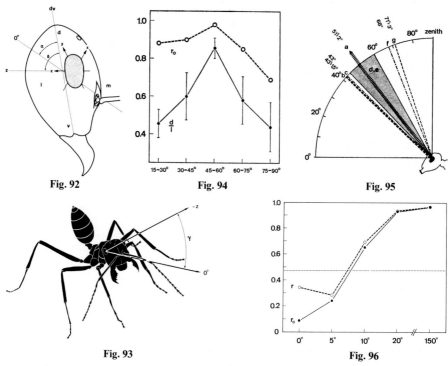

Fig. 92   Fig. 94   Fig. 95

Fig. 93   Fig. 96

Figs. 92–96. Visual coordinates in *Cataglyphis*. **Figs. 92 and 93.** Diagrams showing spatial and anatomical coordinates of the visual system in a running ant (WEHNER, 1975). **Fig. 92.** The major eye axis is
nearly parallel to the morphological dorsoventral axis of the head (*dv*) which, in turn, is somewhat less
than perpendicular to the ommatidial *z*-axis. The horizontal direction 0° lies between the *z*-axis and the
dv axis (or ca 44°). Compare Fig. 93. **Fig. 93.** Posture of running ant, showing relation (γ) of horizon
(0°) to the ommatidial *z*-axis (−*z*). **Figs. 94–96.** Effects of retinal location and area on *Cataglyphis* polarotaxis in the field. (DUELLI, 1975). **Fig. 94.** Changes in accuracy (ordinate) of celestial orientation dependent on elevation angle (abscissa) of a 15° annular almucantar of sky visible to the ants (rest
screened out). Two measures of accuracy are plotted for the five bands tested. One is r_o, the length of
the mean orientation vector (open circles and broken lines); the other (filled circles and continuous lines
and ±S.D.) is the directness of the path estimated from *d* (distance between release point and nest) per
l (length of path taken). Note both curves peak at 45°–60°, but *d* per *l* appears a more sensitive discrimination. **Fig. 95.** Data of Fig. 94 summarized on a frontal view of visual space between the forward horizon and the zenith. *a* indicates the fixation center at 51°±2°, shaded area (d, e) provided "best
orientation." Upper and lower edges of the localized region for polarized sky orientation indicated by
b, c, f, and g. *n* = 20 for each point. **Fig. 96.** Accuracy of orientation as a function of the angular subtent
of a quadratic aperture centered at *a* in Fig. 94. The p = 0.01 level of significance for the vector *n* is
shown by the horizontal dotted line. Thus, highly significant polarotaxis occurs with 10° and larger
apertures. *r* is the mean vector length of the fourth run intervals and r_o is the projection of *r* on the zero
direction

on the angle between the course being followed and the sky patch observed (DUEL-
LI, 1975). A 10° × 10° foveal field, estimated to stimulate 7–19 ommatidia, is adequate for polarotaxis (Fig. 96). Behavioral data indicate that φ and ultraviolet intensity patterns can be perceived independently of *p*. Consequently, a minimum of
three receptor channels would be needed for simultaneous polarization sensitivity
(KIRSCHFELD, 1972). If only two microvillus directions are present in one rhabdom,
more than one ommatidium would be required (DUELLI, 1975).

With such localized sky patches for orientation, *Cataglyphis* turn its body and with it the head and eyes, to bring the image of the informative region into the special retinal area for polarization sensitivity or it turns its body to look at it (Fig. 91 C). Consequently, in order to maintain space constancy, the receptor mapping the polarization pattern must be convoluted with head and body coordinate changes (WEHNER, 1975). In addition, when successive fixations are involved (e.g., looking momentarily at the sky patch), a complex calculation must occur to effect any necessary course correction. Turning and course holding glances at the compass must be ideothetic (i.e., without exteroceptor directional input [DUELLI, 1975]).

b) Compound Eye Organization

α) *Cataglyphis.* Ant eyes are rather similar, in general structure, to those of bees and other hymenopterans (WEHNER, 1976 b). However, ants usually have substantially fewer component ommatidia. A strongly visual species like *Cataglyphis*, for example (Figs. 92 and 93), has only about 1,200 facets in the compound eye of an outdoor worker (HERRLING, 1972; BRUNNERT and WEHNER, 1973). The ommatidium is of the apposition-type, with a long thin fused rhabdom (Fig. 97). Like *Apis*, each retinula has nine cells and rhabdomeres, but there are some differences in detail. Cross sections through the distal half reveal eight retinular cells; similar proximal slices show nine retinular cells. Earlier reports state that *Cataglyphis'* R 1–R 8 comprise alternating cells of quite different size; four large (i.e., R 2, R 4, R 6, R 8) and four small (i.e., R 1, R 3, R 5, R 7) (e.g., BRUNNERT and WEHNER, 1973), with the latter mainly lacking screening pigment granules. More detailed study, however, shows that this Type I retinula is the commonest, but is only one of three kinds present in three corresponding parts of the retina (HERRLING, 1976).

Type I retinulas have a rhabdom about 95 µm long, circular in cross section, and, in their basal third, contain the R 9 rhabdomere. They occupy much of the dorsal two thirds of the retina. Type II retinulas have two unpigmented small cells (i.e., R 1, R 5) and four large pigmented ones (i.e., R 2, R 4, R 6, R 8). R 3 and R 7 are intermediate in size and pigmented, while R 9 has the same features it has in Type I. The rhabdom is longer (i. e., 110 µm) and also circular in cross sections. Type II units occupy the ventral third of the retina.

About 80 ommatidia of Type III occupy the dorsomedial edge of the retina, spreading medially and laterally. The Type III rhabdom is dumbbell-shaped in cross section and only 70–75 µm long. Distally, its cross sectional area is about twice that of Types I or II. As in Type I, four alternate retinular cells are smaller than the others and have fewer screening pigment granules. In the proximal rhabdom, the nine rhabdomeres extend only part way to the basement membrane since, in the basal 15 µm or so, R 9's rhabdomere replaces that of R 3 or R 7. This establishes a short length of optical tiering. Comparison of the locations of these retinular types and the posture of the head with the environmental coordinates indicates that the Type III group is roughly coincident with the retinal area most important for sky polarization mediated homing (DUELLI, 1975).

The pattern of microvillus orientation, which is obviously crucial for polarization sensitivity, is rather complex in the *Cataglyphis* retina (HERRLING, 1976). Extensive analysis of rhabdoms of Types I and II suggest that there are four preferred

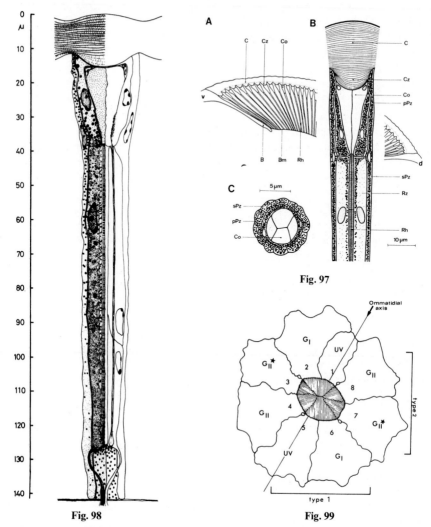

Figs. 97–99. Ommatidial structure in ants. **Fig. 97.** *Cataglyphis* showing **A** a *z*-plane radial section of the compound eye, **B** axial section of distal half of ommatidium, and **C** cross section at the crystalline cone level (WEHNER et al., 1971). *B*, cuticular diaphragm (in part **A**); *Bm*, basement membrane; *C*, cornea; *Co*, crystalline cone; *Cz*, corneal process; *d*, dorsal; *pPz*, primary pigment cell; *Rh*, rhabdom; *Rz*, retinular cell; *sPz*, secondary pigment cells; *v*, ventral. **Fig. 98.** Ommatidium of *Formica* diagramed in axial section. (MENZEL, 1972b). **Fig. 99.** Cross section of *Myrmecia* ommatidium, diagramed in the distal region where R 1–R 8 are present. Ommatidial transverse axis drawn through the small ultraviolet receptors R 1 and R 5; the remaining six cells are three pairs of green receptors. See text for further details. In a sufficiently proximal transverse section, R 9 would appear (see Fig. 98). (MENZEL and BLAKERS, 1975)

directional peaks, about 45° apart, when a local area of the retina is analyzed as a semicircular distribution. In Type III retinulas, the alignment of microvilli is stricter in local areas, at least, and only two orthogonal preferred peaks occur.

Diagonal R 1 and R 5 have the same microvillus direction, whereas R 2–R 4 and R 6–R 8 are at 90°, as is R 9. These orientations have the same relation to the hexagonal x, y, and z facet axes in the right and left eyes. Measurements at different depths along the rhabdom indicate, particularly for Type III, that rhabdomere twisting is not significantly present. This is unlike the honeybee worker, of course, except for the Type d ommatidia, and also unlike the ant *Myrmecia*, which has systematically twisted rhabdoms (MENZEL, 1975b; MENZEL and BLAKERS, 1975).

β) Other Ants. Structural details of other ant eyes may differ considerably from *Cataglyphis* not only in relation to rhabdom twisting. Thus, in the wood ant *Formica polyctena* (MENZEL, 1972a), there are only about 750 ommatidia, rather irregularly arranged with a number of four to seven-sided polygonal facets, in addition to the predominant (i.e., 85%) hexagonal ones. In the central retina, divergence angles of the ommatidia are about 4°.

The retinular cell pattern is rather like that of *Cataglyphis* Type II in that there are two small cells (i.e., R 1 and R 5), six larger ones, and a basal R 9. As in the desert ant, R 9 and its rhabdomere in Types I and II retinulas are added to those of R 1–R 8 in the proximal 0.3 or so of the rhabdom (Fig. 98). The microvillus directions, both within and between the ommatidia, show large variances although there seem, in general, to be three orientation peaks in 180°, ideally 60° apart. No signs of rhabdom twisting were reported.

In the bulldog ant *Myrmecia gulosa*, the fine structure of the ommatidium, twist of the rhabdom, $λ$ selectivity, and polarization sensitivity of its retinular cells have all been studied by MENZEL (1975b, c) and MENZEL and BLAKERS (1975). The basic pattern is closely similar to that described in *Formica* (MENZEL, 1972a, b). The two diagonal small cells and the microvillus pattern in cross section allow R 1–R 8 to be identified (Fig. 99). All diagonal pairs have parallel microvilli. Pairs R 1, R 5 and R 2, R 6 are parallel to each other, while R 3, R 7 and R 4, R 8 are oriented at different intermediate angles, "ideally" differing from each other and from the two aligned pairs by 60°. Two retinular patterns occur in which the cell sequences are clockwise and anticlockwise, respectively.

Selective adaptation of retinular cell screening pigment granules clearly demonstrates that R 1 and R 5 are ultraviolet receptors and the other six green receptors. No selective effect of blue light was found. The green receptors are of two types, 1) one with their microvilli parallel to those of the ultraviolet cells and 2) the other with microvilli at $\pm 60°$ to that axis and having other green cells as their nearest neighbors. This parallels the pattern demonstrated in *Formica* (MENZEL and KNAUT, 1973). Electroretinograms and intracellular recordings from retinular cells supported these conclusions from pigment migration data (MENZEL, 1972b; ROTH and MENZEL, 1972). The receptor potentials yield a $λ_{max}$ at 345 nm for the ultraviolet receptor and one at 510 nm for the green. Although the $λ_{max}$ of R 9 cannot be tested by selective pigment migration, since it lacks such granules, other evidence suggests that it also is an ultraviolet receptor.

γ) Retinular Twisting. In MENZEL and BLAKERS (1975) systematic twisting of the *Myrmecia* retinulas has been described in considerable detail. Two types of ommatidia were reported; one with clockwise the other with anticlockwise twists. Twisting at two rates occurs in both types. One is a sudden substantial angular change of microvillus direction; the other is a steady sustained twist. The functional consequences of both rates of twisting are theoretically the same, namely reduction in polarization sensitivity (Snyder and Menzel, 1975).

Where rather uniform rotations occur between distal and proximal ends of the rhabdom, the clockwise units revolve at 0.5°–0.7° per μm for a total of 50°–60°, whereas the anticlockwise ones turn 1° per μm for a 100° total. Ommatidia with opposite twist directions were reported to occur in about equal numbers and be oriented differently relative to the eye axes (Menzel and Blakers, 1975). At the distal rhabdom tip, the retinular axis (i.e., the microvillus direction of the R 1 and R 5 cells) of the clockwise retinulas make a mean angle of 42° with the z-axis; the anticlockwise ones lie at 71°.

The orientation of R 9 microvilli is reported to differ by an average of 86° from that of the proximal end of the distal ultraviolet cell with which it is in optical series. This could have an important effect on the modulation of polarization sensitivity by filtering (Gribakin, 1972). Furthermore, the angular difference between the facet z-axis and the R 9 microvillus axis direction is different for the two directions of retinular twist (167°$\pm$19° vs. 121°$\pm$29°). A check on the orientation of R 9 microvilli in neighboring pairs of ommatidia showed that half have an average axial difference of 69°, while the other half are parallel (Menzel and Blakers, 1975).

The theoretical consequences of twisting have been quoted above for the bee (C.I.3.b) and are presumably equally valid here. Neither the absolute sensitivity of the organelle as a whole nor that of individual rhabdomeres to unpolarized light are affected by twisting. The polarization sensitivity of a twisted fused rhabdom, however, may be strongly reduced to a degree dependent on the angle of total twist and its dichroic ratio. Thus, a 50°–100° total twist should reduce polarization sensitivity for $\Delta = 10$ from 10 to 3.5 (Snyder and McIntyre, 1975). The effective direction of maximum absorption should also be rotated (McIntyre and Snyder, 1978).

c) Retinular Cell S_p

A further point of interest concerning *Myrmica* is that direct intracellular recordings have yielded the strongest polarization sensitivity (i.e., S_p for one cell was 10; for another 18) so far reported in insects (Menzel, 1975a, b). The previous records in this class were apparently for R 9 in *Apis* where, as described above, S_e's from 3.9 to 9 were measured (Menzel and Snyder, 1974); for a receptor unit in the larval stemma of *Perga*, where $S_{e_{max}}$ was 10 (Meyer-Rochow, 1974); and for the single pigment ultraviolet receptor in the ventral retina of the dragonfly *Hemicordulia*, which had an $S_{e_{max}}$ of 10 (Laughlin, 1976a). With a few exceptions, most other direct retinular recordings in insects have yielded very low S_e for which various explanations have been proposed.

d) Conclusion for Ants

The most striking feature of the high S_e cells of *Myrmecia* is that their λ_{max} is sharply peaked near 500 nm. Yet, practically all current orthodoxies take it for granted that bee and ant polarization sensitivity is predominantly or exclusively dependent on polarized ultraviolet irradiation and specific ultraviolet receptors. In fact, Menzel and Blakers (1975, p. 296) conclude that R 9 in *Myrmecia* is an ultraviolet receptor and seems to be the only retinular cell significantly able to discriminate polarized light.

MENZEL (in lit.) has suggested that the high S_e green cell is only a rare exception and, hence, unimportant. However, no electrophysiological data have yet been presented for R 9 in ants, either with regard to its S_e or its λ_{max} (MENZEL, 1975 b). Consequently, it is difficult to evaluate the relation between the regular retinular cells and the R 9's. This kind of unexpected variation may be similar to the puzzlingly irregular finding in flies of polarization sensitive and insensitive units which seem otherwise the same (see below). Recall also that the published data for high S_p ultraviolet cells are limited in the bee to three units indirectly identified as R 9 (MENZEL and SNYDER, 1974).

5. Flies and Other Dipterans

The visual systems of dipteran insects are amongst the most intensively studied of any organism (FRANCESCHINI and KIRSCHFELD, 1976; POGGIO and REICHARDT, 1976; REICHARDT and POGGIO, 1976; STRAUSFELD, 1976a; McCANN et al., 1977; STARK et al., 1977; TSUKAHARA et al., 1977). Considerable data and insight concerning their polarization sensitivity have often resulted rather incidentally. Nevertheless, our knowledge of their oriented visual behavior in the field is rather sparse. This is perhaps not unexpected considering their small size and often erratic rapid flight.

a) Oriented Free Flying Behavior

In spite of this, visually mediated responses (i.e., fixation, escape, pursuit, flight stability, landing, optomotor course control) have all been studied mainly in the laboratory, but often considered as components of normal field behavior (REICHARDT, 1973; LAND and COLLETT, 1974; COLLETT and LAND, 1975a, b; FERNANDEZ PEREZ DE TALENS and TADDEI FERRETTI, 1975; GÖTZ, 1975; KIRSCHFELD and WENK, 1976). However, possible involvement of polarized light or polarization sensitivity has not been specifically analyzed in such research, even though, for example, the pursuit by male simuliid flies of females silhouetted overhead against strongly polarized twilight sky (KIRSCHFELD and WENK, 1976) no doubt involves some polarized light interaction.

An unusually interesting series of field observations has recently been reported on the natural flight behavior of mosquitos, flies, and other insects correlated with patterns of sky polarization (WELLINGTON, 1974a, 1976a). This research on field behavior stands in marked contrast to the sophisticated physiological and cybernetic approach used in much of the above work on flies. However, the resulting data on dipterans are among the few available for the whole important order. On a qualitative level, they demonstrate a far more general importance of natural polarized light for the behavior of insects than has previously been recognized.

To begin with the mosquito results, one might not expect that the nocturnal or crepuscular behavior usually attributed to these insects would have any relation to natural polarized light. Actually, however, mosquito dispersal flights and short range migrations from rest areas to feeding and ovipositing sites are frequently carried out in open regions under daylight skies. Previous work had proved that such flights are guided by landmarks, but Wellington found that these long roving flights only take place when the zenith sky is substantially polarized.

Mosquitoes of the genera *Aedes* and *Culex*, the species seemed unimportant, have two types of flight under the conditions of these observations made in southwestern Canada. Short range attack flights against the observer were made by resting insects, with or without natural polarized light. Long range roving flights, observed under broken forest canopy or in open clearings, only occurred under certain light conditions. If place and season were chosen for a rather sparse mosquito population, it was possible to follow, in some detail, the long straight courses of the roving flights, once the short range attackers had been eliminated. Documentation consisted of several hundred long flights observed per day at a number of locations and times during the season.

α) *Sky Polarization Dependence.* Two sky conditions, involving changes in polarized light, abruptly terminated the long flights. First, when clouds covered the zenith sky, this flight pattern was no longer observed. Then, when the sun was near the zenith, no such long distance flyers generally were seen for a sustained period. The duration and indeed occurrence of this diurnal inactive period, around local noon, depended on latitude and season. Thus, near the summer solstice, the inactive period was about 2.75 h; decreasing as the summer progressed until, by the end of August, both short and long range flights occurred all day under a cloudless sky.

The duration of the inactive period was shown to coincide, with great precision, with the period during which the sun's elevation angle was 60° or more. No local meteorological factors (e.g., temperature, radiant heating, air movement) were significantly correlated with the noontime pause. In contrast, the sun's altitude hypothesis checked very well with latitudinal, as well as seasonal differences in the sun's course through the sky. Also, a somewhat hazy sky, which would decrease sky polarization and render direct sunlight more diffuse, increases the inactive period to coincide with a solar elevation of 58.5° or greater. When the sun's elevation was less than the critical angle, a cloud covering the sun, but not the zenith, generally did not disrupt long straight flights. Seasonal differences in directional precision of long range flights suggested that, in dispersal flight, the insects were predominantly maintaining East West compass directions.

β) *Extension to Many Other Insects.* There are two additional points of interest in these data: (1) when roving mosquitoes were caught and tested on the ground under a sheet of Polaroid, a 90° rotation of its principal axis evoked a walking turn in the same direction, but when clouds covered the zenith, no response could be elicited by changing the imposed *e*-vector direction; and (2) two aspects of the mosquitoes' behavior pattern were shared by a large range of other kinds of insects observed incidentally.

First, various muscoid flies, sawflies, wasps, hornets, halictine bees, dragonflies, and bumblebees were all noted flying straight courses when the roving mosquitoes were active. These others also became inactive when the rovers did, except for bumblebees which are otherwise known to have strong landmark orientation (Wellington, 1974a). Second, when caught and tested on the ground under a polarizer, all, including *Bombus*, responded to *e*-vector rotation quite like mosquitoes.

Furthermore, later observations made on the dronefly *Eristalis*, as well as some beetles, wasps, and butterflies, (WELLINGTON, 1976b) confirmed and extended the general conclusions drawn from the earlier ones. Both resident and transient insects in this second wide range of groups were shown to have markedly reduced ranges of flight activity correlated with reduced sky polarization in the zenith (Fig. 150).

Obviously, there is an important area of physiological investigation suggested by these field data. The sharpness of the sun elevation cutoff seems particularly striking and may have important diagnostic significance relative to the mechanism of sky polarotaxis (for general discussion, KIRSCHFELD et al., 1975; WEHNER, 1976b). The close similarity of behavior patterns in different mosquito species, also shared with a wide range of other flying insects, implies that explanations derived from further study of these phenomena should have very general importance. Note from Fig. 1 that for an ideal RAYLEIGH sky zenith, p would only be 14% with the sun's zenith angle $= 30°$; for a sky with $p_{max} = 0.7$, the corresponding zenith p would be only 5%, which is considerably below the few known polarization sensitivity thresholds.

b) Compound Eye Organization

Fly (e.g., Diptera, Brachycera) eyes are highly developed, apparently apposition, receptors typically having a large number of ommatidia [e.g., about 3,200 in *Musca* (BRAITENBERG, 1967), about 5,800 in *Calliphora* (WADA, 1974b)] arranged in a strikingly regular convex array (Fig. 100). Facets are located at the intersections of two concentric series of arcs; one dorsal in origin and the other ventral (GEMPERLEIN, 1969). Usually, however, their pattern is described with three axes, appropriate where the packing is hexagonal; x and y for short sectors of these two diagonal arcs and z for horizontal rows, as cited above, for hymenopterans (BRAITENBERG, 1967). The strong regularity of facet arrangement extends internally to incredibly detailed patterning of retinulas (Figs. 101 and 102), rhabdomeres (Figs. 102 and 103), neurommatidia (Figs. 104 and 105), and their interconnections (Figs. 101 and 106) (BRAITENBERG and STRAUSFELD, 1973; STRAUSFELD, 1976a).

α) Typical Ommatidia. Each retinula has eight photoreceptor cells and the corresponding rhabdom is the classic case of an open one. At any given cross section level in the retinula, seven cells are arranged around an intercellular axial space, into which their optically isolated rhabdomeres protrude. Roughly, the rhabdomeres of R 1–R 6 form a peripheral ring-like array and those of R 7 and R 8 comprise a central column thrust axially into the intercellular space by a flange-like extension of their respective cell bodies. These photoreceptor organelles typically have minute diameters [i.e., R 1–R 6 2 μm distally tapering to 1 μm proximally; R 7 and R 8 1 μm (SNYDER, 1973)], but are long. Thus, R 1–R 6 are as much as 200 μm in length, but R 7 was cited at 130 μm and R 8 at 70 μm (Fig. 107). Thus, R 7 is about $^2/_3$ and R 8 $^1/_3$ of the overall rhabdom length (BOSCHEK, 1971).

Obviously, if self absorption were important, e-vector, and λ, discrimination theoretically would be better in the shorter rhabdomeres, although their absolute sensitivity would be less for the same absorption per unit length (SNYDER, 1973,

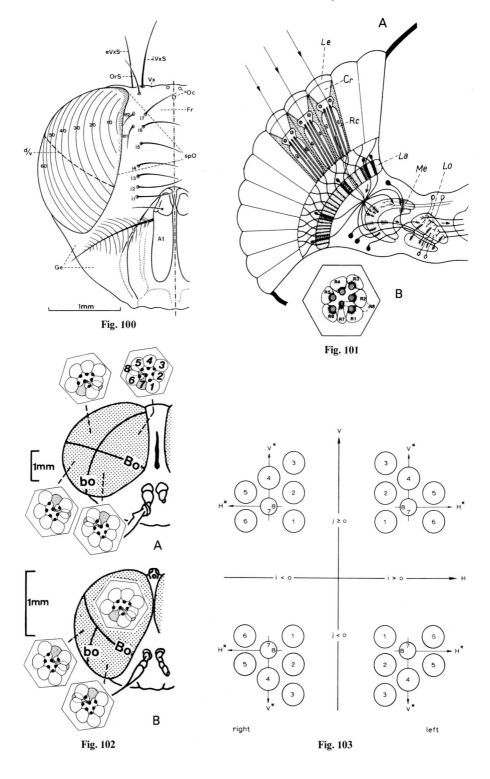

Fig. 100

Fig. 101

Fig. 102

Fig. 103

1975 b). Note also that R 7 and R 8, because of their smaller diameters (SNYDER and PASK, 1973), would admit less light, have higher spatial transmission frequencies, and should have their effective absorption λ_{max} shifted to shorter λ. They may also have special optical behavior arising from the dielectric waveguide properties inherent in their small diameter, greater refractive index than their surround, and the ultraviolet λ_{max} of R 7 (KIRSCHFELD and SNYDER, 1975).

Typically, the rhabdomeres of R 7 and R 8 are in tandem coaxially, in that order. Consequently, R 7 would act as a dichroic and chromatic filter for R 8 (GRIBAKIN, 1975); the fact that the two sets of microvilli in these rhabdomeres are orthogonal could result in a substantial increase in polarization sensitivity. However, recall that fly R 7, with a transverse principal axis, is an exception to the general rule that ϕ_{max} is parallel to rhabdomere microvilli (see below for further discussion).

In each fly rhabdom, the optically isolated rhabdomeres are organized in a trapezoidal pattern, with the parallel sides vertical and the longer one always anterior–medial. As already noted by DIETRICH (1909), the trapezoids in the dorsal and ventral halves of the retina are mirror images so that the acute angle of the figure is oriented dorsally in the dorsal half and ventrally in the ventral half of the retina (Fig. 103).

Using DIETRICH's numbering, R 1–R 3 form the longer parallel side, with R 3 at the apex. The cell body of R 7 is always between R 1 and R 8. Thus, its rhabdomere is supported from the ventral side of the trapezoid in the dorsal retina and from the dorsal side in the ventral. Note that, while the asymmetry readily allows each rhabdomere to be identified, the numbering sequence requires care. In the dorsal half of the right eye, it is counterclockwise, as observed from the outside, whereas in the left eye it is clockwise in the corresponding region; these sequences are reversed in the right and left lower halves.

A further patterning is evident in the location of the cell body of R 8 (Fig. 102). In most of the flies studied physiologically (e.g., *Musca, Calliphora, Eristalis*, and *Drosophila*), it is always located between R 1 and R 2 (WADA, 1975). However, in 24 species in nine families, R 8 occurred regularly between R 5 and R 6 instead of

---

◄ **Figs. 100–103.** Geometry of dipteran compound eyes. **Fig. 100.** Frontal view of right half of ♀*Calliphora* head showing compound eye and ocelli *(Oc)*. Broken line on cornea (d/v) is the border between dorsal and ventral halves of the eye. Arcs of facets are drawn and numbered for every tenth row. *At* = antenna, *spo* = special marginal ocelli discussed in text. (WADA, 1974 b). **Fig. 101.** Dipteran visual system. **A** Diagram showing corneal lens *(Le)*, crystalline cone *(Cr)*, retinular cell *(Rc)*, primary photoreceptor fibers crossing over, and some major interneurons of the lamina *(La)*, medulla *(Me)*, and lobula *(Lo)* (compare Figs. 104–106). **B** Cross section of single ommatidium showing R 1–R 8 and the open rhabdom. For more specific pattern data, see Figs. 102 and 103. (HEISENBERG and BUCHNER, 1977). **Fig. 102.** Comparison of two characteristic dipteran retinal types differing as shown by the presence in the dorsal anterior quadrant of Type A (♀ tabanid) of a retinular pattern absent in Type B (♂ *Rhagio*), where the whole dorsal retina is uniform in this regard. The arcs Bo and bo represent the quadrant boundaries. (WADA, 1975). **Fig. 103.** Rhabdomere patterns seen from outside in four quadrants of a dipteran right eye with a Fig. 102 Type A pattern. Note upper and lower quadrant patterns are mirror images about the horizontal *(H)* axis. The left eye would be a mirror image about the vertical *(V)* axis. The *i* and *j* indices are for assigning matrix locations to ommatidia relative to the *H* and *V* coordinates. (STAVENGA, 1975)

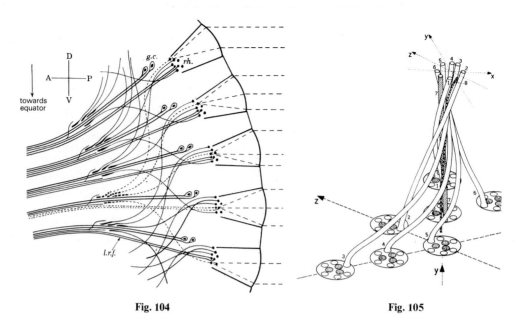

Fig. 104   Fig. 105

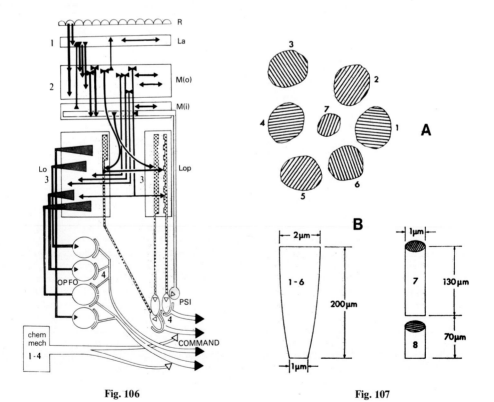

Fig. 106   Fig. 107

its usual location in the higher flies. Thus, in tabanids, the 5/8/6 pattern occurs in both dorsal and ventral anterior quadrants, but, in rhagionid ♂♂'s, it is restricted only to the posterior ventral quadrant.

β) *Special Marginal Ommatidia.* If, as is generally done, R 7 and R 8 are assumed to be critically involved in polarization sensitivity, their geometric patterns may be correlated with processing the relevant information. Furthermore, in certain restricted marginal areas of the fly retina, there are strongly atypical relations between R 1–R 6 and R 7 and R 8 (WADA, 1974a). In all 29 species observed from a wide ranging sample of 13 families, some ommatidia in dorsofrontal margins of the eyes have quite distinctive fine structural features (Fig. 100). These could substantially alter their functional properties from those hypothesized from the typical predominant rhabdom pattern discussed above. The dioptric elements appeared normal.

R 7 and R 8, however, are significantly larger, as shown by their distal tip cross section area. These are greater by factors ranging from 1.3 to 17. Such enlarged rhabdomeres were found in both sexes and were not dependent on the state of light or dark adaptation. Clearly, this larger size could affect all the properties attributed to typical R 7 and R 8, dependent on their tiny diameters. Usually, enlargement of the central column rhabdomeres in marginal ommatidia was accompanied by reduction in the cross sectional areas of the R 1–R 6 rhabdomeres or, in some cases, with their disappearance. Consequently, the operational relations between these two groups of retinular cells must be quite modified in marginal units. In *Calliphora*, for example, the ommatidial population concerned is 3.2% of the total facet count (WADA, 1974b).

Particularly interesting, in relation to polarization sensitivity, is WADA's discovery that, in these dipteran marginal ommatidia, R 7 and R 8 may not be only in tandem, as is typical for most species studied (WADA, 1971, 1974a). In several families of flies, excluding *Musca, Calliphora, Eristalis,* or *Drosophila,* R 7 and R 8 rhabdomeres are, in addition, segmented into alternating sections contributed by the two cells. For each one, their microvilli are parallel, but, in the alternating band, they are orthogonal. Thus, R 7 and R 8 are toothed and partly "in parallel" to one another. In some marginal ommatidia of the tabanid, *Haematopoda,* there are 11 layers in this double unit.

◄ Figs. 104–107. Internal patterns of dipteran visual systems. **Fig. 104.** Diagram illustrating neural superposition in five adjacent ommatidia of a dipteran eye illuminated by parallel light rays. These activate different retinular cells in every ommatidium of a patch of seven, but one of each of the retinular cell series R 1–R 6 converge (shown by broken lines for the cartridge in line with number 4) on a single lamellar *(L)* cartridge and synapse with monopolar cells *(g.c.).* Axons of R 7 and R 8 (lrf) can be seen to pass through the lamina. (HORRIDGE and MEINERTZHAGEN, 1970b). **Fig. 105.** Diagram illustrating distribution of eight axons from one retinula; note R 1–R 6 are systematically distributed to cartridges located under adjacent ommatidia. Three monopolar units (stippled) are shown in each cartridge, as well as the facet pattern axes x, y, and z. (BRAITENBERG, 1967). **Fig. 106.** Diagram summarizing the main channels connecting the retina *(R)* through the optic lobe *(La, M,* and *Lo)* to the protocerebrum in a succession of neuropils (numbered 1–4). Consult original for further details. Compare with Fig. 65 for the decapod crustacean pattern. (STRAUSFELD, 1976b). **Fig. 107.** Diagram showing microvillus pattern **A** of open dipteran rhabdom, as well as shape and relations of its rhabdomeres **B**. Note the strong compression of the axial scale! (SNYDER, 1973)

In various other species reported, there are 3–7. As reviewed above (e.g., for decapod crustaceans) such orthogonal banding should tend optically to optimize polarization sensitivity, λ discrimination, and absolute sensitivity. Nothing is known as yet whether or not these interesting marginal ommatidia function as this suggests or how they contribute to the normal behavioral repertoire of their possessors. In fact, there seems little evidence in the literature that the broadly based detailed analysis by Wada has so far been noticed.

γ) *Neural Superposition*. Another striking feature of the dipteran eye is that, although its dioptric system and screening pigment apparently conform to Exner's apposition type, there are important specialized differences (Kirschfeld, 1973c). Usually, all retinular cells in each ommatidium of the classic type share the same visual field corresponding to the admittance angle of the unit's dioptric system. In contrast, individual retinular cells (i.e., R 1–R 6) in dipterans each have different, but rather precisely oriented, visual fields (Figs. 29, 101, and 104).

Hence, a rather surprising kind of mosaic forming independence may be present in a single ommatidium, as suggested long ago (Dietrich, 1909). Actually, distinct fields for each rhabdomere were first demonstrated optically (Autrum and Wiedemann, 1962; Kuiper, 1962), but axon tracing was required to discover their significance (Trujillo-Cenóz and Melamed, 1966; Braitenberg, 1967; Kirschfeld, 1967, 1969; Horridge and Meinertzhagen, 1970b). Instead of forming a crude "image" within each retinula, optical independence of the rhabdomeres permits them to multiply the sensitivity of the system sixfold. In fact, this summation apparently acts not by increasing the signal strength (i.e., S), but by reducing noise (i.e., N) to $^1/_6$, which correspondingly improves S/N (Scholes, 1969; Smola, 1976).

The convergence Kirschfeld found was that a different rhabdomere in each of six adjacent ommatidia shared the same field of view and corresponded to the bundle of six axons terminating in one cartridge (i.e., neuroommatidium) in the lamina (Trujillo-Cenóz and Melamed, 1966). Another set, having a slightly different field of view, converged on another cartridge and so on until all of R 1–R 6 participated (Figs. 101, 104, and 105). In contrast, R 7 and R 8 are not involved in this neural superposition. Their axons do not terminate or synapse in the lamina, but continue straight through to the medulla (Fig. 106). They are, therefore, long visual axons like those of R 8 in decapod crustaceans (Fig. 67) and R 1, R 5, and R 9 in *Apis* (Fig. 83) and ants (Wehner, 1976b).

δ) *Hypothesis of Two Retinular Subsystems*[9]. Because of their differences, experimental work mainly using optomotor and microspectrophotometric techniques has tested the possibility that the retinula is divided in two subsystems (Kirschfeld and Franceschini, 1968; Kirschfeld, 1973c). In general, R 1–R 6 do seem to comprise a low threshold scotopic component, which also has low contrast transfer. A high threshold photopic component (i.e., 24–48 × less sensitive than the scotopic [Eckert, 1973]) having high contrast transfer is mediated by R 7 and R 8. Strong migration of pigment granules near the rhabdomeres establishes a scotopic pupil-like response for R 1–R 6; an independent photopic "pupil" oper-

---

[9] A somewhat similar duplex system was recently hypothesized for hymenopterans (Wehner, 1976b). Near orientation was proposed to be mediated by R 2–R 4 and R 6–R 8 and far orientation including polarotaxis, by the ultraviolet receptors with long primary axons R 1, R 5, and R 9 (Fig. 83)

ating in a similar manner in R 7 has a threshold 2 log units higher than that for R 1–R 6 (FRANCESCHINI and KIRSCHFELD, 1976).

Such a duality is consistent with the difference in rhabdomere diameters and lengths (Fig. 107); however, the overall system seems to be considerably more complex than that (MORING and JÄRVILEHTO, 1977). Indeed, recent experimental results imply that at least some revision is needed in this duplex hypothesis, including its relation to polarization sensitivity (HEISENBERG and BUCHNER, 1977); however, opinion on this is not unanimous (HARDIE, 1977; KIRSCHFELD et al., 1978).

c) Electrophysiology

α) *Polarization Sensitivity.* Electrophysiological studies in *Calliphora* have demonstrated rather modest polarization sensitivity in the photoreceptor cells. Thus, no *e*-vector discrimination could be observed in the electroretinogram (AUTRUM and STUMPF, 1950), but intracellular recordings demonstrated $S_p = 2.0$ with white or blue (478 nm) light, but not with 603 nm light (BURKHARDT and WENDLER, 1960). Not all impaled retinular cells showed polarization sensitivity. Similar inconsistency was reported for R 1–R 6 by some workers (JÄRVILEHTO and MORING, 1974, 1976; MORING and JÄRVILETHO, 1977), but not by others (MCCANN and ARNETT, 1972; MCCANN et al., 1977). This recent work confirmed low $S_p = 1.4$–2.6 (JÄRVILEHTO and MORING, 1976) or 2.0 (MCCANN et al., 1977). Polarization sensitive retinular cells show faster dark adaptation and better temporal resolution than morphologically similar cells not polarization sensitive (MORING and JÄRVILEHTO, 1977).

Different cells gave a rather wide range of ϕ_{max} (Fig. 108); two perpendicular directions seemed favored by JÄRVILEHTO and MORING (Fig. 109), but three separated by 60° were suggested by the others. No evidence of polarization sensitivity was detected in 1) cartridges (SCHOLES, 1969), 2) monopolar cells (JÄRVILEHTO and MORING, 1976), or 3) sustaining or on–off fibers recorded in the external chiasma (MCCANN et al., 1977). These negative results were interpreted to mean that indiscriminate integration of the R 1–R 6 input does, in fact, occur in the neuroommatidium, as indicated by the morphology (Fig. 109).

β) *Rotating e-Vector.* However, GEMPERLEIN and SMOLA (1973) had previously also found in *Calliphora* that, with a rotating polarizer, the *e*-vector discrimination of retinular cells varied with $d\phi/dt$ reaching a maximum at 18 Hz/π, where S_p doubled its value of 2.07 in the static case. As in crustaceans (YAMAGUCHI, 1967; LEGGETT, 1976; YAMAGUCHI et al., 1976) and beetles (ZOLOTOV and FRANTSEVICH, 1977), this indicates that static *e*-vectors, used in most experiments, may not be an adequate test for significant polarization sensitivity.

For various reasons, the photopic system of R 7 and R 8 has generally been favored as including the operational polarization sensitivity channel and the scotopic system rejected for this function. Evidence supporting such a decision has come from several sources obviously including the electrophysiological results above. In addition, optomotor experiments with *Musca* demonstrate that alternating stripes of polarizer with orthogonal *e*-vectors evoke responses under conditions that suggest the responsible subsystem is R 7 and R 8 and not R 1–R 6 (KIRSCHFELD and REICHARDT, 1970).

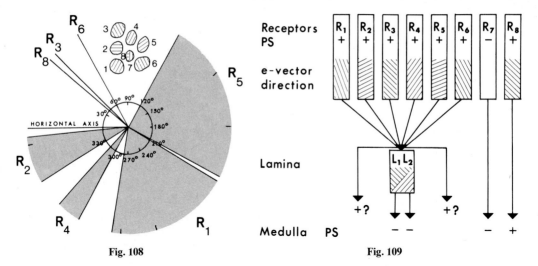

Figs. 108 and 109. Polarization sensitivity in the *Calliphora* compound eye. (JÄRVILEHTO and MORING, 1976). **Fig. 108.** Intracellular recordings from retinular cell somata (R 1–R 6 and R 8) showed R 1–R 6 were inconsistent in their *e*-vector sensitivity, both in its presence and in the location of its ϕ_{max} shown in this diagram. R 1 and R 5, particularly, had a wide range of maximal sensitivities as shown. Small diagram indicates microvillus directions of the eight rhabdomeres present. **Fig.109.** Diagram summarizing retinal polarization sensitivity (Fig. 108) and its implications for more central information processing. Sensitivity to *e*-vector indicated by plus, its absence by a minus. As shown by the hatching in the retinular cell boxes, ϕ_{max} for R 1, R 3, R 6, and R 8 seemed roughly 90° to that in R 2, R 4, and R 5 (compare Fig. 108). $L1$ and $L2$ are laminar interneurons

d) Optomotor Responses

To begin with, the fly response required that, as in the bee but not in *Carcinus*, the stripe *e*-vectors are at $\pm 45°$ to the animal's vertical axis. To discriminate whether or not R 1–R 6 or R 7 and R 8 were specifically involved, black and white optomotor patterns of appropriate angular subtent were used and the ϕ of a linear polarizer, placed between the eye and the moving stripes, was changed systematically.

Both the 12° and 2.8° stripe periods used produced sinusoidal turning response as a function of ϕ, with minima and maxima at $\pm 45°$. With the narrow stripes in both white light or long visible wavelength, the responses were similar and marked by no torque at the minimum. In comparison, using wide stripes and only long wavelengths, the *e*-vector direction did not affect the optomotor response. In white light, the wide stripe response was ϕ sensitive, but the minimal response had a value about 0.5 of the maximum.

When the functional properties of R 7, R 8 are examined, however, their qualifications, including a central role in polarization sensitivity among their other responsibilities, are not yet unambiguous. The optomotor evidence just mentioned and the series, or in a few cases banded, close association of their rhabdomeres with orthogonal microvilli could certainly be interpreted to support such a role. However, there are other data which suggest that R 7 and R 8 have quite different operational characteristics from each other. Hence, the retinular system may have three distinctive channels rather than two. Furthermore, recent, but unpublished, experiments suggest some revision will be required in the interpretation of dipteran optomotor responses in polarized light (HEISENBERG and BUCHNER, 1977).

e) Evidence for Three Retinular Channels

Thus, the *Musca* optomotor experiments, implicating the R 7 and R 8 system in polarization sensitivity, also showed that the responsible component was not ultraviolet sensitive, but had its λ_{max} near 464 nm. In *Drosophila*, R 7 is a single peak ultraviolet cell and R 8 is a double peak ultraviolet–blue receptor (STARK, 1975). Three pigments appear to be present in the *Calliphora* retina; in addition to the typical ultraviolet and green elements generally recognized in flies' R 1–R 6, a blue one has been found, presumably in R 7 and R 8 (ECKERT, 1971; MEFFERT and SMOLA, 1976). In fact, three types of units have now been recorded in this R 7 and R 8 system: ultraviolet, blue, and ultraviolet–blue (SMOLA and MEFFERT, 1977).

In direct recordings from marked R 7 and R 8 in *Calliphora*, R 7 showed no polarization sensitivity to static flashes, but the one case of a marked R 8, whose responses were recorded, was *e*-vector sensitive [10]. Its S_p, also determined with brief flashes, was low at 1.8 (JÄRVILEHTO and MORING, 1976). This, among other things, suggests that the two cells of the R 7 and R 8 system have quite different functions and properties. Perhaps they generally need to be considered separately.

As in the honeybee and ants, the dipteran receptor unit, thought to be responsible for polarization sensitivity, has apparently retreated to a single hard to study element in the depths of the retinula. Unequivocal data are so few that we cannot tell yet whether or not an explanation, so dependent on one "cryptic" cell in each ommatidium, is reasonable. It seems more likely that some interactive mechanism is sharpening and amplifying the basic polarization sensitivity input.

f) Interaction Between R 1–R6 and R 7 and R 8

There is currently considerable evidence for functional coupling of the R 1–R 6 and R 7 and R 8 systems in ways which involve polarization sensitivity. Although the results appear somewhat contradictory, their implications are, nonetheless, important. For example, stimulation of R 7 and R 8 in *Musca*, using fixed linearly polarized light, has been shown to inhibit responses of R 1–R 6 in a neighboring ommatidium [11], given phase shifted periodic stimulation (KIRSCHFELD and LUTZ, 1974). The strength of this inhibition depends strongly (i.e., 1 : 100) on ϕ of the R 7 and R 8 system's stimulus. Already, such strong dynamic effects seem more promising in explaining polarization sensitivity than the many weak static sensitivities previously demonstrated in insects electrophysiologically and by microspectrophotometry. The details of the observed R 7 and R 8 vs. R 1–R 6 interactions were such that this sort of powerful effect could be related not only to polarization sensitivity per se, but also to color and pattern discrimination, as well as light and dark adaptation. Thus, inhibitory action, specifically of R 8 on R 1–

---

[10] $S_p = 2.65$ for R 7 and $S_p = 5.60$ for R 8 were estimated from optical principles (SNYDER, 1973)

[11] Note that movement responses and optomotor responses can be induced by stimulating a single ommatidium (KIRSCHFELD, 1973 c)

R 6[12], has been postulated to account for phototactic responses of *Drosophila* in a T-maze (JACOB et al., 1977). This implies an important correlation between the natural polarized light input and a broad area of insect visual behavior.

g) Effect of φ on Object Fixation.

Some of the most interesting research on dipteran vision has been done on object fixation by flying flies (review, REICHARDT and POGGIO, 1976). This has been studied mainly for azimuth orientation around the vertical axis, but has also been explored for horizontal orientation around the transverse axis (WEHRHAHN and REICHARDT, 1975). Later, it was found that the intensity threshold for fixation of a horizontal stripe coincided with the threshold for the photopic R 7 and R 8 system in *Musca* (WEHRHAHN, 1976). Since optomotor responses mediated by R 7 and R 8 have been found to be dependent on φ (KIRSCHFELD and REICHARDT, 1970; KIRSCHFELD and LUTZ, 1974), the fixation response was also tested for such a dependence (Fig. 110).

Precision of fixation turned out to be systematically correlated with φ; being maximum when the *e*-vector was perpendicular to the eyes' horizontal meridian and minimum when it was parallel to it (Fig. 111). The amplitude of this effect can be gauged by the fact that a 90° rotation of the *e*-vector was equivalent to a $27 \pm 10 \times$ change in light intensity. Here again, polarized light is tied in strongly with one of the basic functions of the insect visual system.

Further, complex evidence for retinal interactions affecting polarization sensitivity among other things has recently been reported from a localized area of *Eristalis*' retina (TSUKAHARA and HORRIDGE, 1977 b). Some anterior retinulas contain receptor cells, believed to be R 1–R 6, which show rather strange properties (e.g., slightly shifting their optic axis with λ). Their spectral response curves are rather flat from 380 nm to 530 nm and they do not subscribe to the principle of univariance (NAKA and RUSHTON, 1966), which means that the number of photons they absorb per unit time is not the only thing which determines their response.

h) Anomalous Retinular Cells

The polarization sensitivity of these unusual retinular cells exhibits the remarkable property that ϕ_{max} depends on λ, with an abrupt shift occurring over a narrow λ-band. One example had ϕ_{max} at about 45° with $\lambda = 474$ nm; a sharp phase shift occurred around 500 nm and at 523 nm ϕ_{max} was at about 150° (Fig. 112). Different cells of this kind exhibit different angular displacements of ϕ_{max}. The overall data suggest that their unorthodox properties are due to interactions with one or more neighboring receptor cells having different ϕ_{max} and λ_{max}. The authors cautiously suggest that the observed effects might be a one-way influence of R 8 on an R 1–R 6 type.

Actually, the situation in the *Eristalis* retina and that of other brachyceran dipterans is considerably more complex than this. As has been well known since BURKHARDT's (1962) intracellular recordings in *Calliphora* retinular cells (JÄRVILEHTO

---

[12] Lateral inhibition, related to reduction in the visual field of lamina monopolar cells, has been found not to be related to R 7 and R 8, but to R 1–R 6 (SMOLA, 1976)

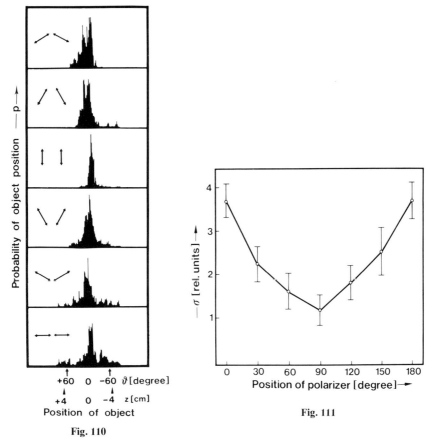

Fig. 110

Fig. 111

Figs. 110 and 111. Dependence of visual fixation accuracy in flying *Musca* on *e*-vector orientation. (WEHRHAHN, 1976). **Fig. 110.** *E*-vector directions of two monocular fields illuminating the eyes near intensity threshold were varied to match the mirror image pattern of the rhabdoms of the two eyes, as shown by the pairs of double-headed arrows. In fixating the fly controls the position of a small horizontal stripe through a closed loop system activated by flight lift induced torque. Best fixation occurred with both fields vertically polarized; worst with horizontal *e*-vectors on both sides. **Fig. 111.** Strong influence of ϕ on precision of orientation is made clear by average values of position histogram half width data (Fig. 110) plotted as a function of ϕ_r and ϕ_1 relative to the horizontal (0°). Best fixation to vertical *e*-vectors was correlated by the author with the microvillus orientation of R7 and R8 in the specific retinal area involved. (WEHRHAHN, 1976)

and MORING, 1976), most fly photoreceptors of the R1–R6 type have distinctly two-peaked responses. One peak is near 360 nm, the other for muscid flies about 490 nm (Fig. 113), and in *Eristalis* near 450 nm. In *Calliphora*, it had been shown (HORRIDGE and MIMURA, 1975) that $\phi_{\max}$ of retinular cells changed with λ and rather abruptly.

Thus, for the ultraviolet peak, $\phi_{\max}$ had a different direction than $\phi_{\max}$ for the green peak by angles that could range from 10° to 90° clockwise or anticlockwise (Fig. 114). The switchover zone was near 400 nm. The authors concluded that two distinct visual pigments were present in each cell, these were presumed to be segre-

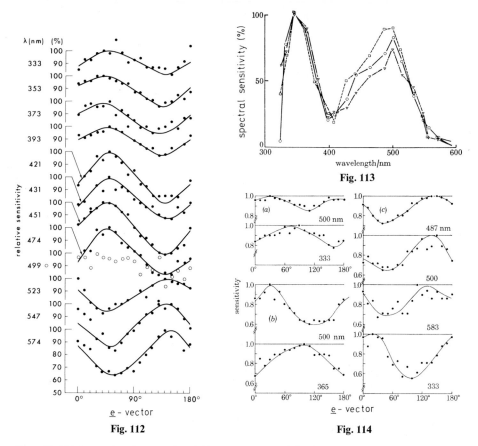

Fig. 113

Fig. 112

Fig. 114

Figs. 112–114. Interactions between ϕ and λ in receptor potentials of dipteran retinular cells. **Fig. 112.** Relative polarization sensitivity of an *Eristalis* unit determined at 12 λ's from 333 nm to 574 nm. Near 500 nm, the major absorption axis shifted about 150°. This was attributed to interaction between unlike neighboring retinular cells. (TSUKAHARA and HORRIDGE, 1977b). **Fig. 113.** Spectral sensitivities of three typical double-peaked retinular cells (350 and 500 nm) in *Calliphora*. (HORRIDGE and MIMURA, 1975). **Fig. 114.** Polarization sensitivities of *Calliphora* units (similar to the one in Fig. 113) showing 60° shifts in ϕ_{max} when stimulus λ was shifted from one absorption peak to the other (Fig. 113). This was attributed to more than one visual pigment segregated in different parts of the rhabdomere having correspondingly different microvillus directions. (HORRIDGE and MIMURA, 1975)

gated at different levels in the same rhabdomere, and the microvillus directions must twist abruptly at the transition depth. Such an hypothesized switch for the fly is reminiscent of the sudden-twist rhabdoms reported to occur in the ant *Myrmecia*, in addition to types gradually rotating clockwise and anticlockwise (MENZEL, 1975c).

In attempting to extend these *Calliphora* results, similar intracellular recordings were made in the retina of *Eristalis* (HORRIDGE et al., 1975). Cells with one, two, or three λ-peaks were encountered, but the typical fly two-peaked receptor potentials predominated. As in *Calliphora*, these two-peaked units had different ϕ_{max}'s at different λ's. Cells presumed to be R7 or R8 did not have high polarization sensitivity. Single peaked retinular cells showed no such dependency of ϕ_{max} on λ. Again, the authors concluded that two or more visual pigments were present in single receptor cells and segregated in rhabdomere regions with different transverse microvillus directions.

Note, however, that TSUKAHARA and HORRIDGE (1977b) did not attribute to two pigments in the same rhabdomere the similar shift in ϕ_{max} with λ observed in the peculiar retinular cells violating invariance. As mentioned above, this was explained as dependent on functional coupling with neighboring cells having different ϕ_{max} and λ_{max}. Still, a third mechanism was proposed to account for the familiar double peaked curve of standard orthodoxly invariant R 1–R 6 cells of *Eristalis* (TSUKAHARA and HORRIDGE, 1977a).

i) Hypothesis for a Sensitizing Pigment

On the basis of chromatic adaptation measurements, they concluded that a modest ultraviolet peak near 360 nm could be only the β peak of a single rhodopsin peaking at 450 nm. The variable, but often pronounced, ultraviolet peak[13] frequently found at the same λ in these cells was thought to depend not on the visual pigment directly, but perhaps on an ultraviolet "antenna" pigment, which is photostable. A single visual pigment hypothesis and the explanation of high ultraviolet sensitivity through an accessory pigment are consistent with the conclusion reached from vitamin A deprivation experiments on *Drosophila* (STARK et al., 1977).

In fact, a dichroic light-stable blue pigment, in addition to the well known photolabile visual pigment, was recently discovered in some, but not all, photopic units of *Musca* (KIRSCHFELD and FRANCESCHINI, 1977; KIRSCHFELD et al., 1977, 1978). Thus, both R 7 and R 8 occur in two forms, pale (i.e., p) without the accessory pigment and yellow (i.e., y) with it. The yellow pigment, perhaps a carotenoid, has a λ_{max} at 456 nm and in situ is itself dichroic with its principal axis perpendicular to the microvillus' axes. Hence, the anomalous orientation of this exceptional rhabdom's dichroism could result from the presence of secondary pigment in the photoreceptor membrane. Some of the seeming conflicts in measurements of polarization sensitivity and spectral sensitivity could also be results of this situation (KIRSCHFELD et al., 1978).

Comparison of the effect of light exposure on the dichroism of R 7 and R 8 is rather spectacular. In those rhabdomeres with the accessory blue pigment, Δ increases as the rhodopsin is isomerized. In the pale rhabdoms, Δ decreases as usual pari passu with bleaching of the visual pigment. Obviously, the presence of such an accessory pigment could have profound effects on polarization sensitivity by decreasing, increasing, or reversing the dichroism established by the rhodopsin system. Isomerization of rhodopsin, with the light linearly polarized parallel to the principal axis of the yellow pigment, was found to be faster than expected on the basis of a simple screening and absorbing model (KIRSCHFELD and FRANCESCHINI, 1977). This suggested that the accessory pigment might act as an antenna pigment absorbing photons and transferring energy so acquired to the photolabile pigment.

---

[13] Strong ultraviolet absorption was attributed to R 7 on the basis of only the physical effect of its small diameter (SNYDER and PASK, 1973)

j) Conclusion for Dipterans

While this interesting hypothesis might seem just a further complication on the way toward understanding the mechanism of polarization sensitivity, it could also, in a broader context, turn out to be an important application in vision of a principle known to be effectively exploited by plants in photosynthesis.

Unfortunately, in attempting to trace the relation of polarization sensitivity through these complex and still unsolved problems of dipteran visual function, we have learned mainly that the polarization sensitivity input channels and those for other parameters are probably interrelated in very elaborate ways (SMOLA, 1976). These may differ in various species, or even in individual retinular cells of the same species. Until they are better understood, the functional relevance of presently available information to polarized light perception is uncertain. The current state of knowledge does, however, indicate a number of crucial experiments which need to be done.

6. Other Insects

a) Compound Eye Organization

The preceding sections have reviewed the three insect types for which there is at least a moderately coherent body of data on their polarization sensitivity. There are, of course, many other kinds for which some direct or indirect data are available (WATERMAN, 1973; WELLINGTON, 1974a, and C.I.5.a.β). Most numerous are studies on the fine structure of compound eyes (Table 1 in GOLDSMITH and BERNARD, 1974; CHU et al., 1975; WACHMANN and SCHRÖER, 1975; HORRIDGE, 1976; HORRIDGE and HENDERSON, 1976; STONE and KOOPOWITZ, 1976[14]; HORRIDGE et al., 1977; KOLB, 1977). These contain relevant information on dioptrics, retinular structure, microvillus pattern, central connectivity, and so on. As demonstrated above, even for more thoroughly studied cases, well educated predictions can be far off target for complex partially known systems like these. Consequently, we should acknowledge the importance and interest of such morphological data meanwhile working toward the experimental pursuit of their functional implications.

b) Dragonflies (Odonata)

However, one exceptional case, the dragonflies, should be discussed further since some multidisciplinary research has, in fact, been done on this interesting group. Odonata are visual predators with relatively enormous well-developed eyes (Fig. 115). In the active flying migratory *Anax junius*, the compound eye has as many as 29,247 ommatidia in the adult (SHERK, 1977). While the influence of sky polarization on their behavior has not been studied, there are a number of reasons to think it may be important.

α) *Possible Oriented Behavior.* For example, active flyers frequently show regular patrolling patterns while seeking prey. These flights are sometimes remarkably

---

[14] In the moth *Galleria*, differential absorption of polarized light by the rhabdom was reported in fixed transverse sections

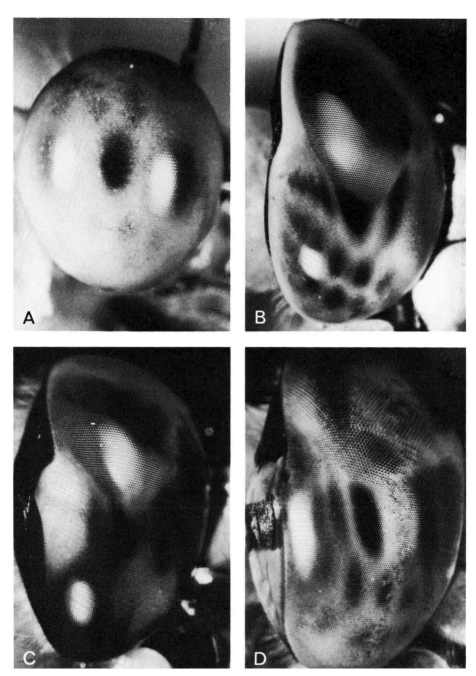

Fig. 115 A–D. Compound eyes of adult odonates seen in external lateral views of the right eye; up is dorsal and right is anterior. **A** *Lestes*, a primitive zygopteran with a relatively simple spheroidal eye. **B** *Aeschna multicolor*, **C** *Somatochlora (a corduliid)* and **D** *Sympetrum* (a libellulid) are examples of more advanced types with variously developed special dorsal eye regions with broader facets, smaller axial divergence, and longer rhabdoms. The dark retinal areas are pseudopupils or accessory pseudopupils. (SHERK, 1978)

straight and coupled by 90°, as well as 180°, sudden shifts of direction. At twilight, I have often observed aeschnids flying repeated linear patrols parallel to the band of strongly polarized skylight in the zenith (Fig. 7). With regard to compound eye structure, specialized retinal areas, defined by facet diameters and intraommatidial angles, are present in most species, but their details vary widely in various types (SHERK, 1977). In addition to those apparently related to predation and horizon stabilization, there are several kinds of dorsal retinal bands which might be specially adapted for looking at the sky polarization, as in *Cataglyphis* (C.I.4.b.α).

β) Compound Eye Organization. The most spectacular and specialized of these is again in *Anax junius* (SHERK, 1977). In its eye, a band shaped high resolution area, along the 56° anterodorsal meridian of the eye, concentrates a large fraction of the whole surface area of the eye into looking at a narrow strip of the visual field (Figs. 116 and 117). Thus, the number of ommatidial axes per square degree reaches a surprising peak of 5.9 in the densest point in this "foveal band." This is nearly 20 × the density of 0.3 found in a roughly symmetrical posterodorsal location. The operational significance of the highly specialized eye region is a matter of considerable interest, but not much data.

Dragonfly ommatidia (Fig. 118) are of the apposition type and have eight retinular cells (HORRIDGE, 1969; EGUCHI, 1971; ARMETT-KIBEL et al., 1977; LAUGHLIN and MCGINNESS, 1978). Our knowledge of their rhabdomere patterns and other relevant details is still incomplete. Consequently, it is difficult to sort out apparent differences, due to lack of information, from real variation among the different genera studied by various researchers. Unfortunately, again, the independent numbering of retinular cells by different investigators has produced four quite different systems; ARMETT-KIBEL et al. (1977, p. 405) tabulate three of them, but LAUGHLIN and MCGINNESS (1978) reporting on still another genus use a fourth and do not cite this 1977 work.

Part of the difficulty may arise from different types of retinulas in the same retina so well documented in crabs (KUNZE, 1968), hymenopterans (Figs. 79 and 81), and dipterans (Figs. 102 and 103). Indeed, quite distinct patterns have been reported in the dorsal and ventral halves of the *Hemicordulia* retina, as cited below. Meanwhile, since I use EGUCHI's illustration (Fig. 117), the following provisional account uses his numbering scheme and electron microscopic data from *Aeschna* (EGUCHI, 1971).

In this genus, as in several others studied, the rhabdom is thin and elongate, partially tiered, asymmetrical, and comprised of rhabdomere microvilli aligned in three main directions 120° apart. The retinular cells share these as follows: R 3, R 4; R 1, R 5; and R 2, R 6, R 7. R 7 has the most distal rhabdomere. Two retinular cells (R 2, R 5) are restricted to the proximal 20% of the retinular axis, where they are the only contributors to the rhabdom and the largest cell bodies in the cross section (Fig. 118 D). In the middle retinular region, cells R 1 and R 6 have the largest cell bodies. Each contributes to the rhabdom a sector about equal to or larger than the one jointly made up of the rhabdomeres of R 3 and R 4 (Fig. 118 C). Only near its distal end does R 7 bear a rhabdomere, its microvilli being parallel to those of R 6 (Fig. 118 A). No rhabdomere was observed in R 8 in *Aeschna* and the presumably corresponding cell (i.e., R 6) in *Sympetrum* (ARMETT-KIBEL et al., 1977).

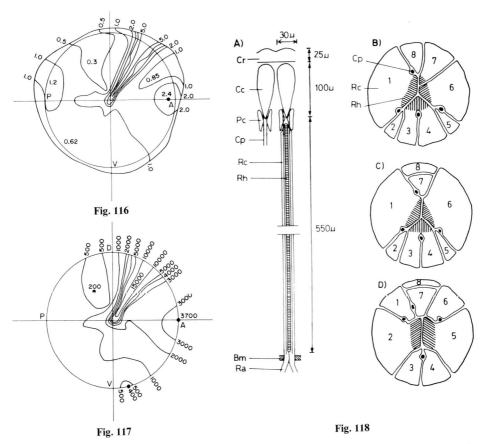

Fig. 116

Fig. 117

Fig. 118

Figs. 116–118. Structure of odonate compound eyes. **Figs. 116 and 117.** Map of anatomical features of the right visual hemisphere of the right eye of *Anax junius*. Axial separation of adjacent ommatidia, as well as their diameters, vary widely and have a systematic distribution. Two consequences of this are shown in the special "foveal" areas where, basically, one of these variables is minimal and the other maximal (SHERK, 1978). **Fig. 116.** Contours mapping the numbers of ommatidial axes within one square degree of visual space over the eye surface. Note that, in the anterodorsal band, this value is nearly 17 × greater than that in the minimum zone; in the anterior horizontal "fovea" it is only 8 × greater. **Fig. 117.** Very similar map produced by contours delimiting the μm² of eye surface devoted to looking at one square degree of visual space. Here, the corresponding ratio for the dorsal fovea vs. the minimum is 75 × and vs. the anterior one is 18.5 ×. **Fig. 118.** Ommatidial structure in the dorsal retina of *Aeschna* (EGUCHI, 1971). A Axial diagram of one complete ommatidium. **B, C,** and **D** Diagrammatic cross sections at distal, medial, and proximal levels of the retinula. Note that the rhabdom is tiered with different retinular cells contributing to the three directional microvillus pattern at various levels. No rhabdomere was observed in R 8. Similar ommatidial patterns have been described for various other dragonfly genera, but, as reviewed in the text, the dorsal retina of *Hemicordulia* is quite modified

Yet, what appears to be the same unit in *Hemicordulia* ("R 1" in LAUGHLIN and McGINNESS, 1978) does have a rhabdomere, but it is described as stunted.

In this genus, the ommatidia of the ventral retina are basically similar to those of *Aeschna* (dorsal half) and some other genera. EGUCHI (1971), ARMETT-KIBEL et al. (1977), LAUGHLIN and McGINNESS (1978) contain more detailed comparisons. But, in *Hemicordulia*, two orientations of this basic pattern have been found and

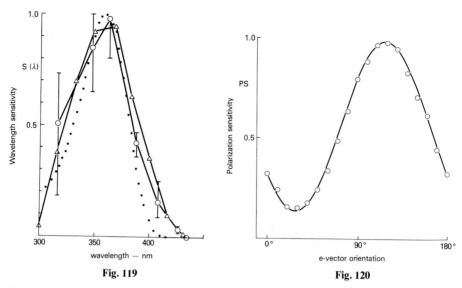

Fig. 119   **Fig. 120**

Figs. 119 and 120. Sensitivities of ultraviolet receptor cells of *Hemicordulia* ventral retina. Indirect evidence suggested these cells were R7 (Fig. 118), which has a distal rhabdomere only. (Laughlin, 1976a). **Fig. 119.** Wavelength sensitivity observed in two experimental series; vertical bars indicate total range of data points. For comparison, points show Dartnall nomogram of a visual pigment with its λ_{max} at 360 nm. **Fig. 120.** Polarization sensitivity of the same cell type shown in Fig. 119. Experimental points from one cell fitted with a curve of the form $PS = a + b \cos^2 \theta$, for which the recorded $S_p = 7.1$. One blue cell, as well as ultraviolet cells, yielded S_p's > 3; others had low S_p

identified by the orthogonal directions of their respective R1 microvilli. This particular retinular cell may be the ultraviolet cell with good polarization sensitivity determined electrophysiologically (Laughlin, 1976a).

A striking break from the *Aeschna* retinular pattern occurs in the highly modified ommatidial types present in *Hemicordulia*'s dorsal retina. Here, R1 and R6–R8 are vestigial, while the remaining four are larger and have rhabdomeres extending throughout the whole 800 µm of these very long retinulas. Note, however, that despite an attribution of "rudimentary" to one or four of them, all eight retinular cells, in both dorsal and ventral ommatidial types, give rise centrally to primary axons.

The significance of *Hemicordulia*'s special dorsal retina is presently somewhat conjectural, but current data and comparisons with other insects suggest that it provides an ultraviolet and blue sensitive area of heightened acuity correlated with crepuscular hunting against a highly polarized sky background (Laughlin and McGinness, 1978).

γ) Retinular Cell Responses. Recent results on *Hemicordulia* (Laughlin, 1976a) resemble earlier odonate data in indicating that there were, in the ventral retina, three light sensitivity peaks corresponding to rhodopsin λ_{max}'s at 350 nm (ultraviolet), 450 nm (blue), and 520 nm (green). Unlike some earlier cases, however, these were recorded separately in three kinds of single pigment receptor cells. Of these, the ultraviolet unit (Fig. 119) had a high $S_p = 7.0 \pm 1.7$ (Fig. 120) and the one blue unit encountered had a more modest $S_p = 3.3$; in *Hemianax*, blue cells were found with $S_p = 3$–6. Because of its distal recording site, the ultraviolet unit was postulated to be R 7, which contributes to the distal 17% of rhabdom length. This was consistent with the fact that the ultraviolet cell's ϕ_{max} was either 0° or 90° to the animal's longitudinal axis, which coincided with observed directions for R 7 microvillus axes.

The single pigment green cells were found to have low polarization sensitivity (i.e., $S_p < 2.5$) at their λ_{max}. Similarly, another category of "linked pigment" cells, which had a broad band response as if at least three rhodopsins were involved, showed $S_p < 2.5$. Complex interactions of polarization sensitivity and λ were evident in these cells. Thus, the ultraviolet single pigment cell apparently acts as a dichroic filter in front of the linked unit and self-absorption did not appear to be involved in the low polarization sensitivity in the long rhabdomeres. Relatively weak polarization sensitivity had been reported earlier for both nymphs and adults of *Anax* and *Libellula* (HORRIDGE, 1969). Various response patterns, relative to wavelength, eye region, and species, are reviewed in EGUCHI's (1971) discussion.

δ) Laminar Monopolar Cell Responses. Recordings from the optic lamina's monopolar cells (LAUGHLIN, 1976c) showed low levels of polarization sensitivity and broad λ sensitivity (i.e., $>40\%$ of the peak response at $\lambda_{max} =$ ca. 500 nm over the whole 317–614 nm range tested; $>75\%$ of the peak response between 400–570 nm). At 524 nm, S_p was only 1.09 ± 0.19, but at 315 nm, S_p was 1.84 ± 0.9, which was rather similar to the responses of the linked pigment retinular units. As in dipterans, convergence of receptor units of different ϕ_{max} and λ_{max} resulted in virtual cancellation of ϕ- and λ-discrimination. There was, however, a signal amplification at the first synapse representing a gain of about $14 \times$.

LAUGHLIN (1976a) suggests that the presence of strong polarization sensitivity in ultraviolet and, perhaps, blue receptors in the ventral retina of dragonflies might be useful over water by providing an artificial horizon from FRESNEL reflection of unpolarized light by the surface. However, the reflection from a natural water surface is much more likely, except with heavy cloud cover, to derive from the polarization of the piece of clear sky visible in the reflection (B.II.1.a.). However, as already mentioned (C.I.2.e.γ), the suggestion that the environmental polarization pattern, whatever its origin, could be used for stabilization of spatial orientation does seem important and deserves experimental study. The additional notion that orientation might be related to sky polarization perceived indirectly in reflection should also be considered. We have already seen (C.I.5.g.) that KIRSCHFELD's and WEHRHAHN's results proved that in dipterans there were strong interactions between ϕ and optomotor, as well as fixation responses.

II. Arthropod "Simple" (Ocellar) Eyes

In addition to compound eyes of widespread occurrence (i.e., crustaceans, insects, xiphosurans, eurypterids, trilobites, a few myriapods), there is an extraordinary range of small ocellar eyes in various arthropod types (BULLOCK and HOR-

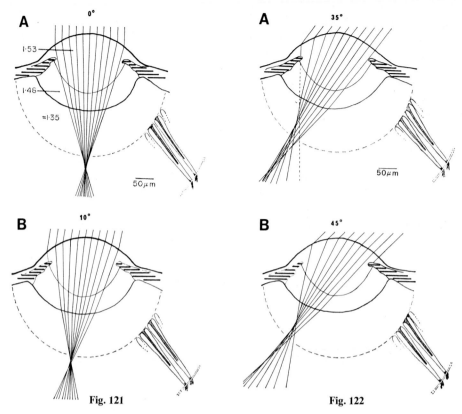

Figs. 121 and 122. Larval lateral ocellus of the sawfly *Perga*. Although the corneal lens is only 0.2 mm in diameter, there is a well developed retina with about 250 retinulas, each bearing an eight part rhabdom. (MEYER-ROCHOW, 1974). **Fig. 121.** Light rays on-axis (**A**, 0°), or nearly so (**B**, 10°), are well focused on the distal photoreceptive layer. **Fig. 122.** Light rays 35° (**A**) or 45° (**B**) off axis are not well focused by the dioptric system. Each rhabdom has microvilli oriented at 0°, 45°, 90°, and 135° in their respective rhabdomeres

RIDGE, 1965). Since these mediate polarization sensitivity in several diverse examples, the relevant functional and structural data are reviewed here.

Such ocelli, unlike compound eyes, have only a single dioptric system, unless it is absent altogether, projecting light onto a minute retina (Figs. 121 and 122). In some cases (e.g., the lateral ocelli of lepidopteran larvae), the whole organ rather resembles an ommatidium isolated from a compound eye, but in others (e.g., the dorsal [median] ocelli of pterygote insects), the ocellus is more like a miniature camera eye with a subspherical corneal, or cellular, lens and a many-celled retina with up to several hundred photoreceptor cells.

Even some of the lateral ocelli of cicindelid beetle larvae have several thousand receptor cells and a single dorsal ocellus of *Periplaneta* has more than 10,000 receptor cells (WEBER and RENNER, 1976). Reports that the image focused by ocellar lenses usually lies behind the retina (Figs. 121 and 122) are often cited as evidence that directional information and good visual acuity are not the forte of these eyes. However, this leaves a reasonable explanation of the hundreds or thousands of primary receptor cells, often present, somewhat in doubt. Recent data for the salticid spider *Plexippus* actually demonstrate better acuity and absolute threshold for its posterior lateral eyes than insect compound eyes several times as large (HARDIE and DUELLI, 1978).

Clearly, where the ommatidium-like ocelli form clusters, their strict discrimination from compound eyes may become difficult, particularly in comparison with divided or reduced compound eyes [e.g., in apterygote insects (PAULUS, 1972, 1975, 1977)]. Similarly, the distinction, except for size, may not be so obvious between an araneid ocellus, which projects excellent images into its multicellular retina, and a "proper" camera eye, usually considered to be restricted to vertebrates, cephalopods, and alciopid polychaetes (WALD and RAYPORT, 1977).

On the other hand, naupliar eyes of crustaceans usually are unambiguously simple (WATERMAN, 1961 a; ELOFSSON, 1963, 1965, 1966). There are often three minute contiguous ocelli; two dorsolateral and one anteroventral (Fig. 49). Each may have only two or three rhabdomere bearing photoreceptor cells partly surrounded by screening and reflecting pigment. Often, special dioptric components are completely lacking. However, careful comparative study shows that there are, in fact, four different types of naupliar eyes in various crustacean taxa. In addition, two, three, or four other presumed photoreceptors (i.e., frontal organs) are more or less intimately associated with the naupliar eye (Fig. 49) in three of these four types (ELOFSSON, 1966).

Consequently, the combinations of putative photoreceptors mediating visual responses in crustaceans are complex and largely unexplored physiologically. Even the usually simple structure of naupliar eyes has become elaborately evolved in three or four families of pelagic copepods, exemplified by *Copilia, Pontella*, and *Sapphirina* (VAISSIÈRE, 1961; ELOFSSON, 1969).

As usually defined, both compound eyes and camera eyes are always on the anterior part of the head and almost universally in a bilaterally symmetrical single transverse pair. Simple eyes in arthropods are also on the head, but often include a median unpaired unit in addition to paired, sometimes numerous, lateral ones. Thus, the dorsal ocelli of larval and nymphal hemimetabolous insects and adult pterygote insects generally are often three in number (i.e., one median, two paired lateral) and located in the frontal region of the head.

In crustaceans, as mentioned, there often may be one median ventral, plus two dorsal lateral units, but three, five, or seven simple eyes have been cited as the basic configuration in different groups (ELOFSSON, 1966). Ocelli of spiders commonly comprise four pairs with different visual fields and those of scorpions sometimes six pairs. The lateral ocelli of holometabolous insect larvae may reach six or seven pairs, clustered on either side of the head.

Sometimes ocelli occur in addition to well developed compound eyes (e.g., many crustaceans, insects, xiphosurans). Here, they presumably function as supplemental or auxillary visual organs. In other arthropods, they are *the* eyes (e.g., arachnids, copepods, adult thoracican barnacles, larval holometabolous insects, most myriapods). As in compound eyes, electron microscopy has revealed a fascinating array of fine structural details in simple eyes (EAKIN, 1972). Microvilli and rhabdomeres, almost without exception, form the organizational basis of arthropod photoreceptive membranes.

Yet, the regularity of their arrangement and patterns of association into rhabdoms, where present, vary greatly. At present, the functional implications of their structure remain largely conjectural. Recent investigations of simple eye physiology have been limited mainly to a few insect dorsal ocelli (GOODMAN, this Handbook, Vol. VII/6C), the naupliar eyes of adult thoracican barnacles, and *Limulus* median dorsal ocelli and ventral eyes. Almost none have been tested for their polarization sensitivity.

Because of the scarcity of relevant sensory physiology and the great diversity of arthropod and, indeed, other invertebrate simple eyes, a detailed review is not appropriate here. Instead, the main evidence for polarization sensitivity in specific cases will be briefly presented. These cases involve naupliar eyes of crustaceans, both types of insect ocelli, and the anteromedian eyes (i.e., *Hauptaugen*) and probably other eyes of certain spiders.

1. Naupliar Eyes of Crustaceans

In an important survey of arthropod orientation mechanisms, JANDER (1965) concluded that simple naupliar eyes of crustaceans are not capable of mediating polarotaxis, or even transverse phototactic responses (e.g., the dorsal light reflex). In particular, no polarization sensitivity was found in a number of cyclopoid copepods or *Artemia* developmental stages before the compound eyes were differentiated (STOCKHAMMER, 1959). Nor could JANDER evoke any polarization sensitive orientation in three copepods tested (i.e., *Macrocyclops*, *Cyclops*, and *Labidocera*). Both STOCKHAMMER and JANDER concluded that naupliar eyes are not polarization sensitive.

a) Oriented Behavior

However, in a more extensive sample of copepods (i.e., 16 spp.) using several types of experimental protocol, UMMINGER (1968a, b, 1969) demonstrated polarotaxis in seven species, in as many genera, from four different orders of the subclass (Table I). To begin with, a freshwater calanoid *Cyclops vernalis* was shown, in the laboratory, to have strong preferential orientation to the plane of polarization (UMMINGER, 1968a). Its behavior suggested an important role for underwater polarization in diurnal vertical migration and other oriented behavior. Thus, polarotactic responses were shown to depend, in complex ways, on the time of day and the ratio of downward to horizontal light intensities.

When this ratio was large, the animals oriented perpendicularly to the *e*-vector of a vertical beam at all times in the light phase of a 12 h light: 12 h dark cycle. However, when the ratio was small, a diurnal rhythm was released in the polarotaxis (Fig. 123). Near the laboratory dawn (i.e., 0–1 h in L) and dusk (i.e., 11–12 h in L) orientation was highly significantly centered at 90°; near the laboratory noon (i.e., 5.5–6.5 h in L). polarotaxis was also highly significant, but parallel, to the *e*-vector. During the interim periods (i.e., 1–5.5 h L and 6.5–11 h L), average orientation was random and, presumably, in transition between parallel and perpendicular polarotaxis. In unpolarized light, neither time of day nor radiance distribution had significant effects on orientation behavior.

Table 1. Relation of polarotaxis to copepod ecology (UMMINGER, 1968b)

Species	Polaro-tactic	Medium	Habitat	Vertical migration	Food habits	Eye structure
Calanoida						
Labidocera aestiva	Yes	SW	Pelagic	Yes	Omnivore	Complex
Pontella meadii	Yes	SW	Pelagic	—	Omnivore	Complex
Centropages hamatus	Yes	SW	Pelagic	Yes	Omnivore	Complex
Diaptomus shoshone	Yes	FW	Pelagic	Yes	Predator	Simple
Pseudodiaptomus coronatus	No	SW	Pelagic	Yes	Probably herbivore	Simple
Acartia tonsa	No	SW	Pelagic	Yes	Omnivore	Simple
Eucalanus monachus	No	SW	Pelagic	—	Probably herbivore	Simple
Cyclopoida						
Cyclops vernalis	Yes	FW	Littoral	—	Predator	Simple
Corycaeus speciosus	No	SW	Pelagic	Yes	Predator	Complex
Oncaea venusta	No	SW	Pelagic	—	Probably herbivore	Simple
Oithona similis	No	SW	Littoral	Yes	Predator	Simple
Oithona nana	No	SW	Pelagic	Yes	Herbivore	Simple
Oithona spinirostris	No	SW	Pelagic	Yes	Predator	Simple
Harpacticoida						
Tisbe furcata	Yes	SW	Littoral	—	Herbivore	Simple
Euterpina acutifrons	No	SW	Pelagic	—	Scavenger	Simple
Caligoida						
Caligus rapax	Yes	SW	Pelagic	—	Exoparasite	Complex

A horizontal polarization pattern added to the usual lateral illumination had the effect of providing spatial reference for *Cyclops'* orientations. In its presence, the animals swam vertically up or down at dawn and dusk, as well as horizontally around noon. Predominantly vertical swimming occurred, but no rhythmic changes were present, if the downward light intensity was significantly greater than the horizontal. When graduated light intensity changes, roughly simulating dawn and dusk, were also added to a relatively uniform radiance distribution, as well as horizontal polarization of the lateral light, still another behavior pattern emerged.

Under these conditions, *Cyclops* effectively underwent a diurnal vertical migration in the experimental vessel. At dawn, the vertical movement was mainly downward and, at dusk, upward. These directional effects of the sign of ΔI could be induced at any time during the L phase. Hence, they overrode the endogenous behavioral rhythm shown to be present otherwise. In the simulated diurnal migrations, therefore, polarized light was necessary for two reasons.

First, in combination with an appropriate radiance distribution, it released the endogenous rhythm which became evident in shifts from parallel or perpendicular orientation relative to the *e*-vector. Second, the orientation of the polarization plane in lateral illumination determined the transverse orientation of the copepod's longitudinal body axis while swimming. Finally, the gradual waxing and waning of I somehow released the basis for a cyclic pattern by establishing the sign of the vertical movement vectors at dawn and dusk. These experiments thus appeared to

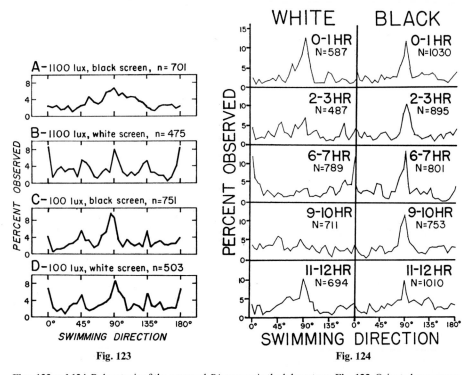

Figs. 123 and 124. Polarotaxis of the copepod *Diaptomus* in the laboratory. **Fig. 123.** Oriented responses to overhead *e*-vector under various conditions of illumination. Swimming directions relative to the *e*-vector at 0° are plotted on the abscissa. **A** Rather broad perpendicular orientation to *e*-vector at high light intensity with black surround. **B, C,** and **D.** Four peaked (0°, 45°, 90°, and 135°) orientation at high intensity with a white surround (which provides a more natural ratio of vertical to horizontal irradiance) and at low intensity with either black or white surround. This light contrast response is similar to that of *Daphnia* (JANDER and WATERMAN, 1960) and the mite *Arrenurus* (UMMINGER, 1969). **Fig. 124.** Correlation of polarotaxis and diurnal rhythm of *Diaptomus* locomotion. When there was a white surround (left column), swimming was preferentially perpendicular to the *e*-vector in the first and last hours of the 12:12 LD cycle. At 6–7 h (noon) of the 12 h light period, it was predominantly parallel to the polarization plane. Between these times, orientation was random. In relation to submarine polarization, this diurnal polarotactic behavior pattern could play an important role in the copepod's diurnal vertical migration. Note that with a black surround (right column), polarotaxis was at 90° during the whole light period (UMMINGER, 1968a)

have remarkable relevance to the normal behavior of such copepods and, perhaps, other zooplankton in nature. They also suggest the complex and rather surprising interactions, which may have to be discovered before even relatively simple behavior patterns can be understood.

In extending such experiments to other copepods, nine species tested showed no polarotaxis under conditions similar to those used for *Cyclops* (UMMINGER, 1968 b). The remaining six species (Table I) did orient in polarized light, but no differential effects of time of day or conditions of illumination were detected in these tests. Three patterns of *e*-vector orientation were observed: 1) *Labidocera* oriented parallel to the *e*-vector of a vertical beam; 2) *Centropages, Diaptomus,* and *Caligus* preferred perpendicular polarotaxis, whereas 3) *Pontella* and *Tisbe* showed orientation peaking at 0°, 45°, 90°, and 135°.

However, the specificity of these response differences is not certain since further study of *Diaptomus'* polarotaxis demonstrated that four peaked responses like those found for *Pontella* and *Tisbe*, as well as a wide range of other organisms, also occurred in this copepod under appropriate stimulus conditions (UMMINGER, 1969). More specifically, *Diaptomus'* behavior resembled that of *Daphnia* (JANDER and WATERMAN, 1960) in showing a light contrast reaction and intensity effect in the following way (Fig. 124). In the former, reducing the contrast between vertical and horizontal radiance intensities converts a 90° orientation to the *e*-vector to one with multiple peaks, as specified. Also, if the overall light stimulus was reduced from a high intensity to a more moderate one still having the same directional contrast, a similar transformation from one to four peaks occurred.

Perhaps, less clear is how to interpret the failure to elicit polarotaxis in 9 of 16 species tested. Most of these (e.g., *Diaptomus* initially) were not tested as extensively as *Cyclops*. Hence, the probable interactions of accessory factors may not have been discovered. Yet, quite closely related species, as cited above, may have different eye structure, channel connectivity, behavior patterns, etc. and, indeed, UMMINGER (1968 b) was well aware of this. Comparing polarization sensitivity with the ecology and eye structure of the 16 spp. (Table I) at least indicates whether or not any correlations were apparent.

Thus, most of the polarotactic species are pelagic, but so are seven of the nine which seemed to lack polarization sensitivity. Three of the nine species, tabulated as undertaking vertical migration, showed polarotaxis; the other six did not. UMMINGER concluded that there was some positive correlation between predatory or omnivorous feeding and polarotaxis, as well as suggestive evidence from rhabdom fine structure that polarization sensitivity occurred where two orthogonal channels of dichroic sensitivity were implied by the microvillus pattern.

b) Ocellar Organization

Typically, the naupliar eye is a small median structure in the head (Figs. 125 and 126). In *Cyclops vernalis*, evidence for an orthogonal microvillus pattern was found in electron micrographs (EM) of the dorsal ocelli. Their microvilli were shown to be normal to the optic axis of the rhabdom and, at least in some contiguous rhabdomeres, regularly oriented in two perpendicular sets, presumably belonging to different retinular cells. Earlier fine structural study of another copepod's (i.e., *Macrocyclops*) eyes disclosed that its dorsal ocelli contain nine retinular cells each; the median ventral ocellus only five (FAHRENBACH, 1964). Their rhabdomeres comprise axial microvilli perpendicular to the optic axis. The microvillus pattern of the rhabdom is not clear, but, in the diagram of one dorsal ocellus (Fig. 126), the three sets of microvilli shown all appear to be parallel.

In *Sapphirina* (ELOFSSON, 1969), microvilli of some of the receptor cells of its naupliar eye were found to be perpendicular to the optic axis; others, however, had these elements parallel to the optic axis. The latter orientation, as ELOFSSON suggested, would not yield any selective dichroic absorption; nor would it yield efficient isotropic absorption either. Although *Sapphirina* has not been tested for its

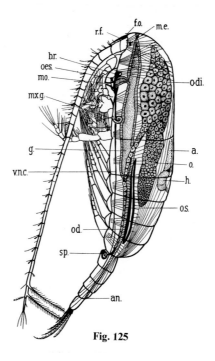

Fig. 125

Figs. 125 and 126. Median naupliar eye (ocellus) of copepods. **Fig. 125.** Lateral diagrammatic view of a ♀ *Calanus* showing location of median eye (no compound lateral eyes are present in this large important group). (MARSHALL and ORR, 1955). **Fig. 126.** Frontal section of naupliar eye in adult *Macrocyclops*. Left is anterior; right is adjacent to the protocerebrum. Seven of the nine retinular cells present are shown, including three rhabdomeres with their microvilli in the plane of section. (FAHRENBACH, 1964)

polarization sensitivity, the probable absence of such an ability was predicted from its microvillus pattern.

While the behavioral and fine structural data available so far seem rather inadequate to support more than tentative conclusions, there are two further points of interest to be made about the seven copepod species which do have polarization sensitivity (Table I). Clearly, this visual capacity is not a special adaptation of either standard unspecialized naupliar eyes (i.e., *Diaptomus* and *Cyclops*) or variously specialized complex ocellar eyes (i.e., *Labidocera*, *Pontella*, *Centropages*, and *Caligus*). Other genera with either simple or complex types failed to exhibit this oriented behavior.

Similarly, this sample tested also is interesting because at least one representative of four major systematic groups showed polarotactic behavior. Both of these considerations suggest that polarization sensitivity may be a rather basic potentiality for copepods. Its further correlation with transverse phototaxis, and therefore spatial orientation, and a normal role in diurnal vertical migration deserve further study, especially because copepods are, in fact, a highly evolved group of more than 4,500 spp. and of great ecological importance in the sea.

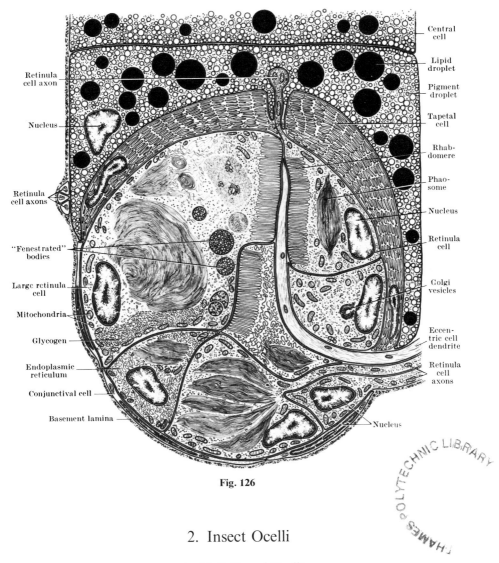

Fig. 126

2. Insect Ocelli

a) Adult Dorsal Ocelli

These minute photoreceptors have, for a long time, proved elusive in their adaptive and phylogenetic significance (GOODMAN, 1970). Their seeming erratic occurrence has been puzzling, although fairly good correlation exists between their presence and well developed flight. Hypotheses about their importance as stimulatory organs or elements in basic rhythmic or neurosecretory systems have been repeatedly discussed, but have not yet achieved broad experimental support.

The physiological responses of ocelli imply that they provide signals to the brain relative to environmental light levels and their changes. Ocellar involvement in a feedback control of phototaxis was proposed by JANDER and BARRY (1968). In addition, there have been persistent, if somewhat controversial, suggestions that orientation to polarized light in the sky is somewhat dependent on dorsal ocelli in some insects.

α) *Oriented Behavior*. To begin with, adult fleshflies *Sarcophaga* were reported capable of polarotactic orientation using blue sky to maintain a course (WELLING-TON, 1953). Outdoor directional orientation was judged to be normal with the ocelli intact, even when the compound eyes were covered. It was also normal with the compound eyes intact and the ocelli eliminated. With regard to the honeybee, however, VON FRISCH (summary, 1965, pp. 412–413) had concluded that the ocelli were neither necessary for nor capable of *e*-vector discrimination in sky light. Experiments had shown that covering the ocelli did not disorient dancing bees using the sky for direction finding. More cogently, polarotaxis was eliminated in *Apis* with their compound eyes, but not their ocelli covered. These results led VON FRISCH to suggest that the *Sarcophaga* results needed replication.

On the other hand, behavioral experiments proved that covering worker bees' ocelli substantially shortened the active collecting period at both morning and evening twilight, compared with normal hive mates (LINDAUER and SCHRICKER, 1963; SCHRICKER, 1965). This is, at least, consistent with the possibility that the more sensitive upwardly directed ocelli were deriving orientational information from sky polarization after light levels had fallen well below those needed for this purpose by the compound eye.

Experiments paralleling those on *Sarcophaga* were soon reported for adult sawflies *Neodiprion* (Hymenoptera) (GREEN, 1954). As later confirmed for mosquitoes (WELLINGTON, 1974a), sawflies on the ground usually responded to Polaroid filter rotation only with clear overhead sky. Qualitative evidence that the dorsal ocelli could function alone in polarotaxis was reported, but, like the *Sarcophaga* data, needed quantitative confirmation.

Experiments to duplicate the *Sarcophaga* results with another fly (i.e., *Lucilia*), although not published in detail, were reported to be negative (GOODMAN, 1970). Furthermore, microvilli of single ocellar retinular cells of flies were described as having multiple directions (TOH et al., 1971). Consequently, the notion of ocellar involvement in polarotaxis has been in need of further positive behavioral data. These have now been obtained in another hymenopteran.

Twenty years after his dipteran paper, WELLINGTON (1974b), on the basis of field experiments on a western bumblebee of the genus *Bombus*, concluded that its ocelli had polarization sensitivity. Furthermore, they could function either alone or in collaboration with the compound eyes to produce a natural polarized light compass response. At twilight, this ocellar capacity was responsible for extending the dawn and dusk orienting abilities in the bumblebee in a manner resembling that reported earlier for *Apis*. In *Bombus*, the homing behavior observed with different sky conditions, the details of flight experiments with partial or complete screening of the compound eyes, and comparisons of ground responses to Polaroid rotation, as well as the behavior of normal control bees, all seemed to provide coherent support for the hypothesis.

As with WELLINGTON's (1974a) field studies on polarotaxis in mosquitoes (C.I.5.a.), the *Bombus* data demonstrate the apparent general importance of polarized light to insects flying straight courses when landmarks are either not available or not being used. Of course, the participation of dorsal ocelli in such behavior still does not provide a solution to the vexing general problem of ocellar function because, as WELLINGTON pointed out, polarized light direction finding also has been shown to be quite feasible for anocellate insects.

β) *Ocellar Organization.* Several important features of dorsal ocellar structure have already been mentioned. Some additional points need to be raised here, but as polarization sensitivity has not been measured directly in this type of eye, only a few suggestive details will be cited (for recent reviews see PATTERSON, 1976; GOODMAN, this Handbook, Vol. VII/6C). Clearly, if rhabdom dichroism is involved, the fine structure of rhabdomeres and rhabdoms will provide at least a preliminary basis for evaluation. Actually, a wide range of photoreceptor membrane organization has been reported.

For example, in the worker honeybee, ocellar rhabdoms were found to be plate-like structures comprising two apposed rhabdomeres arising on the lateral surface from a contiguous pair of retinular cells (TOH and KUWABARA, 1974). Rhabdoms derived like these from two cells have been described not only in hymenopteran, but also homopteran ocelli (WEBER and RENNER, 1976). In *Apis*, the microvilli were perpendicular to the plate surface in both rhabdomeres and seemed closely parallel within the whole structure. No comment was made on the distribution of rhabdom orientation in the retina, which contained about 400 of these two-celled retinulas. In one electron micrograph, however, cross sections of about 10 retinulas showed the plates roughly lined up $\pm 30°$ to one plane.

In dragonflies, the rhabdoms are tripartite, with three retinular cells each contributing microvilli to two of the three plate-like flanges (CHAPPELL and DOWLING, 1972). The organelle was Y-shaped in cross section and the microvilli appeared highly regularly arranged perpendicular to the optic axis and the plane of the rhabdom arm they comprise. Hence, each rhabdomere contains two sectors of microvilli well aligned in each set, but at an angle of $100°-140°$ for a given retinular cell. This would, presumably, largely cancel any dichroism present separately in each arm of its rhabdomere in that cell.

In the fleshfly *Boettcherisca* (Fig. 127), each retinular cell formed multiple rhabdomeres on several lateral faces of its distal end (TOH et al., 1971). As a result, the "rhabdom" was distributed throughout the retina in a somewhat irregular network of mostly hexagonal or pentagonal meshes. Comparable net-like or tubular rhabdoms have also been found in ocelli of Ephemeroptera and Neuroptera, as well as Diptera (WEBER and RENNER, 1976). In the fly, the microvilli of a given rhabdomere segment were all quite regular and parallel, as well as being normal to the optic axis. Their different orientation on variously oriented surfaces of a single receptor cell, however, would obviously reduce or cancel whatever dichroism they have, based on membrane fine structure.

Another interesting peculiarity is that microvilli of facing rhabdomeres do not extend only part way across the rhabdom, as is usual. Here, they reach all the way across, but longitudinally share the length of the system with adjacent cells by being toothed, like decapod crustacean rhabdomeres. Hence, microvilli from different cells are interdigitated (Fig. 128). In the fly case, however, the alternate layers of ocellar microvilli (i.e., only 2–3 present in the short axial extent of the rhabdom)

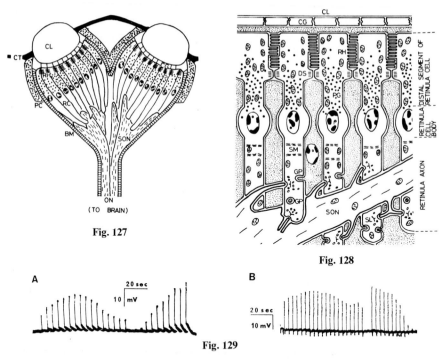

Figs. 127–129. Adult and larval ocelli of insects. **Fig. 127.** Diagram of the two lateral ocelli of the adult blowfly *Boettcherisca* showing relations between dioptric elements, the rhabdom bearing retina, the synaptic plexus below it, and the parallel ocellar nerves. *BM*, basement membrane; *CG* corneagenous cell; *CL*, corneal lens; *CT*, cuticle; *DS*, desmosome; *GP*, fine glial process; *ON*, optic nerves; *PC*, pigment cell; *PG*, pigment granule; *RC*, retinular cell; *SL*, synaptic locus; *SM*, septate membrane; *SON*, distal process of second order neuron. (Toн et al., 1971). **Fig. 128.** Diagram of receptor and synaptic region of an ocellus in Fig. 127 showing toothed rhabdomeres, synapses between retinular cell axes, and a large second order neuron, as well as prominent glial cells (stippled) from which fine processes project into the retinular axon. Further study (Toн and Kuwabara, 1975) has demonstrated more complex synaptic patterns, including feedback synapses from interneurons onto regular retinular axons. (Toн et al., 1971). **Fig. 129.** Intracellular receptor potentials from the larval ocellus (stemma) of the sawfly *Perga* (see Figs. 121 and 122) responding to flashes at 4 s intervals. **A** First series shows angular sensitivity data obtained with 3° vertical displacement of the stimulus between flashes; second series is response–intensity calibration in steps over 7.5 density units. Acceptance angles were 4.5°–25° in light adapted state; somewhat larger when dark adapted. **B** First series shows response amplitude modulation induced by 10° *e*-vector rotation between flashes; second series response–intensity calibration over 3.5 log units. Most retinular cells were found highly sensitive to *e*-vector direction. Mean S_p was 6.1 ± 2.1 S.D., with maximum S_p observed being 10. (Meyer-Rochow, 1974)

are apparently parallel rather than perpendicular, as in various compound eyes, including dipterans, cited above.

A rather extreme example of a multidirectional microvillus pattern in individual retinular cells has been reported for the sphingid moth *Manduca* (Dickens and Eaton, 1974). There, the ocellar rhabdomere is within the parent cell, lining an invaginated cavity with an omnidirectional array of microvilli.

A retinular pattern, somewhat more like that in compound eyes, was reported for *Periplaneta* ocelli (Weber and Renner, 1976). As many as seven retinular cells, but fewer on the average, may contribute to each rhabdom. The microvilli were generally perpendicular to the optic axis; within rhabdomeres, they often appeared in regular parallel array, whereas, between neighboring rhabdomeres, orthogonal relations were not infrequently observed. Two λ-specific systems have been identified in the ocellar retinas of the honeybee, mantids, dragonflies, and a moth (EATON, 1976); one peaking at 360 nm, the other at 500–530 nm. Spectral sensitivities of dorsal ocelli have been widely tested; in *Calliphora* for instance the ocellar receptors differ in their sensitivities from those so far known in the compound eye (KIRSCHFELD and LUTZ, 1977).

The actively flying dragonfly *Anax junius* has been reported to have, in addition, a blue receptor (i.e., $\lambda_{max} = 440$ nm) (CHAPPELL and DEVOE, 1975). The presence of a reverse PURKINJE effect and chromatic adaptation in *Anax* suggested that the ocelli might function in the analysis of sky light, especially at dawn and dusk, as discussed above, for the dorsal half of the *Hemicordulia* retina. Again, the strong zenith polarization, which is a prominent feature of the twilight sky, could be important here, as in *Bombus*.

Another aspect of most known dorsal ocelli, that has seemed to contraindicate directional or image forming capabilities, is the marked convergence between primary visual fibers and the relatively few secondary units with which they synapse. Typically, stimulation gives rise to hyperpolarization and, hence, inhibition of ongoing spontaneous activity in the post-synaptic units (PARRY, 1947). Ordinarily, these synapses are within the ocellus, but, in recently discovered lepidopteran ocelli, the primary axons run to the protocerebrum before synapsing (EATON, 1975).

Obviously, these are fascinating visual systems, but, so far, we have little direct information about their possible polarization sensitivity. However, the electrophysiological demonstration of strong differential responses to *e*-vector orientation in an insect lateral ocellus (next section) makes it quite likely that similar responses also will be found in dorsal ocelli.

b) Larval Ocelli (Stemmata)

α) *Oriented Behavior.* Not long after VON FRISCH's first publication on bee polarotaxis, oriented behavior to *e*-vector, both in the field and laboratory, was reported for late instar hymenopteran and lepidopteran larvae (WELLINGTON et al., 1951). The insects involved were 1) sawfly (i.e., *Neodiprion*) larvae whose eyes, at the stage in point, were one pair of tiny stemmata, each rather like a dorsal ocellus, and 2) caterpillars of two moth species whose eyes were six pairs of stemmata, each resembling an ommatidium.

These experiments were later extended until essentially similar behavior had been demonstrated in arctiid, geometrid, lasiocampid, nymphalid, and tortricid caterpillars [15], in addition to the hymenopteran larvae (SULLIVAN and WELLINGTON, 1953; WELLINGTON et al., 1954; WELLINGTON, 1955). The lepidopteran larvae, especially, were highly sensitive to sky polarization, which they could use menotactically to maintain straight courses over the ground in a given direction.

Clouds or smoke which passed over the zenith sector of the sky produced characteristic disruption of such straight line paths. Polarizers held over the animals in-

---

[15] Similar qualitative field data also were reported for a lymantriid caterpillar (DOANE and LEONARD, 1975)

duced corresponding course changes on rotation of their e-vector, especially through angles of 90°. Interesting interactions were demonstrated at various temperatures and "light compass reactions" to the sun's disk itself were concluded to be thermally, rather than photically, mediated. In any case, polarotaxis was stronger than phototaxis in the oriented field behavior of these caterpillars, as in the case of *Cataglyphis* adults.

Similar orientation also was reported for a variety of adult insects, (i.e., coccinellid and curculionid beetles, sarcophagid flies, and diprionid hymenopterans), but was not documented. Note that WELLINGTON's (1974a) more recent field data for flying insects, especially mosquitoes, reaffirms the polarotactic importance of clear blue sky, particularly the area within zenith angles of 0° and 30° (C.I.5.a.α).

β) Ocellar Organization and S_p. Like dorsal ocelli, stemmata have a rather wide range of structural patterns, as mentioned above. The only case where ocellar polarization sensitivity has been electrophysiologically demonstrated is in the larval stemmata (Figs. 121 and 122) of the Australian sawfly *Perga* (MEYER-ROCHOW, 1974). Here, the head bears one pair of minute lateral ocelli; the corneal lens was only about 0.2 mm in diameter, the retina 0.6–0.7 mm.

About 250 retinulas, each made up of eight photoreceptor cells bearing parallel microvilli axially, comprise the sensory mosaic. The resulting eight rhabdomeres, their microvilli are perpendicular to the optic axis, form a central rhabdom shaped in cross section like a maltese cross. Four retinular cells, with peripheral rhabdomeres at the end of the cross arms, have parallel microvilli in opposite cells, but orthogonal sets in adjacent cells. The other four inner retinular cells have four sets of microvilli, also in opposite orthogonal pairs, but at oblique angles to the first four. Hence, microvilli in a single ommatidium are oriented at about 0°, 45°, 90°, and 135°; the overall retinal mosaic was not reported except to say that it was less regular than is usual for a compound eye.

Intracellular recordings showed that receptor potentials (Fig. 129) were typical arthropod depolarizing responses (MEYER-ROCHOW, 1974). Although both ultraviolet and green units were presumed present, only the latter should have been activated by the ultraviolet-free stimulus used. The mean S_p of nine cells tested was 6.1 ± 2.1, whereas the two most sensitive had S_p's of 10, among the largest recorded in insects (C.I.4.c.). Again, it is noteworthy that this high polarization sensitivity was obtained in the green and not in the ultraviolet.

Note that although larval and adult behavior, ocellar structure, and electrophysiology have not all been studied in the same sawfly species, nevertheless, both *Neodiprion*, on which field and laboratory experiments have been done (α. above), and *Perga* are at least in the same wasp family. Consequently, this case provides a unique, reasonably coherent, example of polarization sensitivity in insect simple eyes.

3. Arachnid Ocelli

The four major lines of arthropods [i.e., Uniramia (including insects), Crustacea, Trilobita, and Chelicerata] differ so fundamentally that the assemblage has surely been heterogeneous since the Cambrian (CISNE, 1974). It is, therefore, not surprising that chelicerates differ from crustaceans and insects in a number of important respects. However, they do share many characteristics, including a broad range of simple ocellar eyes and the rare presence in recent species of lateral compound eyes as in xiphosurans.

Polarization sensitivity among the chelicerates has been reported only in arachnids, and there only in mites (Acari) and spiders (Araneae). Only for spiders, however, does any substantial and coherent information exist, and even there our knowledge is still not profound.

a) Acari

α) *Oriented Behavior*. In their first report on polarotaxis in *Daphnia* and other cladocerans, BAYLOR and SMITH (1953) casually mentioned that a freshwater mite, among other arthropods, spontaneously oriented like *Daphnia* at 90° to the *e*-vector in a vertical light beam. Later, two species of *Arrenurus*, also freshwater forms, were found to show four preferential orientation directions [i.e., the usual 0°, 45°, 90°, and 135° pattern (Fig. 130)] to polarized light (JANDER and WATERMAN, 1960).

A quite different oriented response (i.e., a broad single peak towards the light) to a differential radiance distribution showed that phototaxis and polarotaxis were independent processes. In addition, changing the ratio of vertical to horizontal illumination evoked a light contrast reaction in the *Arrenurus* polarotaxis similar to that in *Daphnia* (JANDER and WATERMAN, 1960) and *Diaptomus* (UMMINGER, 1969).

The red spider mite *Tetranychus*, crawling over the ground in clear sunlight, was found to react to the rotation of a polarizer held over it with a corresponding temporary course change (HUSSEY and PARR, 1963). Believing this to demonstrate behavior similar to that of insect larvae (C.II.2.b.α), the authors suggest that straight walking, during dispersal in this mite under clear skies, was a polarotaxis. Later experiments, however, were interpreted merely as responses to differences in external reflected light intensities resulting from different *e*-vector directions (MCENROE, 1971).

β) *Ocellar Organization*. Electron microscopy of the paired double ocelli of this species (Fig. 131) demonstrated that 17 rhabdomeres were present on the 15 retinular cells on each side; three of the anterior eyes' components had two rhabdomeres each. Some of these bore microvilli differently aligned along their proximal distal extent and others had them radially arranged in a fanlike pattern. However, some rhabdomeres comprised rather strictly parallel microvilli (MILLS, 1974) and, hence, might provide a dichroic analyzer of the usual pattern.

Probably the *Arrenurus* data, demonstrating a distinction between the mechanisms of polarotaxis and phototaxis, are the only observations, so far, that warrant a further look at this group in the present context. It would be of considerable interest to confirm the convergence of a similar orienting mechanism in the dispersal of forms so different morphologically and physiologically as mites, caterpillars, and adult mosquitoes.

b) Araneae

α) *Oriented Behavior*. The first evidence of polarization sensitivity in spiders was published by PAPI (1955 a, b) about the same time as GÖRNER (1958, 1962) was

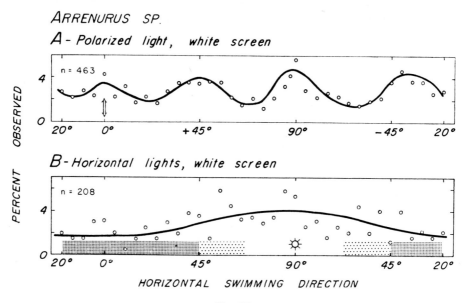

Fig. 130

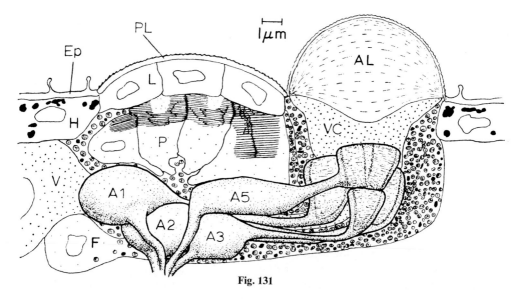

Fig. 131

Figs. 130 and 131. Mite polarotaxis and eye structure. **Fig. 130.** Comparison of polarotaxis **A** and phototaxis **B** in the freshwater mite *Arrenurus*. Multimodal response (0°, ±45°, and 90°) to overhead *e*-vector at 0°; broad single peak response to horizontal light and dark sectors without polarized light, as diagramed. (Jander and Waterman, 1960). **Fig. 131.** Medial section of the double anterior eye of the mite *Tetranychus* showing anterior and posterior lenses (*AL* and *PL*), their corresponding retinular cells (*A* and *P*), and rhabdoms. Vitreous and pigment cell bodies (*V* and *F*) are displaced from the vitreous body *(VC)* and pigmented cytoplasm. (Mills, 1974)

starting to work on the topic with VON FRISCH. PAPI found that in a lycosid spider *Arctosa*, orientation to a familiar shoreline was a well developed field behavior, as in many animals that live on river banks or beaches (HERRNKIND, 1972). This has been discussed above for various crabs (C.I.2.a.*β*), but was also studied for beach amphipods and isopods about the same time as the spider field research (reviewed in PARDI, 1957; HERRNKIND, 1972).

A spider thrown onto the water would quickly run over the surface, by a course perpendicular to the shoreline, back to the place where it had been captured. Such behavior was dependent on a clear sky; with overcast, pilotage was used as the animals proceeded to the nearest shore rather than to their original site. If no landmark was visible, they were disoriented under cloudy skies. Accurate returns were found in areas shaded from direct sunlight, but open to the blue sky.

Tests with polarizing filters demonstrated that sky polarization was, in fact, the cue for the shoreline orientation when the sun could not be seen. Hence, a menotaxis was involved in this behavior and the direction steered from the observed *e*-vector was the one learned by the spider to be perpendicular to its habitual shoreline.

Hence, specimens taken from variously oriented shorelines spontaneously chose appropriately different compass directions. In addition, they were capable of time compensating this astromenotaxis, as VON FRISCH and KRAMER had shown could be done by bees and birds. Thus, *Arctosa* in the laboratory would "accept" a fixed artificial light source as the sun and adjust its geographic orientation so that a constant heading would have been maintained, had the reference been moving like the sun. Comparative experiments on three species of *Arctosa* showed that the accuracy of the astromenotaxis was correlated to the habits and habitat of the different spiders (PAPI, 1959).

β) Ocellar Functional Organization. Spider eyes are of two structural and functional sorts (Fig. 132). The principal or primary eyes (i.e., one pair; also called the anterior median eyes) appear black as they lack a tapetum, have their rhabdoms distally located, and are the only eyes known to mediate polarotaxis, but others show peripheral polarization sensitive responses. Anterior median eyes have moveable retinas, are capable of detailed image formation, have small visual fields, function at moderate distances, and are used for object fixation. Principal eyes have more than one type of visual pigment with regard to λ_{max}. Two pigments were reported in a lycosid, one ultraviolet (i.e., 360 nm) and the other green (i.e., 510 nm) (DEVOE, 1972), and two retinular cell types (i.e., λ_{max}'s at 370 nm and 532 nm) in *Phidippus*, a salticid.

Four retinular cell types were found (YAMASHITA and TATEDA, 1976) in another salticid *Menomerus* (i.e., λ_{max}'s 360 nm, 480–500 nm, 520–540 nm, and 580 nm), where some support was inferred for the segregation of different types in four retinal layers as earlier proposed on optical grounds (LAND, 1969). In contrast to the three deeper layers (i.e., 1, 2, and 3), LAND suggested that the most superficial (i.e., 4) might be the site of polarization sensitivity. However, neither the anterior median eyes of salticids nor the spiders themselves have yet been tested with this parameter. Lycosids, agelenids, and tarantulas have, however, been found to be polarization sensitive.

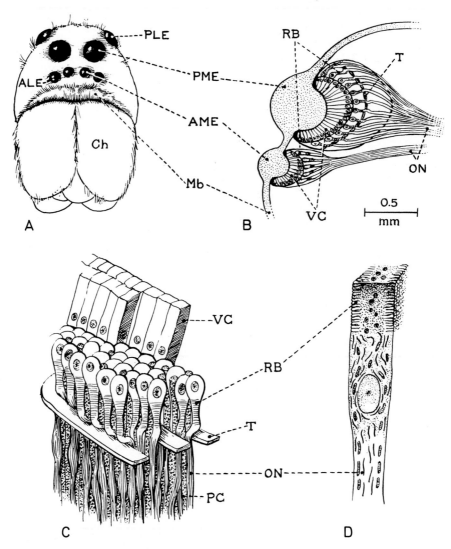

Fig. 132 A–D. Structure of wolf spider *(Lycosa)* eyes. **A** Frontal view of the head showing four pairs of ocelli (*AME*, anterior median; *ALE*, anterior lateral; *PME*, posterior median; and *PLE*, posterior lateral) (*n*, chelicerae; *mb*, arthrodial membrane). **B** Diagram of AME and PME as seen in parasagittal section. *Rb*, rhabdoms; *VC*, vitreous cells; *T*, tapetum; and *ON*, optic nerves. **C** Schematic perspective view of the PME retina showing vitreous cell *(VC)*, rhabdom *(RB)*, and pigment cell *(PC)*. **D** Part of retinular cell of AME showing two rhabdomeres distally. (DeVoe et al., 1969)

In contrast the other type of ocelli, the accessory or secondary set (i.e., three pairs) usually possess a tapetum which produces a characteristic eyeshine and has distinctive structural features in various species (HOMANN, 1971), but is absent in salticids. They function at short ranges, have poor spatial resolution, large visual fields, function in movement perception and operate in phototactically regulating the line of sight of the anterior median eyes. Unlike the principal eyes, the secondary pairs are monochromatic in the lycosids and salticids studied (DeVoe, 1972; Yamashita and Tateda, 1976; Hardie and Duelli, 1978).

Field experiments on *Arctosa*, in which various pairs of eyes were covered, demonstrate the predominant role of the anterior median eyes in orientation to the sky (Magni et al., 1965). This was nearly normal with only anterior median eyes functional, severely disturbed with only anterior median eyes covered, and random if only a single pair of secondary eyes were left uncovered. Recordings of electroretinograms from the various eye types showed, as expected, that *e*-vector position modulated the response amplitude of anterior median eyes to 100 ms flashes presented every 10 s (Fig. 133).

Curiously, the plane of polarization also affected the posterior median eyes (PME) in *Arctosa*, but not the anterior (ALE) and posterior (PLE) lateral pairs. In both median types, maximum response occurred with longitudinal *e*-vector orientation. It was concluded, with the support of some control experiments, that ocellar receptor cells were polarization sensitive, with major and minor axes in specific eye meridians. In the salticid *Plexippus*, retinal cells of posterior lateral eyes have been found in intracellular recordings to show a modest $S_e = 2.33 \pm 0.83$ (Hardie and Duelli, 1978). Note that the λ_{max} for these cells is at about 535 nm, far from the ultraviolet.

In the wolf spider *Lycosa*, the anterior median eyes' rhabdoms were found to comprise two rhabdomeres borne distally by adjacent retinular cells (Melamed and Trujillo-Cenóz, 1966). The retina of such an ocellus had about 450 photoreceptor cells; only 200–250 were inferred for *Agelena* (Schröer, 1974). In the central part of the retina, the rhabdom pattern was irregular with five-faced distal ends of retinular cells, bearing three rhabdomeres with microvilli, oriented in different directions. However, in the marginal retina, the rhabdomeric part of the receptor was four-sided and bore two sets of mutually parallel microvilli on opposite faces (Fig. 134).

In addition, microvillus orientation in neighboring rhabdoms was primarily tangential and radial and, therefore, nearly perpendicular. Such a fine structural pattern suggests a sort of inverse fovea with a peripheral polarization sensitive zone. Note, however, that the radial tangential orientation of the presumed analyzers would not establish a simple two channel orthogonal input. Obviously, adding all the radial, or tangential, inputs would cancel out *e*-vector discrimination, at least optically, if the system is radially symmetrical.

In the funnel spider *Agelena* (Schröer, 1974, 1976), however, the distribution of similar types of retinular cells has been reported to be different; there, only a ventral area of the retina has the type expected, from its fine structure, to have good polarization sensitivity. Retinular cells with two or more sets of microvilli oriented in more than one direction, and, therefore, likely to have weak or no significant polarization sensitivity, occurred in the central and dorsal retinal areas of the main eyes.

In both of these spider families, certain parts of anterior median eyes' photoreceptor membranes appeared to be specifically organized to provide polarization sensitivity, while other areas were not. Similar analysis of microvillus pattern in rhabdomeres of anterior median eyes of *Argiope*, an orb web building form from still another spider family (Argiopidae), implies that no polarization sensitive re-

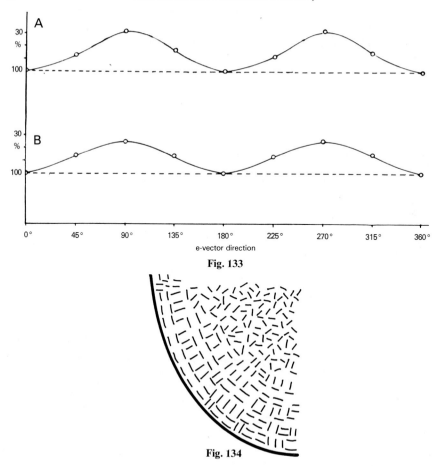

Fig. 133

Fig. 134

Figs. 133 and 134. Anterior median eyes of lycosid spiders. **Fig. 133.** Variation in ERG amplitude recorded as a function of *e*-vector orientation. **A** Response from anterior median eye. **B** Response from posterior median eye. (MAGNI et al., 1965). **Fig. 134.** Rhabdom distribution pattern showing parallel or perpendicular orientation of peripheral units vis á vis retinal radii and their random alignment centrally. (MELAMED and TRUJILLO-CENÓZ, 1966)

gions should be present in this case (UEHARA et al., 1977). There, web vibrations, perceived by mechanoreceptors, were observed to provide the major modality for orientation.

III. Mollusk Eyes

1. Camera Eyes of Octopus and Other Cephalopods

The capacity of cephalopods to discriminate the plane of polarization was first reported by MOODY and PARRISS (1960, 1961). Strong development of this sensory capacity seemed rather surprising for a camera eye, yet it certainly is in keeping with the old knowledge that some mollusk retinas contain rhabdoms (GRENACHER,

1886) and the general correlation, reviewed in the introduction to Sect. C, between rhabdoms and polarization sensitivity discovered in arthropods beginning in 1948 and 1949.

a) Behavioral Responses

Octopus in aquaria were trained with a technique used by BOYCOTT and YOUNG (1950) for shape discrimination. Both food reward and shock punishment were used to condition the animals to discriminate *e*-vector orientations differing by 90° (MOODY and PARRISS, 1961). *Octopus* could easily learn to discriminate 0° from 90°, as well as 45° from 135°. The experimental technique did not scrupulously exclude the possibility that the observed discrimination was mediated by differential scattering in the medium or selective reflection from the bottom, as well as other factors.

However, the authors argued that such intensity artifacts were unlikely to be the effective stimulus. This was directly proved by other experiments which eliminated possible dependence on surface reflections (ROWELL and WELLS, 1961) and provided stimulus substitutions which demonstrated discrimination learning independent of extraocular clues (MOODY, 1962). Hence, octopus' polarization sensitivity must be intraocular.

Experiments on juveniles of two decapod cephalopods *Euprymna* and *Sepioteuthis*, spontaneously orienting in a vertical beam of linearly polarized light, evoked preferential swimming directions remarkably similar to those of many arthropods (JANDER et al., 1963). Four peaks were present in 180° at 0°, 45°, 90°, and 135°, relative to the *e*-vector direction (Figs. 135 and 136). These responses were not evoked by horizontal intensity patterns simulating those produced by differential light scattering. When both *e*-vector and horizontal intensity patterns were presented simultaneously, the former predominated in determining oriented responses. Hence, it was concluded that the observed polarotaxis depended on a specific visual submodality involving intraocular *e*-vector perception.

b) Retinal Organization

As already mentioned, the retina of cephalopods is a mosaic of receptor cells (Figs. 25, 26, and 137), each typically bearing two lateral rhabdomeres on opposite surfaces of a roughly rectangular terminal segment (WOLKEN, 1958; MOODY and PARRIS, 1961; ZONANA, 1961; YAMAMOTO et al., 1965; COHEN, 1973a). In species with the most highly developed eyes and vision (e.g., *Octopus*), as well as certain squids, the cellular pattern and rhabdomeres show a remarkably regular pattern of orthogonally oriented elements. These are predominantly parallel to the eye's vertical and horizontal axes, as they are frequently in arthropods.

The retina itself is unusually simple, as interneurons are not present. Nevertheless, there are numerous collaterals arising from the receptor cells in its plexiform layer (COHEN, 1973b), where cholinergic synaptic and, perhaps, gap junction contacts are made with neighboring units (TASAKI et al., 1974). The rectangular pattern, evident in the retina itself, has been elegantly demonstrated by J.Z.YOUNG (1971) to be reflected in the organization of underlying elements in the optic lobe (Fig. 138).

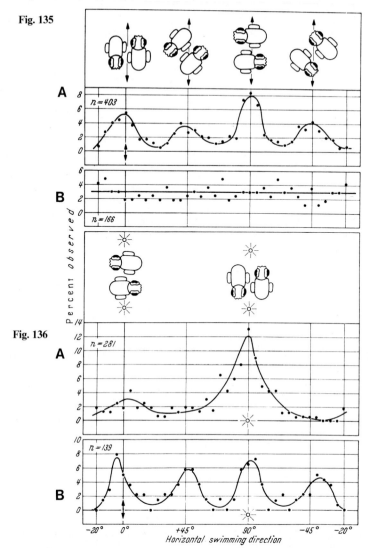

Figs. 135 and 136. Polarotaxis and phototaxis in juveniles of the sepiolid cephalopod *Euprymna* swimming in a vertical light beam. (JANDER et al., 1963). **Fig. 135. A** Directional preferences relative to the *e*-vector at 0° in polarized overhead light. Four significant peaks. **B** Control with overhead beam unpolarized. No significant preference. **Fig. 136. A** Overhead light unpolarized plus two horizontal lights at 90° and 270° evoked strong positive phototaxis and weak negative phototaxis. **B** Same horizontal illumination with overhead beam linearly polarized at 0°. Polarotaxis with four peaks overrode phototaxis as if the horizontal lights were not there (not significantly different from Fig. 135A)

Note that such a precise mosaic of repeated receptor and neuronal unit patterns is not only typical of strongly visual mollusks and arthropods, but is also striking in teleosts (e.g., ALI and ANCTIL, 1976). The possible relevance of this retinal regularity for vertebrate polarization sensitivity is considered below. Certainly, the latter is different generally, both in principle and in detail, from that in rhabdom-bearing eyes.

While the cephalopod retinular cell pattern frequently forms four-part rhabdoms from two pairs of orthogonal rhabdomeres (Figs. 26 and 137), a given receptor cell in the squid *Loligo* may participate in rhabdoms comprising microvilli from one to eight other cells (COHEN, 1973a). Consequently, the actual patterning may differ considerably from an ideal diagram. Serial sections demonstrate, however, that the microvillus pattern and directions are quite stable along the length of the outer segment. Direct measurements of rhabdom dichroism in *Loligo* yielded a recordsetting and widely quoted $\Delta = 6$, briefly reported in an abstract (HAGINS and LIEBMAN, 1963), although later microspectrophotometry in octopus has apparently not rivaled this (see below).

c) Rhabdom Dichroism

The dichroism of the dark adapted octopus *Eledone* retina (TÄUBER, 1973) coincides with the absorption spectrum of the rhodopsin present (Fig. 139), as in crustaceans (WATERMAN et al., 1969). Adaptation to polarized light at 475 nm changes some rhodopsin to acid metarhodopsin and shifts the dichroism λ_{max} towards longer λ's. If the adapting illumination is polarized parallel to the microvillus axis, the dichroism spectrum increases over the whole visible range, but, when ϕ is perpendicular to that, dichroism decreases.

These data show that metarhodopsin is also anisotropic and has its ϕ_{max} in the same direction as the rhodopsin in the membrane. Hence, net dichroism of the rhabdom could depend on both metarhodopsin and rhodopsin. In *Eledone*, the Δ estimated for rhodopsin was about 2.0 and that for metarhodopsin was about 1.6 (TÄUBER, 1975). This difference was suggested to result from a $15°$ tilt of the metarhodopsin dipole. The screening effect of the metarhodopsin was estimated to be small for short rhabdomeres or cases with small fractional light absorption (ISRAELACHVILLI et al., 1976).

Conversely, if rhabdom length were greater or most of the light absorbed, the metarhodopsin may significantly decrease or increase the polarization sensitivity relative to the level established by rhodopsin alone. As photoreversible thermostable metarhodopsins are characteristic of crustaceans and insects (GOLDSMITH, 1972, 1977; LANGER, 1973), as well as cephalopods, where they were discovered, interrelations of their absorption and dichroism spectra may be important for rhabdomeric polarization sensitivity generally.

d) Electrophysiology

Selective polarized light adaptation of the ERG in *Octopus* (TASAKI and KARITA, 1966a) demonstrated, as it did in the crab *Cardisoma* (WATERMAN and HORCH, 1966), that there were two, and only two, polarization sensitivity channels in the retina. Their orientation coincided with that of the two main directions of microvilli in the rhabdoms (i.e., vertical and horizontal). Essentially similar results were obtained in the squid *Ommastrephes* (TASAKI and KARITA, 1966b). Intracellular recordings from octopus retinular cells directly demonstrated that all units recorded fell into one of two classes (Fig. 140), with their ϕ_{max} either vertical or horizontal (SUGAWARA et al., 1971).

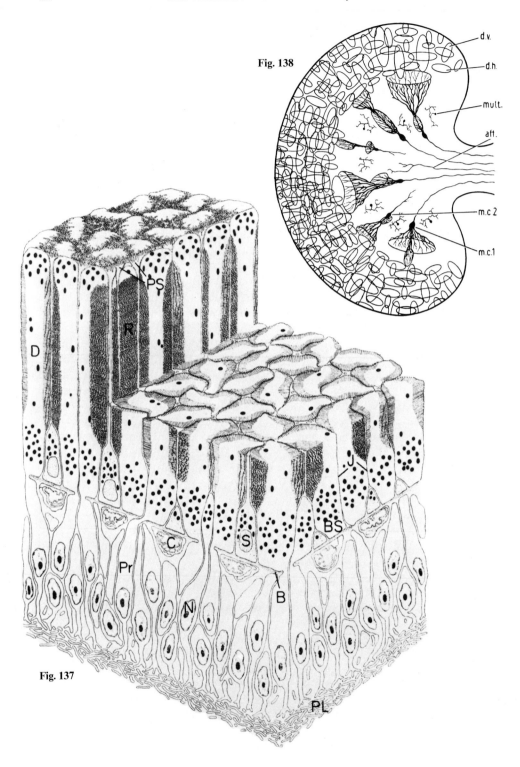

Fig. 138

Fig. 137

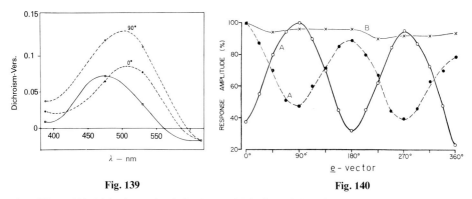

Fig. 139   Fig. 140

Figs. 139 and 140. Dichroism and polarization sensitivity in cephalopod visual cells. **Fig. 139.** Spectral distribution of retinal dichroism (solid curve) in octopus *(Eledone)* coincides with its rhodopsin absorbance. As in arthropods, the visual pigment here is the molecular basis of polarization sensitivity. After 15 s light adaptation at 475 nm (e-vector parallel to microvilli yielded 0° dashed curve; e-vector perpendicular to microvilli yielded 90° dashed curve), changes due to selective bleaching and formation of acid metarhodopsin are apparent. (TÄUBER, 1973). **Fig. 140.** Response amplitudes of two different *Octopus* retinular cells (curves A) compared to ERG amplitude (curve B) as a function of stimulus e-vector direction relative to 0° the direction of the normal horizontal axis of the eye. (SUGAWARA et al., 1971)

Compared with arthropods, our general knowledge of cephalopod visual systems is rather elementary. There has been some analysis of optic nerve spikes, but, so far, none directly relevant to the animal's strongly developed polarization sensitivity.

2. Molluskan Simple Eyes

In addition to the spectacular camera eyes of cephalopods, the mollusks also have a broad range of smaller ocellar eyes varying in number, location, and structure in the several other classes (CHARLES, 1966). Differential behavioral responses to e-vector direction were reported some years ago for gastropods (WATERMAN,

---

◄ **Figs. 137 and 138.** *Octopus* visual system. **Fig. 137.** Block of retina shown schematically. Two rhabdomeres are borne on opposite lateral surfaces of each photoreceptor cell (Figs. 25 and 26). Four such elements (typically) with two orthogonal microvillus directions form a rhabdom *(R)*. In addition to its rhabdomere, each receptor cell is seen to have a distal segment *(D)*, a pigmented basal spindle *(BS)*, and, below the basement membrane *(B)*, a proximal section *(Pr)* which contains the nucleus *(N)*, among other organelles. Special membrane junctions *(J)* are present between adjacent receptor cells in the spindle area. Probably, there are several classes of receptor cells in addition to the two differing in their microvillus orientation, but not much is known about it. Supporting cells *(S)* lie between receptor cells and a rich blood supply *(C)* is present under B. The proximal retinal plexus (shown very sketchily here) comprises fine collaterals from the primary visual axons which, themselves, pass directly through it to the optic nerve and fine terminal branches from efferent axons running out the optic nerve (for details see YOUNG, 1962). (YAMAMOTO et al., 1965). **Fig. 138.** Horizontal section of the optic lobe showing its cortical region constituting a "deep retina" analogous to the neuroommatidial (cartridge) layer of arthropod laminas. In this layer, where most primary optic fibers terminate after penetrating the convex outer surface of this lobe, the ellipses indicate the predominantly vertical and horizontal dendritic fields of some of the bipolar interneurons. This geometry obviously correlates with vertical and horizontal dichroism of the rhabdomeres (Figs. 137, 139, and 140) and certain properties of the animal's visual discrimination. (YOUNG, 1960)

1966a, for references). However, these were demonstrated to arise either from differential reflection from nearby substrate surfaces or from a selective refraction–reflection mechanism at the ocular surface.

Consequently, no inherent polarization sensitivity has been demonstrated in noncephalopod mollusks. It is not certain whether or not this has, in fact, ever been carefully tested. Certainly, mollusks flourish in many of the habitats occupied by polarization sensitive arthropods. Hence, their basic orientation needs appear similar. From a comparative point of view, one might expect inherent *e*-vector discrimination to be most critical adaptively to littoral species like many snails and free swimming pelagic forms (e.g., heteropods, pteropods).

There has been considerable important research in recent years on the eyes of various mollusks like *Aplysia, Hermissenda, Strombus, Tritonia, Lima,* and *Pecten* (for references, WATERMAN, 1975 b). The simple eye of *Strombus,* for example, was found to have some functional similarities to typical insect dorsal ocelli. The primary receptors depolarize on light stimulus, are nonspiking, and apparently exert a synaptic inhibitory effect on the second order cells by hyperpolarizing them (GILLARY, 1977). In fine structure, the retinas of gastropods and pelecypods were shown to be quite different from those of cephalopods (HUGHES, 1970; EAKIN, 1972; KATAOKA, 1975). Often the microvilli present on the surface of visual cells are terminal brush-like or even mop-like aggregates with little evidence for the highly regular parallel alignment normal to the optic axis characteristic of known dichroic rhabdomeres.

Mollusk eyes are also quite different from arthropod eyes in frequently having cells with photoreceptor membranes obviously derived from ciliary elements rarely even detected in rhabdom-bearing eyes. The pallial ocelli of *Pecten* and *Lima,* for example, have two retinas. The distal receptor layer is hyperpolarizing and contains photoreceptor membranes associated with cilia (MCREYNOLDS and GORMAN, 1974). The proximal retina, which is depolarizing, has its receptor membrane in the form of irregular tufts of microvilli. In various gastropods, microvillus membranes unrelated to cilia predominate, but there is considerable variability in the presence of presumed receptor cells with ciliary membranes (HUGHES, 1970). Thus, the fine structural evidence, too, does not encourage high expectations that strongly dichroic rhabdomeric elements are present in these simple eyes.

IV. Vertebrate Photoreceptors

As emphasized in the introduction, man as a vertebrate and mammal is little aware of the ubiquitous partial polarization of light in his environment. Under special conditions or just with careful observation, we can perceive the presence of strong linear polarization and the orientation of its *e*-vector by means of HAIDINGER's or BOEHM's brushes. Recently, optical evidence of an entoptic pattern resembling the former has been presented for the rhesus monkey (HOCHHEIMER, 1978), but, in general, our anthropocentric point of view tends to discount the possibility of any vertebrates making adaptive use of natural polarized light.

Nevertheless, evidence has been accumulating for some time that fishes (Figs. 141–146), amphibians, reptiles, and birds can discriminate polarized light and, in certain cases, use it for orientation (for review, WATERMAN, 1975 a, b). Yet, most of the data are rather fragmentary or quantitatively so weak that not much analysis of mechanism or significance has yet proved feasible. One basic difficulty with achieving this goal may be the general fact that vertebrates, in behavioral experiments, seem less likely than many invertebrates (e.g., insects) to respond consistently in a stereotyped way to repeatedly presented simple stimulus configurations.

On the other hand, the kind of elegant quantitative results obtainable with fish showing the dorsal light reflex (VON HOLST, 1950) may suggest that the blame may be more with the insight of the experimenter than in the capabilities of the experimental subjects. In any case, the scope of this volume and fairly recent reviews just cited warrant only a brief reference here to some current developments in vertebrate polarization sensitivity.

1. Camera Eyes

Exquisitely well developed eyes are the rule in most vertebrates. In many species, including man, they account for a substantial fraction of the whole exteroceptor input. Yet, they clearly lack any obvious intraocular polarizer which could serve to discriminate input polarization. It is well known, since the classic work of W.J.SCHMIDT, that the receptor membranes are optically isotropic for light propagated along their optic axis, but have dichroic ratios between 2.0 and 4.55 (Fig. 145) for transverse light (HÁROSI and MACNICHOL, 1974a; HÁROSI, 1975; LIEBMAN, 1975).

The explanation for this normal pattern of outer segment dichroism is, of course, the characteristic multiple disc structure of rod and cone photoreceptor membranes (Fig. 28). Because of restrictions in the orientation of visual pigment chromophores, their dichroism is only evident when the organelles' discs are examined edge on. Normally, this is never done in the eye by direct illumination because of the system's geometry.

Recently, however, a rather startling exception to the previously accepted universal rule has been discovered in certain cones in the anchovy retina (FINERAN and NICOL, 1976, 1978). In at least two species of *Anchoa*, two types of novel cones occurred, both having their receptor lamellae rotated about 90° so that they are edge-on to the incident light. If the visual pigment molecules are oriented, as in normal rod and cone disc membranes, these special cones would be dichroic, with absorption being at least 2–3 × greater for photons vibrating parallel to the lamellae, compared with those perpendicular (HÁROSI and MACNICHOL, 1974a). Interestingly, the two types of novel cones (Fig. 146) have their disc lamellae aligned in an orthogonal pattern.

One type (i.e., long cones) has horizontal lamellae, whereas the bifid cone, which had its membrane system split into two parts diverging distally by an angle of about 20°, has vertical lamellae. All, or nearly all, of the light reaching one long cone outer segment must first pass through parts of two bifid cones. Thus, filtering

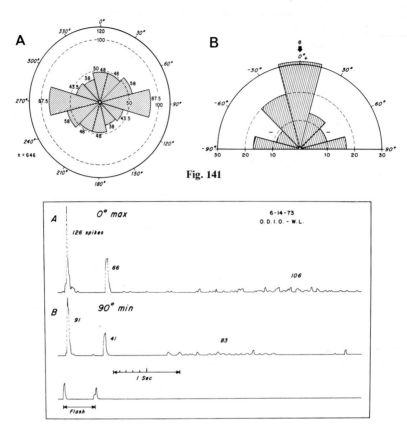

Fig. 141

Fig. 142

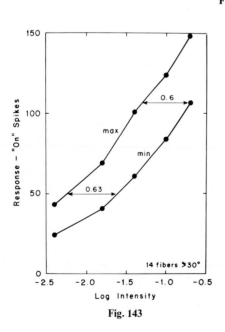

Fig. 143

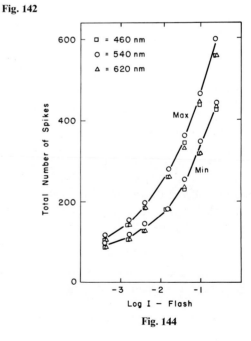

Fig. 144

in this tiered system should have important effects on long cone polarization sensitivity. The cones themselves are arranged in parallel vertical rows separated by rods. Hence, with their alternate orthogonal orientation, lamellae of the two types would establish a remarkably regular dichroic mosaic. Only morphological studies of this very special retinal system have been published so far and none of its behavioral or electrophysiological properties are yet known. Obviously, they should be of great interest.

In other kinds of fish with an ordinary outer segment fine structure, selective scattering, rather than dichroism, of polarized light by the retina is the most likely hypothesis to account for behavioral and optic tectum polarization sensitivity (WATERMAN and AOKI, 1974). However, direct evidence for such a mechanism has yet to be obtained. Also, progress has been slow in efforts to obtain stronger behavioral responses to *e*-vector direction in order to learn more of mechanism and adaptive significance in fishes.

Meanwhile, some new data have been reported on bird sensitivity to the plane of polarization. Previous positive results were restricted to rather limited evidence that homing pigeons could discriminate a moving from a stationary *e*-vector (KREITHEN and KEETON, 1974). Both behavioral and electrophysiological experiments now add further support for pigeon *e*-vector discrimination and its usefulness in azimuth orientation, at least in the laboratory (DELIUS et al., 1976).

In SKINNER box training experiments, homing pigeons readily learned to peck at a key located at a particular azimuth angle relative to overhead linear polarization. Significant correct orientation was learned in one to nine training sessions by different birds whether or not the correct keys were at 0°, 45°, or 90° to the plane of polarization. During their 22 nd through 25 th trials, all five trained birds yielded $p < 0.01$ for no learning.

The nature of the task learned proved that, by examining overhead polarization, the pigeon could make significantly better than random directional choices to achieve the food reward. Care was taken to control artifacts in the experimental setup and human subjects proved unable to make the correct choices, even when they were deliberately briefed on HAIDINGER's brushes, possible *e*-vector related intensity cues, and other factors.

Electroretinogram recordings demonstrated changes in the shape of the *b*-wave as a function of *e*-vector direction. These were not mimicked by differences in

◄ **Figs. 141–144.** Polarization sensitivity in fish. **Fig. 141.** Spontaneous directional responses of the half-beak teleost *Zenarchopterus* to an imposed overhead *e*-vector at 0°. **A** Series of underwater experiments in which 90° orientation predominated. (WATERMAN and FORWARD, 1972). **B** Series of experiments at the air–water interface in which 0° orientation was strongly preferred. (FORWARD et al., 1972). **Figs. 142–144.** *E*-vector discrimination by single optic tectum units in the goldfish. **Fig. 142.** Spike responses (summed for eight pairs of 500 ms flashes polarized at 0° or 90°). On, off, and delayed off responses are obvious; corresponding numbers are spike counts. Obviously the unit was more sensitive to horizontal (0°) *e*-vectors. Intensity response curves for 13 neurons indicate that mean S_p was 8.2. (WATERMAN and HASHIMOTO, 1974). **Fig. 143.** Demonstration that mean S_p for 14 tectal units maintained a value of about 4 (indicated by the horizontal separation of the maximum and minimum curves over the intensity range tested; Fig. 142). (WATERMAN and AOKI, 1974). **Fig. 144.** Demonstration of lack of selective effect of λ on S_p in a single tectal unit tested (as in Fig. 142) over the intensity and λ ranges indicated. (WATERMAN and AOKI, 1974)

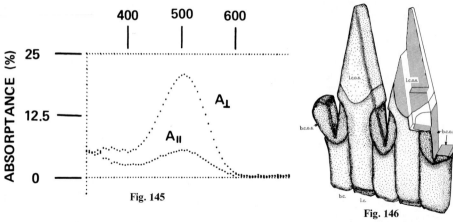

Figs. 145 and 146. Normal dichroism and special cone structure in vertebrate retinas. **Fig. 145.** Micro-spectrophotometric measurements (means of 32 bidirectional scans averaged at 5 nm intervals) on 38 rhodopsin containing rods demonstrating dichroism to transverse illumination with major absorbance occurring with the e-vector perpendicular to the ROS optic axis; computed $\Delta = 3.9$–4.9. With illumination parallel to the rod optic axis absorbance is, of course, isotropic in contrast to a rhabdomeric system (Figs. 27 and 28) (HÁROSI and MACNICHOL, 1974b). **Fig. 146.** Apparently dichroic special cone types from the retina of the anchovy *(Anchoa)*. Long cones *(l.c.)* and short bifid cones *(b.c.)* alternate in rows (vertically oriented in the eye) separated by rods. Both cone types have their photoreceptor lamellae parallel to the incident light and, hence, should be operationally dichroic (Fig. 145). Their respective lamellar orientation planes are orthogonal: vertical in bifid cones *(b.c.o.s.)* and horizontal in long cones *(l.c.o.s.)*, as shown at the right. Each bifid cone's outer segment precedes, in optical series, two long cone outer segments. Conversely, each long cone outer segment would seem to receive most of its light through half outer segments of two short cones. Obviously, the short cones should act as polarization filters, but nothing is known about their possible color filtering. Note that the wedge-like open space projecting down between adjacent long cones and actually dividing the bifid cone outer segments almost in half are in vivo filled with a process of a pigment epithelium cell having mirror like reflecting platelets isolating the cone outer segment triplets. (FINERAN and NICOL, 1978)

stimulus light intensity, but were intensified if the polarized beam was directed onto the lower retina which might normally be expected to "look at" the sky. The authors suggested that an intraretinal analyzer is present and speculated whether or not double cones might be particularly involved.

We had earlier wondered whether or not the regularly arranged twin cones of the teleost eye could be responsible for the marked polarization sensitivity (Figs. 142–144) recorded in the goldfish optic tectum (WATERMAN and AOKI, 1974; WATERMAN and HASHIMOTO, 1974). However, neither a wide range of light intensities nor wavelengths had selective effects on the S_p of the tectal cells. Consequently, it seemed rather unlikely that a mechanism dependent exclusively on cones could be responsible in that case.

Naturally, the possibility that homing pigeons, like a number of arthropods, could use natural polarization as a directional clue is exciting. It was already clear that the orientational repertoire used to achieve their remarkable homing performance depends on several sensory mechanisms (KEETON, 1974). No doubt, the possible adaptive significance of polarization sensitivity for migrating birds, not to mention fishes and marine mammals, is a real challenge to ongoing research on animal orientation and navigation.

2. Extraocular Photoreceptor Mechanisms

There is more than a remote possibility that the pineal or other vertebrate midbrain photoreceptors could be involved in the polarization sensitivity of at least lower vertebrates (e.g., fish, amphibians, reptiles). Most directly, polarotaxis in the newt *Ambystoma* was reported to be independent of the eyes, but dependent on some midbrain receptor (ADLER and TAYLOR, 1973). Earlier experiments on another newt *Taricha* and the cricket frog *Acris* showed that celestial orientation, as well as entrainment of circadian rhythms, could be mediated by extraocular photoreceptors (TAYLOR and FERGUSON, 1970).

The possibility of pineal polarization sensitivity was made more probable by the demonstration of organized membrane structures resembling vertebrate cone outer segments in this organ in fishes, amphibians, and reptiles (DODT, 1973). In view of the strong dichroism of retinal outer segments in transverse illumination (Fig. 145), similar *e*-vector discrimination would be expected of their pineal counterparts (HAMASAKI and EDER, 1977). Work has been reported "in progress" on the role of these structures in polarization sensitivity.

Note that in various fish behavioral responses to *e* vector direction midbrain participation has generally not been excluded or controlled. However, we are certain in the goldfish that the optic tectum's polarization sensitivity was mediated exclusively through the retina, since it alone was being illuminated (WATERMAN and AOKI, 1974; WATERMAN and HASHIMOTO, 1974).

D. Conclusions

As mentioned above (A.III.), a really adequate treatment of polarization sensitivity should not just summarize the known facts, but also should generate a central model for mechanisms around which a comparative analysis could be organized. Ideally, such an analysis should range, hierarchically, through all levels from optical input through sensory perception to the resulting adaptive behavior and its consequences. Clearly, the present account falls short of such ambitious aims on several counts.

To begin with, it concentrates mainly on the major animal groups which have been studied. It doesn't attempt to survey all the less perfectly known cases. More importantly, neither does it essay the systematic cross group synthesis that ultimately will prove most interesting. Our present state of knowledge seems too imperfect and our ideas of mechanism, as well as significance, so speculative that an attempt to do so would seem ill-advised, or even pretentious. Instead, it seems preferable to conclude by underlining some doubtful or paradoxical aspects of current knowledge whose resolution may accelerate progress towards a more effective understanding.

One striking general point is that the natural behavior of animals dependent on polarized light is a seamless part of their overall adaptedness. Hence, our dissection of it into rather simple components (e.g., polarotaxis, patterns of microvillus organization, channels of information processing) may, with its very plethora of intriguing detail, delude us into a false sense of understanding. Subjects such as this are no doubt rather vulnerable to the usual limitations of reductionism. The ultimate biological test of the fine structure, molecular biology, microspectrophotometry, and electrophysiology is their contribution to understanding the overall fitness of the organisms concerned.

I. Biological Purpose

This, of course, leads us to the question of the biological purpose of polarization sensitivity. Some understanding, or at least formulation, of this problem may allow us now to think more effectively about appropriate experiments required and possible models of mechanism. Later, when the field is more coherently developed, comparisons of the actual means used and an assessment of their importance will become possible.

From its discovery in hymenopterans, polarization sensitivity has been generally recognized as a potentially important means of using the polarization of scattered sunlight as a compass. Such direction finding can obviously aid the animal in homing, foraging, or migrating from one place to another. Another possibility is that natural polarization in the sky or underwater could be coupled to motor output in such a way that, quite in contrast, it provides a stable reference for station keeping.

We know that maintenance of a particular location, or sphere of action or territory, is fundamental to optimal functioning in most animals. Thus, systematic programs of swimming or flying, steered from the diurnally shifting polarization pattern, might be used in maintaining a fixed locus in space. Underlying this is an even more fundamental function, namely that of monitoring stable angular relations of the animal's body axes to environmental coordinates. Such a fixed reference platform, usually horizontal with dorsal side up, underlies practically all normal locomotion and other behavior. As mentioned above, reflex stabilization of this sort could be provided by scattering polarization, particularly in aerial and pelagic habitats where the extent of natural polarization in the visual field is large and the availability of other useful directional reference data is low.

A third important possibility is the potential improvement in visual contrast offered by polarization sensitivity. This has been suggested several times for underwater vision, where contrast is at a premium (LYTHGOE and HEMMINGS, 1967; LYTHGOE, 1972; LURIA and KINNEY, 1974). It also may well be functionally important in dorsally directed retinal regions of dragonflies, dipterans, and other predatory or aerial mating types. Here, acuity is of prime importance. Another related application, again repeatedly evoked for aerial and terrestrial forms, is the possibility of glare control from reflecting surfaces through appropriately oriented polarizers (B.II.3.).

Clearly, the sensory requirements of these three or four major types of use could be quite different. Corresponding behavioral responses also would be quite distinctive. In planning and executing experiments, as well as in devising models as possible aids in analysis, such selective requirements need to be kept in mind.

For example, the obvious importance in some cases, at least, of e-vector rotation is a matter of fresh interest. In *Calliphora*, even in retinular cells, an increase to 2 × its static value was observed in S_e using optimal rotation rates (GEMPERLEIN and SMOLA, 1973). In the beetle *Geotrupes*, interneurons of several classes responding to rotating e-vector have been found, but S_e was rather low (i.e., near 2) (ZOLOTOV and FRANTSEVICH, 1977). In crayfish, a crab, and a stomatopod, any significant e-vector sensitivity at the optic nerve level required its rotation, even if it is very slow. This has two major implications that need to be pursued. To begin with, the persistently low S_p's found in visual cells and second order interneurons in insects with good polarotactic behavior has been surprising.

Perhaps, failure to find polarization sensitivity at all, or at appreciable levels in such cases, may have resulted from failure to use a suitably rotating or otherwise moving plane of polarization. This certainly seems to explain our own earlier failure to detect polarization sensitivity in decapod crustacean optic fibers, despite extensive search (reviewed in WATERMAN, 1977). The dependence of this sensory capability on a changing stimulus would certainly be consistent with much else we know about compound eye function and, indeed, with the responses of many other kinds of visual system.

Eye or eyestalk jitter, head turning, and minor or major changes in locomotor direction (e.g., rapid circling of bee dances) would provide practically ubiquitous sources of visual input rotation. Obviously, the stimulating or amplifying effect of movement on polarization sensitivity would reinforce the importance of environmental e-vectors in the visual stabilization of spatial position. It is also clearly relevant to the unsolved problem of instantaneous vs. sequential e-vector discrimination.

II. Polarization Perception

Another desideratum about which we have little clue, as yet, is the question of what an animal perceives in natural polarized light. Presumably, if polarization vision is analogous to color vision, ϕ should be its most characteristic dimension. If so, we can wonder what it may look[16] like. How many just noticeable differences does it encompass? Is perceptual "absolute ϕ" possible? Must a pattern be present?

What kind of "imagery" is correlated with a complex polarized field like the sky or submarine polarization? Clearly, at the stimulus level, the distribution of ϕ will be superimposed on those of p and I, as well as λ. But how will they appear? Again, if a color vision analogy holds, some rather special discriminatory capabilities may emerge. For an extended color field like LAND's "color mondrian," it is clear that the perceived experience is not that expected from the processing of quantal catches by three kinds of YOUNG-HELMHOLTZ receptors at a "point" in the retina.

---

[16] Our own poor polarization sensitivity, emphasized in the introduction, doesn't help us much here. HAIDINGER's brushes combine a faint color system (i.e., blue and yellow) and a small cross-like image; BOEHM's brushes are achromatic, but appear as an entoptic pattern with moving light and dark sectors. Both phenomena are only noticed under rather special viewing conditions

Instead, it seems to result from comparisons of three corresponding lightnesses integrated over the whole retinal area stimulated (McCANN et al., 1976). Obviously, such comparisons would seem difficult for an animal without some standard against which to measure input or sensitivity. Perhaps, for polarization sensitivity as for color sensitivity, the photoregeneration of retinal pigments, which seems quite general in rhabdom-bearing eyes so far studied, may establish a suitable receptor baseline (HÖGLUND et al., 1973).

Certainly it is a prominent feature of much of the above review that the most recent contributions, instead of providing general explanations, have tended to devaluate earlier relatively simple hypotheses while substituting more elaborate, even somewhat byzantine, new ones. For example, it seems clear that the usually expected adaptive correlation between spectral irradiance and spectral sensitivity has to be reevaluated. The crucial significance of quantal excitation of photochemical systems has, of course, been long appreciated. Yet, the marked dependence of spectral irradiance curves on whether or not power units or quantal rate units are used has only recently become obvious to the visual physiologists.

No serious analysis has yet been made of its implications, for example, in the classic orientation of the honeybee to sky polarization. A rather loose correlation has usually been assumed between the known dependence of this behavior on blue and ultraviolet radiation and the λ^4 dependency of polarization by RAYLEIGH scattering. Consequently, most people have been quick to conclude that only ultraviolet receptors are required in the e-vector sensing mechanism. Nevertheless, the largest value of S_p (i.e., $= 18$) reported for insects was for a retinular cell in the ant *Myrmecia*, having its $\lambda_{max} = 500$ nm. This was reported by MENZEL (1975a, b) who originally hypothesized that the short ultraviolet receptor R9 is the only polarization detector in the bee retinula. The latter conclusion was also generalized to ants (MENZEL, 1975b; MENZEL and BLAKERS, 1975).

Furthermore, the demonstration (VAN DER GLAS, 1977b, 1978) in the honeybee worker that rather normal oriented dances can be obtained using an unpolarized overhead blue–green and purple colored sector pattern instead of sky or dichroic filter polarization provides an interesting challenge to the hypothesis that only R9, with its ultraviolet λ_{max} and apparently high S_e, is involved in polarization sensitivity. More established workers in this field have yet to acknowledge much weight in this challenge partly, no doubt, because the relevant publications may be somewhat opaque. Of itself, however, that does not seem to be an adequate basis for hypothesis rejection.

Several lines of evidence suggest that polarization sensitivity in the worker bee must involve at least some retinal localization effects and interactions of other wavelengths in addition to ultraviolet. We have also seen that λ_{max} for e-vector discrimination in *Daphnia*, crayfish, the jumping spider *Plexippus*, and cephalopods is not in or near the ultraviolet range.

Another hypothesis (VAN DER GLAS, 1978) challenges the common assumption that instantaneous unambiguous e-vector discrimination is basic to polarized light menotaxis (KIRSCHFELD, 1972, 1973a; BERNARD and WEHNER, 1977). This so-called "break-model" for polarotaxis assumes that mirror symmetry of sky polarization (Figs. 147–149) allows a bee, or any other animal using sky and, presumably, underwater polarization as a compass, very simply to sense the sun's azimuth

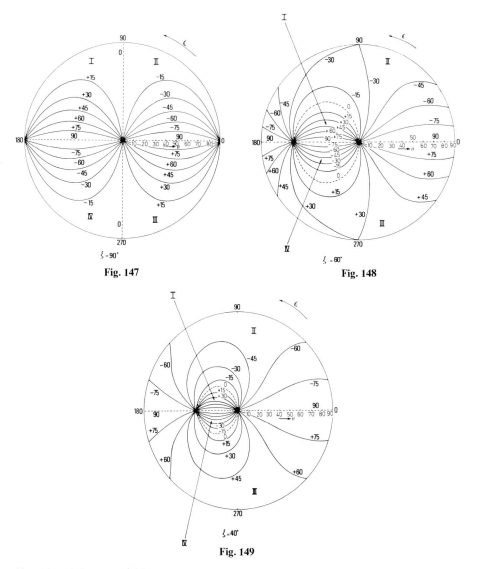

Fig. 147

Fig. 148

Fig. 149

Figs. 147–149. Patterns of ϕ in the sky calculated for RAYLEIGH scattering of sunlight when the zenith angle of the sun (θ_s) is respectively 90° (sun's location 180°; antisun at 0°, Fig. 147), 60° (Fig. 148), and 40° (Fig. 149). From the zenith in the center, sky points have as coordinates *(1)* angular relation to the sun's azimuth at 180° and *(2)* zenith distances from 0°–90°. Curves in the circle are loci of the given directions of ϕ measured from the vertical (negative for clockwise variations; positive for anticlockwise). Note that $\phi = 90$° (horizontal) at all points on the solar meridian and deviates symmetrically to the right and left of the sun's bearing. Note also that only when the sun is on the horizon or in the zenith is the polarization pattern symmetrical in the sky halves bisected by the solar meridian. Thus, at sunrise, the broken lines for the meridian at 90°–270° divide the sky into equal halves, so that I, II, III, IV are symmetrical quadrants (Fig. 147). At other times of day (except when θ_s—0°), I and IV, as well as II and III, are symmetrical to each other, but I, II and III, are symmetrical to each other (Figs. 148 and 149). A sky compass could unambiguously determine the sun's bearing (except when θ_s is 0° or 90°) if it bisected the ϕ symmetry and discriminated sectors I from II and III from IV (VAN DER GLAS, 1977a). Neutral points and "negative" polarization are not included in these figures, but appear in Figs. 6, 9, and 10 from the sign reversal of ϕ at the sun's vertical. The effectiveness of this mechanism depends on the fact that the arrangement of e-detectors in bees, and a number of other arthropods, also has mirror image symmetry in the two eyes (Dietrich, 1909; Stockhammer, 1956; Braitenberg, 1967; Kunze, 1968; Menzel and Snyder, 1974; Herrling, 1976).

Dancing on a horizontal comb surface, symmetrical polarized light stimulation would occur in the animal's right and left eyes only at the moment when its longitudinal axis coincides with the sun's bearing, or its opposite. Distinction between the azimuths of sun and antisun could depend on asymmetries between the corresponding sky quadrants, except when the sun's zenith angle is either $0°$ or $90°$ (Figs. 2 and 147). Note also that, for restricted sky areas, this ϕ-symmetry model could be valid only when the area concerned includes the solar vertical.

Another more general ϕ-symmetry model has also been proposed by van der Glas (1978), in which a reference plane related to ommatidial geometry in the eyes is defined so that 1) different head positions. 2) different tilts of the walking, dancing or flying reference planes and 3) various solar azimuth angles can all be accomodated. The original should be consulted for details. An interesting consequence of this hypothesis involving direction finding by equalizing polarization pattern input to the two eyes is that it is reminiscent of a classical tropotaxis and earlier suggested mechanisms of polarotaxis (Waterman, 1966d; Reichardt and Poggio, 1976). In such cases, bilaterally asymmetrical sensory input induces a corrective turning tendency which becomes zero when symmetry is achieved.

If such a model is valid, astromenotaxis, using polarized light patterns, presumably would then be not much more complex in its information processing demands than a direct sun compass. Nevertheless, we still have to solve the fundamental channeling problem of how e-vector patterns are discriminated. If sequential, rather than instantaneous, e-vector determination is involved, are three differently oriented dichroic receptor units a minimum requirement for polarotaxis?

Note that the results of von Frisch's experiments (1965, p. 418), in which he painted over the dorsal cornea of one eye of foraging workers, could be interpreted as supporting a ϕ-symmetry model. Those experimental bees, which returned to the hive and danced, did not produce normal waggle dances. In contrast, painting over the ventral sector of one eye had no disruptive effect on normal dancing behavior. On the other hand, monocular menotaxis by sky polarized light has been demonstrated in the field for *Cataglyphis* (Duelli, 1975). Consequently, a two eye mechanism is not necessary in this ant. However, in the field, *Cataglyphis* apparently maintains ideothetic course control between looks (i.e., about every 40 cm of the course) at the sky patch it is using as a compass. Since these fixations are described as comprising successive fixes by each eye, some sort of sequential binocular comparison ordinarily may be used, even if it is not required.

III. Number of Channels

Certainly, in many insects and most crustaceans and cephalopods, the predominance of two orthogonal microvillus directions within rhabdoms is striking. The occasional three directional case (e.g., cockroaches, locusts, dragonflies) does not happen to be in animals like *Apis*, *Daphnia*, and *Octopus*, where polarization sensitivity has appeared to be so strong as to demand some explanation. As discussed above (C.I.3.), BERNARD and WEHNER (1977) have compared the polarization discrimination capabilities of one, two, and three channel systems.

Actually, their plots demonstrating the degree of confusion inherent in two channel vs. three channel model systems are instructive. They show that, indeed, the latter has less ambiguity than the former. Yet the families of confusion curves generated in the second order neurons for a three channel system are qualitatively quite similar to those for only two. Consequently, the sizes and specific distributions of just noticeable differences will still be dependent on the angles between the polarization sensitive channels and the characteristics of the subsequent processing system.

We know in color discrimination that trichromats surely lose less λ input information than dichromats, but a tetrachromat could discriminate color mixtures which look identical to a normal human eye. Furthermore, there is an infinite number of properly selected combinations of three optical inputs which cannot be discriminated by a trichromatic mechanism, even though they range widely in λ_{max}, purity, and intensity.

With regard to primate λ discrimination, only four color opponent comparisons are apparently made in the processing system, and two of these are redundant (DE VALOIS, 1973; MARROCCO and DE VALOIS, 1977). Hence, only two, rather than the possible three, primary color input comparisons appear to be used in hue discrimination. Two nonopponent blue units are also commonly encountered. In the bee, only two types of color opponent cells have been found in the medulla; both of these involved antagonism between ultraviolet vs. blue and green. Predominant were cells excited by ultraviolet and inhibited by blue and green. The other type inhibited by ultraviolet and excited by blue and green occur rarely (KIEN and MENZEL, 1977). The bee system is, consequently, also redundant, but has only one pair of opponent color channels.

More directly related to polarization sensitivity, the available data on input information processing (YAMAGUCHI, 1967; LEGGETT, 1978) in decapod and stomatopod crustaceans give no evidence of polarization channel opponency comparable to that of primates and bees. Thus, crayfish and stomatopod optic nerve fibers seem to be transmitting the sum of inputs of the two orthogonal dichroic receptor systems. In an opponent contrast system, one would presumably expect isolation of two or more polarization sensitive channels by cancelling out intensity and other stimulus input parameters.

Failure to find opponency units relevant to polarization sensitivity may be evidence that the appropriate neurons have not yet been recorded. On the other hand polarization sensitivity as suggested in several places above may depend more on imaging of some sort rather than point for point *e*-vector discrimination. In that case some sort of holographic hypothesis (PRIBRAM, 1978) or spatio-temporal transfer function (BRODIE et al., 1978) may be required to explain processing of visual input for polarization sensitivity.

The whole problem of discrimination and orientation ambiguities emphasizes the likely importance, at least analytically, of the multiple peak orientation often found for polarotaxis (JACOBS-JESSEN, 1959; JANDER and WATERMAN, 1960; VAN der Glas, 1975). Better data on the dynamics of polarotaxis should indicate how the accuracy of orientation is, in fact, related to the neutral angles. In turn, such information should be used to correlate the occurrence of multiple peaks with the structural and functional data on the number, as well as the distribution, of the channels present. As discussed in several places above, polarotaxis with preferential orientation at 0°, 45°, 90°, and 135° relative to the e-vector has been well documented in animals with visual systems as diverse as copepods, *Daphnia*, crabs, hymenopterans, and squid.

Yet, one important caveat about multiple peak orientation is that it may largely be a response pattern generated under laboratory or otherwise artificial conditions. Indeed, available evidence indicates that *Cataglyphis* or *Aedes* orienting from sky polarized light follow a single directional course at a given period. They do not normally oscillate between widely different basitactic headings. Similarly, it is apparently rather difficult or impossible with dancing honeybee workers to obtain four peaks over 180° when the insects are just using the sky for direction finding (Michael Brines, personal communication). Hence, multiple peaks, in this case, may be more important in suggesting analytical clues to the nature of polarization sensitivity than in any natural operational function. However, in the crab *Ocypode*, four peak orientation was found in oriented responses to the blue sky (Fig. 53).

IV. Future Progress

At some risk of advocating folly, several research areas most likely to yield future progress may be suggested in conclusion. Probably the most important ones can be included under two general headings. To begin with, we desperately need to have more direct data on operational e-vector channels in the visual system. While our knowledge of receptor cell responses leaves something to be desired, especially with regard to crucial R 7, R 8, and R 9 in arthropods, data on polarization sensitivity in various orders of visual interneurons are even less satisfactory.

There seems to be no evidence yet for high polarization sensitivity in insect interneurons and apparently no data at all at this level in cephalopods. Surely, the various cases cited, particularly for dipterans, where certain types of interaction in the processing system induce marked gain in S_p need to be pursued further. In addition, the crustacean and insect results obtained with rotating e-vector have been referred to above, but the experiments so far published seem to be only in an exploratory stage.

For compound eyes, it is a matter of some interest to know which visual parameters can be effectively analyzed by one ommatidium. In the crayfish, bee, and ant, the different classes of wavelength discriminating cells occur in a characteristic pattern in each retinula, even though the properties of different retinal areas (e.g., dorsal vs. ventral) may be distinct. However, we also know that the visual field of higher order visual interneurons may be very large at the retina and movement perception models usually involve more than one ommatidium. How about polarization sensitivity?

Obviously, the current models for the bee eye require at least two neighboring ommatidia with differently oriented R 9 rhabdomeres. On the other hand, the sub-

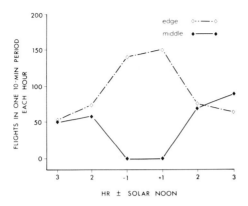

Fig. 150. Effect of degree of zenith polarization of flight paths of a variety of insects (flies, beetles, wasps, and butterflies) across and around an open lawn on a clear midsummer day. Confirming and extending earlier observations, primarily on mosquitoes (WELLINGTON, 1974a), long flights across the open area were virtually stopped during a period ± 1 h relative to local noon when zenith sky polarization was at a minimum. During that same period, flights around the edges of the open area were maximal. (WELLINGTON, 1976b)

stantial role of ultraviolet in insect vision and particularly their polarization sensitivity now seems rather exceptional. Available evidence for *Daphnia*, crayfish, spiders, squids, and fishes indicates that their polarization sensitivity does not have its λ_{max} in the ultraviolet, but rather at wavelengths significantly longer than 400 nm.

This reemphasizes the importance of sophisticated quantitative study of oriented behavior in nature as the second major type of research required (Fig. 150). Such work is needed not only in relation to the underlying visual physiology, but also to the relevance of laboratory behavioral data. Differences between laboratory and field behavior could be dependent on one or the other, or both, of two rather poorly understood factors. One is the potentially crucial role of secondary stimuli or the physiological state of the experimental animal in releasing responses to the "primary" stimuli we happen to have chosen to study.

The other is the possibility that some aspects of the stimulus configuration not obvious to us are, in fact, the determinants of orientation for the organisms (VAN DER GLAS' color hypothesis). Both careful experimentation and good fortune are requisites in unraveling such involved problems. Still, another relevant matter is the cybernetic mechanism whereby menotactic or compass responses are derived from underlying basitactic oriented responses. In other words, how does the central nervous system command of the moment find expression through the basic mechanism?

This has given rise to considerable discussion (JANDER, 1963b; MITTELSTAEDT, 1966; SCHÖNE, 1975; EDRICH, 1977), but clearly needs more quantitative experimental study than it has yet received. As already mentioned for *Cataglyphis*, this steering information is intermittent and requires complex periodic integration with other sensory inputs. Again, an effective study of polarotaxis dynamics would obviously be very helpful.

Even though this review has not wrapped up the subject, it may, nonetheless, serve some useful functions. One of these is to demonstrate, in specific detail, what a wealth of biological and environmental relevance is encapsulated in one apparently special, or perhaps even exotic, aspect of sensory physiology. In so doing, it has disclosed a surprising range of unknown factors, poorly understood data, and important unsolved problems. In the present state of high interest in polarization sensitivity, these may challenge us to turn out the kind of work needed to attain effective progress. Several key areas seem ripe for forearmed and well informed assault.

E. Acknowledgements

The author's research is currently being supported by grants from the United States National Institutes of Health (EY 00405) and the Research Committee of the National Geographic Society. Thanks are due to many friends and colleagues for helpful discussion and exchange of ideas during the incubation of this review. Gary Bernard, Michael Brines, Nils Jerlov, George Kattawar, Kuno Kirschfeld, William McFarland, Randolf Menzel, Allan Snyder, and Rüdiger Wehner should be especially thanked. The expert help of Mabelita Campbell in preparing the manuscript and bibliography and of Stanley D. Poole in assembling the figures is also gratefully acknowledged.

References

Adler, K., Taylor, D. H.: Extraocular perception of polarized light by orienting salamanders. J. Comp. Physiol. **87**, 203–212 (1973)

Ali, M. A., Anctil, M.: Retinas of fishes. Berlin-Heidelberg-New York: Springer 1976

Altevogt, R.: Wirksamkeit polarisierten Lichtes bei *Uca tangeri*. Naturwissenschaften **50**, 697–698 (1963)

Altevogt, R.: Lichtkompaß- und Landmarkendressuren bei *Uca tangeri* in Andalusien. Z. Morphol. Ökol. Tiere **55**, 641–655 (1965)

Altevogt, R., Hagen, H., von: Über die Orientierung von *Uca tangeri* Eydoux im Freiland. Z. Morphol. Ökol. Tiere **53**, 636–656 (1964)

Arago, D. F. J.: Mémoire sur une modification rémarquable qu'éprouvant les rayons lumineux dans leur passage à travers certains corps diaphanes d'optique. Mem. Inst. (Paris) **1**, 93–134 (1811)

Armett-Kibel, C., Meinertzhagen, I. A., Dowling, J. E.: Cellular and synaptic organization in the lamina of the dragon-fly *Sympetrum rubicundum*. Proc. R. Soc. Lond. (Biol.) **196**, 385–413 (1977)

Autrum, H., Stumpf, H.: Das Bienenauge als Analysator für polarisiertes Licht. Z. Naturforsch. **5b**, 116–122 (1950)

Autrum, H., Thomas, I.: Comparative physiology of colour vision in animals. In: Handbook of sensory physiology, Vol. VII/3A: Central processing of visual information (ed. R. Jung), pp. 661–692. Berlin-Heidelberg-New York: Springer 1973

Autrum, H., Wiedemann, I.: Versuche über den Strahlengang im Insektenauge (Appositionsauge). Z. Naturforsch. **17b**, 480–482 (1962)

Autrum, H., Zwehl, V. von: Die spektrale Empfindlichkeit einzelner Sehzellen des Bienenauges. Z. Vergl. Physiol. **48**, 357–384 (1964)

Bainbridge, R., Waterman, T. H.: Polarized light and the orientation of two marine Crustacea. J. Exp. Biol. **34**, 342–364 (1957)

Bainbridge, R., Waterman, T. H.: Turbidity and the polarized light orientation of the crustacean *Mysidium*. J. Exp. Biol. **35**, 487–493 (1958)

Batschelet, E.: Statistical methods for the analysis of problems in animal orientation and certain biological rhythms. Washington, D.C.: Am. Inst. Biol. Sciences 1965

Baumgärtner, H.: Der Formensinn und die Sehschärfe der Bienen. Z. Vergl. Physiol. 7, 56–143 (1928)

Baylor, E. R., Hazen, W. E.: The analysis of polarized light in the eye of *Daphnia*. Biol. Bull. **123**, 233–242 (1962)

Baylor, E. R., Kennedy, D.: Evidence against a polarizing analyzer in the bee eye. Anat. Rec. **132**, 411 (1958) (Abs.)

Baylor, E. R., Smith, F. E.: The orientation of Cladocera to polarized light. Am. Naturalist **87**, 97–101 (1953)

Baylor, E. R., Smith, F. E.: Diurnal migration of plankton crustaceans. In: Recent advances in invertebrate physiology (ed. B. T. Scheer), pp. 21–35. Eugene: University of Oregon 1957

Baylor, E. R., Smith, F. E.: Extraocular polarization analysis in the honeybee. Anat. Rec. **132**, 411–412 (1958) (Abs.)

Baylor, E. R., Smith, F. E.: Bees and polarized light. Final Report, Department of Navy, Office of Naval Research. Ann Arbor: University of Michigan Office of Research Administration 1961

Beardsley, G. F., Jr.: The polarization of the near asymptotic light field in sea water. Ph.D. thesis, 119 pp. Massachusetts Institute of Technology, 1966

Bernard, G. D.: Physiological optics of the fused rhabdom. In: Photoreceptor optics (eds. A. W. Snyder, R. Menzel), pp. 78–97. Berlin-Heidelberg-New York: Springer 1975

Bernard, G. D., Wehner, R.: Functional similarities between polarization vision and color vision. Vision Res. **17**, 1019–1028 (1977)

Birukow, G.: Menotaxis im polarisierten Licht bei *Geotrupes silvaticus* Panz. Naturwissenschaften **40**, 611–612 (1953)

Birukow, G.: Photo-geomenotaxis bei *Geotrupes silvaticus* Panz. und ihre zentralnervöse Koordination. Z. Vergl. Physiol. **36**, 176–211 (1954)

Björn, L. O.: Why are plants green? Relationships between pigment absorption and photosynthetic efficiency. Photosynthetica **10**, 121–129 (1976)

Bohn, H., Täuber, U.: Beziehungen zwischen der Wirkung polarisierten Lichtes auf das Elektroretinogramm und der Ultrastruktur des Auges von *Gerris lacustris* L. Z. Vergl. Physiol. **72**, 32–53 (1971)

Boschek, C. B.: On the fine structure of the peripheral retina and lamina ganglionaris of the fly, *Musca domestica*. Z. Zellforsch. **118**, 369–409 (1971)

Boycott, B. B., Young, J. Z.: The comparative study of learning. In: Physiological mechanisms in animal behavior. Symp. Soc. Exp. Biol., Vol. 4, pp. 432–453. New York: Academic Press 1950

Braitenberg, V.: Patterns of projection in the visual system of the fly. I. Retina lamina projections. Exp. Brain Res. **3**, 271–298 (1967)

Braitenberg, V., Strausfeld, N. J.: Principles of the mosaic organization in the visual system's neuropil of *Musca domestica* L. In: Handbook of sensory physiology, Vol. VII/3 A. Central processing of visual information (ed. R. Jung), pp. 631–659. Berlin-Heidelberg-New York: Springer 1973

Brines, M. L.: Skylight polarization patterns as cues for honey bee orientation, physical measurements, and behavioral experiments. Ph.D. thesis, 264 pp. Rockefeller University, 1978

Brodie, S. E., Knight, B. W., Ratliff, F.: The spatiotemporal transfer function of the *Limulus* lateral eye. J. Gen. Physiol. **72**, 167–202 (1978)

Brooks, J. L.: Cladocera. In: Freshwater biology, 2nd Ed (ed. W. T. Edmonson), pp. 587–656. New York-London: Wiley 1959

Brun, R.: Die Raumorientierung der Ameisen und das Orientierungsproblem im Allgemeinen. Jena: Fischer 1914

Brunnert, A., Wehner, R.: Fine structure of light and dark adapted eyes of desert ants, *Cataglyphis bicolor*. J. Morphol. **140**, 15–30 (1973)

Bruno, M., Barnes, S. N., Goldsmith, T. H.: The visual pigment and visual cycle of the lobster, *Homarus*. J. Comp. Physiol. **120**, 123–142 (1977)

Buikema, A. L., Jr.: Oxygen consumption of the cladoceran, *Daphnia pulex*, as a function of body size, light, and light acclimation. Comp. Biochem. Physiol. **42 A**, 877–888 (1972)

Buikema, A. L., Jr.: Some effects of light on the energetics of *Daphnia pulex* and implications for the significance of vertical migrations. Hydrobiologia **47**, 43–58 (1975)

Bullock, T. H., Horridge, G. A.: Structure and function in the nervous systems of invertebrates, Vol. II. San Francisco-London: Freeman 1965

Burkhardt, D.: Spectral sensitivity and other response characteristics of single visual cells in the arthropod eye. Symp. Soc. Exp. Biol. **16**, 86–109 (1962)

Burkhardt, D., Wendler, L.: Ein direkter Beweis für die Fähigkeit einzelner Sehzellen des Insektenauges, die Schwingungsrichtung polarisierten Lichtes zu analysieren. Z. Vergl. Physiol. **43**, 687–694 (1960)

Burton, P. R., Stockhammer, K. A.: Electron microscopic studies of the compound eye of the toadbug, *Gelastocoris oculatus*. J. Morphol. **127**, 233–258 (1969)

Bush, B. M. H., Wiersma, C. A. G., Waterman, T. H.: Efferent mechanoreceptive responses in the optic nerve of the crab *Podophthalmus*. J. Cell. Comp. Physiol. **64**, 327–346 (1964)

Butler, R., Horridge, G. A.: The electrophysiology of the retina of *Periplaneta americana* L. 2. Receptor sensitivity and polarized light sensitivity. J. Comp. Physiol. **81**, 279–288 (1973)

Cassier, P.: Le phototropisme du criquet migrateur (note préliminaire). Bull. Soc. Zool. Fr. **85**, 165–174 (1960)

Chandrasekhar, S.: Radiation transfer. Oxford: Clarendon Press 1950

Chandrasekhar, S., Elbert, D. D.: The illumination and polarization of the sunlit sky on Rayleigh scattering. Trans. Am. Phil. Soc. **44**, 643–728 (1954)

Chappell, R. L., DeVoe, R. D.: Action spectra and chromatic mechanisms of cells in the median ocelli of dragonflies. J. Gen. Physiol. **65**, 399–419 (1975)

Chappell, R. L., Dowling, J. E.: Neural organization of the median ocellus of the dragonfly. J. Gen. Physiol. **60**, 121–165 (1972)

Charles, A. H.: Sense organs (less Cephalopods). In: Physiology of Mollusca, Vol. II (eds. K. M. Wilbur, C. M. Yonge), pp. 455–521. New York: Academic Press 1966

Chen, H. S., Rao, C. R. N.: Polarization of light on reflection by some natural surfaces. Br. J. Appl. Phys. (J. Phys. D) Ser. 2., **1**, 1191–1200 (1968)

Chu, H., Norris, D. M., Carlson, S. D.: Ultrastructure of the compound eye of the diploid female beetle, *Xyleborus ferrugineus*. Cell Tissue Res. **165**, 23–36 (1975)

Cisne, J. L.: Trilobites and the origin of arthropods. Science **186**, 13–18 (1974)

Clark, L. B.: The visual acuity of the fiddler-crab, *Uca pugnax*. J. Gen. Physiol. **19**, 311–319 (1935)

Clarke, D., Grainger, J. F.: Polarized light and optical measurement. Oxford-New York: Pergamon Press 1971

Cohen, A. I.: An ultrastructural analysis of the photoreceptors of the squid and their synaptic connections. I. Photoreceptive and non-synaptic regions of the retina. J. Comp. Neurol. **147**, 351–378 (1973 a)

Cohen, A. I.: An ultrastructural analysis of the photoreceptors of the squid and their synaptic connections. II. Intraretinal synapses and plexus. J. Comp. Neurol. **147**, 379–398 (1973 b)

Collett, T. S., Land, M. F.: Visual control of flight behaviour in the hoverfly *Syritta pipiens* L. J. Comp. Physiol. **99**, 1–66 (1975 a)

Collett, T. S., Land, M. F.: Visual spatial memory in a hoverfly. J. Comp. Physiol. **100**, 59–84 (1975 b)

Coulson, K. L.: Effect of surface reflection on the angular and spectral distribution of skylight. J. Atmosph. Sci. **25**, 759–770 (1968)

Coulson, K. L.: The polarization of light in the environment. In: Planets, stars, and nebulae (ed. T. Gehrels), pp. 444–471. Tucson: University of Arizona Press 1974

Cox, C. S.: Refraction and reflection of light at the sea surface. In: Optical aspects of oceanography (eds. N. G. Jerlov, E. Steemann Nielsen), pp. 51–75. London-New York: Academic Press 1974

Crozier, W. J., Mangelsdorf, A. F.: A note on the relative photosensory effect of polarized light. J. Gen. Physiol. **6**, 703–709 (1924)

Dartnall, H. J. A.: Assessing the fitness of visual pigments for their photic environments. In: Vision in fishes (ed. M. A. Ali), pp. 543–563. New York-London: Plenum Press 1975

Daumer, K.: Reizmetrische Untersuchung des Farbensehens der Bienen. Z. Vergl. Physiol. **38**, 413–478 (1956)

Daumer, K., Jander, R., Waterman, T. H.: Orientation of the ghost-crab *Ocypode* in polarized light. Z. Vergl. Physiol. **47**, 56–76 (1963)

Delius, J. D., Perchard, R. J., Emmerton, J.: Polarized light discrimination by pigeons and an electroretinographic correlate. J. Comp. Physiol. Psychol. **90**, 560–571 (1976)

DeValois, R. L.: Central mechanisms of color vision. In: Handbook of sensory physiology, Vol. VII/3A: Central processing of visual information (ed. R. Jung), pp. 209–253. Berlin-Heidelberg-New York: Springer 1973

DeVoe, R. D.: Dual sensitivities of cells in wolf spider eyes at ultraviolet and visible wavelengths of light. J. Gen. Physiol. **59**, 247–269 (1972)

DeVoe, R. D., Small, R. J. W., Zvargulis, J. E.: Spectral sensitivities of wolf spider eyes. J. Gen. Physiol. **54**, 1–32 (1969)

Dickens, J. C., Eaton, J. L.: Fine structure of ocelli in sphinx moths. Tissue Cell **6**, 463–470 (1974)

Dietrich, W.: Die Facettenaugen der Dipteren. Z. Wiss. Zool. **92**, 465–539 (1909)

Doane, C. C., Leonard, D. E.: Orientation and dispersal of late-stage larvae of *Porthetria dispar* (Lepidoptera: Lymantriidae). Can. Entomol. **107**, 1333–1338 (1975)

Dodt, E.: The parietal eye (pineal and parietal organs) of lower vertebrates. In: Handbook of sensory physiology, Vol. VII/3B: Central processing of visual information (ed. R. Jung), pp. 113–140. Berlin-Heidelberg-New York: Springer 1973

Downing, H. C.: The hydraulic suspension of the *Daphnia* eye, a new kind of universal joint? Vision Res. **14**, 647–652 (1974)

Duelli, P.: The relation of astromenotactic and anemomenotactic orientation mechanisms in desert ants, *Cataglyphis bicolor* (Formicidae, Hymenoptera). In: Information processing in the visual systems of arthropods (ed. R. Wehner), pp. 281–286. Berlin-Heidelberg-New York: Springer 1972

Duelli, P.: Astrotaktisches Heimfindevermögen tragender und getragener Ameisen (*Cataglyphis bicolor* Fabr., Hymenoptera, Formicidae). Rev. Suisse Zool. **80**, 712–719 (1973)

Duelli, P.: A fovea for *e*-vector detection in the eye of *Cataglyphis bicolor* (Formicidae, Hymenoptera). J. Comp. Physiol. **102**, 43–56 (1975)

Duelli, P., Wehner, R.: The spectral sensitivity of polarized light orientation in *Cataglyphis bicolor* (Formicidae, Hymenoptera). J. Comp. Physiol. **86**, 37–53 (1973)

Duntley, S. Q.: Light in the sea. J. Opt. Soc. Am. **53**, 214–233 (1963)

Duntley, S. Q.: Underwater visibility and photography. In: Optical aspects of oceanography (eds. N. G. Jerlov, E. Steemann Nielsen), pp. 135–149. London-New York: Academic Press 1974

Eakin, R. M.: Structure of invertebrate photoreceptors. In: Handbook of sensory physiology, Vol. VII/1. Photochemistry of vision (ed. H. J. A. Dartnall), pp. 625–684. Berlin-Heidelberg-New York: Springer 1972

Eakin, R. M., Brandenburger, J. L.: Osmic staining of amphibian and gastropod photoreceptors. J. Ultrastruct. Res. **30**, 619–641 (1970)

Eaton, J. L.: Electroretinogram components of the ocellus of the adult cabbage looper moth *Trichoplusia ni*. J. Insect Physiol. **21**, 1511–1515 (1975)

Eaton, J. L.: Spectral sensitivity of ocelli of adult cabbage looper moth *Trichoplusia ni* (Noctuidae). J. Comp. Physiol. **109**, 17–24 (1976)

Eckert, B.: Orientujíci vliv polaisovanéko světla no perloočky. Česk. Biol. **2**, 76–80 (1953) [Abs.: Ber. Wiss. Biol. **89**, 198 (1954)]

Eckert, H.: Die spektrale Empfindlichkeit des Komplexauges von *Musca* (Bestimmung aus Messungen der optomotorischen Reaktion). Kybernetik **9**, 145–156 (1971)

Eckert, H.: Optomotorische Untersuchungen am visuellen System der Stubenfliege *Musca domestica* L. Kybernetik **14**, 1–23 (1973)

Eckert, M.: Hell-Dunkel-Adaptation in aconen Appositionsaugen der Insekten. Zool. Jb. Physiol. **74**, 102–120 (1968)

Edrich, W.: Interaction of light and gravity in the orientation of the waggle dance of honey bees. Anim. Behav. **25**, 342–363 (1977)

Edrich, W., Helversen, O. von: Polarized light orientation of the honey bee: the minimum visual angle. J. Comp. Physiol. **109**, 309–314 (1976)

Edwards, A. S.: The structure of the eye of *Ligia oceanica* L. Tissue Cell **1**, 217–228 (1969)

Eguchi, E.: The structure of rhabdom and action potentials of single retinula cells in crayfish. Ph.D. thesis, 25 pp. Kyushu University (Japan) 1964

Eguchi, E.: Rhabdom structure and receptor potentials in single crayfish retinular cells. J. Cell. Comp. Physiol. **66**, 411–429 (1965)

Eguchi, E.: Fine structure and spectral sensitivities of retinular cells in the dorsal sector of compound eyes in the dragonfly *Aeschna*. Z. Vergl. Physiol. **71**, 201–218 (1971)

Eguchi, E., Waterman, T. H.: Fine structure patterns in crustacean rhabdoms. In: The functional organization of the compound eye (ed. C. G. Bernhard), pp. 105–124. Oxford: Pergamon Press 1966

Eguchi, E., Waterman, T. H.: Cellular basis for polarized light perception in the spider crab, *Libinia*. Z. Zellforsch. **84**, 87–101 (1968)

Eguchi, E., Waterman, T. H.: Orthogonal microvillus pattern in the eighth rhabdomere of the rock crab *Grapsus*. Z. Zellforsch. **137**, 145–157 (1973)

Eguchi, E., Waterman, T. H.: Freeze-etch and histochemical evidence for cycling in crayfish photoreceptor membranes. Cell Tissue Res. **169**, 419–434 (1976)

Eguchi, E., Waterman, T. H., Akiyama, J.: Localization of the violet and yellow receptor cells in the crayfish retinula. J. Gen. Physiol. **62**, 355–374 (1973)

Elofsson, R.: The nauplius eye and frontal organs in Decapoda (Crustacea). Sarsia **12**, 1–68 (1963)

Elofsson, R.: The nauplius eye and frontal organs in Malacostraca (Crustacea). Sarsia **19**, 1–54 (1965)

Elofsson, R.: The nauplius eye and frontal organs of the non-Malacostraca (Crustacea). Sarsia **25**, 1–128 (1966)

Elofsson, R.: The ultrastructure of the nauplius eye of *Sapphirina* (Crustacea: Copepoda). Z. Zellforsch. **100**, 376–401 (1969)

Elofsson, R., Dahl, E.: The optic neuropiles and chiasmata of Crustacea. Z. Zellforsch. **107**, 343–360 (1970)

Elterman, L.: Relationship between vertical attenuation and surface meteorological range. Appl. Opt. **9**, 1804–1810 (1970)

Emlen, S.T.: Migration: orientation and navigation. In: Avian biology, Vol. 5 (eds. D.S. Farner, J.R. King), pp. 129–219. New York: Academic Press 1975

Fahrenbach, W. H.: The fine structure of a nauplius eye. Z. Zellforsch. **62**, 182–197 (1964)

Fernández, H. R., Nickel, E. E.: Ultrastructural and molecular characteristics of crayfish photoreceptor membranes. J. Cell Biol. **69**, 721–732 (1976)

Fernández-Morán, H.: Fine structure of the light receptors in the compound eyes of insects. Exp. Cell Res. [Suppl.] **5**, 586–644 (1958)

Fernandez Perez de Talens, A., Taddei Ferretti, C.: Landing and optomotor responses of the fly *Musca*. In: The compound eye and vision of insects (ed. G. A. Horridge), pp. 490–501. Oxford: Clarendon Press 1975

Fesenkov, V. G. (ed.): Scattering and polarization of light in the atmosphere. Akad. Nauk Kazakhskoi. Washington: Translation by Israel Program for Scientific Translation. U.S. Department of Commerce and National Science Foundation 1965

Fineran, B. A., Nicol, J. A. C.: Novel cones in the retina of the anchovy *(Anchoa)*. J. Ultrastruct. Res. **54**, 296–303 (1976)

Fineran, B. A., Nicol, J. A. C.: Studies on the photoreceptors of *Anchoa mitchilli* and *A. hepsetus* (Engraulidae) with particular reference to the cones. Philos. Trans. R. Soc. Lond. [Biol.] **283**, 25–60 (1978)

Forward, R. B., Jr.: Light and diurnal vertical migration: photobehavior and photophysiology of plankton. Photochem. Photobiol. Rev. **1**, 157–209 (1975)

Forward, R. B., Jr., Horch, K. W., Waterman, T. H.: Visual orientation at the water surface by the teleost *Zenarchopterus*. Biol. Bull. **143**, 112–126 (1972)

Franceschini, N.: Sampling of the visual environment by the compound eye of the fly: fundamentals and applications. In: Photoreceptor optics (eds. A. W. Snyder, R. Menzel), pp. 98–125. Berlin-Heidelberg-New York: Springer 1975

Franceschini, N., Kirschfeld, K.: Le contrôle automatique du flux lumineux dans l'oeil composé des Diptères. Biol. Cybern. **21**, 181–203 (1976)

Frantsevich, L., Govardovski, V., Gribakin, F., Nikolajev, G., Pichka, V., Polanovsky, A., Shevchenko, V., Zolotov, V.: Astroorientation in *Lethrus* (Coleoptera, Scarabaeidae). J. Comp. Physiol. **121**, 253–271 (1977)

Fresnel, A. J.: Mémoire sur la diffraction de la lumière. Ann. Chim. (Paris) **1**, 239–281 (1816)

Frisch, K. von: Gelöste und ungelöste Rätsel der Bienensprache. Naturwissenschaften **35**, 38–43 (1948)

Frisch, K. von: Die Polarisation des Himmelslichtes als orientierender Faktor bei den Tänzen der Bienen. Experientia **5**, 142–148 (1949)

Frisch, K. von: Die Sonne als Kompaß im Leben der Bienen. Experientia **6**, 210–221 (1950)

Frisch, K. von: Die Fähigkeit der Bienen, die Sonne durch die Wolken wahrzunehmen. Sitzungsber. 1953, Bayer. Akad. Wiss., Math. Naturw. Kl., 197–199 (1954)

Frisch, K. von: Tanzsprache und Orientierung der Bienen. Berlin-Heidelberg-New York: Springer 1965

Frisch, K. von: Honeybees: do they use direction and distance information provided by their dancers? Science **158**, 1072–1076 (1967)

Frisch, K. von: Decoding the language of the bee. Science **185**, 663–668 (1974)

Frisch, K. von, Kupelwieser, H.: Über den Einfluß der Lichtfarbe auf die phototaktischen Reaktionen niederer Krebse. Biol. Zentr. **33**, 517–552 (1913)

Frisch, K. von, Lindauer, M.: Himmel und Erde in Konkurrenz bei der Orientierung der Bienen. Naturwissenschaften **11**, 245–253 (1954)

Frisch, K. von, Lindauer, M., Daumer, K.: Über die Wahrnehmung polarisierten Lichtes durch das Bienenauge. Experientia **16**, 289–301 (1960)

Gehrels, T. (ed.): Planets, stars, and nebulae. Tucson: University of Arizona Press 1974 a

Gehrels, T.: Introduction and overview. In: Planets, stars, and nebulae (ed. T. Gehrels), pp. 3–44. Tucson: University of Arizona Press 1974 b

Gemperlein, R.: Grundlagen zur genauen Beschreibung von Komplexaugen. Z. Vergl. Physiol. **65**, 428–444 (1969)

Gemperlein, R., Smola, V.: Die Wirkung linear polarisierten Lichtes auf die Sehzellen von *Calliphora erythrocephala*. J. Comp. Physiol. **87**, 285–292 (1973)

Gillary, H. L.: Electrical potentials from the eye and optic nerve of *Strombus*: effects of electrical stimulation of the optic nerve. J. Exp. Biol. **66**, 159–171 (1977)

Giulio, L.: Elektroretinographische Beweisführung dichroitischer Eigenschaften des Komplexauges bei Zweiflüglern. Z. Vergl. Physiol. **46**, 491–495 (1963)

Glas, H. W. van der: Polarization induced colour patterns: a model of the perception of the polarized skylight by insects. I. Tests in choice experiments with running honey bees *Apis mellifera*. Neth. J. Zool. **25**, 476–505 (1975)

Glas, H. W. van der: Polarization induced colour patterns: a model of the perception of the polarized skylight by insects. II. Experiments with direction trained dancing bees, *Apis mellifera*. Neth. J. Zool. **26**, 383–413 (1976)

Glas, H. W. van der: Models for unambiguous *e*-vector navigation in the bee. J. Comp. Physiol. **113**, 129–159 (1977 a)

Glas, H. W. van der: Die Bienenorientierung auf unpolarisierte Farbenmuster, die das Polarisationsmuster am Himmel imitieren. Verh. Dtsch. Zool. Ges. **1977**, 235 (1977 b)

Glas, H. W. van der: Mechanisms of *e*-vector orientation in the honeybee. Ph.D. thesis, 186 pp, University of Utrecht 1978

Goldsmith, T. H.: Fine structure of the retinulae in the compound eye of the honeybee. J. Cell Biol. **14**, 489–494 (1962)

Goldsmith, T. H.: The natural history of invertebrate visual pigments. In: Handbook of sensory physiology, Vol. VII/1. Photochemistry of vision (ed. H. J. A. Dartnall), pp. 685–719. Berlin-Heidelberg-New York: Springer 1972

Goldsmith, T. H.: The polarization sensitivity-dichroic absorption paradox in arthropod photoreceptors. In: Photoreceptor optics (eds. A. W. Snyder, R. Menzel), pp. 392–409. Berlin-Heidelberg-New York: Springer 1975

Goldsmith, T. H.: The spectral absorption of crayfish rhabdoms: pigment, photo-product, and pH sensitivity. Vision Res. **18**, 463–473 (1978)

Goldsmith, T. H., Bernard, G. D.: The visual system of insects. In: The physiology of the Insecta, 2 nd Ed., Vol. II (ed. M. Rockstein), pp. 165–262. New York-San Francisco-London: Academic Press 1974

Goldsmith, T. H., Fernández, H. R.: Comparative studies of crustacean spectral sensitivity. Z. Vergl. Physiol. **60**, 156–175 (1968)

Goldsmith, T. H., Philpott, D. E.: The microstructure of the compound eyes of insects. J. Biophys. Biochem. Cytol. **3**, 429–440 (1957)

Goldsmith, T. H., Wehner, R.: Restrictions of rotational and translational diffusion of pigment in the membranes of a rhabdomeric photoreceptor. J. Gen. Physiol. **70**, 453–490 (1977)

Goodman, L. J.: The structure and function of the insect dorsal ocellus. Adv. Insect Physiol. **7**, 97–195 (1970)

Görner, P.: Die optische und kinästhetische Orientierung der Trichterspinne *Agelena labyrinthica* (Cl.). Z. Vergl. Physiol. **41**, 111–153 (1958)

Görner, P.: Die Orientierung der Trichterspinne nach polarisiertem Licht. Z. Vergl. Physiol. **45**, 307–314 (1962)

Götz, K. G.: Hirnforschung am Navigationssystem der Fliegen. Naturwissenschaften **62**, 468–475 (1975)

Gould, J.L.: The dance-language controversy. Q. Rev. Biol. **51**, 211–244 (1976)

Govardovskii, V.I.: (Possible adaptive significance of the position of the visual-pigment absorption maximum.) J. Evol. Biochem. Physiol. **8**, 5–12 (1972)

Green, G.W.: The functions of the eyes and antennae in the orientation of adults of *Neodiprion lecontei* (Fitch). Can. Entomol. **86**, 371–376 (1954)

Grenacher, H.: Abhandlungen zur vergleichenden Anatomie des Auges. I. Die Retina der Cephalopoden. Abh. Naturforsch. Ges. Halle **16**, 207–256 (1886)

Gribakin, F.C.: The types of photoreceptor cells of the compound eye of the honeybee relative to their spectral sensitivities. (Russian). Tsitologiia **11**, 308–314 (1969)

Gribakin, F.C.: The distribution of the long wave photoreceptors in the compound eye of the honey bee as revealed by selective osmic staining. Vision Res. **12**, 1225–1230 (1972)

Gribakin, F.C.: Functional morphology of the compound eye of the bee. In: The compound eye and vision of insects (ed. G.A. Horridge), pp. 154–176. Oxford: Clarendon Press 1975

Griffin, D.R.: Bird navigation. In: Recent studies in avian biology (ed. A. Wolfson), pp. 154–197. Urbana: University of Illinois Press 1955

Griffin, D.R.: The physiology and geophysics of bird navigation. Q. Rev. Biol. **44**, 255–276 (1969)

Groot, C.: On the orientation of young sockeye salmon *(Oncorhynchus nerka)* during their seaward migration out of the lakes. Behaviour [Suppl.] **14**, 1–198 (1965)

Grundler, O.J.: Elektronenmikroskopische Untersuchungen am Auge von *Apis mellifera*. Zulassungsarbeit zur wissenschaftlichen Prüfung für das Lehramt an Gymnasien. University of Würzburg 1971

Grundler, O.J.: Elektronenmikroskopische Untersuchungen am Auge der Honigbiene *(Apis mellifica)*. I. Untersuchungen zur Morphologie und Anordnung der neun Retinulazellen in Ommatidien verschiedener Augenbereiche und zur Perzeption linear polarisierten Lichtes. Cytobiologie **9**, 203–220 (1974)

Hagins, W.A., Liebman, P.A.: The relationship between photochemical and electrical processes in living squid photoreceptors. Abstracts of the 7th Annual Meeting of the Biophysical Society (New York) ME6 1963

Hallberg, E.: The fine structure of the compound eyes of mysids (Crustacea: Mysidacea). Cell Tissue Res. **184**, 45–65 (1977)

Hamasaki, D.J., Eder, D.J.: Adaptive radiation of the pineal system. In: Handbook of sensory physiology, Vol. VII/5. The visual system in vertebrates (ed. F. Crescitelli), pp. 497–548. Berlin-Heidelberg-New York: Springer 1977

Hardie, R.C.: Electrophysiological properties of R7 and R8 in dipteran retina. Z. Naturforsch. **32c**, 887–889 (1977)

Hardie, R.C., Duelli, P.: Properties of single cells of posterior lateral eyes of jumping spiders. Z. Naturforsch. **33c**, 156–158 (1978)

Hárosi, F.I.: Absorption spectra and linear dichroism of some amphibian photoreceptors. J. Gen. Physiol. **66**, 357–382 (1975)

Hárosi, F.I., MacNichol, E.F., Jr.: Visual pigments of goldfish cones: spectral properties and dichroism. J. Gen. Physiol. **63**, 279–304 (1974a)

Hárosi, F.I., MacNichol, E.F., Jr.: Dichroic microspectrophotometer: a computer-assisted, rapid, wavelength-scanning photometer for measuring linear dichroism in single cells. J. Opt. Soc. Am. **64**, 903–918 (1974b)

Harris, J.E., Wolfe, U.K.: A laboratory study of vertical migration. Proc. R. Soc. Lond. [Biol.] **144**, 329–354 (1955)

Harris, W.A., Ready, D.F., Lipson, E.D., Hudspeth, A.J.: Vitamin A deprivation and *Drosophila* photopigments. Nature **266**, 648–650 (1977)

Hartline, H.K., Graham, C.H.: Nerve impulses from single receptors in the eye. J. Cell. Comp. Physiol. **1**, 277–295 (1932)

Hasler, A.D.: Underwater guideposts. Madison-Milwaukee-London: University of Wisconsin Press 1966

Hays, D., Goldsmith, T.H.: Microspectrophotometry of the visual pigment of the spider crab *Libinia emarginata*. Z. Vergl. Physiol. **65**, 218–232 (1969)

Hazen, W.E., Baylor, E.R.: Behavior of *Daphnia* in polarized light. Biol. Bull. **123**, 243–252 (1962)

Heberdey, R.F.: Der Farbensinn helladaptierter Daphnien. Biol. Zentr. **56**, 207–216 (1936)

Heberdey, R.F.: Das Unterscheidungsvermögen von *Daphnia* für Helligkeiten farbiger Lichter. Z. Vergl. Physiol. **31**, 89–111 (1949)

Heisenberg, M., Buchner, E.: The role of retinula cell types in visual behavior of *Drosophila melanogaster*. J. Comp. Physiol. **117**, 127–162 (1977)

Helversen, O. von, Edrich, W.: Der Polarisationsempfänger im Bienauge: ein Ultraviolettrezeptor. J. Comp. Physiol. **94**, 33–47 (1974)

Herrling, P. L.: Measurements on the arrangement of ommatidial structures in the retina of *Cataglyphis bicolor* (Formicidae, Hymenoptera). In: Information processing in the visual systems of arthropods (ed. R. Wehner), pp. 49–53. Berlin-Heidelberg-New York: Springer 1972

Herrling, P. L.: Regional distribution of three ultrastructural retinula types in the retina of *Cataglyphis bicolor* Fabr. (Formicidae, Hymenoptera). Cell Tissue Res. **169**, 247–266 (1976)

Herrnkind, W. F.: Adaptive visually-directed orientation in *Uca pugilator*. Am. Zool. **8**, 585–598 (1968)

Herrnkind, W. F.: Orientation in shore-living arthropods, especially the sand fiddler crab. In: Behavior of marine animals, Vol. I (eds. H. E. Winn, B. L. Olla), pp. 1–59. New York: Plenum 1972

Hesse, R.: Untersuchungen über die Organe der Lichtempfindung bei niederen Thieren. VII. Von den Arthropodenaugen. Z. Wiss. Zool. **70**, 347–473 (1901)

Hockheimer, B. F.: Polarized light retinal photography of a monkey eye. Vision Res. **18**, 19–23 (1978)

Höglund, G., Hamdorf, K., Rosner, G.: Trichromatic visual system in an insect and its sensitivity control by blue light. J. Comp. Physiol. **86**, 265–279 (1973)

Højerslev, N., Zaneveld, J. R. V.: A theoretical proof of the existence of the submarine asymptotic daylight field. Københavns Univ. Inst. Fysisk Oceanog. Rep. **34**, 1–16 (1977)

Holst, E. von: Quantitative Messung von Stimmungen im Verhalten der Fische. In: Physiological mechanisms in animal behaviour. Symp. Soc. Exp. Biol. **4**, 143–172 (1950)

Homann, H.: Die Augen der Araneae. Anatomie, Ontogenie und Bedeutung für die Systematik (Chelicerata, Arachnida). Z. Morphol. Tiere **69**, 201–272 (1971)

Horridge, G. A.: Perception of polarization plane, colour and movement in two dimensions by the crab, *Carcinus*. Z. Vergl. Physiol. **55**, 207–224 (1967)

Horridge, G. A.: Unit studies on the retina of dragonflies. Z. Vergl. Physiol. **62**, 1–37 (1969)

Horridge, G. A.: The ommatidium of the dorsal eye of *Cloeon* as a specialization for photoreisomerization. Proc. R. Soc. Lond. [Biol.] **193**, 17–29 (1976)

Horridge, G. A.: Insects which turn and look. Endeavour (N.S.) **1**, 7–17 (1977)

Horridge, G. A., Giddings, C.: Movement on dark-light adaptation in beetle eyes of the neuropteran type. Proc. R. Soc. Lond. [Biol.] **179**, 73–85 (1975)

Horridge, G. A., Henderson, I.: The ommatidium of the lacewing *Chrysopa* (Neuroptera). Proc. R. Soc. Lond. [Biol.] **192**, 259–271 (1976)

Horridge, G. A., Meinertzhagen, I.: The exact neural projection of the visual fields upon the first and second ganglia of the insect eye. Z. Vergl. Physiol. **66**, 369–378 (1970a)

Horridge, G. A., Meinertzhagen, I. A.: The accuracy of the patterns of connexions of the first- and second-order neurons of the visual system of *Calliphora*. Proc. R. Soc. Lond. [Biol.] **175**, 69–82 (1970b)

Horridge, G. A., Mimura, K.: Fly photoreceptors. I. Physical separation of two visual pigments in *Calliphora* retinula cells 1–6. Proc. R. Soc. Lond. [Biol.] **190**, 211–224 (1975)

Horridge, G. A., McLean, M., Stange, G., Lillywhite, P. G.: A diurnal moth superposition eye with high resolution *Phalaenoides tristifica* (Agaristidae). Proc. R. Soc. Lond. [Biol.] **196**, 233–250 (1977)

Horridge, G. A., Mimura, K., Tsukahara, Y.: Fly photoreceptors. II. Spectral and polarized light sensitivity in the drone fly *Eristalis*. Proc. R. Soc. Lond. [Biol.] **190**, 225–237 (1975)

Hughes, H. P. I.: A light and electron microscope study of some opisthobranch eyes. Z. Zellforsch. **106**, 79–98 (1970)

Hulburt, E. O.: The polarization of light at sea. J. Opt. Soc. Am. **24**, 35–42 (1934)

Hussey, N. W., Parr, W. J.: Dispersal of the glasshouse red spider mite *Tetranychus urticae* Koch (Acarina, Tetranychidae). Entomol. Exp. Appl. **6**, 207–214 (1963)

Hutchinson, G. E.: A treatise on limnology. In: Geography, physics, and chemistry, Vol. I, 1015 pp. New York: Wiley and Sons 1957

Ioannides, A. C., Horridge, G. A.: The organization of visual fields in the hemipteran acone eye. Proc. R. Soc. Lond. [Biol.] **190**, 373–391 (1975)

Israelachvili, J. N., Sammut, A. A., Snyder, A. W.: Birefringence and dichroism of photoreceptors. Vision Res. **16**, 47–52 (1976)

Ivanoff, A.: Polarization measurements in the sea. In: Optical aspects of oceanography (eds. N. G. Jerlov, E. Steemann Nielsen), pp. 151–175. London: Academic Press 1974

Ivanoff, A., Waterman, T.H.: Factors, mainly depth and wavelength, affecting underwater polarized light. J. Mar. Res. **16**, 283–307 (1958a)

Ivanoff, A., Waterman, T.H.: Elliptical polarization of submarine illumination. J. Mar. Res. **16**, 255–282 (1958b)

Jacob, K.G., Willmund, R., Folkers, E., Fischbach, K.F., Spatz, H.C.: T-maze phototaxis of *Drosophila melanogaster* and several mutants in the visual systems. J. Comp. Physiol. **116**, 209–225 (1977)

Jacobs-Jessen, U.F.: Zur Orientierung der Hummeln und einiger anderer Hymenopteren. Z. Vergl. Physiol. **41**, 597–641 (1959)

Jander, R.: Die optische Richtungsorientierung der roten Waldameise *(Formica rufa)*. Z. Vergl. Physiol. **40**, 162–238 (1957)

Jander, R.: Grundleistung der Licht- und Schwereorientierung von Insekten. Z. Vergl. Physiol. **47**, 381–430 (1963a)

Jander, R.: Insect orientation. Ann. Rev. Entomol. **8**, 95–114 (1963b)

Jander, R.: Die Phylogenie von Orientierungsmechanismen der Arthropoden. Verh. Dtsch. Zool. Ges. Jena (Zool. Anz. Suppl.), 266–306 (1965)

Jander, R.: Interaction of light and gravity orientation in *Daphnia pulex*. Fortschr. Zool. **23**, 174–184 (1975)

Jander, R., Barry, C.K.: Die phototaktische Gegenkopplung von Stirnocellen und Facettenaugen in der Phototropotaxis der Heuschrecken und Grillen (Saltatoptera: *Locusta migratoria* und *Gryllus bimaculatus*). Z. Vergl. Physiol. **57**, 432–458 (1968)

Jander, R., Waterman, T.H.: Sensory discrimination between polarized light and light intensity patterns by arthropods. J. Cell. Comp. Physiol. **56**, 137–160 (1960)

Jander, R., Daumer, K., Waterman, T.H.: Polarized light orientation by two Hawaiian decapod cephalopods. Z. Vergl. Physiol. **46**, 383–394 (1963)

Järvilehto, M., Moring, J.: Polarization sensitivity of individual retinula cells and neurons of the fly *Calliphora*. J. Comp. Physiol. **91**, 387–397 (1974)

Järvilehto, M., Moring, J.: Spectral and polarization sensitivity of identified retinal cells of the fly. In: Neuronal principles in vision (eds. F. Zettler, R. Weiler), pp. 214–226. Berlin-Heidelberg-New York: Springer 1976

Jerlov, N.G.: Optical oceanography. Amsterdam-London-New York: Elsevier 1968

Jerlov, N.G.: Marine optics. Amsterdam-Oxford-New York: Elsevier 1976

Jerlov, N.G., Steemann Nielsen, E.: Optical aspects of oceanography. London: Academic Press 1974

Kalmus, H.: Responses of insects to polarized light in the presence of dark reflecting surfaces. Nature **182**, 1526–1527 (1958)

Kataoka, S.: Fine structure of the retina of a slug *Limax flavus* L. Vision Res. **15**, 681–686 (1975)

Kattawar, G.W., Plass, G.N.: Asymptotic radiance and polarization in optically thick media: ocean and clouds. Appl. Opt. **15**, 3166–3178 (1976)

Kattawar, G.W., Plass, G.N., Guinn, J.A., Jr.: Monte Carlo calculations of the polarization of radiation in the earth's atmosphere-ocean system. J. Phys. Oceanog. **3**, 353–372 (1973)

Keeton, W.T.: The orientational and navigational basis of homing in birds. Adv. Study Behavior **5**, 47–132 (1974)

Kerz, M.: Wahrnehmung polarisierten Lichtes durch *Eupagurus*. Experientia **6**, 427 (1950)

Kien, J., Menzel, R.: Chromatic properties of interneurons in the optic lobes of the bee. J. Comp. Physiol. **113**, 35–53 (1977)

Kirschfeld, K.: Die Projektion der optischen Umwelt auf das Raster der Rhabdomere im Komplexauge von *Musca*. Exp. Brain Res. **3**, 248–270 (1967)

Kirschfeld, K.: Absorption properties of photopigments in single rods, cones and rhabdomeres. In: Processing of optical data by organisms and machines (ed. W. Reichardt), pp. 116–136. New York-London: Academic Press 1969

Kirschfeld, K.: Aufnahme und Verarbeitung optischer Daten im Komplexauge von Insekten. Naturwissenschaften **58**, 201–209 (1971)

Kirschfeld, K.: Die notwendige Anzahl von Rezeptoren zur Bestimmung der Richtung des elektrischen Vektors linear polarisierten Lichtes. Z. Naturforsch. **27b**, 578–579 (1972)

Kirschfeld, K.: Vision of polarized light. Symposium Proceedings of the 4th International Biophysical Congress Moskow, 1973a, pp. 289–296

Kirschfeld, K.: Optomotorische Reaktionen der Biene auf bewegte „Polarisations-Muster". Z. Naturforsch. **28c**, 329–338 (1973b)

Kirschfeld, K.: Das neurale Superpositionsauge. Fortschr. Zool. **21**, 229–257 (1973c)

Kirschfeld, K., Franceschini, N.: Optische Eigenschaften der Ommatidien im Komplexauge von *Musca*. Kybernetik **5**, 47–52 (1968)

Kirschfeld, K., Franceschini, N.: Photostable pigments within the membrane of photoreceptors and their possible role. Biophys. Struct. Mech. **3**, 191–194 (1977)

Kirschfeld, K., Lutz, B.: Lateral inhibition in the compound eye of the fly, *Musca*. Z. Naturforsch. **29c**, 95–97 (1974)

Kirschfeld, K., Lutz, B.: The spectral sensitivity of the ocelli of *Calliphora* (Diptera). Z. Naturforsch. **32c**, 439–441 (1977)

Kirschfeld, K., Reichardt, W.: Optomotorische Versuche an *Musca* mit linear polarisiertem Licht. Z. Naturforsch. **25b**, 228 (1970)

Kirschfeld, K., Snyder, A.W.: Waveguide mode effects, birefringence and dichroism in fly photoreceptors. In: Photoreceptor optics (eds. A.W. Snyder, R. Menzel), pp. 56–77. Berlin-Heidelberg-New York: Springer 1975

Kirschfeld, K., Wenk, P.: The dorsal compound eye of simuliid flies: an eye specialized for the detection of small, rapidly moving objects. Z. Naturforsch. **31c**, 764–765 (1976)

Kirschfeld, K., Lindauer, M., Martin, H.: Problems of menotactic orientation according to the polarized light of the sky. Z. Naturforsch. **30c**, 88–90 (1975)

Kirschfeld, K., Franceschini, N., Minke, B.: Evidence for a sensitising pigment in fly photoreceptors. Nature **269**, 386–390 (1977)

Kirschfeld, K., Feiler, R., Franceschini, N.: A photostable pigment within the rhabdomeres of fly photoreceptors no. 7. J. Comp. Physiol. **125**, 275–284 (1978)

Klotsche, K.: Beiträge zur Kenntnis des feineren Baues der Cladoceren *(Daphnia magna)*. Jena. Z. Naturwissenschaften **50**, 601–646 (1913)

Kolb, G.: The structure of the eye of *Pieris brassicae* L. (Lepidoptera). Zoomorphol. **87**, 123–146 (1977)

Kondratyev, K.Y.: Radiation in the atmosphere. New York-London: Academic Press 1969, 912 pp

Korte, R.: Durch polarisiertes Licht hervorgerufene Optomotorik bei *Uca tangeri*. Experientia **21**, 98 (1965)

Korte, R.: Untersuchungen zum Sehvermögen einiger Dekapoden insbesondere von *Uca tangeri*. Z. Morphol. Ökol. Tiere **58**, 1–37 (1966)

Kramer, G.: Orientierte Zugaktivität gekäfigter Singvögel. Naturwissenschaften **37**, 188 (1950)

Kreithen, M.L., Keeton, W.T.: Detection of polarized light by the homing pigeon, *Columba livia*. J. Comp. Physiol. **89**, 83–92 (1974)

Kuiper, J.W.: The optics of the compound eye. Symp. Soc. Exp. Biol. **16**, 58–71 (1962)

Kullenberg, G.: Observed and computed scattering functions. In: Optical aspects of oceanography (eds. N.G. Jerlov, E. Steemann Nielsen), pp. 25–49. London-New York: Academic Press 1974

Kunze, P.: Die Orientierung der Retinalzellen im Auge von *Ocypode*. Z. Zellforsch. **90**, 454–462 (1968)

Kunze, P., Boschek, C.B.: Elektronenmikroskopische Untersuchung zur Form der achten Retinulazelle bei *Ocypode*. Z. Naturforsch. **23b**, 568–569 (1968)

Land, M.F.: Structure of the retinae of the principal eyes of jumping spiders (Salticidae: Dendryphantinae) in relation to visual optics. J. Exp. Biol. **51**, 443–470 (1969)

Land, M.F., Collett, T.S.: Chasing behaviour of houseflies *(Fannia canicularis)*. J. Comp. Physiol. **89**, 331–357 (1974)

Langer, H.: Nachweis dichroitischer Absorption des Sehfarbstoffes in den Rhabdomeren des Insektenauges. Z. Vergl. Physiol. **51**, 258–263 (1965)

Langer, H.: Grundlagen der Wahrnehmung von Wellenlänge und Schwingungsebene des Lichtes. Verh. Dtsch. Zool. Ges. Göttingen **30**, 195–233 (1966)

Langer, H. (ed.): Biochemistry and physiology of visual pigments. New York-Heidelberg-Berlin: Springer 1973

Langer, H., Thorell, B.: Microspectrophotometric assay of visual pigments in single rhabdomeres of the insect eye. In: The functional organization of the compound eye (ed. C.G. Bernhard), pp. 145–149. Oxford: Pergamon Press 1966

Laughlin, S.B.: The sensitivities of dragonfly photoreceptors and the voltage gain of transduction. J. Comp. Physiol. **111**, 221–247 (1976a)

Laughlin, S. B.: Adaptations of the dragonfly retina for contrast detection and the elucidation of neural principles in the peripheral visual system. In: Neuronal principles in vision (eds. F. Zettler, R. Weiler), pp. 175–193. Berlin-Heidelberg-New York: Springer 1976b

Laughlin, S. B.: Neural integration in the first optic neuropile of dragonflies. IV. Interneuron spectral sensitivity and contrast coding. J. Comp. Physiol. **112**, 199–211 (1976c)

Laughlin, S., McGinness, S.: The structures of dorsal and ventral regions of a dragonfly retina. Cell Tissue Res. **188**, 427–447 (1978)

Laughlin, S. B., Menzel, R., Snyder, A. W.: Membranes, dichroism, and receptor sensitivity. In: Photoreceptor optics (eds. A. W. Snyder, R. Menzel), pp. 237–259. Berlin-Heidelberg-New York: Springer 1975

Leggett, L. M. W.: Polarized light-sensitive interneurones in a swimming crab. Nature **262**, 709–711 (1976)

Leggett, L. M. W.: Some visual specializations of a crustacean eye. Ph.D. thesis, 140 pp. Australian National University 1978

Liebman, P. A.: Birefringence, dichroism, and rod outer segment structure. In: Photoreceptor optics (eds. A. W. Snyder, R. Menzel), pp. 199–214. Berlin-Heidelberg-New York: Springer 1975

Lindauer, M., Martin, H.: Die Schwereorientierung der Bienen unter dem Einfluß des Erdmagnetfeldes. Z. Vergl. Physiol. **60**, 219–243 (1968)

Lindauer, M., Schricker, B.: Über die Funktion der Ocellen bei den Dämmerungsflügen der Honigbiene. Biol. Zentralbl. **82**, 721–725 (1963)

Locket, N. A.: Adaptations to the deep-sea environment. In: Handbook of sensory physiology, Vol.-VII/5. The visual system in vertebrates (ed. F. Crescitelli), pp. 67–192. Berlin-Heidelberg-New York: Springer 1977

Lopresti, V., Macagno, E. R., Levinthal, C.: Structure and development of neuronal connections in isogenic organisms' lamina neuroblasts. Proc. Natl. Acad. Sci. USA **71**, 1098–1102 (1974)

Lüdtke, H.: Retinomotorik und Adaptationsvorgänge im Auge des Rückenschwimmers (*Notonecta glauca* L.). Z. Vergl. Physiol. **35**, 129–152 (1953)

Lundgren, B.: On the polarization of the daylight in the sea. Københavns Univ. Inst. Fysisk Oceanog. Rep. **17**, 1–34 (1971)

Lundgren, B., Højerslev, N.: Daylight measurements in the Sargasso Sea. Københavns Univ. Inst. Fysisk Oceanog. Rep. **14**, 1–33 (1971)

Luria, S. M., Kinney, J. A. S.: Linear polarising filters and underwater vision. Undersea Biomed. Res. **1**, 371–378 (1974)

Lythgoe, J. N.: The adaptation of visual pigments to the photic environment. In: Handbook of sensory physiology, Vol. VII/1. Photochemistry of vision (ed. H. J. A. Dartnall), pp. 566–603. Berlin-Heidelberg-New York: Springer 1972

Lythgoe, J. N., Hemmings, C. C.: Polarized light and underwater vision. Nature **213**, 893–894 (1967)

Macagno, E. R., Levinthal, C.: Computer reconstruction of the cellular architecture of the *Daphnia magna* optic ganglion. Proc. EM Soc. Am. 33 ann. Meeting 1975 (ed. G. W. Bailey), pp. 284–285. Baton Rouge: Claitor's 1975

Macagno, E. R., Lopresti, V., Levinthal, C.: Structure and development of neuronal connections in isogenic organisms: variations and similarities in the visual system of *Daphnia magna*. Proc. Natl. Acad. Sci. USA **70**, 57–61 (1973)

Magni, F., Papi, F., Savely, H. E., Tongiorgi, P.: Research on the structure and physiology of the eyes of a lycosid spider. III. Electroretinographic responses to polarized light. Arch. Ital. Biol. **103**, 146–158 (1965)

Malus, E. L.: Sur une propriété de la lumière réfléchie par les corps diaphanes. Soc. Philom. Bull. (Paris) **1**, 266–269 (1808)

Marrocco, R. T., DeValois, R. L.: Locus of spectral neutral point in monkey opponent cells depends on stimulus luminance relative to background. Brain Res. **119**, 465–470 (1977)

Marshall, S. M., Orr, A. P.: Biology of a marine copepod. Edinburgh-London: Oliver and Boyd 1955

Mayrat, A.: Premiers résultats d'une étude au microscope électronique des yeux des Crustacés. C.R. Acad. Sci. [D] (Paris) **255**, 766–768 (1962)

McCann, G. D., Arnett, D. W.: Spectral and polarization sensitivity of the dipteran visual system. J. Gen. Physiol. **59**, 534–558 (1972)

McCann, G. D., Fargason, R. D., Shantz, V. T.: The response properties of retinula cells in the fly *Calliphora erythrocephala* as a function of the wavelength and polarization properties of visible and ultraviolet light. Biol. Cybern. **26**, 93–107 (1977)

McCartney, E.J.: Optics of the atmosphere. New York-London-Sydney-Toronto: Wiley 1976

McEnroe, W.D.: Eyes of the female two spotted spider mite, *Tetranychus urticae*. III. Analysis of polarized light. Ann. Ent. Soc. Am. **64**, 879–883 (1971)

McFarland, W.N., Munz, F.W.: The visible spectrum during twilight and its implications to vision. In: Light as an ecological factor: II (eds. G.C. Evans, R. Bainbridge, O. Rackham), pp. 249–270. Oxford-Edinburgh-Melbourne: Blackwell 1975

McIntyre, P., Snyder, A.W.: Light propagation in twisted anisotropic media: application to photoreceptors. J. Opt. Soc. Am. **68**, 149–157 (1978)

McReynolds, J.S., Gorman, A.L.F.: Ionic basis of hyperpolarizing receptor potential in scallop eye: increase in permeability to potassium ions. Science **183**, 658–659 (1974)

Meffert, P., Smola, U.: Electrophysiological measurements of spectral sensitivity of central visual cells in eye of blowfly. Nature **260**, 342–344 (1976)

Melamed, J., Trujillo-Cenóz, O.: The fine structure of the visual system of *Lycosa* (Araneae; Lycosidae). Z. Zellforsch. **74**, 12–31 (1966)

Menzel, R.: The fine structure of the compound eye of *Formica polyctena*, functional morphology of a hymenopteran eye. In: Information processing in the visual systems of arthropods (ed. R. Wehner), pp. 37–47. Berlin-Heidelberg-New York: Springer 1972a

Menzel, R.: Feinstruktur des Komplexauges der roten Waldameise, *Formica polyctena* (Hymenoptera, Formicidae). Z. Zellforsch. **127**, 356–373 (1972b)

Menzel, R.: Polarized light sensitivity in arthropods. In: Light as an ecological factor: II (eds. G.C. Evans, R. Bainbridge, O. Rackam), pp. 289–303. Oxford-London-Edinburgh-Melbourne: Blackwell 1975a

Menzel, R.: Polarization sensitivity in insect eyes with fused rhabdoms. In: Photoreceptor optics (eds. A.W. Snyder, R. Menzel), pp. 372–387. Berlin-Heidelberg-New York: Springer 1975b

Menzel, R.: Optical and electrical coupling in an ommatidium with fused rhabdom. Verh. Dtsch. Zool. Ges. **1974**, 33–36 (1975c)

Menzel, R., Blakers, M.: Functional organization of an insect ommatidium with fused rhabdom. Cytobiologie **11**, 279–298 (1975)

Menzel, R., Blakers, M.: Colour receptors in the bee eye-morphology and spectral sensitivity. J. Comp. Physiol. **108**, 11–33 (1976)

Menzel, R., Knaut, R.: Pigment movement during light and chromatic adaptation in the retinula cells of *Formica polyctena* (Hymenoptera, Formicidae). J. Comp. Physiol. **86**, 125–138 (1973)

Menzel, R., Snyder, A.W.: Polarized light detection in the bee, *Apis mellifera*. J. Comp. Physiol. **88**, 247–270 (1974)

Meyer-Rochow, V.B.: A crustacean-like organization of insect rhabdoms. Cytobiologie **4**, 241–249 (1971)

Meyer-Rochow, V.B.: The eyes of *Creophilus erythrocephalus* F. and *Sartallus signatus* Sharp (Staphylinidae: Coleoptera). Light-, interference-, scanning electron- and transmission electron microscope examinations. Z. Zellforsch. **133**, 59–86 (1972)

Meyer-Rochow, V.B.: Structure and function of the larval eye of the sawfly, *Perga* (Hymenoptera). J. Insect Physiol. **20**, 1565–1591 (1974)

Meyer-Rochow, V.: Larval and adult eye of the western rock lobster, *Panulirus longipes*. Cell Tissue Res. **162**, 439–457 (1975)

Miller, W.H.: Morphology of the ommatidia of the compound eye of *Limulus*. J. Biophys. Biochem. Cytol. **3**, 421–428 (1957)

Miller, W.H., Snyder, A.W.: The tiered vertebrate retina. Vision Res. **17**, 239–255 (1977)

Mills, L.R.: Structure of the visual system of the two-spotted spider-mite, *Tetranychus urticae*. J. Insect Physiol. **20**, 795–808 (1974)

Mittelstaedt, H.: Die Regelungstheorie als methodisches Werkzeug der Verhaltensanalyse. Naturwissenschaften **48**, 246–254 (1961)

Mittelstaedt, H.: Grundprobleme der Analyse von Orientierungs-Leistungen. Max-Planck-Gesellschaft für Förderung der Wissenschaften, Jahrbuch, pp. 121–151 (1966)

Mittelstaedt, H.: Kybernetik der Schwereorientierung. Verh. Dtsch. Zool. Ges. 1971, 185–200 (1972)

Moody, M.F.: Evidence for the intraocular discrimination of vertically and horizontally polarized light by *Octopus*. J. Exp. Biol. **39**, 21–30 (1962)

Moody, M.F.: Photoreceptor organelles in animals. Biol. Rev. **39**, 43–86 (1964)

Moody, M.F., Parriss, J.R.: The discrimination of polarized light by *Octopus*: a behavioural and morphological study. Z. Vergl. Physiol. **44**, 268–291 (1961)

Morel, A.: Optical properties of pure water and pure sea water. In: Optical aspects of oceanography (eds. N. G. Jerlov, E. Steemann Nielsen), pp. 1–24. London-New York: Academic Press 1974

Moring, J., Järvilehto, M.: Dark recovery of polarized light sensitive and insensitive receptor cells in the retina of the fly. J. Comp. Physiol. **122**, 215–226 (1977)

Mote, M. I.: Polarization sensitivity. A phenomenon independent of stimulus intensity or state of adaptation in retinular cells of the crabs *Carcinus* and *Callinectes*. J. Comp. Physiol. **90**, 389–403 (1974)

Muller, K. J.: Photoreceptors in the crayfish compound eye: electrical interactions between cells as related to polarized light sensitivity. J. Physiol. (Lond.) **232**, 573–595 (1973)

Munz, F. W., McFarland, W. N.: The significance of spectral position in the rhodopsins of tropical marine fishes. Vision Res. **13**, 1829–1874 (1973)

Munz, F. W., McFarland, W. N.: Evolutionary adaptations of fishes to the photic environment. In: Handbook of sensory physiology, Vol. VII/5. The visual system in vertebrates (ed. F. Crescitelli), pp. 193–274. Berlin-Heidelberg-New York: Springer 1977

Naka, K. I., Rushton, W. A. H.: S-potentials from colour units in the retina of fish (Cyprinidae). J. Physiol. (Lond.) **185**, 536–555 (1966)

Nässel, D. R.: The retina and retinal projection on lamina ganglionaris of the crayfish *Pacifastacus leniusculus* (Dana). J. Comp. Neurol. **167**, 341–360 (1976a)

Nässel, D. R.: The fine structure of photoreceptor terminals in the compound eye of *Pandalus* (Crustacea). Acta Zool. **57**, 153–160 (1976b)

Nässel, D. R.: Types and arrangement of neurons in the crayfish optic lamina. Cell Tissue Res. **179**, 45–75 (1977)

Nässel, D. R., Waterman, T. H.: Golgi EM evidence for visual information channelling in the crayfish lamina ganglionaris. Brain Res. **130**, 556–563 (1977)

Nilsson, H. L., Elofsson, R.: A layered rhabdom in an isopod (Crustacea). A case of convergent development. Z. Mikrosk.-Anat. Forsch. **91**, 415–420 (1977)

Nosaki, H.: Electrophysiological study of color encoding in the compound eye of crayfish, *Procambarus clarkii*. Z. Vergl. Physiol. **64**, 318–323 (1964)

O'Day, W. T., Fernández, H. R.: Vision in the lanternfish *Stenobrachius leucopsarus* (Myctophidae). Marine Biol. **37**, 187–195 (1976)

Papi, F.: Ricerche sull'orientamento astronomica di *Arctosa perita* (Latr.) (Araneae Lycosidae). Pubbl. Staz. Zool. Napoli **27**, 76–103 (1955a)

Papi, F.: Astronomische Orientierung bei der Wolfspinne *Arctosa perita* (Latr.) Lycosidae. Z. Vergl. Physiol. **37**, 230–233 (1955b)

Papi, F.: Sull'orientamento astronomico in specie del gen. *Arctosa* (Araneae Lycosidae). Z. Vergl. Physiol. **41**, 481–489 (1959)

Pardi, L.: L'orientamento astronomico degli animali: risultati e problemi attuali. Boll. Zool. **24**, 473–523 (1957)

Parker, G. H.: The histology and development of the eye in the lobster. Bull. Mus. Comp. Zool. Harvard **20**, 1–60 (1890)

Parker, G. H.: The compound eyes in crustaceans. Bull. Mus. Comp. Zool. (Harvard) **21**, 45–140 (1891)

Parker, G. H.: The retina and optic ganglion in decapods especially in *Astacus*. Mitth. Zool. Sta. Neapel **12**, 1–73 (1895)

Parry, D. A.: The function of the insect ocellus. J. Exp. Biol. **24**, 211–219 (1947)

Patterson, J. A.: Neuronal architecture and function in the ocellar system of the locust. In: Neural principles in vision (eds. F. Zettler, R. Weiler), pp. 334–353. Berlin-Heidelberg-New York: Springer 1976

Paulus, H. F.: Zum Feinbau der Komplexaugen einiger Collembolen, eine vergleichend-anatomische Untersuchung (Insecta, Apterygota). Zool. Jb. Anat. **89**, 1–116 (1972)

Paulus, H. F.: The compound eyes of apterygote insects. In: The compound eye and vision of insects (ed. G. A. Horridge), pp. 3–19. Oxford: Clarendon Press 1975

Paulus, H. F.: Das Doppelauge von *Entomobrya muscorum* Micolet (Insecta, Collembola). Zoomorphol. **87**, 277–293 (1977)

Perrelet, A.: The fine structure of the retina of the honey bee drone. Z. Zellforsch. **108**, 530–562 (1970)

Perrelet, A., Bauer, H., Fryder, V.: Fracture faces of an insect rhabdom. J. Microscopie **13**, 97–106 (1972)

Phillips, E. F.: Structure and development of the compound eye in the honey bee. Proc. Acad. Nat. Sci. Philadelphia **57**, 123–157 (1905)

Poggio, T., Reichardt, W.: Visual control of orientation behaviour in the fly. Part II. Towards the underlying neural interactions. Q. Rev. Biophys. **9**, 377–438 (1976)

del Portillo, J.: Beziehungen zwischen den Öffnungswinkeln der Ommatidien, Krümmung und Gestalt der Insektenaugen und ihrer funktionellen Aufgabe. Z. Vergl. Physiol. **23**, 100–145 (1936)

Preisendorfer, R. W.: Hydrologic optics, Vol. I, pp. 50–53, Vol. III, pp. 19–24. Honolulu: U.S. Department of Commerce, National Oceanic and Atmospheric Administration 1976

Pribram, K. H.: Consciousness and neurophysiology. Fed. Proc. **37**, 2271–2274 (1978)

Ramus, J., Lemon, F., Zimmerman, C.: Adaptation of light-harvesting pigments to downwelling light and the consequent photosynthetic performance of the eulittoral rockweeds *Ascophyllum nodoseum* and *Fucus vesiculosus*. Marine Biol. **42**, 293–303 (1977)

Reichardt, W.: Nervous processing of sensory information. In: Theoretical and mathematical biology (eds. T. II. Waterman, H. J. Morowitz), pp. 344–370. New York: Blaisdell 1965

Reichardt, W.: Musterinduzierte Flugorientierung. Verhaltens-Versuche an der Fliege *Musca domestica*. Naturwissenschaften **60**, 122–138 (1973)

Reichardt, W., Poggio, T.: Visual control of orientation behaviour in the fly. Part. I. A quantitative analysis. Q. Rev. Biophys. **9**, 311–375 (1976)

Rensing, L., Bogenschütz, H.: Vorzugsrichtungen von *Corixa punctata* Illig. in polarisiertem Licht. Zool. Jahrb. Abt. Allg. Zool. Physiol. **72**, 123–135 (1966)

Ribi, W. A.: The neurons of the first optic ganglion of the bee *(Apis mellifera)*. Adv. Anat. Embryol. Cell Biol. **50**, 1–43 (1975)

Ringelberg, J., Flik, B. J. A., Buis, R. C.: Contrast orientation in *Daphnia magna* and its significance for vertical plane orientation in the pelagic biotope in general. Neth. J. Zool. **25**, 454–475 (1975)

Robert, P., Scheffer, D., Médioni, J.: Réactions oculo-motrices de la Daphnie (*Daphnia pulex* DeGeer) en réponse à des lumières monochromatiques d'égale énergie. Sensibilité visuelle et sensibilité dermatoptique. C. R. Soc. Biol. (Paris) **152**, 1000–1003 (1958)

Rodieck, R. W.: The vertebrate retina. San Francisco: Freeman 1973

Röhlich, P., Törö, I.: Fine structure of the compound eye of *Daphnia* in normal, dark- and strongly light-adapted state. In: The structure of the eye. II. Symposium (ed. J. W. Rohen), pp. 175–186. Stuttgart: Schattauer 1965

Roth, H., Menzel, R.: ERG of *Formica polyctena* and selective adaptation. In: Information processing in the visual systems of arthropods (ed. R. Wehner), pp. 177–181. Berlin-Heidelberg-New York: Springer 1972

Rowell, C. H. F., Wells, M. J.: Retinal orientation and the discrimination of polarized light by octopuses. J. Exp. Biol. **38**, 827–831 (1961)

Rozenberg, G. V.: Twilight. New York: Plenum Press 1966

Rutherford, D. J., Horridge, G. A.: The rhabdom of the lobster eye. Q. J. Microsc. Sci. **106**, 119–130 (1965)

Santschi, F.: Observations et remarques critiques sur le méchanisme de l'orientation chez les fourmis. Rev. Suisse Zool. **19**, 303–338 (1911)

Santschi, F.: Les différentes orientations chez les fourmis. Rev. Zool. Afr. **11**, 111–144 (1923)

Schinz, R. H.: Structural specialization in the dorsal retina of the bee, *Apis mellifera*. Cell Tissue Res. **162**, 22–34 (1975)

Schneider, L., Langer, H.: Die Struktur des Rhabdoms im „Doppelauge" des Wasserläufers *Gerris lacustris*. Z. Zellforsch. **99**, 538–559 (1969)

Schneider, L., Langer, H.: Electron microscopic investigations on the structure of the photoreceptor cells in the compound eye of *Ascalaphus macaronius* (Insecta: Neuroptera). (Preliminary note). In: Photoreceptors optics (eds. A. W. Snyder, R. Menzel), pp. 410–412. Berlin-Heidelberg-New York: Springer 1975

Scholes, J.: The electrical responses of the retinal receptors and the lamina in the visual system of the fly *Musca*. Kybernetik **6**, 149–162 (1969)

Schöne, H.: Menotaktische Orientierung nach polarisiertem und unpolarisiertem Licht bei der Mangrovekrabbe *Goniopsis*. Z. Vergl. Physiol. **46**, 496–514 (1963)

Schöne, H.: Orientation in space: Animals. In: Marine ecology, Vol. II (ed. O. Kinne), pp. 499–560. London-New York: Wiley 1975

Schöne, H., Schöne, H.: Eyestalk movements induced by polarized light in the ghost crab, *Ocypode quadrata*. Science **134**, 675–676 (1961)

Schönenberger, N.: The fine structure of the compound eye of *Squilla mantis* (Crustacea, Stomatopoda). Cell Tissue Res. **176**, 205–233 (1977)

Schricker, B.: Die Orientierung der Honigbiene in der Dämmerung, zugleich ein Beitrag zur Frage der Ocellenfunktion bei Bienen. Z. Vergl. Physiol. **49**, 420–458 (1965)

Schröer, W. D.: Zum Mechanismus der Analyse polarisierten Lichtes bei *Agelena gracilens* C.L. Koch (Araneae, Agelenidae). I. Die Morphologie der Retina des vorderen Mittelauges. Z. Morphol. Tiere **79**, 215–231 (1974)

Schröer, W. D.: Polarisationsempfindlichkeit rhabdomerialer Systeme in den Hauptaugen der Trichterspinne *Agelena gracilens* (Arachnidae: Araneae: Agelenidae). Ent. Germ. **3**, 88–92 (1976)

Schulz, H.: Über die Bedeutung des Lichtes im Leben niederer Krebse. Z. Vergl. Physiol. **7**, 488–552 (1928)

Seitz, G.: Nachweis einer Pupillenreaktion im Auge der Schmeißfliege. Z. Vergl. Physiol. **69**, 169–185 (1970)

Sekera, Z.: Polarization of skylight. In: Handbuch der Physik, Vol. 48 (ed. S. Flügge), pp. 288–328. Berlin-Göttingen-Heidelberg: Springer 1957

Sekera, Z., Coulson, K. L., Deirmendjian, D., Fraser, R. S., Seaman, C.: Investigation of polarization of skylight. Final Report Contract No. AI 19 (122)–239. Los Angeles, University of California, Department of Meteorology 1955, 133 pp

Shaw, S. R.: Polarized light responses from crab retinula cells. Nature **211**, 92–93 (1966)

Shaw, S. R.: Interreceptor coupling in ommatidia of drone honeybee and locust compound eyes. Vision Res. **9**, 999–1029 (1969a)

Shaw, S. R.: Sense-cell structure and interspecies comparisons of polarized light absorption in arthropod compound eyes. Vision Res. **9**, 1031–1040 (1969b)

Sherk, T. E.: Development of the compound eyes of dragonflies (Odonata). III. Adult compound eyes. J. Exp. Zool. **203**, 61–79 (1978)

Shurcliff, W. A.: Polarized light, production and use. Cambridge: Harvard University Press 1962

Skrzipek, K. H., Skrzipek, H.: Die Anordnung der Ommatidien in der Retina der Biene (*Apis mellifera* L.). Z. Zellforsch. **139**, 567–582 (1973)

Skrzipek, K.-H., Skrzipek, H.: The ninth retinula cell in the ommatidium of the worker honey bee (*Apis mellifica* L.). Z. Zellforsch. **147**, 589–593 (1974)

Smith, F. E., Baylor, E. R.: Color responses in the Cladocera and their ecological significance. Am. Nat. **87**, 49–55 (1953)

Smith, F. E., Baylor, E. R.: Bees, *Daphnia* and polarized light. Ecol. **41**, 360–363 (1960)

Smith, R. C.: Structure of solar radiation in the upper layers of the sea. In: Optical aspects of oceanography (eds. N. G. Jerlov, E. Steemann Nielsen), pp. 95–119. London-New York: Academic Press 1974

Smola, U.: Voltage noise in insect visual cells. In: Neural principles in vision (eds. F. Zettler, R. Weiler), pp. 194–213. Berlin-Heidelberg-New York: Springer 1976

Smola, U., Meffert, P.: Spectral sensitivity of central visual cells in eye of blowfly *Calliphora erythrocephala*. Verh. Dtsch. Zool. Ges. 282 (1976)

Snyder, A. W.: Polarization sensitivity of individual retinula cells. J. Comp. Physiol. **83**, 331–360 (1973)

Snyder, A. W.: Light absorption in visual photoreceptors. J. Opt. Soc. Am. **64**, 216–230 (1974)

Snyder, A. W.: Optical properties of invertebrate photoreceptors. In: The compound eye and vision of insects (ed. G. A. Horridge), pp. 179–235. Oxford: Clarendon 1975a

Snyder, A. W.: Photoreceptor optics – theoretical principles. In: Photoreceptor optics (eds. A. W. Snyder, R. Menzel), pp. 38–55. Berlin-Heidelberg-New York: Springer 1975b

Snyder, A. W.: Acuity of compound eyes, physical limitations and design. J. Comp. Physiol. **116**, 161–182 (1977)

Snyder, A. W., Laughlin, S. B.: Dichroism and absorption by photoreceptors. J. Comp. Physiol. **100**, 101–116 (1975)

Snyder, A. W., McIntyre, P.: Polarization sensitivity of twisted fused rhabdoms. In: Photoreceptor optics (eds. A. W. Snyder, R. Menzel), pp. 388–391. Berlin-Heidelberg-New York: Springer 1975

Snyder, A. W., Menzel, R. (eds.): Photoreceptor optics. Berlin-Heidelberg-New York: Springer 1975

Snyder, A. W., Pask, C.: Spectral sensitivity of dipteran retinula cells. J. Comp. Physiol. **84**, 59–76 (1973)

Snyder, A. W., Menzel, R., Laughlin, S. B.: Structure and function of the fused rhabdom. J. Comp. Physiol. **87**, 99–135 (1973)

Snyder, A. W., Stavenga, D. G., Laughlin, S. B.: Spatial information capacity of compound eyes. J. Comp. Physiol. **116**, 183–207 (1977)

Sommer, E., Wehner, R.: The retina-lamina projection in the visual system of the bee, *Apis mellifera*. Cell Tissue Res. **163**, 45–61 (1975)

Stark, W.S.: Spectral selectivity of visual response alterations mediated by interconversions of native and intermediate photopigments in *Drosophila*. J. Comp. Physiol. **96**, 343–356 (1975)

Stark, W.S., Ivanyshyn, A.M., Greenberg, R.M.: Sensitivity and photopigments of R 1–R 6, a two-peaked photoreceptor, in *Drosophila, Calliphora*, and *Musca*. J. Comp. Physiol. **121**, 289–305 (1977)

Stavenga, D.G.: Optical qualities of the fly eye – an approach from the side of geometrical, physical and waveguide optics. In: Photoreceptor optics (eds. A.W. Snyder, R. Menzel), pp. 126–144. Berlin-Heidelberg-New York: Springer 1975

Stearns, S.C.: Light responses of *Daphnia pulex*. Limn. Oceanogr. **20**, 564–570 (1975)

Steemann Nielsen, E.: Light and primary production. In: Optical aspects of oceanography (eds. N.G. Jerlov, E. Steemann Nielsen), pp. 361–388. London-New York: Academic Press 1974

Sterba, G.: Die neurosekretorischen Zellgruppen einiger Cladoceren (*Daphnia pulex* und *magna, Simocephalus vetulus*). Zool. Jb. Abt. Anat. **76**, 303–310 (1957)

Stockhammer, K.: Zur Wahrnehmung der Schwingungsrichtung linear polarisierten Lichtes bei Insekten. Z. Vergl. Physiol. **38**, 30–83 (1956)

Stockhammer, K.: Die Orientierung nach der Schwingungsrichtung linear polarisierten Lichtes und ihre sinnesphysiologischen Grundlagen. Ergeb. Biol. **21**, 23–56 (1959)

Stone, A.C., Koopowitz, H.: The ultrastructural organization of the visual system of the wax moth *Galleria mellonella*: the retina. Cell Tissue Res. **174**, 519–531 (1976)

Stowe, S., Ribi, W.A., Sandeman, D.C.: The organization of the lamina ganglionaris of the crabs *Scylla serrata* and *Leptograpsus variegatus*. Cell Tissue Res. **178**, 517–532 (1977)

Strausfeld, N.J.: Atlas of an insect brain. Berlin-Heidelberg-New York: Springer 1976a

Strausfeld, N.J.: Mosaic organizations, layers, and visual pathways in the insect brain. In: Neural principles in vision (eds. F. Zettler, R. Weiler), pp. 245–279. Berlin-Heidelberg-New York: Springer 1976b

Sugawara, K., Katagiri, Y., Tomita, T.: Polarized light responses from octopus single retinular cells. J. Fac. Sci. Hokkaido Univ. Ser. VI Zool. **17**, 581–586 (1971)

Sullivan, C.R., Wellington, W.A.: The light reactions of larvae of the tent caterpillars, *Malacosoma disstria* Hbn., *M. americanum* (Fab.), and *M. pluviale* (Dyar). (Lepidoptera: Lasiocampidae). Can. Entomol. **85**, 297–310 (1953)

Tasaki, K., Karita, K.: Intraretinal discrimination of horizontal and vertical planes of polarized light by octopus. Nature **209**, 934–935 (1966a)

Tasaki, K., Karita, K.: Discrimination of horizontal and vertical planes of polarized light by the cephalopod retina. Jpn. J. Physiol. **16**, 205–216 (1966b)

Tasaki, K., Tsukahara, Y., Watanabe, M., Suzuki, H.: Lateral inhibition in the retina of the octopus. Proceedings of the International Union of Physiological Science (New Delhi), **11** (1974), (Abs.)

Täuber, U.: Octopus rhodopsin *in situ:* microphotometric measurements of orientational and spectral changes. In: Biochemistry and physiology of visual pigments (ed. H. Langer), pp. 313–317. Berlin-Heidelberg-New York: Springer 1973

Täuber, U.: Analyse des Polarisationszustandes des aus dem Rhabdomer austretenden Lichtes. J. Comp. Physiol. **95**, 169–183 (1974)

Täuber, U.: Photokinetics and dichroism of visual pigments in the photoreceptors of *Eledone (Ozoena) moschata*. In: Photoreceptor optics (eds. A.W. Snyder, R. Menzel), pp. 296–315. Berlin-Heidelberg-New York: Springer 1975

Taylor, D.H., Ferguson, D.E.: Extraoptic celestial orientation in the southern cricket frog *Acris gryllus*. Science **168**, 390–392 (1970)

Timofeeva, V.A.: Spatial distribution of the degree of polarization of natural light in the sea. Bull. (Izv.) Acad. Sci. U.S.S.R., Geophys. Ser. **12**, 1843–1851 (1962)

Timofeeva, V.A.: Optics of turbid waters. In: Optical aspects of oceanography (eds. N.G. Jerlov, E. Steemann Nielsen), pp. 177–219. London-New York: Academic Press 1974

Toh, Y., Kuwabara, M.: Fine structure of the dorsal ocellus of the worker honeybee. J. Morphol. **143**, 285–306 (1974)

Toh, Y., Kuwabara, M.: Synaptic organization of the fleshfly ocellus. J. Neurocytol. **4**, 271–287 (1975)

Toh, Y., Tominaga, Y., Kuwabara, M.: The fine structure of the dorsal ocellus of the fleshfly. J. Electron Microsc. (Tokyo) **20**, 56–66 (1971)

Treviño, D. L., Larimer, J. L.: The responses of one class of neurons in the optic tract of crayfish *(Procambarus)* to monochromatic light. Z. Vergl. Physiol. **69**, 139–149 (1970)

Trujillo-Cenóz, O., Bernard, G. D.: Some aspects of the retinal organization of *Sympycnus lineatus* Loew (Diptera, Dolichopodidae). J. Ultrastruct. Res. **38**, 149–160 (1972)

Trujillo-Cenóz, O., Melamed, J.: Compound eye of dipterans: anatomical basis for integration. An electron microscope study. J. Ultrastruct. Res. **16**, 395–397 (1966)

Tsukahara, Y., Horridge, G. A.: Visual pigment spectra from sensitivity measurements after chromatic adaptation of single dronefly retinula cells. J. Comp. Physiol. **114**, 233–251 (1977a)

Tsukahara, Y., Horridge, G. A.: Interaction between two retinula cell types in the anterior eye of the dronefly *Eristalis*. J. Comp. Physiol. **115**, 287–298 (1977b)

Tsukahara, Y., Horridge, G. A., Stavenga, D. G.: Afterpotentials in dronefly retinula cells. J. Comp. Physiol. **114**, 253–266 (1977)

Tyler, J. E.: Radiance distribution as a function of depth in an underwater environment. Bull. Scripps Inst. Oceanog. Univ. Calif. **7**, 363–412 (1960)

Tyler, J. E.: Estimation of per cent polarization in deep oceanic water. J. Mar. Res. **21**, 102–109 (1963)

Tyler, J. E.: Heuristic arguments for the pattern of polarization in deep ocean water. In: Planets, stars, and nebulae (ed. T. Gehrels), pp. 434–443. Tucson: University of Arizona Press 1974

Uehara, A., Toh, Y., Tateda, H.: Fine structure of the eyes of orbweavers *Argiope amoena* L. Koch (Araneae: Argiopidae). I. The anteromedial eyes. Cell Tissue Res. **182**, 81–91 (1977)

Umminger, B. L.: Polarotaxis in copepods. I. An endogenous rhythm in polarotaxis in *Cyclops vernalis* and its relation to vertical migration. Biol. Bull. **135**, 239–251 (1968a)

Umminger, B. L.: Polarotaxis in copepods. II. The ultrastructural basis and ecological significance of polarized light sensitivity in copepods. Biol. Bull. **135**, 252–261 (1968b)

Umminger, B. L.: Polarotaxis in copepods. III. A light contrast reaction in *Diaptomus shoshone* Forbes. Crustaceana **16**, 202–204 (1969)

Vaissière, R.: Morphologie et histologie comparées des yeux des Crustacés Copépodes. thesis, University of Paris 1961, 25 pp

Varela, F. G., Porter, K. R.: Fine structure of the visual system of the honeybee *(Apis mellifera)*. J. Ultrastruct. Res. **29**, 236–259 (1969)

Varela, F. G., Wiitanen, W.: The optics of the compound eye of the honeybee *(Apis mellifera)*. J. Gen. Physiol. **55**, 336–358 (1970)

Verkhovskaya, I. N.: The influence of polarized light on the phototaxis of certain organisms. Bull. Moscow Nat. Hist. Soc., Biol. Sect. **49**, 101–113 (1940)

Via, S. E., Forward, R. B. F.: The ontogeny and spectral sensitivity of polarotaxis in larvae of the crab *Rhithropanopeus harrisi* (Gould). Biol. Bull. **149**, 251–266 (1975)

Viaud, G.: Recherches expérimentales sur le phototropisme des Daphnies. Publs. Fac. Lettres Strasbourg **84**, 1–196 (1938)

Vowles, D. M.: Sensitivity of ants to polarized light. Nature **165**, 282–283 (1950)

Vowles, D. M.: The orientation of ants. I. The substitution of stimuli. J. Exp. Biol. **31**, 341–355 (1954a)

Vowles, D. M.: The orientation of ants. II. Orientation to light, gravity and polarized light. J. Exp. Biol. **31**, 356–375 (1954b)

Vries, H. de, Kuiper, J. W.: Optics of the insect eye. Ann. N.Y. Acad. Sci. **74**, 196–303 (1958)

Vries, H. de, Spoor, A., Jielof, R.: Properties of the eye with respect to polarized light. Physica **19**, 419–432 (1953)

Wachmann, E.: Vergleichende Analyse der feinstrukturellen Organisation offener Rhabdome in den Augen der Cucujiformia (Insecta, Coleoptera), unter besonderer Berücksichtigung der Chrysomelidae. Zoomorphol. **88**, 95–131 (1977)

Wachmann, E., Schröer, W. D.: Zur Morphologie der Dorsal- und Ventralaugen des Taumelkäfers *Gyrinus substriatus* (Steph.) (Coleoptera, Gyrinidae). Zoomorphol. **82**, 43–61 (1975)

Wada, S.: Ein spezieller Rhabdomerentyp im Fliegenauge. Experientia **27**, 1237–1238 (1971)

Wada, S.: Spezielle randzonale Ommatidien der Fliegen (Diptera: Brachycera): Architektur und Verteilung. Z. Morphol. Tiere **77**, 87–125 (1974a)

Wada, S.: Spezielle randzonale Ommatidien von *Calliphora erythrocephala* Meig. (Diptera, Calliphoridae): Architektur der zentralen Rhabdomeren-Kolumne und Topographie im Komplexauge. Int. J. Insect Morphol. Embryol. **3**, 397–424 (1974b)

Wada, S.: Morphological duality of the retinal pattern in flies. Experientia **31**, 921–923 (1975)

Wald, G., Rayport, S.: Vision in annelid worms. Science **196**, 1434–1439 (1977)

Wald, G., Seldin, E.: Spectral sensitivity of the common prawn, *Palaemonetes vulgaris.* J. Gen. Physiol. **51**, 694–700 (1968)

Waterman, T. H.: A light polarization analyzer in the compound eye of *Limulus.* Science **111**, 252–254 (1950)

Waterman, T. H.: Polarized light navigation by arthropods. Trans. N.Y. Acad. Sci. **14**, 11–14 (1951)

Waterman, T. H.: Polarization patterns in submarine illumination. Science **120**, 927–932 (1954a)

Waterman, T. H.: Polarized light and angle of stimulus incidence in the compound eye of *Limulus.* Proc. Natl. Acad. Sci. USA **40**, 258–262 (1954b)

Waterman, T. H.: Polarization of scattered sunlight in deep water. Deep Sea Res. **3** [Suppl.], 426–434 (1955)

Waterman, T. H.: Polarized light and plankton navigation. In: Perspectives in marine biology (ed. A. A. Buzzati-Traverso), pp. 429–450. Berkeley: University of California Press 1958

Waterman, T.H.: Interaction of polarized light and turbidity in the orientation of *Daphnia* and *Mysidium.* Z. Vergl. Physiol. **43**, 149–172 (1960)

Waterman, T.H.: Light sensitivity and vision. In: The physiology of Crustacea, Vol. II (ed. T.H. Waterman), pp. 1–64. New York: Academic Press 1961a

Waterman, T. H.: Polarized light and orientation by aquatic arthropods. Proceedings of the 3rd International Congress on Photobiology, pp. 214–216. Amsterdam: Elsevier 1961b

Waterman, T. H.: The analysis of spatial orientation. Ergeb. Biol. **26**, 98–117 (1963)

Waterman, T. H.: Specific effects of polarized light on organisms. In: Environmental biology (eds. P. L. Altman, D.S. Dittmer), pp. 155–165. Bethesda: Fed. Am. Soc. Exp. Biol. 1966a

Waterman, T. H.: Polarotaxis and primary photoreceptor events in Crustacea. In: The functional organization of the compound eye (ed. C. G. Bernhard), pp. 493–511. Oxford: Pergamon 1966b

Waterman, T. H.: Information channeling in the crustacean retina. Proceedings of the Symposium on Information Processing in Sight Sensory Systems, 1965 (ed. P. W. Nye), pp. 48–56. Pasadena: California Institute of Technology 1966c

Waterman, T. H.: Systems analysis and the visual orientation of animals. Am. Sci. **54**, 15–45 (1966d)

Waterman, T. H.: Visual direction finding by fishes. In: Animal orientation and navigation (eds. S. R. Galler, K. Schmidt-Koenig, G. J. Jacobs, R. E. Belleville), pp. 437–456. Washington: National Aeronautics and Space Administration 1972

Waterman, T. H.: Responses to polarized light: Animals. In: Biology data book, Vol. II (eds. P. L. Altman, D.S. Dittmer), pp. 1272–1289. Bethesda: Fed. Amer. Soc. Exp. Biol. 1973

Waterman, T. H.: Polarimeters in animals. In: Planets, stars, and nebulae (ed. T. Gehrels), pp. 472–494. Tucson: University of Arizona Press 1974a

Waterman, T. H.: Underwater light and the orientation of animals. In: Optical aspects of oceanography (eds. N. G. Jerlov, E. Steemann Nielson), pp. 415–443. London: Academic Press 1974b

Waterman, T. H.: Natural polarized light and *e*-vector discrimination by vertebrates. In: Light as an ecological factor: II (eds. G. C. Evans, R. Bainbridge, O. Rackham), pp. 305–335. Oxford: Blackwell 1975a

Waterman, T. H.: Expectation and achievement in comparative physiology. J. Exp. Zool. **194**, 309–343 (1975b)

Waterman, T. H.: The optics of polarization sensitivity. In: Photoreceptor optics (eds. A. W. Snyder, R. Menzel), pp. 339–371. Berlin-Heidelberg-New York: Springer 1975c

Waterman, T. H.: The bridge between visual input and central programming in crustaceans. In: Identified neurons and behavior in arthropods (ed. G. Hoyle), pp. 371–386. New York: Plenum 1977

Waterman, T. H., Aoki, K.: *E*-vector sensitivity patterns in the goldfish optic tectum. J. Comp. Physiol. **95**, 13–27 (1974)

Waterman, T.H., Chace, F.A., Jr.: General crustacean biology. In: The physiology of Crustacea, Vol. I (ed. T.H. Waterman), pp. 1–33. New York: Academic Press 1960

Waterman, T.H., Fernández, H.R.: *E*-vector and wavelength discrimination by retinular cells of the crayfish *Procambarus.* Z. Vergl. Physiol. **68**, 154–174 (1970)

Waterman, T. H., Forward, R. B., Jr.: Field demonstration of polarotaxis in the fish *Zenarchopterus.* J. Exp. Zool. **180**, 33–54 (1972)

Waterman, T. H., Hashimoto, H.: *E*-vector discrimination by the goldfish optic tectum. J. Comp. Physiol. **95**, 1–12 (1974)

Waterman, T. H., Horch, K. W.: Mechanism of polarized light perception. Science **154**, 467–475 (1966)

Waterman, T. H., Westell, W. E.: Quantitative effect of the sun's position on submarine light polarization. J. Mar. Res. **15**, 149–169 (1956)

Waterman, T. H., Wiersma, C. A. G.: The functional relation between retinal cells and optic nerve in *Limulus*. J. Exp. Zool. **126**, 59–86 (1954)

Waterman, T. H., Wiersma, C. A. G.: Electrical responses in decapod crustacean visual systems. J. Cell. Comp. Physiol. **61**, 1–16 (1963)

Waterman, T. H., Wiersma, C. A. G., Bush, B. M. H.: Afferent visual responses in the optic nerve of the crab, *Podophthalmus*. J. Cell. Comp. Physiol. **63**, 135–156 (1964)

Waterman, T. H., Fernández, H. R., Goldsmith, T. H.: Dichroism of photosensitive pigment in rhabdoms of the crayfish *Orconectes*. J. Gen. Physiol. **54**, 415–432 (1969)

Weber, G., Renner, M.: The ocellus of the cockroach, *Periplaneta americana* (Blattariae). Receptory area. Cell Tissue Res. **168**, 209–222 (1976)

Wehner, R.: Optische Orientierungsmechanismen im Heimkehr-Verhalten von *Cataglyphis bicolor* Fab. (Formicidae, Hymenoptera). Rev. Suisse Zool. **75**, 1076–1085 (1968)

Wehner, R.: Visual orientation performances of desert ants *(Cataglyphis bicolor)* toward astromenotactic directions and horizon landmarks. In: Animal orientation and navigation (eds. S. R. Galler, K. Schmidt-Koenig, G. J. Jacobs, R. E. Bellville), pp. 421–436. Washington: National Aeronautics and Space Administration 1972

Wehner, R.: Space constancy of the visual world in insects. Fortschr. Zool. **23**, 148–160 (1975)

Wehner, R.: Polarized-light navigation by insects. Sci. Am. **235**, 106–115 (1976a)

Wehner, R.: Structure and function of the peripheral pathway in hymenopterans. In: Neuronal principles in vision (eds. F. Zettler, R. Weiler), pp. 280–333. Berlin-Heidelberg-New York: Springer 1976b

Wehner, R., Bernard, G. D.: Die Bestimmung der *E*-Vektor-Richtung partiell linear polarisierten Lichts bei Hymenopteren. Verh. Dtsch. Zool. Ges. **1976**, 252 (1976)

Wehner, R., Duelli, P.: The spatial orientation of desert ants, *Cataglyphis bicolor*. Experientia **27**, 1364–1366 (1971)

Wehner, R., Eheim, W. P., Herrling, P. L.: Die Rastereigenschaften des Komplexauges von *Cataglyphis bicolor* (Formicidae, Hymenoptera). Rev. Suisse Zool. **78**, 722–737 (1971)

Wehner, R., Bernard, G. D., Geiger, E.: Twisted and non-twisted rhabdoms and their significance for polarization detection in the bee. J. Comp. Physiol. **104**, 225–245 (1975)

Wehrhahn, C.: Evidence for the role of receptors R 7/8 in the orientation behaviour of the fly. Biol. Cybern. **21**, 213–220 (1976)

Wehrhahn, C., Reichardt, W.: Visually induced height orientation of the fly *Musca domestica*. Biol. Cybern. **20**, 37–50 (1975)

Weiler, R., Huber, M.: The significance of different eye regions for astromenotactic orientation in *Cataglyphis bicolor*. In: Information processing in the visual systems of arthropods (ed. R. Wehner), pp. 287–294. Berlin-Heidelberg-New York: Springer 1972

Wellington, W. G.: Motor responses evoked by the dorsal ocelli of *Sarcophaga aldrichi* Parker, and the orientation of the fly to plane polarized light. Nature (Lond.) **172**, 1177 (1953)

Wellington, W. G.: Solar heat and plane polarized light versus the light compass reaction in the orientation of insects on the ground. Ann. Entomol. Soc. Am. **48**, 67–76 (1955)

Wellington, W. G.: Changes in mosquito flight associated with natural changes in polarized light. Can. Entomol. **106**, 941–948 (1974a)

Wellington, W. G.: Bumblebee ocelli and navigation at dusk. Science **183**, 550–551 (1974b)

Wellington, W. G.: A special light to steer by. Nat. Hist. **83** (10), 46–53 (1974c)

Wellington, W. G.: Mountain cloud barriers to the dispersal of alpine mosquitoes. Bull. Am. Meteorol. Soc. **57**, 283–284 (1976a) (Abs.)

Wellington, W. G.: Applying behavioral studies in entomological problems. In: Perspectives in forest entomology (eds. J. F. Anderson, H. K. Kaya), pp. 87–97. New York-San Francisco-London: Academic Press 1976b

Wellington, W. G., Sullivan, C. R., Green, A. W.: Polarized light and body temperature level as orientation factors in the light reactions of some hymenopterous and lepidopterous larvae. Can. J. Zool. **29**, 339–351 (1951)

Wellington, W. G., Sullivan, C. R., Henson, W. R.: The light reactions of larvae of the spotless fall webworm *Hyphantria textor* Harr. (Lepidoptera: Arctiidae). Can. Entomol. **86**, 529–541 (1954)

Wenner, A. M.: The bee language controversy. Educational Programs Improvement 1971

Whitney, L. V.: The angular distribution of characteristic diffuse light in natural waters. J. Mar. Res. **4**, 122 (1941)

Wiersma, C. A. G., Bush, B. M. H., Waterman, T. H.: Efferent visual responses of contralateral origin in the optic nerve of the crab, *Podophthalmus*. J. Cell. Comp. Physiol. **64**, 309–326 (1964)

Wolken, J. J.: Retinal structure. Mollusc cephalopods: *Octopus*, *Sepia*. J. Biophys. Biochem. Cytol. **4**, 835–838 (1958)

Wolken, J. J., Gallik, G. J.: The compound eye of a crustacean: *Leptodora kindtii*. J. Cell Biol. **26**, 968–973 (1965)

Wolken, J. J., Capenos, J., Turano, A.: Photoreceptor structures. J. Biophys. Biochem. Cytol. **3**, 441–448 (1957)

Woodcock, A. E. R., Goldsmith, T. H.: Spectral responses of sustaining fibers in the optic tract of crayfish *(Procambarus)*. Z. Vergl. Physiol. **69**, 117–133 (1970)

Yamaguchi, T.: Mechanism of polarized light perception and its neural processes through the optic nerves in crayfish. Zool. Mag. **76**, 443 (1967), (Abs.)

Yamaguchi, T., Katagiri, Y., Ochi, K.: Polarized light responses from retinula cells and sustaining fibers in the mantis shrimp. Biol. J. Okayama Univ. **17**, 61–66 (1976)

Yamamoto, T., Tasaki, K., Sugawara, Y., Tonosaki, A.: Fine structure of the *Octopus* retina. J. Cell Biol. **25**, 345–359 (1965)

Yamashita, S., Tateda, H.: Spectral sensitivities of jumping spider eyes. J. Comp. Physiol. **105**, 29–41 (1976)

York, B., Wiersma, C. A. G.: Visual processing in the rock lobster (Crustacea). Prog. Neurobiol. **5**, 127–166 (1975)

Young, J. Z.: The visual system of *Octopus*. I. Regularities in the retina and optic lobes of *Octopus* in relation to form discrimination. Nature **186**, 836–844 (1960)

Young, J. Z.: The retina of cephalopods and its degeneration after optic nerve section. The optic lobes of *Octopus vulgaris*. Philos. Trans. R. Soc. Lond. [Biol.] **245**, 1–58 (1962)

Young, J. Z.: The anatomy of the nervous system of *Octopus vulgaris*. Oxford: Clarendon 1971

Young, S.: Directional differences in the color sensitivity of *Daphnia magna*. J. Exp. Biol. **61**, 261–267 (1974)

Young, S., Downing, A. C.: The receptive fields of *Daphnia* ommatidia. J. Exp. Biol. **64**, 185–202 (1976)

Zaneveld, J. R.: New developments of the theory of radiative transfer in the oceans. In: Optical aspects of oceanography (eds. N.G. Jerlov, E. Steemann Nielsen), pp. 121–134. London-New York: Academic Press 1974

Zolotov, V., Frantsevich, L.: Orientation of bees by the polarized light of a limited area of the sky. J. Comp. Physiol. **85**, 25–36 (1973)

Zolotov, V. V., Frantsevich, L. I.: Polarized light sensitive interneurons in insects. Neirofiziologiya **7**, 397–401 (1977)

Zonana, H. V.: Fine structure of the squid retina. Hosp. Johns Hopkins Bull. **109**, 185–205 (1961)

Note Added in Proof

In the 2 years since the above was completed (June, 1978) a considerable number of important relevant publications in this area have appeared or are in press. Nearly all the major contributions relate to insects and deal with various behavioral, structural, and electrophysiological aspects of polarization sensitivity as well as polarotaxis. New data on the honeybee are prominent in these contributions and suggest that progress in solving the untidy problem of sensory mechanisms underlying worker bees' polarotaxis may be emerging. In turn this could lead to a more effective understanding of how polarization sensitivity contributes to the resourceful orientation and navigation of this key species. But before reviewing this rather exciting part of current research some recent results in the more compacted (and perhaps somewhat existential) topic of dipteran polarization sensitivity should be discussed. Although very little generally accepted behavioral work in this insect group exists, substantial progress is being made in understanding basic mechanisms of their open rhabdom structure and function.

Thus, considerable new electrophysiological work has been done on functional properties of the various retinular cells in fly eyes, particularly R 7 and R 8 (e.g., HARDIE et al., 1979; SMOLA and MEFFERT, 1978). These results are important in correlating detailed microspectrophotometric, fine structural, and receptor cell response properties of these well-studied eyes. Yet they are rather disappointing in terms of polarization sensitivity. Indeed, their general impact is to demonstrate that the dipteran retinula is considerably more complex than had been previously appreciated (HARDIE et al., 1979).

Extensive and technically impressive intracellular recording of R 7 in *Calliphora* and *Musca* demonstrated significant sensitivity to *e*-vector orientation in most cases. High values of S_p were not observed in the so-called UV type R 7 cells and measurements of the relationship between λ and S_p in these authors' UV type R 7 revealed maximum polarization sensitivity in all cases near 455 nm but never any obvious sensitivity to the *e*-vector in ultraviolet. Note, however, that 455 nm is near the λ_{max} for blue-sky polarization as well as the λ_{max} of the photostable pigment contained in R 7 y rhabdomeres.

In these cells maximum responses to polarized stimuli were found with the *e*-vector parallel to the microvillus axis of the corresponding rhabdomere even though maximum extinction by the rhabdomere of R 7 had previously been demonstrated perpendicular to the microvillus orientation. However, mainly low S_p's between 1 and 2 have been recorded for individual photoreceptor cells. Polarization sensitivity of R 8 was tested in a few cases only, and further work is required to characterize it effectively.

However function may be organized in fly retinulas, polarization sensitivity has not yet been found to be an outstanding component. Thus our understanding of dipteran polarization sensitivity and polarotaxis has scarcely evolved over the past 2 years except to reinforce the need for a fresh breakthrough, perhaps relating to certain special ommatidia like the marginal ones studied in morphological detail by WADA references given previously (1971, 1974a, b, 1975).

The first report of intracellular recording from *Cataglyphis* eyes opens up a fresh prospect of coordinating field behavior and sensory mechanism in a manner rarely possible (MOTE and WEHNER, 1980). Three types of cell were recorded from ocelli as well as from the compound eye. One had its λ_{max} in the ultraviolet around 350 nm while a second was most sensitive near 505 nm. The third class showed a broad λ sensitivity suggesting that this category arises from electrical coupling between the other two receptor cell types. S_p's ranging from 1.6 to 6.0 were found in 90% of the cells recorded. The notion that the third cell type (UV-VIS) actually represented recording from coupled UV and VIS cell types was supported by the finding of phase difference in polarization sensitivity as a function of λ.

Happily, this recent period has been much more productive for the polarization sensitivity of the honeybee where renewed and more sophisticated experiments have been carried out on celestial orientation. The waggle dance observed in enclosed hives with controlled illumination has been intensively studied in several laboratories to provide a better analysis of the sky light (and other) parameters involved in the polarized light compass. Based on the assumption that small (10°) isolated areas of natural blue sky (or the same aperture polarized 100% by a rotatable polarizer transmitting and polarizing in the ultraviolet as well as the visible) provide a visual stimulus valid for analyzing normal sky-oriented behavior, some provocative experiments have been performed and reported by ROSSEL et al. (1978).

Using trained bees on a horizontal comb dance orientation was measured as a function of (1) the elevation angle of such a single *e*-vector stimulus area and (2) its azimuthal deviation from the sun's bearing. When stimulus *e*-vectors were vertical, bidirectional responses differing by 180° were always obtained; one of these preferred directions was oriented approximately toward the trained feeding azimuth. When stimulus *e*-vectors were horizontal, only a single goal-oriented response was evoked.

At intermediate *e*-vector orientations, the bees danced in directions clearly influenced in a nonlinear manner by changes in the polarization plane. The smooth symmetrical functions obtained experimentally were interpreted as indications of the workers' internal, somewhat generalized, map of sky polarization. While this might seem rather cerebral for an insect, the map compass problem is certainly a fundamental one for animal navigation in general.

Of further interest in this work was the fact that the correlation of the bee's map (so determined) with the natural sky polarization was better near the zenith than the horizon. This is consistent with WELLINGTON's data (cited previously) demonstrating the critical importance of zenith polarization for insects steering straight courses from the sky. It is also consistent with VON FRISCH's classic demonstration that the dorsal part of the bee's eye is essential for orientation to sky polarization. Current research on important implications of such localization is cited in the following.

In a rather similar experimental setup bee waggle dances have been ingeniously used to demonstrate that specialization both of peripheral photoreceptor channels and of central integrating mechanisms occurs for various components of celestial orientation (EDRICH et al., 1979). Thus, sunlight and blue skylight were shown to have distinctly different orienting effects in experiments in which interaction with gravity responses was used to provide specific action spectra for sun compass responses and for polarization-dependent orientation. These experiments were done on a variably inclined flat dance surface under a dome which provided an unpolarized 2.3° spot stimulus of variable wavelength and intensity. This spot stimulus was located 45° from the dome's zenith and in a plane perpendicular to the tilt plane; alternatively, a polarized stimulus directly dorsal to the dancing bees was centered at the dome's zenith point.

In this situation sun compass reactions were found to depend entirely on the eye's blue ($\lambda_{max} = 450$ nm) and green ($\lambda_{max} = 550$ nm) receptors; ultraviolet receptors ($\lambda_{max} = 350$ nm) contribute nothing to directional sunlight (or artificial sunlight) orientation unless the ultraviolet stimulus is polarized. Therefore, sun compass responses and polarotaxis are qualitatively different. Similarly, classical phototaxis, when coupled in this manner with gravity-geotaxis, seems qualitatively different from sun compass orientation. An interesting additional point emerging from these experiments is that the inherent 180° ambiguity of single *e*-vector orientation could be resolved correctly by dancing bees with an asymmetrical gravity stimulus.

When the 2.3° spot at 45° zenith distance in the above setup was restricted to ultraviolet wavelengths and was unpolarized, the bee dances were oriented but the preferred direction was displaced by 180°. Hence, they were directed toward the bearing of the antisun. Action spectra determined from the variance in dance orientation occurring on a horizontal plane illuminated by completely unpolarized stimulus showed that sun orientation was evoked between 410 nm and 600 nm with peaks at 450 nm and 550 nm (Edrich et al., 1979). Antisun orientation appeared below 410 nm, reaching a very strong negative peak near 359 nm. For a fixed feeding site both sun and antisun orientation were time compensated, which is of course an important point for celestial navigation in general (e.g., Gould, 1980). Edrich and his colleagues conclude that with $\phi = 0°$, a patch of ultraviolet also acts as a direction indicator which worker bees interpret as lying on the sun's meridian (the only locus of $\phi = 0°$ in a clear sky) and in the antisun's bearing.

This demonstration of strong wavelength dependence in celestial orientation of various kinds raises some questions concerning the interpretation of the Rossel et al. (1979) results. Since they were using ultraviolet-transmitting polarizers the amount of ultraviolet in the stimulus may have been an important variable in addition to the e-vector orientation which was the one being deliberately considered. When Polaroid filters transmitting small amounts of ultraviolet are used (von Frisch [1965], reference given previously, and van der Glas [1979, in lit.]) results different from those reported by Rossel et al. (1979) were found.

Antisun orientation in bee dances responding to unpolarized ultraviolet light has also been independently observed by Brines and Gould (1979) in experiments systematically testing more celestial stimulus parameters than those above. According to their results, bees not only use relative ultraviolet content and degree of polarization to distinguish between sun and sky, but also depend on the size of the light stimulus. A second conclusion, which is supported also by the data of Rossel et al. (1979), is that in choosing between two sky meridians which have the same e-vector directions at the same zenith angle the bee workers choose the one further from the sun's bearing. A third operational decision which Brines and Gould induce is that when the two ambiguous directions implied by the e-vector pattern are equidistant from the sun the bees choose the right-hand one. These three behavioral rules relative to sky polarized light are interpreted as part of the larger set of conventions required for the sender and receiver of the dance language to communicate effectively.

A theoretical model of bee polarotaxis has been developed by Frantsevitch (1979), which is more general than the simplified empirical equation proposed by Rossel et al. (1979). In fact, according to the Frantsevitch model, their equation is the exact solution for the case where the single observed sky area lies in the region of maximum sky polarization, i.e., near the solar meridian and 90° from the sun. This again raises the point just mentioned that variable ultraviolet content of the stimulus may have prevented the dance behavior observed by Rossel et al. (1979) from being a response purely to e-vector direction. Frantsevitch's analysis suggests that the solar azimuth (or its celestial longitude) is estimated by the bees from the vector sum averaged over the retinal map of visible sky area.

Evidence that wavelength patterns within a relatively restricted stimulus area may strongly affect bee orientation is amply provided in the response of workers dancing on a horizontal plane surface in a covered hive in some of VAN DER GLAS's experiments (1980). In this series a 17.7° zenith area of the hive's dome-like cover is illuminated with an unpolarized cross-shaped pattern of two orthogonal color bars which are ingeniously made to grade smoothly and alternately from quadrants of one color to neighboring quadrants of the other color. Such a Maltese cross-shaped color pattern might be likened to the human entoptic pattern of Haidinger's brushes discussed previously. Color boundary patterns were also used by VAN DER GLAS in parallel experiments in which each of the two colors has its characteristic azimuth direction. Again the stimulus is unpolarized.

When these patterns have colors of short wavelength bees are well oriented, but they signal directions relative to the antisun. Hence, such unpolarized color stimuli like the smaller unpolarized ultraviolet areas tested by EDRICH et al. (1979) provide good compass directional information to the bees, but their orientation is transposed by 180°. Note that control experiments by VAN DER GLAS using analogous intensity gradients of bee white prove that the observed strong orientation to color gradient stimuli depends specifically on λ and not on apparent brightness patterns.

While VAN DER GLAS concludes that more than one receptor type must be involved in his color pattern-evoked bee dances, it is not yet clear how this is to be reconciled with various kinds of evidence proving that e-vector orientation in *Apis* can be effected exclusively with its ultraviolet receptors. On the other hand, completely unpolarized ultraviolet stimuli may also evoke strongly oriented responses. Further publication of VAN DER GLAS' unorthodox but stimulating ideas and more experiments like those of BRINES and GOULD (1979), in which the multidimensional contributions of sky irradiance are explored in more detail, should improve our understanding of this λ-dependent interaction.

Some important new work from WEHNER's department in Zürich, still largely unpublished may well provoke the progress needed to understand the sensory mechanisms basic to these problems of bee polarization sensitivity and polarotaxis. Briefly put, this current work transfers attention from most of the bee retina where elaborate but theoretically adequate hypotheses are required to explain polarization sensitivity to a localize special area.

As we have seen, most of the retina is believed (but not unanimously [RIBI, 1979, 1980]) to comprise twisted rhabdoms in retinulas with eight long and one short retinular cell. The new shift in attention is directed to the small fraction (ca. 2.5% of the whole eye where nontwisted ommatidia with nine long retinular cells lie near its dorsomedial margin. Structural (SOMMER, 1979), electrophysiological (LABHART, 1980), and behavioral (WEHNER et al., unpublished) evidence combine to support the notion that this special area comprising only about 140 of the 5,500 ommatidia in the whole retina is the primary site of the e-vector discrimination required for the polarotaxis discovered by VON FRISCH.

Consistently high polarization sensitivity (up to $S_p = 10$) has been found intracellularly in the exclusively ultraviolet-sensitive retinular cells of these dorsally marginal retinulas (LABHART, 1980). Curiously, the polarization sensitivities of the

---

[1]   Estimated as 1% by SCHINZ, 1975, cited above

green cells even in their nontwisted retinulas, were consistently low (av. $S_p = 1.8$). Mapping the e-vector sensitivities of these cells demonstrates a regular fan-shaped pattern of ϕ_{max} orientation in each eye. In the middorsal (zenith-directed) area maximum sensitivity of two ultraviolet cells R 1 and R 5 parallels the transverse plane of the head, whereas ϕ_{max} for R 9 is parallel to the sagittal plane; in both the anterior and posterior regions of the long R 9 area these three ultraviolet cells have their maximum sensitivities displaced 90° from the above.

Clearly the two main populations of ommatidia have orthogonal ultraviolet polarization sensitivities, whereas ommatidia in intermediate zones of the fan have transitional orientations. Hence different flight directions relative to the sun's azimuth will result in distinctive stimulation patterns evoked by overhead sky polarization in the dorsal marginal cells. The e-vector pattern could be "perceived" with one fixed look, but 180° ambiguity would result when the sun is at or near the horizon, or at all times with courses steered at 0° or 180° to the sun's bearing.

The visual fields of these dorsal marginal ommatidia are considerably larger than those found in most of the retina and also show curious intensity response curves. The composite visual field covered by them collectively in both compound eyes defines a quite specific upward-looking elliptical area centered on the zenith and having its major axis (about 90° in angular extent) anteroposteriorly oriented. The minor axis covers about 40°.

The eyes' polarization sensitivity has recently been reported in the desert ant *Cataglyphis* (Räber, 1979; Wehner and Räber, 1979) to be centered in retinal regions which look at the overhead sky in much the same way as the honeybee's long R 9 ommatidia according to Sommer's results. This would seem to be at variance with the earlier reports that best orientation is provided in this ant's compound eye by an area about 50° above the forward horizon (Figs. 94, 95). However, Herrling (1976, cited previously) thinks the correlation between his special type III retinulas on the dorsomedial eye margin and the area of optimal polarization sensitivity is rather good. No doubt Räber's thesis (1979), which the author has not yet seen, may explain these relations more consistently.

Curiously, in both *Apis* and *Cataglyphis*, these dorsal marginal visual fields are heterolateral in that the one belonging to the left eye maps a sky area subtending the right side of the animal, and vice versa. Among other things this recent hymenopteran work clearly suggests the importance of reevaluating van der Glas's hypotheses regarding the sky pattern discrimination and Wellington's field data on the crucial importance of zenith sky polarization for insect compass navigation in general. If such a reexamination in the honeybee is fruitful it may provide the key for a much more general understanding of polarotaxis.

References Added in Proof

Brines, Michael L., Gould, J.L.: Bees have rules. Science **206**, 571–573 (1979)

Edrich, Wolfgang, Neumeyer, C., Helversen, O. von: "Anti-sun orientation" of bees with regard to a field of ultraviolet light. J. Comp. Physiol. **134**, 151–157 (1979)

Frantsevich, L.I.: Theoretical model of polarotaxis. Vestnik Zoologii Kiev 1979 (5). 1–10 (1979)

van der Glas, H.W.: Orientation of bees, *Apis mellifera*, to unpolarized colour patterns, simulating the polarized zenith skylight pattern. J. Comp. Physiol. (in press) (1980)

Gould, J. L.: Sun compensation by bees. Science **207**, 545–547 (1980)

Hardie, R. C., Franceschini, N., McIntyre, P. D.: Electrophysiological analysis of fly retina. II. Spectral and polarisation sensitivity in R 7 and R 8. J. Comp. Physiol. **133**, 23–39 (1979)

Labhart, T.: Specialized photoreceptors at the dorsal rim of the honeybee's compound eye: polarizational and angular sensitivity. J. Comp. Physiol. (in press) (1980)

Mote, M. I., Wehner, R.: Functional characteristics of photoreceptors in the compound eye and ocellus of the desert ant, *Cataglyphis bicolor*. J. Comp. Physiol. **137**, 63–71 (1980)

Räber, F.: Retinatopographie und Sehfeldtopologie des Komplexauges von *Cataglyphis bicolor* (Formicidae, Hymenoptera). Diss., Univ. Zürich. (1979)

Ribi, W. A.: Do the rhabdomeric structures in bees and flies really twist? J. Comp. Physiol. **134**, 109–112 (1979)

Ribi, W. A.: New aspects of polarized light detection in the bee in view of non-twisting rhabdomeric structures. J. Comp. Physiol. **137**, 281–285 (1980)

Rossel, S., Wehner, R., Lindauer, M.: E-vector orientation in bees. J. Comp. Physiol. **125**, 1–12 (1979)

Smola, U., Meffert, P.: The spectral sensitivity of the visual cells R 7 and R 8 in the eye of the blowfly *Calliphora erythrocephala*. J. Comp. Physiol. **133**, 41–52 (1978)

Sommer, E. W.: Untersuchungen zur topografischen Anatomie der Retina und zur Sehfeldtopologie im Auge der Honigbiene, *Apis mellifera* (Hymenoptera) PhD. thesis, Univ. Zürich (1979)

Wehner, R., Räber, F.: Visual spatial memory in desert ants, *Cataglyphis bicolor* (Hymenoptera: Formicidae). Experientia **35**, 1569–1571 (1979)

Chapter 4

Optics and Vision in Invertebrates

M. F. LAND, Brighton, Great Britain

With 65 Figures and 6 Tables

Contents

A. Introduction

Like cameras, eyes provide spatially resolved images of the surroundings, and it is tempting to make the same sort of judgments about the capabilities and quality of a particular kind of eye that one would when buying a new camera. For example: This instrument is better than that because it has a large lens so that it can be used in dim light, the optics are well corrected so that all of the image is as sharp as possible, the format is sufficiently large that the graininess of the film will not limit its performance, and it contains a sufficient number of adjustments (shutter speed, F-stop, focus), preferably of an automatic kind, so that it can be used over a wide range of distances and light intensities. These are not unfair criteria, in general, to apply to the enormous variety of eyes a zoologist encounters among different groups of animals; but before making or seeking to make relative judgments of merit, one has to ask on the animal's behalf the same questions a shopper would ask himself. Do I need it? Can I afford it? Is it so big as to be cumbersome? There is clearly no point in, for example, an earthworm possessing an eye providing vast amounts of information that its brain cannot handle and its way of life does not require. Equally, though, no flying predator would succeed unless its eyesight was good enough to follow small objects at high speeds, and that inevitably means that it must possess large "expensive" eyes.

The study of animal eyes is in part a study of different kinds of optical invention since, like men themselves, animals have produced in the course of evolution almost every conceivable type of optical system, involving curved surfaces, lenses, mirrors, and light-guides. There are even some devices, like the inhomogeneous lenses of fish and cephalopods, and the mirror eyes of crustaceans, whose interesting and useful optical properties have yet to be duplicated by optical engineers.

Eyes, however, are never optical inventions of a straightforward kind; they always embody in their design complicated compromises between different competing factors – bulk versus resolution, resolution versus light-gathering power, and so on. Some of these compromises are of a strictly physical nature. For example: What is the ideal aperture for an eye of a particular size, given that resolution gets worse at large apertures because of lens defects and also at small apertures because of diffraction? Problems of this kind are worth examining to see the extent to which nature and physical theory agree. Often the results are surprising, and the discovery of anomalies and apparent deficiencies may lead to inquiries which show that what one took to be an oversight of nature turns out to be a more subtle compromise than one suspected. This is no less true for the eyes of invertebrate animals than it is for the human eye, about which HELMHOLTZ wrote in 1868: "... the eye has every possible defect that can be found in an optical instrument, and even some which are peculiar to itself; but they are all so counteracted, that the inexactness of the image which results from their presence very little exceeds, under ordinary conditions of illumination, the limits which are set to the delicacy of sensation by the dimensions of the retinal cones."

Compared with the relatively standard pattern of vertebrate eyes, those of invertebrates present an enormous diversity. They vary greatly in size, the method of formation of the image, resolving power and sensitivity, and this variety is a reflection partly of the different evolutionary histories of the different kinds of eye and partly of the different visual needs of the animals that bear them. It would be wrong, however, to regard even the simple eyecups of flatworms as less successful, evolutionarily, than the large and sophisticated compound eyes of a dragon-fly or the fish-like eyes of an octopus. It is more profitable to regard each as being a perfected compromise suited to the requirements of the life-style of the animal in question than it is to classify some as "primitive" and others as "advanced." It is true that some eyes are capable of supplying more information than others, but at a higher cost in terms of the space they take up and the metabolic energy they require.

In this chapter I have set out to do two things. First, in Sect. B, the various physical factors that determine and limit the performance of eyes are discussed in general terms. Particular emphasis is laid on two properties of eyes, their resolving power ($\mathscr{R}$) and sensitivity $\mathscr{S}$ as defined in Table 1. I have deliberately omitted much discussion of either colour vision or polarization sensitivity, not because they are unimportant but because they are basically attributes of photoreceptors rather than of eyes themselves. These aspects of vision are dealt with elsewhere in this handbook by MENZEL (Vol. VII/6A, Chap. 9) and by WATERMAN (this Vol., Chap. 3). Section B is based heavily on the seminal account of eye design by BAR-

Table 1. Definitions of principal symbols

Symbol	Explanation
A	Diameter of the aperture of an optical system.
f	Principal focal length, or posterior nodal distance, of an optical system (Figs. 7, 45 and 64).
F-number	f/A (as in photography). Its reciprocal A/f is referred to as the relative aperture.
d	Receptor diameter.
p	Centre-to-centre receptor separation.
$\Delta\varrho$	Acceptance angle of a receptor in object space. Geometrically equal to d/f (rad) but in practice slightly wider because of image degradation and wave guide properties of the receptor.
$\Delta\phi$	Angular receptor spacing. Equal to p/f (rad) in simple eyes, and A/r in apposition compound eyes, where r is the local radius of curvature of the eye (Fig. 45).
x	Receptor length.
k	Natural extinction coefficient of photopigment in situ (B.II.5).
v	Angular spatial frequency of a grating object (rad^{-1}) (Fig. 9).
$\mathscr{R}$	Resolving power of an eye, defined as the highest spatial frequency v that can be transmitted by the receptor mosaic. Equal to $1/(2\Delta\phi)$, or $\lambda f/2p$ in simple eyes and superposition eyes and $r/2A$ in apposition compound eyes (Eq. 16, 20, 21, 28, 37, 38). "Resolution" is used loosely throughout.
$\mathscr{S}$	Sensitivity of an eye, defined as the amount of light energy absorbed per second by a single receptor when imaging an extended object of unit luminance. $\mathscr{S} = \left(\dfrac{\pi}{4}\right)^2 \left(\dfrac{A}{f}\right)^2 d^2(1-e^{-kx})$, for all types of eye (Eq. 15). Units are area; i.e. $\mathscr{S}$ also signifies the equivalent area of a totally absorbing surface outside the eye, receiving light from a source of unit luminance subtending one steradian at the surface.

LOW (1964) and the more general account by PIRENNE (1967). Since then there have been important contributions to the subject by KIRSCHFELD (1974, 1976), which compare in detail the way these principles apply to both simple and compound eyes, and by SNYDER et al. (1977a, b) who have developed a particularly satisfying and rigorous approach to the question of how eyes can maximize the amount of information they can extract from the environment. This is set out by SNYDER (1979) in Part A of this Vol. Chap. 5.

One reason for giving an outline of optical principles in Sect. B is to provide a basis for interpreting, and to some extent judging, the range of invertebrate eye types given in Sect. C. This is essentially a catalogue in which the different sorts of optical systems that have evolved are described and compared. I have not attempted a complete survey of all eyes, but hope to have presented a reasonably full account of all eye types, the themes around which eyes themselves are variations. Section C is inevitably based on a wide range of sources, as all existing textbook accounts are at best partial. However, many of the old anatomical studies are excellent and in some ways more informative than more recent studies. I would cite particularly GRENACHER's book (1879) on arthropod eyes and the comprehensive and accurate papers of HESSE, published between 1898 and 1908. BULLOCK and HORRIDGE (1965) have performed the excellent service of bringing together much of the older literature, as has EAKIN (1972) who provides a comprehensive review of photoreceptor ultrastructure. Comparative reviews that both overlap and supplement this chapter can be found in PLATE (1924), BUDDENBROCK (1952), DUKE-ELDER (1958), HESSE (1935), MILNE and MILNE (1959), WEALE (1974), and WOLKEN (1971, 1974). Compound eyes have been the subject of intense study over the past 2 decades, and general references are given at the beginning of Sect. C.III.

Finally, at the end of Sect. C, there is a short section that attempts to relate eye evolution to the evolution of visual capabilities. This is purposely brief, and for an exploration of the much wider subject of the uses to which visual information is put, the reader is referred to the chapter by WEHNER (this Handbook, Vol. VII/6C, Chap. 4).

B. Design of Eyes

I. Optical Limits to Vision

All eyes must meet two requirements: They must obtain enough light from the environment for the receptors to provide a usable neural signal, and they must provide resolution, that is, they must split up the light reaching them according to its direction of origin. Three properties of light are of special importance for the way eyes have evolved to attain these requirements.

First, light is *quantal* in nature, which means that there is a minimum unit of energy capable of being absorbed and hence detected. Furthermore, energy quanta (photons) emanating from a source are randomly distributed in time, so that tasks such as movement perception that involve the detection of differences in brightness between two or more sources will require the capture of many photons – enough to obtain a statistically reliable estimate of the average numbers coming from each. These considerations suggest that the more light an eye can trap, the better.

Secondly, light is a *wave form*, with a wavelength range in air between about 0.35 µm (ultraviolet) and 0.8 µm (deep red). Waves show interference phenomena and several of these are relevant to eye design. Perhaps the most important is diffraction occurring at apertures, such as the pupils of eyes. Light passing through one part of an aperture interferes with that passing through other regions, resulting in an interference pattern on the retina that tends to degrade the quality of the image. This effect is particularly serious where apertures are small, for example, in compound eyes where each receptor unit has its own, very small, optical system, and in such eyes diffraction is frequently the major factor limiting resolution . A second consequence of interference phenomena is that there is a practical minimum limit to the diameter a receptive structure can have. If they are too narrow (less than about 1 µm, see Sect. B.III.2), light tends to travel around their outside and so is not absorbed. This in turn means that a minimum area of retina is needed to resolve a given number of points in space, so that in general, better resolution requires a larger eye. Constructive interference also plays a major role in the optical mechanism of reflecting surfaces (Sect. C.II.5), which are never made of metal in animals but of plates whose thicknesses are typically about one-fourth of the wavelength of light.

Finally, of course, light travels along *rays*, or can be considered to do so when the objects with which it interacts are large compared with its wavelength. It is this property that makes the imaging of external objects possible. Rays from single sources can be selected by shadowing out all others or redirected to a common focus by refraction or reflection. A survey of the ways animals achieve this is the subject of Sect. C. The remainder of this section will be devoted to a more detailed study of the physical factors that limit sensitivity and resolution in all types of eye.

II. Absolute Sensitivity

1. Photon Capture and the Probability of Seeing

The quantal nature of light means that at relatively low levels of illumination, individual receptors will be receiving either one or no photons at all, and since these photon captures are randomly distributed in time it is obvious that in any short period the amount of information a receptor can transmit is extremely limited. The most it can announce is that the part of the environment imaged on it is not totally dark. It cannot indicate how dark, unless its signal is averaged over a long period of time, and the fact that it has *not* received a photon does not mean that its sector of the world is lightless, merely that no photon reached the receptor. This point is made very well by Fig. 1, which is taken from PIRENNE (1967). In other words, at low light levels the signals transmitted by single receptors – even if they faithfully record every photon that reaches them – are highly ambiguous in nature, or, to use the familiar analogy, "noisy." It cannot be argued that animals only see at light levels well above that at which these statistical considerations apply; in humans, for example, the absolute threshold for vision occurs when a large field has a luminance of about $3 \cdot 10^{-6}$ candela $\cdot$ m^{-2}, and when this is translated into photons absorbed per rod, it works out at about one every 40 min. It is only when the background is reflecting or emitting light at 10^3–10^4 times this level (corresponding to moonlight when we see fairly well) that individual receptors begin to receive photons at a rate of more than one per second (WALD et al., 1962). At higher levels still, well into what we think of as daylight vision, our resolution – both spatial and temporal – continues to improve as it becomes possible for the nervous system to reduce both the number of receptors whose signals it must pool and also the time interval over which it must sample, while still maintaining a statistically reliable signal.

2. Reliability of the Signal

The question of how much light is required depends on the task being performed, but basically the problems can be put in statistical terms. For example: "How many photons must each of two receptors capture before it is possible for them to signal that one source is brighter than another, with a reliability of (e.g.) 95%, when the relative brightness difference ($\Delta I/I$) is actually 10%." This is the sort of task

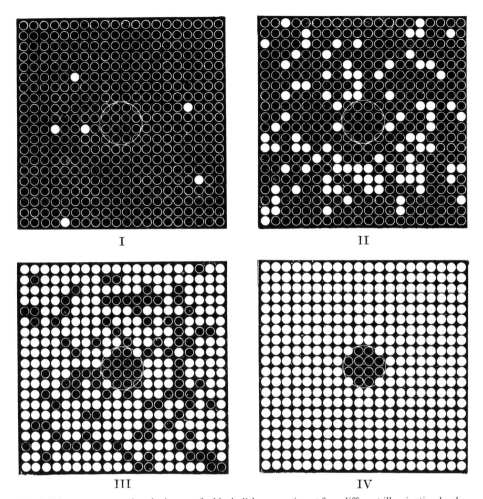

Fig. 1. Diagram representing the image of a black disk on a retina at four different illumination levels. The small circles represent receptors, and those that have received a photon in a fixed time period appear light. The situation in I approximately represents the situation in the human retina at the absolute threshold of vision. The black disk only becomes unambiguously detectable at light levels 2–3 log units higher than this because of the scarcity of photon captures. (PIRENNE, 1967)

visual systems are confronted with when working in the vicinity of their useful threshold.

The statistics of photon capture follow a Poisson distribution (because they represent the sampling of a very small population from a very large universe), and this is described by the equation:

$$P(n|s) = \frac{s^n e^{-s}}{n!}, \tag{1}$$

where P $(n|s)$ is the probability of n events occurring if the average number is s. An important feature of such distributions is that the scatter of n, expressed as the

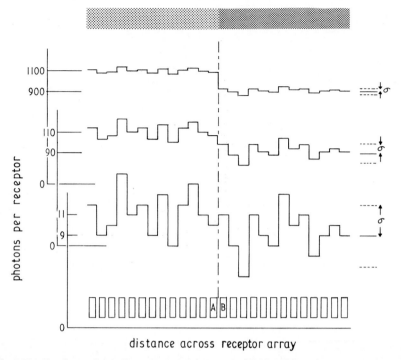

Fig. 2. How luminance level affects the detectability of small brightness differences. The abscissa represents distance across a retina, and the three graphs show the magnitude of the variations in receptor photon counts when the average number of photons caught is 10 (bottom), 100, and 1,000. The stripe at the top represents a step change in luminance of 20%. At the lowest light level this is completely lost in the photon "noise." With 10 times more light the difference is detectable but only by averaging across the receptor array, and with 10 times more light again it is clearly detectable by the two adjacent receptors A and B. σ is the standard deviation of photon counts and is equal to the square root of the average count

standard deviation σ, is equal to the square root of the average number s. This means that, although the scatter increases as s increases, the *relative* scatter ($\sigma/s = \sqrt{s}/s = 1/\sqrt{s}$) *decreases* as s increases (see BARLOW, 1964). This simply means that the "signal-to-noise ratio" of a photoreceptor improves as the amount of light available, and hence s increases (Fig. 2).

Provided that the average number in a sample is greater than about 20, the Poisson distribution can be approximated by a normal (Gaussian) distribution, and ordinary statistical methods can be used. If two samples, n_1 and n_2, differ by at least 1.96 standard deviations, the probability that this is due to chance is only 5%, or to put it another way, the reliability of the difference is 95%. For 80% reliability, the corresponding deviation (R) would be 1.28 σ; for 90%, 1.65 σ; and for 99%, 2.58 σ. In general terms, we can write that the condition for a sample difference to be accepted as real, with a given reliability, is that

$$n_1 - n_2 \geqslant R\sigma_{\mathrm{diff}} , \qquad (2)$$

Table 2. Number of photons required to distinguish different relative intensities

Relative intensity difference ($\Delta I/I$)	Reliability			
	80%	90%	95%	99%
0.003	3.64×10^5	6.05×10^5	8.54×10^5	1.48×10^6
0.01	3.28×10^4	5.45×10^4	7.68×10^4	1.33×10^5
0.03	3.64×10^3	6.05×10^3	8.54×10^3	1.48×10^3
0.1	328	545	768	1,330
0.3	36	61	85	148

where σ_{diff} is the standard deviation of the difference, given by $\sqrt{(\sigma_1^2 + \sigma_2^2)}$. If n_1 and n_2 are similar to each other and to the average sample size s, σ_{diff} becomes $\sqrt{2}\,\sigma^2$, or $\sqrt{2}\,s$.

To calculate s, the sample size needed to make a particular discrimination, we can replace the actual sample difference by its average value. That is to say, we can assume that $(n_1 - n_2)/s$ is the same as the real relative brightness difference $(\Delta I/I)$. Equation 2 can now be rewritten in the form:

$$\frac{\Delta I}{I} \geq \frac{R\sqrt{2s}}{s}, \quad or, \quad s \geq 2\left(\frac{R}{\Delta I/I}\right)^2. \tag{3}$$

This now gives the minimum number of photons required per receptor, and when applied to the problem that introduced this section ($R = 1.96$, $\Delta I/I = 0.1$), s comes to 768. The numbers of photon captures needed for the discrimination of other differences, with other degrees of reliability, are given in Table. 2.

3. Photon Capture and Resolution

The calculations above assume that receptors can signal the captures of single photons. In man the famous experiments of HECHT et al. (1942) showed that this was almost certainly true for rods. In invertebrates the evidence was for a long time less clear-cut, although the results of electrophysiological studies on *Limulus* (FUORTES , 1969) and squid receptors (HAGINS, 1965) and behavioural studies on flies (REICHARDT, 1965, 1969) were at the very least compatible with the suggestion that single photon captures are effectively transduced. However, in 1977, LILLY-WHITE showed unambiguously that in fully dark-adapted locust receptors, single photons produced depolarizing "bumps" in membrane potential of millivolt size and with a probability of occurrence of at least 0.59.

The sample size, i.e. the number of photons available to the nervous system in making a discrimination, is the product of three quantities: the retinal illuminance (E_r), the area of retina (a) over which the photons are counted, and the time (t) available for the task. Hence:

$$s = K \cdot E_r \cdot a \cdot t, \tag{4}$$

where K is a constant, less than unity, representing the proportion of incident photons that are actually absorbed. Given even the most favourable assumptions, some photons will pass between receptors or pass through them without being absorbed.

Consider an animal living in a constant dim environment. It needs to make reliable distinctions between objects whose brightnesses differ by, for instance, 10%. E_r is now fixed by the ambient light level and the optical properties of the eye (see Sect. 4), and s is fixed by the nature of the task (Sect. 2). This means that a and t are reciprocally related. The animal may increase the retinal area devoted to viewing the stimulus (either by having larger receptors or pooling the signals from many), in which case it can reduce the sampling time (t). As a larger sampling area means a reduction in the fineness of detail that can be resolved, this statement is equivalent to saying that the animal really has a choice between good *spatial* resolution, but at the expense of *temporal* resolution, or vice versa.

It is commonly pointed out that insects have poor spatial resolution because of the optical limitations of compound eyes (Sect. C.III.3), but it is almost certainly true that in the rapid fliers (Diptera, Hymenoptera, Odonata, etc.) the equation is tipped in favour of temporal resolution. The total reaction time of a fly chasing another, for example, is less than 30 ms (LAND and COLLETT, 1974) compared with 125–200 ms for the generation of a human eye movement (ROBINSON, 1968). Similarly, the flicker fusion frequency in the blowfly is about 300 Hz (AUTRUM, 1950) compared with 90–100 Hz for the human electroretinogram (BROWN, 1965).

There is only one way that both good spatial and temporal resolution can be achieved – by having a large eye. A large retinal area a can then be devoted to a small region of space, and t can be kept short. Thus, one finds large eyes not only in nocturnal or deep aquatic animals (moths, lobsters, many fish) where retinal illuminance (E_r) is inevitably low, but also in fast-moving animals that operate in daylight (dragon-flies, hoverflies and, of course, birds). Probably the largest eyes of all are found in deep-sea squid, whose predatory life-style requires the exercise of high temporal and spatial resolution in dim light (Sect. C.II.3.).

4. Amount of Light Reaching the Retina

Except at very high light levels, it is an advantage for retinal receptors to capture as many of the available photons as possible, and this section examines those features of eye design that determine the amount of light reaching the receptors. A good discussion is given by KIRSCHFELD (1974).

Figure 3 represents a camera-type eye viewing an extended surface of luminance L candela m^{-2}.[1] Such a surface emits L lumens per m^2 into each unit solid angle (steradian, sr). If the pupil of the eye has an area S_a and is situated at a dis-

---

[1] 1 candela $\cdot$ m^{-2} = 1 lumen $\cdot$ m^{-2} $\cdot$ steradian (sr)$^{-1}$ = 0.314 millilambert = 1.46 $\cdot$ 10^{-3} watt $\cdot$ m^{-2} $\cdot$ sr^{-1} = 4.08 $\cdot$ 10^{15} photons $\cdot$ s^{-1} $\cdot$ m^{-2} $\cdot$ sr^{-1}, for yellow-green light of wavelength 555 nm. The interconversion of photometric units (lumen, etc.) to radiometric units (watt, photon $\cdot$ s^{-1}, etc.) is only straightforward when dealing with human vision, because the photometric units are all based on the spectral sensitivity of a "standard human observer." To apply these units in research, the reader should consult a good textbook of photometry

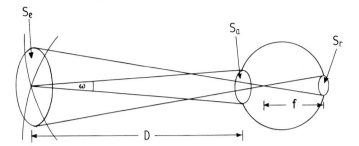

Fig. 3. Diagram illustrating the way retinal illuminance can be calculated. Details in the text

tance D from the surface, then the solid angle (ω) it subtends at the surface will be S_a/D^2 (from the definition of solid angle) and the total flux passing through it (F_a in lumen) will be given by:

$$F_a = \frac{L \cdot S_e \cdot S_a}{D^2},\tag{5}$$

where S_e is the area of the surface.

The light from the pupil is imaged onto the retina over an area S_r, so that the retinal illuminance (E_r in lumen m^{-2}) is given by:

$$E_r = \frac{F_a}{S_r}.\tag{6}$$

However, from the geometry of Fig. 3, it can be seen that the solid angle subtended by the source at the eye is the same as that subtended by the patch of retina that images it at the nodal point, i.e.:

$$\frac{S_e}{D^2} = \frac{S_r}{f^2},\tag{7}$$

where f is the posterior nodal distance or principal focal length of the eye (see Fig. 7). Substitution of Eq. (7) into Eq. (5) gives

$$F_a = \frac{L \cdot S_a \cdot S_r}{f^2}\tag{8}$$

and from Eq. (6) this gives the retinal illuminance as

$$E_r = \frac{L \cdot S_a}{f^2}.\tag{9}$$

If the pupil is circular, S_a can be replaced by $\frac{\pi}{4} A^2$, A being the pupil diameter.

The retinal illuminance then becomes

$$E_r = L \cdot \frac{\pi}{4} \cdot \frac{A^2}{f^2}. \tag{10}$$

Equation (10) states that for *extended* sources – parts of the surroundings rather than stars or distant luminescent animals – the brightness of the retinal image is proportional to the luminance of the source and the square of the aperture diameter and inversely proportional to the square of the focal length. In photographic terms, $(A/f)^2$ is related to the *F-number* of the lens, which is f/A, and Eq. (10) expresses the well-known result that different lenses with the same *F-number* transmit the same amount of light to the film. *Image brightness is thus not related to the absolute size of an eye, but to a feature of its shape: the ratio of aperture diameter to focal length.* The other feature of Eq. (10) worth mentioning is that E_r is not dependent on the distance of the surface. *Surfaces of the same luminance will appear equally bright, whatever their distance.*

This is *not* true for point sources, where all the flux entering the eye can be assumed to come from and be imaged onto one point. The visibility of such objects is proportional only to the flux entering the eye (F_a, Eq. 5). The intensity of the source, I in candelas, replaces $L \cdot S_e$, the product of luminance and area, giving:

$$F_a = \frac{I \cdot S_a}{D^2}. \tag{11}$$

The rate at which photons reach the retina is now related to source intensity and the absolute area of the pupil and is inversely proportional to the square of the distance.

5. Amount of Light Absorbed by Receptors

Ultimately, the accuracy of the spatial and temporal information an eye can transmit to the brain depends on the numbers of photons absorbed by each receptor or pooled group of receptors (Sect. 3). This is clearly related to the retinal illuminance (E_r, Eq. 10) and also to the size and shape of the receptors. The light flux F_p (lumen) entering a photoreceptor will be the product of retinal illuminance and the surface area the receptor presents to the incident light, i.e.:

$$F_p = E_r \cdot \frac{\pi}{4} \cdot d^2, \tag{12}$$

where d is the diameter of a receptor, which is assumed to have a circular cross-section.

An ideal receptor would absorb all the light reaching its distal surface. Strictly, this is impossible because absorption by pigment molecules attenuates light exponentially: a constant length of receptor absorbs a constant *fraction* of the light reaching it (Lambert's Law), and what remains can never be reduced to zero.

The fraction of light that is absorbed by a length x of receptor is given by:

$$\frac{F_{abs}}{F_{inc}} = (1 - e^{-kx}),\tag{13}$$

where k is the absorption coefficient, and F_{inc} and F_{abs} are the incident and absorbed light fluxes. The coefficient k is the fraction of light absorbed in a defined short length, and this length can be conveniently taken to be 1 μm.

There is an alternative and frequently used way of defining absorption, which is by specifying the *optical density* of the structure. This is a logarithmic measure of absorption, which means that optical densities are additive; a structure twice as long as another of the same composition has twice its optical density. Optical density (D) is defined as $\log_{10}$ (incident flux/transmitted flux), or $-\log_{10} T$ where T is the transmittance. Since the absorbed flux is the incident flux minus the transmitted flux:

$$D = \log_{10}\frac{F_{inc}}{F_{tra}} = \log_{10}\frac{F_{inc}}{F_{inc} - F_{abs}} = -\log_{10}(1 - F_{inc}/F_{abs}).$$

But since from Eq. (13), $(1 - F_{abs}/F_{inc}) = e^{-kx}$, we have:

$$D = -\log_{10} e^{-kx}, \quad \text{or,} \quad D = kx \log_{10} e.$$

The quantity D/x is the optical density per unit length, or specific absorbance of the structure, and is equal to $k \log_{10} e$, or $0.4343 k$. Correspondingly, $k\,(\mu m^{-1}) = 2.3 D\,(\mu m^{-1})$.

Provided the value of k is known, we can ask: "How long should a receptor be to absorb 95%, for example, of the incident light?" Equation (13) then gives a set of paired values of k and x such that $e^{-kx} = 0.05$. For fly rhabdomeres, KIRSCHFELD (1969 a) estimated k to be about 0.005 μm^{-1}, and for 95% absorption this requires a length (x) of 600 μm, which is longer than the rhabdomeres of flies (~ 200 μm), but not as long as in dragon-flies where they can reach 1 mm. Probably the most accurate estimate of k in a rhabdomeric receptor is from the lobster *Homarus* (BRUNO et al., 1977). They estimate that for axial unpolarized light the density per μm is 0.0029, or $k = 0.0067$. This means that a lobster rhabdom 240 μm long absorbs 80% of the light reaching it. For an equivalent flux capture, vertebrate receptors can be much shorter. DENTON and WYLLIE (1955) found the density of frog rods to be about 0.015 μm^{-1} ($k = 0.035$), and this value will give 95% absorption in a length of only 86 μm. This value for k is typical for vertebrates (DENTON and NICOL, 1964), and the fivefold difference between this and the lobster value is presumably due to the much more open packing of membranes in rhabdoms compared with the contiguous plates in rods (Fig. 4).

The final equation which summarizes all the important properties of an eye that affect the amount of light absorbed by single receptors can be obtained by combining Eqs. (10), (12), and (13). If $F_{p(abs)}$ is the flux absorbed per receptor, we have:

$$F_{p(abs)} = L \cdot \left(\frac{\pi}{4}\right)^2 \cdot \left(\frac{A}{f}\right)^2 \cdot d^2 \cdot (1 - e^{-kx}).\tag{14}$$

If the units of L are photons·s^{-1}·m^{-2}·sr^{-1}, then the units of $F_{p(abs)}$ are photons per second. The implications of this equation are that an eye capable of securing the maximum number of photons per receptor should have a large relative aperture

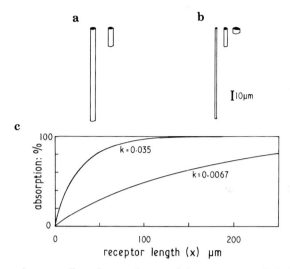

Fig. 4a–c. Effects of receptor dimensions on the rate of photon capture. **a** Relative lengths of a rhab-domeric receptor and a vertebrate rod (right) both of which capture 50% of the light reaching them (scale on b). **b** Three rhabdomeric receptors (2-, 4-, and 8-μm diameter) each of which will absorb the same *number* of photons when the retinal illuminance is the same. **c** The relation between absorption and receptor length for vertebrate rods (upper curve) and lobster rhabdoms (lower curve)

(A/f) and wide receptors *(d)* which are long enough to absorb a large proportion of the light reaching them. There is usually a price to be paid, in terms of resolution or size, for having either a large aperture or large receptors, but this can best be considered in Sect. B.IV, after limits to resolution have been discussed.

Equation (14) can be applied to most kinds of eye, and it is interesting that the values obtained for $F_{p(abs)}$ are quite similar in eyes of quite different optical types and evolutionary histories, provided the animals bearing them inhabit similar photic environments. For example, the value of A/f is very similar in man with a wide-open pupil (0.5) and in a bee (0.42), even though the facets of a bee's eye are only about 1/280 th the diameter of the human pupil, and since the human cone and bee rhabdom are of similar diameter (~ 2 μm), the flux per receptor (F_p) will be almost the same when both are looking at surfaces of the same luminance (KIRSCHFELD, 1974). An estimate of the photon flux per receptor is readily obtained. A white card at sunset has a luminance of about 1 cd·m^{-2}, which is equivalent to $4.08 \cdot 10^{15}$ photons·s^{-1}·m^{-2}·sr^{-1} for a wavelength of 555 nm (i.e., this is the number available to an eye whose spectral sensitivity is similar to that of a human eye in daylight). The luminance and photon radiance of surfaces under other illumination conditions is given in Table 3. If, then, $A/f = 0.5$, $d = 2.10^{-6}$ m and all the photons reaching a receptor are absorbed $[(1 - e^{-kx}) = 1]$, $F_{p(abs)}$ comes to 2,517 photons per second. Table 2 indicates that this is sufficient to distinguish two surfaces differing in brightness by between 3% and 10%, with 90% reliability, if the sampling time is 1 s. The difference between bee and human is that we could in principle make this judgment about surfaces subtending about 1′ of arc at the eye, whereas in the bee the equivalent spatial separation is more like 1°.

6. Comparisons of Sensitivity

It is not possible to put an exact figure to the absolute sensitivity of an eye, because the minimum amount of light required varies with the kind of task being undertaken. Other things being equal, fine discrimination of detail requires more light than coarse judgments of the presence of objects, and rapid activities such as flight require more light to coordinate them than slower ones like crawling, for reasons already discussed. Similarly, different numbers of receptors may be involved in different tasks; wide-field movement detectors, concerned in optomotor responses, are common in insects, and clearly they receive a total input from a much larger region of space than small-field neurons concerned with tracking or identifying objects.

The total size of the photon sample (s, Eq. 4) is obviously greater in the wide-field units, and one would accordingly expect them to continue to function at lower light levels than small-field units. For these reasons the term "absolute sensitivity" is one that must be interpreted with caution. Nevertheless, it is possible to compare eyes in terms of their sensitivity, provided one assumes that the nervous systems they supply have comparable tasks to perform. This is because, as discussed in Sect. 2 and 3, similar tasks require similar minimum numbers of photons per detector for their performance. An appropriate measure of sensitivity is then the number of photons absorbed per receptor, per unit of luminance in the visual field being imaged. This is then simply given by $F_{p(abs)}/L$ in Eq. (14), i.e.:

$$\text{Sensitivity } (\mathscr{S}) = \left(\frac{\pi}{4}\right)^2 \cdot \left(\frac{A}{f}\right)^2 \cdot d^2 \cdot (1 - e^{-kx}). \tag{15}$$

On this basis, the definition of $\mathscr{S}$ is the ratio of the number of photons absorbed per receptor to the number emitted per steradian by 1 m² of an extended source. The differences in sensitivity attainable as a result of increases in relative aperture (A/f), receptor diameter (d) and length (x) can be quite substantial. For example, the nocturnal spider *Dinopis rufus* was estimated to have an absolute sensitivity greater than that of a diurnal spider *Phidippus johnsoni* by a factor of more than 2,000 (BLEST and LAND, 1977), and KIRSCHFELD (1974), using a measure essentially similar to Eq. (15), estimated that the eyes of nocturnal moths are more sensitive than those of diurnal bees by a factor of around 1,000 (Table 6, Sect. C.IV).

To what extent do these differences compensate for the differences in brightness of objects during the day and at night? Table 3, which shows the luminance of objects under various conditions, indicates that the compensation is only partial; the luminance of a scene in sunlight is about a million times greater than in moonlight, and a sensitivity increase of 3 log units still leaves a 1,000-fold difference. On this basis one would expect a comparable visual performance from a bee in room light and a moth in moonlight. Each would then be receiving about 10^4 photons/s per receptor. It is worth noting that the moth eye (a superposition compound eye) and the camera-type eye of the spider *Dinopis* both represent extreme adaptations to low light conditions (Sects. C.II.4 and C.III.4), and their light-gathering power probably cannot be improved upon without an even greater sacrifice of angular resolution than has already been made.

Table 3. Luminance of a white card under various illumination conditions

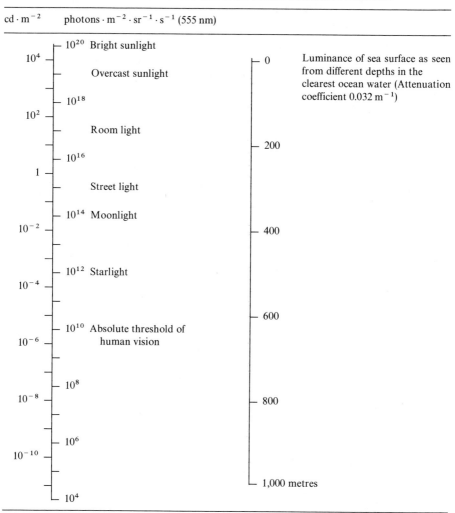

$cd \cdot m^{-2}$ $photons \cdot m^{-2} \cdot sr^{-1} \cdot s^{-1}$ (555 nm)

III. Resolution

We have seen that at low light levels the factors leading to good vision are those that produce a high photon catch per receptor, i.e. a high relative aperture (A/f), and receptors that are both wide and long. These are not necessarily the conditions for good spatial resolution when eyes are operating in the middle or upper parts of their "working range," where photon availability is no longer the limiting factor. Optimal resolution now becomes a matter of producing a high definition image, and matching it to a retina whose "grain" – to borrow the photographers' term – is fine enough to exploit it.

It is convenient to tackle the problem in two parts. First, how is resolution affected by making the receptor mosaic as fine as possible, and a related question: Is there a limit to the fineness that can be attained? Second, what are the conditions that lead to good image formation? These can again be divided into two types: the *diffraction limit* which is absolute and related only to aperture diameter and practical limits set by the inevitable imperfections of optical systems – the *aberrations*. These are often overcome to various degrees by eyes, allowing the image quality to approach that set by diffraction, although the biological solutions are not always the same as those available in optical technology.

1. Resolution and Receptor Size

Receptors, or optically or neurally coupled groups of receptors, represent pools for light reaching the retina within which no further resolution is possible. The angle subtended in space by a single receptor is thus an important measure of resolution. The reciprocal of this angle in minutes of arc is often referred to as the (anatomical) *acuity*. A slightly more useful measure is the reciprocal of the angle subtended by *two* receptors, since this represents the highest spatial frequency in the object that the eye can be expected to detect; the assumption here is that a minimum of two receptors is required to indicate each period of a grating object, one to detect the light and one the dark component (Fig. 5). At this limit the subtense of two receptors at the nodal point of the eye is the same as the subtense of one period of the object grating at the eye, so that we can define an eye's *resolving power* ($\mathcal{R}$) as the spatial frequency (v) of a just-resolved grating:

$$\mathcal{R} = \frac{D}{P} = \frac{f}{2p}, \tag{16}$$

where P is the distance between two stripes in a grating at a distance D from the eye, f is the first focal length (posterior nodal distance) and p is the receptor sep-

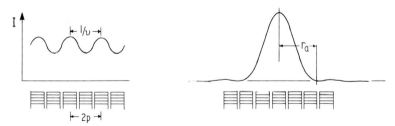

Fig. 5. Left: The receptor separation in the retina limits the highest spatial frequency (v cycles per radian) that an eye can resolve. Two receptors are needed to resolve one period of the highest spatial frequency component of the image, so that if the receptor separation is p and the focal length of the eye is f the mosaic will resolve spatial frequencies up to $v = f/2 p$. This is used as the definition of anatomical resolving power in Eq. (16). Right: If the quality of the image is limited by diffraction, all the information in the image can be extracted by a receptor array in which 2.44 receptors occupy the radius (r_A) of the Airy diffraction pattern from a point source: see Sect. B.III.3. (Based on KIRSCHFELD, 1976)

aration. If receptors are contiguous, as they are in many eyes (most simple eyes in annelids, molluscs, and arachnids), p is the same as the receptor diameter d used in the equations in Sect. II; however, for the moment it is useful to preserve the distinction.

One important implication of Eq. (16) is that if the receptors could be made very small, so could the focal length – and hence the size – of the eye, without the angular resolution being compromised. If, on the other hand, there is a practical lower limit to the width (d) or separation (p) of receptors, then there must also be a lower limit to the size of eyes capable of a particular resolution.

2. Lower Limit to Receptor Size

The optical behaviour of very narrow fibres such as photoreceptors cannot be accounted for simply in terms of geometrical optics; when their diameter begins to approach the wavelength of light, they start to behave as *waveguides*, where, because of interference effects, the light distribution within the fibre becomes non-uniform. These non-uniformities take the form of a family of geometrical patterns known as waveguide *modes*, whose cross-sections are constant along the length of the fibre. SNYDER (1975 a, b) has studied modes in photoreceptors in great detail, and the most important conclusions can be summarized as follows:

1) Only a fraction of the light power of a particular mode is contained within the fibre; the remainder propagates along the fibre, but outside it, and may therefore be absorbed by the surrounding medium or by adjacent receptors. The latter causes "optical cross-talk" which will reduce the quality of the neural signal, compared with the quality of the optical image.

2) The number of modes that can propagate down a fibre, and the fraction of light in each mode within the fibre, are specified by a single dimensionless parameter V, where

$$V = \frac{\pi d}{\lambda} \sqrt{(n_1^2 - n_2^2)}. \tag{17}$$

λ is the wavelength of light in vacuum, d is the fibre diameter, and n_1 and n_2 are the refractive indices of the fibre and its surroundings. The importance of waveguide effects increases as V becomes smaller, so that when $V = 1$ almost all the light travels outside the fibre. This reduces to about 50% when $V = 2$, even though only one mode is present, and to about 10% when $V = 7$ and several modes coexist in the fibre. At about this point $(V > 7)$, geometrical optics provide a reasonable approximation again to the fibre's behaviour, and it is probably only for $V < 2$–3 that waveguide effects are so serious that cross-talk between receptors begins to degrade the resolution available in the image (Fig. 6).

The important point here is that receptors for which V is less than 2 would be of little value, and so, depending on the refractive index difference, there is a lower useful limit to the receptor diameter. There are few estimates of refractive indices of invertebrate receptors, and the uncertainties involved in their measurement are considerable, but the careful study of KIRSCHFELD and SNYDER (1975) puts the value between 1.37 and 1.40 for fly rhabdomeres. This is slightly less than the re-

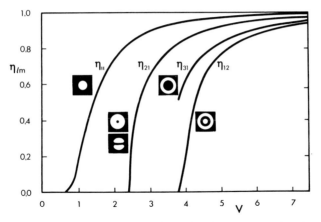

Fig. 6. Light passes down narrow receptors in the form of modes – transverse interference patterns with a characteristic appearance as shown. Only a fraction (η) of the light energy lies within the receptor, and this depends on the value of the wave guide parameter (V, Eq. 17) and on which modes are present. The graph shows the values of η for several of the modes present in the narrowest fibres. (KIRSCHFELD and SNYDER, 1975)

fractive index of vertebrate receptors – about 1.41 for rods and 1.39 for cones (SIDMAN, 1957). If the index of extracellular space is taken to be 1.34, the receptor diameter for which $V=2$ comes to between 0.8 and 1.1 μm for fly rhabdomeres in blue-green light (500 nm). Thus, there is a physical limit to the useful minimum diameter of a photoreceptor, and this is about 1 μm. This also corresponds closely to the narrowest actually observed, which are probably the central rhabdomeres of fly ommatidia whose diameter is slightly less than 1 μm.

It follows from this that there is a fundamental minimum limit to the size of a simple eye capable of resolving a given spatial frequency, $v=\mathscr{R}$. If receptors are contiguous, $p=d=1$ μm, and Eq. (16) can be written: $f=2\mathscr{R}$ (μm). Thus, the smallest eye capable of resolving a grating with a 1′ period ($\mathscr{R}=3{,}440$) would need a focal length of at least 6.9 mm, and for a 1° period, 120 μm. These limits are never quite reached in practice, usually because the receptors are somewhat wider than the 1-μm minimum. Compound eyes of comparable resolution are nearly always larger than simple eyes, but for rather different reasons (Sect. C.III.3).

3. Diffraction Limit

Light which enters one part of the aperture of an eye is capable of interfering with light entering through another region, the waves tending either to reinforce or destroy each other when they reach the image plane. An image is thus not just the simple geometrical image that can be constructed by drawing rays, but an interference (diffraction) pattern as well (Fig. 7), and the effect of the inevitable peaks and troughs of intensity is always to degrade the quality of the geometrical image. A poor-quality image means that the receptors will receive a pattern of light whose contrast is low compared with the contrast of the object and, consequently, is less

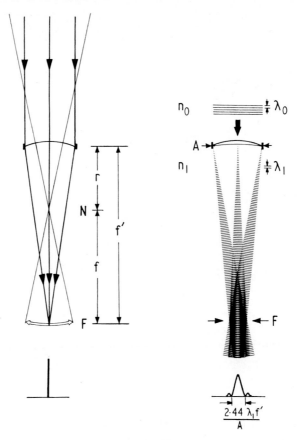

Fig. 7. Image formation according to ray optics (left) and wave optics (right). In ray optics a point-source object forms a point image in the focal plane (F). The size of the image of extended sources can be worked out from the angle the source subtends at the nodal point of the eye (N) which, in the case of a simple refracting surface, is situated at the centre of curvature of that surface. In wave optics, a plane wave front from a point source is converted by the refracting surface into a spherical wave front of shorter wavelength $\left(\lambda_1 = \dfrac{n_0}{n_1}\lambda_0\right)$ converging on F. As each point on this wave front can be thought of as initiating waves, the result is an interference pattern in the region of the image (the Airy pattern) which has approximately the form shown. Since the ratio of the second focal length (f') to the principal focal length or posterior nodal distance (f) is the same as the ratio of the refractive indices ($n_1 : n_0$), the diameter of the Airy pattern can be written as either $2.44 \, \lambda_1 f'/A$, or $2.44 \, \lambda_0 f/A$. f and f' can be found from Eq. (23)

detectable. We need to know the extent to which this image degradation is a problem in eye design, the circumstances which make it a real limit to resolution, and what can be done about it.

There are two well-known kinds of diffraction pattern which act as useful guides to image quality. The first is the *Airy disk*. This is the diffraction pattern corresponding to the image of a point source, and it consists of a patch of light surrounded by light and dark rings of sharply decreasing intensity (Fig. 7). The angle

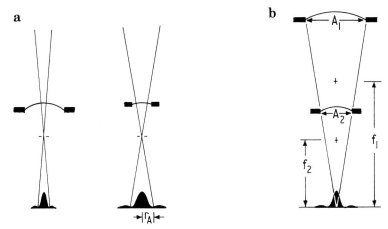

Fig. 8. a The angular size of the Airy diffraction pattern on the retina increases, and hence resolution decreases, when the aperture of the eye is reduced (Eq. 18). **b** The actual size of the Airy pattern on the retina is the same for optical systems with the same *F-number* (f/A in Eq. 19). (Based on KIRSCHFELD, 1976)

θ subtended by the radius of the disk at the nodal point, from the first dark ring to the centre, is given by:

$$\theta = 1.22 \frac{\lambda}{A} \text{ (radians)} . \tag{18}$$

λ and A having their usual meanings. The important point here is that θ gets smaller, and so resolution improves, the wider the aperture (A) of the pupil (Fig. 8). A criterion often applied to optical systems (the *Rayleigh criterion*) states that two point sources can only be resolved if the geometrical image of the first is at least as far from the other as the first dark ring of the Airy disk, and although this seems somewhat arbitrary – and rather unlike the task that most animals are usually faced with – it does in fact work well in practice. Thus, if θ is 1 min of arc (1/3,440 radian) and λ is 560 nm, A would need to be 1.99 mm, which is almost exactly the pupil diameter of a human eye in normal daylight. The actual size on the retina of a radius of the Airy disk (r_A) is given by substituting r_A/f for θ in Eq. (18) (Fig. 8 b):

$$r_A = 1.22 \frac{\lambda \cdot f}{A}. \tag{19}$$

For a human, with $f = 16.7$ mm and $A = 2$ mm, r_A is approximately 5 µm, or about twice the spacing of foveal cones. This agreeable match leads one to expect similar correspondences amongst the diverse range of invertebrate eyes (see Fig. 5).

The second way of assessing optical performance is very similar to the first, but is less arbitrary and more useful; it is the *contrast transfer function* of the optical system. It was originally devised for the study of camera lenses, but has also been applied profitably to eyes (see WESTHEIMER, 1964, 1972). If an eye, or any other optical system, images a grating whose contrast remains the same but whose stripes decrease progressively in their spacing, there comes a point at which the contrast

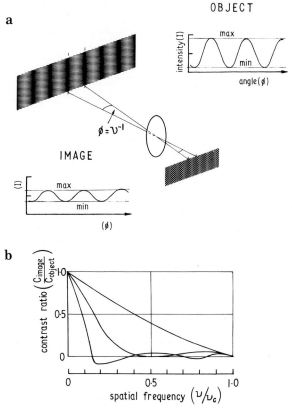

Fig. 9. a All optical systems reduce the contrast of the image compared with that of the object. This is partly due to diffraction and partly to aberrations, and the extent of image degradation is greatest at high spatial frequencies (v large, ϕ small). Contrast is defined as $\left(\dfrac{I_{max} - I_{min}}{I_{max} + I_{min}}\right)$. **b** The contrast transfer function of an optical system is the ratio of image–to–object contrast, for sinusoidally modulated gratings covering all spatial frequencies (v). In any optical system there is a "cut-off" frequency (v_c), set by diffraction at the aperture and given by λ/A, above which there is no contrast in the image. The upper curve shows the contrast transfer in a perfect optical system, and the lower curves optical systems that are out of focus by different amounts. (**b** adapted from BORN and WOLF, 1965)

of the stripes in the image reaches zero. This is the *spatial cut-off frequency* (in cycles per radian) and is given simply by:

$$v_c = \frac{A}{\lambda},\tag{20}$$

where A and λ are in the same units (see Fig. 9). Aside from the factor of 1.22, v_c is the same as $1/\theta$, the limit to spatial frequency implied by the Rayleigh criterion. The overall relation between object and image contrast – the transfer function – is determined by the grating frequency v, and in the ideal case of a square pupil with no aberrations, the relation is linear (Fig. 9 b). The presence of defects in the optical system alters this precise relation so that some spatial frequencies are enhanced at the expense of others, or the whole high frequency end of the function is flattened, but nevertheless the limit v_c remains unalterably set by diffraction at the aperture.

4. Diffraction and Aperture Size

In an eye where other defects are not important, one might expect the limit to resolvable spatial frequency set by diffraction to be the same as that set by the spacing of the receptor mosaic, i.e. v_c in Eq. (20) should equal $\mathscr{R}$ in Eq. (16). This gives the following relation:

$$\frac{f}{2p} = \frac{A}{\lambda} \quad \text{or} \quad \frac{A}{f} = \frac{\lambda}{2p}. \tag{21}$$

This means that in an eye where the receptor separation is p, there is a fixed value for the relative aperture (A/f) above which diffraction is unimportant. Taking 1 μm as the minimum practicable receptor separation (see Sect. 2) and 500 nm as the wavelength (λ), A/f is 0.25; or put another way, the eye should have an *F-number* not exceeding 4 (see also KIRSCHFELD, 1976). If the receptor spacing is greater than 1 μm, A/f can be smaller (or the *F-number* greater) without diffraction becoming the limiting factor. In fact, nearly all invertebrate eyes, simple and compound, have *F-numbers* less than 4, so that diffraction is not often the factor that limits resolution. However, as Fig. 9 b shows, image contrast is only 50% of object contrast when the spatial frequency of the stimulus is 0.4 v_c, and if this, rather than zero contrast, is taken as a more reasonable limit, one would expect *F-numbers* of 2 or less in eyes with receptors of minimal size. This is, in fact, more closely in accord with *F-numbers* typically observed.

5. Light Trapping by Receptors

In the last section, it was suggested that there might be a lower useful limit to the relative aperture (A/f) of an optical system, which depended on the receptor diameter or spacing. There are good reasons for thinking that there may also be an upper limit.

A receptor, or any other cylindrical structure of higher refractive index than its surroundings, will trap light entering it by total internal reflection, provided that the cone of light reaching it is narrow (Fig. 10). For an interface between two media, the angle of incidence above which total internal reflection occurs is given by:

$$\sin i_T = \frac{n_2}{n_1}, \tag{22}$$

where n_1 is the higher refractive index inside the cylinder. If n_2 is cytoplasm (~ 1.34) and n_1 is in the range 1.37–1.41, typical of photoreceptors, then i_T will be between 78° and 73°. The maximum width of the entry cone a receptor will accept will be approximately equal to twice $(90-i_T)°$, i.e. between 24° and 36°. For light not to pass between receptors, the cone of light supplied by the pupil, whose width is given

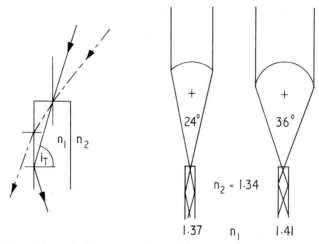

Fig. 10. Left: Light will be retained in a receptor by total internal reflection provided that the angle rays initially make with a normal to the receptor wall is greater than the critical angle (i_T) given by $\sin^{-1} n_2/n_1$. Right: Approximate sizes of the cones of light that will be accepted by receptors of different refractive indices, corresponding roughly to those of rhabdomeric receptors (left) and vertebrate rods. If the optical system supplies wider cones than these, light will pass between receptors and spoil the image

by $2 \tan^{-1} (A/2f')$, should not exceed these values. Where the optical system is a lens with water on both faces, $f' = f$ and these angles correspond to *F-numbers* (i.e. f/A) in the range 2.35–1.54. For a corneal lens with air in front, $f' \sim 1.34 f$, and the corresponding *F-numbers* are smaller, 1.75–1.15. For most invertebrates, it is likely that the higher limits apply (n_1 low), so that one might not expect to find many eyes with *F-numbers* much lower than 2. There certainly are exceptions: the nocturnal spider *Dinopis*, for example, has an *F-number* of about 0.6, and image-forming light must pass between receptors since there is no screening pigment (Sect. C.II.4.b). Presumably the need to acquire photons in very dim light is greater than the requirement for good resolution. The cephalopod molluscs, with *F-numbers* of around 1.3, also have a potential problem, but they tend to have both a mobile iris and retinal screening pigment and so are in a position to trade increased resolution for decreased sensitivity, and vice versa (Sect. C.II.3).

6. Image Defects

There are many reasons why a spherical surface, lens, or other optical device may produce a worse image than that implied by the diffraction limit. Classically, these are the lens aberrations (spherical aberration, coma, astigmatism, field curvature, distortion, and chromatic aberration, to which should be added defects of focus; see Born and Wolf, 1965). The only ones that are of any importance in eyes are spherical aberrations, chromatic aberrations and defects of focus. This is because all the rest concern rays making large angles with the optical axis and do not apply to systems like eyes with more or less spherical symmetry. Interestingly, their deleterious effects are all lessened by decreasing the relative aperture (A/f) of the optical system, whereas other features of optical design – diffraction and light capture – are both improved by increasing it. The causes and consequences of each type of aberration will be examined in turn.

a) Spherical Aberration

This defect arises from the fact that only rays close to the axis are brought to a focus at the gaussian focal point, given by the simple equations for refraction (or reflection) at spherical surfaces. Rays further from the axis are focussed progressively nearer to the refracting surface. Let us consider the image formed by a single spherical surface separating air and a material of refractive index 1.4 (roughly the situation in the eyes of spiders or the ocelli of some insect larvae). In such a system the focal point for rays parallel with and close to the axis will be situated at a distance f' from the surface where

$$f' = nf = \frac{rn}{n-1}, \tag{23}$$

in which r is the radius of curvature of the surface. Note that if the outside medium is not air $(n=1)$, then n in this equation must be replaced by the ratio of external and internal indices, e.g. n_1/n_0 in Fig. 7. With $n=1.4$, $f'=3.5\ r$. As can be seen from Fig. 11 a, rays parallel to the axis but at a distance (a) from it are focussed closer to the surface, and it is easy to show from the geometry of the figure that in the limiting case of a ray just grazing the surface $(a=r)$, the focus is located at a point whose distance from the front surface is r $[1+\tan(\sin^{-1} 1/n)]$, i.e. at 2.02 r or 1.48 r in front of the focus. Rays from intermediate zones intersect the axis at various positions between these extreme foci, and for values of a/r less than about 0.8 the deviation of the focal point from the gaussian focus is proportional to a^2. Figure 11 b shows that the intersection of rays from all zones of the surface (in this case for $a/r=0.9$ as the extreme ray) results in a circle of least confusion at C, whose position according to geometrical optics is such as to divide the line joining the gaussian focus (F) and marginal focus (M) in the ratio 3:1. The radius of the circle of confusion can be found by constructing the point of intersection of the marginal ray with a plane through C perpendicular to the axis, and the sizes and positions of the geometrical blur circles determined in this way are shown in Fig. 11 c.

We can now answer the question: "What is the maximum focal length and aperture a simple optical system can have, without requiring some kind of correction for spherical aberration?" It is reasonably accurate to say that spherical aberration becomes important when the size of the blur circle is larger than the size of the Airy disk due to diffraction, which is given by Eq. (19). Whilst this decreases with increasing relative aperture, the diameter of the blur circle increases, approximately as the cube of A/f. Plotting the sizes of the blur circles as a function of A/f (i.e. 0.8 a/r when n is 1.4) for different focal lengths and comparing these with the Airy disk diameters gives the results shown in Fig. 11 d. The intersections of the curves show that spherical aberration becomes important at smaller apertures as the eyes increase in focal length (or size) so that for an eye of focal length 100 μm, A/f can be as large as 0.56 $(F/1.8)$, but that when $f=1$ mm, this is reduced to 0.33, and to

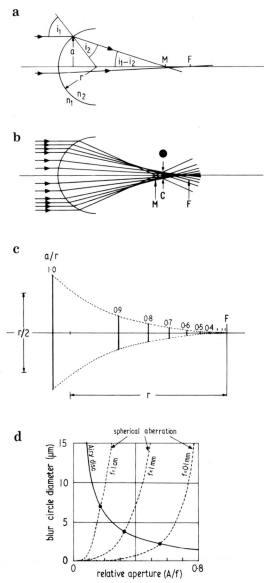

Fig. 11 a–d. Spherical aberration. **a** Construction for locating the focal point for rays at a distance from the axis. **b** Scale construction showing the extent of aberration produced by a spherical surface ($n=1.4$, air on the left) with a semi-aperture (a) equal to 0.9 radii. F is the focus for rays close to the axis, and M the focus of the marginal ray. The circle of least confusion is at C, and its actual size is indicated by the black dot. **c** Sizes of the circles of least confusion (blur circles) and their positions relative to the Gaussian focal point (F), expressed in terms of the radius (r) of the refracting surface for different aperture sizes. When the refracting surface is a full hemisphere ($a/r=1$), the blur circle is more than a radius in front of the focal point, and more than half a radius in diameter. **d** With increasing relative aperture, the size of the diffraction blur circle decreases (Airy disk, Fig. 7), but that due to spherical aberration increases dramatically. The points represent the smallest blur circles attainable with uncorrected simple eyes of different focal lengths. Note that the longer the focal length the smaller the optimum aperture

0.18 when $f = 1$ cm. At the same time, the diameter of the optimal blur circle increases slightly from about 2 µm up to 7 µm for the 1 cm eye. The implication is that spherical aberration is virtually non-existent for the ommatidia of compound eyes because these have focal lengths less than 100 µm; it becomes important enough to limit slightly either resolution or aperture in eyes like those of spiders with focal lengths in the range 100 µm–1 mm and, in larger "corneal" eyes, it is a defect that must either be overcome optically or else necessitates the use of quite small apertures, with a corresponding loss of retinal illuminance.

The largest eyes in invertebrates, those of the cephalopod molluscs, do have lenses that are corrected for spherical aberration (Sect. C.II.3). The trick they employ is a lens whose refractive index changes systematically from the centre (high) to the periphery. An alternative would be to use aspherical surfaces; the human cornea, for example, is not spherical and aspherical surfaces are employed as condenser lenses of high aperture in photographic enlargers and projectors. The problem here is that such surfaces can only correct for aberration along one axis, and since most eyes cover wide angles, the image will in general be worse with an aspherical lens or cornea over most of the image. The only serious suggestion that aspherical surfaces are used in this way in invertebrates comes from a most unlikely source – the fossilized remains of the eyes of trilobites. CLARKSON and LEVI-SETTI (1975) found that the outer part of each ommatidial lens consisted of oriented calcite ($n = 1.66$), often still preserved after several hundred million years, but that the inner part consisted of another material, possibly chitin, which has disappeared in the fossils and been replaced. The interesting feature of these "doublets" is the configuration of the surface between the two parts, which very closely resembles a Cartesian oval, a shape which produces no spherical aberration itself and which is also capable of correcting the aberration of another spherical surface. There is, of course, no way of knowing exactly how these eyes functioned in life, but the wide aperture of the lenses ($F/1.1$ in water) and their comparatively large diameter ($A \sim 250$ µm) indicate that spherical aberration would have been severe enough to warrant correction.

b) Chromatic Aberration

All transparent materials have a higher refractive index for shorter wavelengths than for longer ones, and this means that at a spherical surface blue light is refracted more than red, and so comes to a focus closer to the surface. The difference in focal length can be found by applying Eq. (23) which gives:

$$f'_R - f'_B = \frac{r n_R}{n_R - 1} - \frac{r n_B}{n_B - 1} \simeq \frac{f'}{n} \left(\frac{n_B - n_R}{n - 1} \right), \tag{24}$$

where the suffixes R and B refer to red and blue light, and no suffix indicates the focal length or refractive index for light in the middle of the spectrum (typically taken as that of the yellow sodium D line). The expression in brackets in Eq. (24) is the dispersive power of the medium, which for water or aqueous solutions is about 0.029, taken between wavelengths 434 and 656 nm. This value is probably appropriate to most biological materials except those which are dry or crystalline.

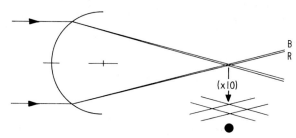

Fig. 12. Chromatic aberration. Scale construction to show the divergence of the red and blue ray at a spherical interface $(n=1.4)$. The circle of least confusion is shown much enlarged. Note that this is a very much less severe defect than uncorrected spherical aberration (Fig. 11 b)

As with spherical aberration, the existence of different foci gives rise to a circle of least confusion as the best image of a point source, situated in this case halfway between the blue and red focal points. From the geometry of Fig. 12, its radius (r_c) is given by:

$$r_c = \frac{A}{4f'}(f'_R - f'_B), \quad \text{or, from Eq. (24),} \quad r_c = \frac{A}{4n}\left(\frac{n_B - n_R}{n-1}\right). \tag{25}$$

The size of the blur circle is thus proportional to the absolute diameter of the aperture A. With $n=1.4$, and the dispersive power taken as that of water, the blur circle diameters for apertures of 100 μm, 1 mm, and 1 cm are 1.04, 10.4, and 104 μm, respectively. In reality these dimensions can be halved, since the visual pigments of photoreceptors have a half-width sensitivity of roughly 100 nm, and so each only "sees" between a third and a half of the calculated blur circle.

This calculation shows that as with spherical aberration, small eyes or the single ommatidia of insects whose facet diameters ($\sim A$) rarely exceed 50 μm will not be troubled by chromatic aberration and that this defect only becomes important when the pupil diameter is 0.5 mm or more, implying a focal length (f) of 1–2 mm. The only invertebrates that are likely to have a serious problem with chromatic aberration are the cephalopod molluscs, whose eyes can attain a prodigious size (up to 37-cm diameter; see Sect. C.II.3). Even here, however, the problem is not as great as it appears because most of the larger cephalopods are squid from deep waters where the residual daylight is so nearly monochromatic (blue $\sim$475 nm) that chromatic aberration will be almost irrelevant.

There are no known instances of eyes which correct for chromatic aberration in the way we do in instruments, i.e. by using compound lenses with components having different dispersive powers; indeed, the fact that the human eye, which does suffer significantly from chromatic aberration, is no better than an equivalent system containing an air/water interface (HARTRIDGE, 1950) is a strong argument for believing that this cannot be done with biological materials. However, where extreme resolution is important, *and* the eye contains receptors sensitive to different wavelength ranges, one way of minimizing chromatic aberration would be to have a layered retina in which the receptors sensitive to short wavelengths lie in front of those sensitive to longer wavelengths. This appears to be the situation in fish (EBERLE, 1967) and amongst invertebrates in jumping spiders (Figs. 31 c and 32).

In these animals the principal eyes have at least two and probably four visual pigments (DeVoe, 1975; Yamashita and Tateda, 1976), and they have a four-layered retina (Eakin and Brandenburger, 1971) in which the separation of the layers corresponds well to the longitudinal separation of the foci for wavelengths spanning the visible spectrum. There is a good case here for supposing that a good focus for all wavelengths has been achieved not by correcting the optics but by organizing the retina in such a way as to cope with the optical imperfections.

c) Depth of Focus and Accommodation

A relation well-known to photographers is that between the depth in object space over which the image can be said to be "in focus" and the aperture and focal length of the lens, the smaller the aperture and the shorter the focal length, the greater the depth of focus. For this reason it is common to find that very short focal lenses (on 8 mm cine cameras, for example) are not provided with a focussing adjustment because it is not necessary; the image is adequately resolved over the whole range of object distances ordinarily required – from a metre or so to infinity. The same is true of eyes. There is a need for some arrangement to change the focal point of the optical system in large eyes, but not in small ones, and it is of some interest to establish how large an eye must be before a mechanism of accommodation comes to be of value.

In an eye where a single spherical surface forms the image, the distance of an object from the eye (U) which is conjugate with an image at a distance V from the refracting surface is given by:

$$\frac{n}{V} - \frac{1}{U} = \frac{n-1}{r} = \frac{1}{f} = \frac{n}{f'}, \tag{26}$$

where n is the refractive index of the interior of the eye, r is the radius of curvature of the surface, and f and f' are the first and second focal lengths. The object is assumed to be in air, and a Cartesian (right positive) sign convention is used. This expression can be used to find the distance in object space that produces a blur circle on the retina whose diameter does not exceed a permitted amount (e.g. twice the receptor separation) when objects at infinity are also in focus. From Fig. 13, if an object at infinity forms an image at X and one at the "near point" is imaged at Y, the diameter of the blur circle will be $A(V-f')/f'$ when the object is either at infinity or at the near point. Making this equal to $2p$, where p is the receptor separation, gives $V = f'(2p+A)/A$. Substituting for V in Eq. (26) gives:

$$U = \frac{f'(2p+A)}{n} \frac{}{2p} \simeq \frac{fA}{2p}. \tag{27}$$

This formula indicates that the nearest object plane that can be considered to be in focus becomes more distant in direct proportion to the focal length of the eye and to its absolute aperture. The same equation holds for a lens in water. If we consider three eyes, each with receptor separations of 2 μm and relative apertures (A/f) of 0.5, but with focal lengths of 100 μm, 1 mm, and 1 cm, their correspond-

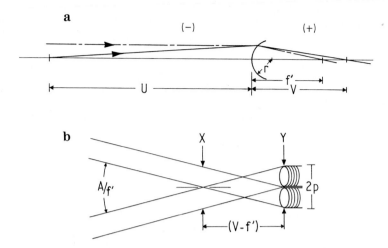

Fig. 13a, b. Change in focus with change in object distance. **a** A scale diagram of the amount by which the image is shifted when an object moves from infinity to a distance of $4f$ in front of the refracting surface. **b** A possible, rather stringent criterion for estimating the depth of focus of an eye which lacks an accommodation mechanism (Eq. 27). The eye can be said to be in focus if the blur circle on the retina does not exceed the width of two receptors. X and Y represent the focal points for objects at infinity and the "near point," respectively

ing near points will be 1.25 mm, 12.5 cm, and 12.5 m (notice that if the relative aperture is constant, the near point recedes as the square of f). The conclusions to be drawn are that compound eyes (f is less than 100 μm) have an in-focus image for virtually all distances, eyes with focal lengths of ~ 1 mm may or may not need a focussing mechanism, depending on whether they are called upon to resolve very fine detail at distances of a few centimetres, but larger eyes – like those of cephalopods – must have an accommodation mechanism if they are to resolve clearly at distances of a few body lengths as well as at infinity.

An important assumption made here is that the retina can be regarded as occupying a single plane of negligible depth. This will be true if the receptors are indeed short (less than about 10 μm) or if they are long but are optically isolated from each other. Optical isolation, which can be achieved either by surrounding each receptor with pigment or by the receptor itself acting as a light guide (see Sect. 5) means that the image "seen" by the receptor is the image present in the plane of their distal tips. If such mechanisms are not present, the image will be blurred because the cone of light will pass obliquely through a number of receptors.

As a postscript to this section, it has to be said that the arguments used here are all based on geometrical optics, rather than on a full diffraction optics theory of image defects, which would be more accurate but much more laborious (cf. BORN and WOLF, 1965). It does mean that the kinds of estimates of image quality presented here tend to be rather more "pessimistic" than they would be using more rigorous optics. This, however, is not too serious a drawback since the main concern has been to try to establish limits of eye performance, rather than actual working conditions.

IV. Conclusions and Compromises

1. Eye and Brain

The important properties of an eye, as far as its ability to collect and transmit information about the visual world is concerned, are very largely specified by its spatial resolving power (Eq. 16) and by its sensitivity (Eq. 15). The former determines the fineness with which the external world is sampled, and the latter the size, in terms of photons per unit time, of each such sample. This information – samples of photons in "bins" corresponding to different directions – is the material the brain has to deal with.

A preliminary task of the nervous system, before using visual information to direct actions, recognize objects, construct memories and so on, is to decide how these spatially allocated photon counts are best handled. There are four possibilities (excluding colour and polarization) indicated by Eqs. (3) and (4). If the eye secures for each receptor a large number of photon captures, these samples can be used as follows:

1) to make fine judgements of brightness between adjacent surfaces ($\Delta I/I$ small in Eq. 3) by making use of small differences in receptor signals.
2) to increase the statistical reliability of a particular judgement by only accepting large differences in signal as real (R large in Eq. 3).
3) to decrease the sampling time of the visual process by dividing the signal into smaller temporal units (t small, Eq. 4). This would mean that rapid movements are not interpreted as lack of contrast – a "blur" in a photograph – such as would occur if the time spent by an object within the field of view of a receptor was much less than the sampling (or integration) time of that receptor. Fast-moving animals need short sampling times and so need eyes that are able to supply their receptors with greater numbers of photons than do slower moving animals performing otherwise similar visual "tasks" (SNYDER, 1977).
4) to increase the effective size of each sample by pooling, neurally, the signals from several receptors. The enlarged sample (increased a, Eq. 4) can then be used to improve the performance of any of the functions 1–3 above, but this pooling does inevitably mean a decrease in spatial resolving power as each photon bin, within which no further resolution is possible, has been widened.

By studying an eye on its own, there is no way of telling what compromise has been struck between these four possibilities of contrast resolution, signal reliability, temporal and spatial resolution. Optical and anatomical measurements can indicate, for a particular eye, how much information is available at a particular light level, but not the way it is used.

2. Information Capacity of Eyes

The spatial resolving power of an eye, as determined from the receptor spacing, is only a useful indication of the resolution an eye is likely to attain under circumstances where each receptor has a very high photon capture rate. At low light levels where this is not true, a different kind of measure of resolution is required which somehow manages to marry the concepts of anatomical resolving power and the statistical uncertainties resulting from photon noise. This has been provided in the idea of the *information capacity* of an eye, worked out by Snyder et al. (1977a) for human eyes and Snyder et al. (1977b) for compound eyes. The information capacity is quantified by determining the number of different "pictures" the photoreceptor array can reconstruct, the quality of a reconstructed scene being determined by a combination of *both* the spatial density of the receptors in the array viewing it *and* the number of different intensity levels that each receptor is able to reliably distinguish. The actual measure used by Snyder et al. (1977a, b), in keeping with the usual conventions of information theory, is the product of the number of photoreceptors per square degree of object field and the natural logarithm of the number of distinguishable intensity levels. Many of the steps in their argument have already been dealt with in Sect. B.II and III. However, these authors have provided the only fully quantitative account of the way an eye's performance ought to vary with light intensity, and more important, how its performance can be optimized to provide the maximum information over a range of different light levels. The most important conclusions from these studies are, first, that optical factors (diffraction, minimum receptor size) are likely to provide the fundamental limit to resolution only during bright daylight. At all lower levels there is more information to be gained by increasing receptor size and thereby lowering spatial resolving power in the interests of obtaining a higher photon flux per receptor. Second, they show that for an eye of known optical characteristics, there is only one receptor spacing that is appropriate for extracting the maximum information at a particular light level. The corollary of this is that an eye which is to work over a wide range of ambient intensities *ought* to possess a range of receptor diameters. Snyder et al. (1977a) estimate that in the human eye a 100-fold range in effective photoreceptor diameter is required to optimize information extraction over the roughly million-fold range in light level spanning day and night vision. Generally speaking, eyes do not possess a range of photoreceptor diameters, and so this matching of light level to the appropriate size of light capture unit must be done by neural pooling. This is an important and general conclusion, and although such pooling is not yet well documented in invertebrates, as in vertebrates it is, one would nevertheless expect to find pooling mechanisms present, especially in species that are active over a range of illumination conditions.

Although "information capacity" is an important conceptual tool for deciding on the best compromise between fine-detail resolution and contrast resolution in an eye of given dimensions, it is somewhat unwieldy as a way of describing an eye's performance, and it is difficult to use when making comparisons between eye types. The separate concepts of spatial resolving power and absolute sensitivity are still valuable for describing the relative capabilities of eyes, especially when these eyes differ in size and structure.

3. Eye Size, Sensitivity, and Resolution

The evolution of eyes in the direction of either greater sensitivity or greater resolution requires an increase in size. Equations (15) and (16) are reproduced here

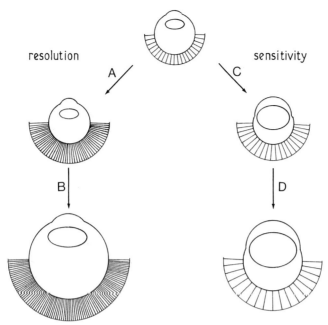

resolution   sensitivity

A   C

B   D

Fig. 14 A–D. Ways in which the resolving power and sensitivity of eyes can be increased. **A** Resolving power can be increased without an increase in focal length by reducing the receptor diameter to a minimum. If a decrease in sensitivity is to be avoided, this will entail an increase in receptor length. **B** Further resolution can only be gained by increasing the size of the eye. Doubling resolution requires a doubling of the focal length. For unchanged sensitivity receptor size and the relative aperture of the eye stay the same. **C** Sensitivity can be increased initially by increasing the aperture of the optical system and lengthening the receptors. **D** A further increase without resolution loss requires an increase in receptor diameter, coupled with an increase in focal length. Doubled sensitivity means an increase in focal length of 2

for convenience because they show why this is so.

$$\mathcal{S} = \left(\frac{\pi}{2}\right)^2 \cdot \left(\frac{A}{f}\right)^2 \cdot d^2 \cdot (1 - e^{-kx}), \tag{15}$$

$$\mathcal{R} = \frac{f}{2p} \simeq \frac{f}{2d}. \tag{16}$$

Suppose the sensitivity of an eye is to be increased by a factor of 10 without loss of resolution (meaning that it can supply the same spatial and contrast information, but at a 1 log unit lower ambient light level). Then from Eq. (15) either A must be increased, f decreased or d increased (the receptor length x is assumed to be already maximal). However, the ratio of f to d is fixed by the required resolving power; so if one is changed the other must change reciprocally. The aperture A can be increased on its own, but not to a value much greater than $0.5 f$, if the receptors are to trap light efficiently, and in any case it cannot physically be larger than $2 f$. Thereafter, the only way an increased sensitivity can be achieved is for A, f, and d to increase together. Sensitivity then increases in proportion to the square of any of the three dimensions, so that a 10-times sensitivity increase must mean an increase in linear size of the eye of $\sqrt{10}$, or 3.16 times (Fig. 14).

Resolving power, on the other hand, can be increased simply by increasing the focal length f. This must be accompanied by a corresponding increase in A if sensitivity is to be preserved, but all this means is that the relative proportions of the eye stay the same. Decreasing d (and increasing A proportionately) is a possible alternative, but since there is a lower limit to the diameter of a receptor (Sect. B.III.2), this is of limited value. Generally, resolution should be directly proportional to linear eye size, when sensitivity changes are not involved. Incidentally, this statement is *not* true for apposition compound eyes (Sect. C.III.3.d), where an increase in resolution requires an increase in both the size *and* number of individual facets, so that size has to increase as the square of resolving power (Barlow, 1952).

4. Summary

The main conclusions of Sect. B are collected here so that they can serve as a basis for making comparisons between the different types of eye discussed in the next section. Most of the conclusions apply to both simple and compound eyes, but there are some important differences, and these are discussed further in Sect. C.III.

1) The main properties of an eye, as far as its ability to transmit visual information is concerned, are summarized by its sensitivity (Eq. 15) and spatial resolving power (Eq. 16). Both high sensitivity and high resolution necessitate a large eye. Eyes specialized for high sensitivity in dim light will have large apertures (*F-numbers* as great as 0.5) and long, large-diameter receptors. Eyes specialized for high resolution in bright light will have smaller apertures (*F-numbers* of 1.5 or more) and narrow receptors whose diameter approaches the limit of 1–2 μm imposed by waveguide optics. Where an animal is active under both diurnal and nocturnal conditions, its eyes should either contain receptors of widely varying diameters, or more likely, neural arrangements for pooling signals from different sized areas of retina.

2) High sensitivity characteristics in an eye might mean that it is used for the detection of relatively high contrast objects under very dim conditions, or for making small contrast differences detectable under brighter conditions, or that it is a "high-speed" eye with a shorter receptor sampling time. These different possibilities cannot be distinguished on the basis of eye anatomy.

3) In simple (camera-type) eyes, diffraction at the pupil does not normally limit resolution, although in apposition compound eyes it may. Of the other possible image defects, spherical aberration does require correction if the eye has a focal length of 1 mm or more, but there are ways of minimizing this defect (Sect. C.II.3.a). Chromatic aberration cannot be removed optically in biological lenses; it can, however, be made less important if receptors sensitive to different wavelengths lie in different planes, and its consequences are in any case lessened by the narrow wave band that photopigment molecules accept. It is unimportant in compound eyes. Focussing mechanisms are necessary in eyes with focal lengths longer than about 1 mm if the image is to be sharp at different distances. Again, they are not needed in compound eyes where each ommatidial lens has a short (~ 0.1 mm) focal length.

C. Survey of Optical Mechanisms

I. Optical Principles

The discussions of sensitivity and resolution in Sect. B relied on the assumption that eyes possess optical arrangements capable of producing resolved images. This section explores the ways such images are actually produced. Figure 15 is a summary diagram containing nine different mechanisms capable of producing spatially resolved images on an array of receptors; all exist in different invertebrates and, with minor modifications, they probably represent the totality of such mechanisms. They are classified here according to the optical principle involved. *A* and *B* rely simply on the *shadowing* effect of dark pigment to restrict the angle over which each receptor can receive light. *C–F* employ a *refracting* mechanism. This is a lens in *C* where the eye operates in water, and an air/tissue corneal interface in *D* which represents a terrestrial simple eye. *E* is an apposition compound eye which, like *D*, employs corneal refraction, and *F* is a superposition compound eye where light from many facets is combined to form the image. In *G* and *H* the image is formed by *reflection;* the simple eye shown in *G* forms an image on a retina concentric with a concave mirror, and in *H* a superposition-type image is formed by large numbers of small reflectors oriented radially. In *I* the ray selection is by *total internal reflection*, in which light guides of only slightly higher refractive index than the surroundings each accept light from a restricted angle. The phylogenetic occurrence of the different types of eye is shown in Table 4, and their optical properties are discussed in detail in later parts of this section. The scheme outlined here differs from all previous ones in that it incorporates eyes with reflecting optics *(G–I)* which are discoveries or rediscoveries of the last few years.

The physical classification given in Fig. 15 cuts across the more usual division of eyes into *simple* or "camera-like" *(A, C, D, G)* where a single optical system supplies the image for all receptors, and *compound (B, E, F, H, I)* where each eye contains many distinct optical systems. However, the simple/compound division does remain useful, partly because the two classes of eye are superficially very different and partly also because they tend to occur in separate phylogenetic groups, simple eyes being typical of annelids, molluscs, arachnids and, of course, vertebrates, and compound eyes typical of crustacea and insects, although there are many exceptions. In the discussion that follows, the simple and compound eye distinction is retained.

II. Simple Eyes

1. Pigment Cups

The simplest imaginable eye, if one excludes the intracellular eyespots of some protozoa, is a simple cup of pigment nearly enclosing a small number of receptors (Fig. 15A). Eyes of this type are found in several phyla, and include the eyespots of some medusae (Coelenterata), flatworms (Turbellaria), leeches and many

Table 4. Phylogenetic distribution of the types of eye shown in Fig. 15

	A Pigment cups with lens ineffective or absent	B Multiple pigment tubes	C Aquatic lens eye	D Corneal lens in air	E Apposition compound eye	F Refracting superposition	G Simple reflector eye	H Reflecting superposition	I Apposition eye using total internal reflection	Notes, and relevant parts of Section C
Coelenterata	S									Cubomedusae especially
Platyhelminthes	S									(A) II. 1
Other Acoelomata	S									
Annelida										
Polychaeta	M	S	S		S					(B, E)III.2; (C)II.3.b.α
Oligochaeta										Unicellular eye spots
Hirudinea	M									(A)II.1
Mollusca										
Gastropoda	M		S	S						(C)II.3.b.β
Lamellibranchiata	S				S		S			(E)III.2; (G)II.5.c
Cephalopoda	S		M							(A)II.2; (C)II.3.b.γ
Arthropoda										
Onychophora			S							(D)II.4.b.α
Trilobita					M					(E)III.2
Crustacea										Very mobile compound eyes in Cladocera
Branchiopoda	M				M					
Ostracoda	M				S		S			(G)II.5.c
Copepoda	M		S				S			(C)II.3.c
Branchiura	M				M					
Cirripedia	M				M					Compound eyes in larvae only
Malacostraca					S	S		S	S	(F)III.4.d; (H)III.4.e; (I)III.3.i. Apposition eyes in Isopoda and Brachyura
Myriapoda				M	S					(D, E)III.2
Insecta										
Apterygota					M					(E)III.2
Pterygota				M	M	S				(D)II.4.b.β;(E)III.3;(F)III.4
Arachnida				M	S					(D)II.4.b.γ;(E)III.3.a
Echinodermata	S	S								Simple and compound eyespots in Asteroidea
Chordata	M		M	M						Eyespots in some Protochordata; camera-type eyes in Vertebrata

S = some,   M = most

polychaetes (Annelida), as well as in a few molluscs, echinoderms, prochordates and in some of the minor phyla. The best known examples of this type of eye are probably those of flatworms (HESSE, 1897; TALIAFERRO, 1920; RÖHLICH and TÖRÖK, 1961). In *Planaria maculata* each of the two eyes is composed of a pigment cup about 45 μm wide and 25 μm deep, with an unpigmented aperture 30 μm

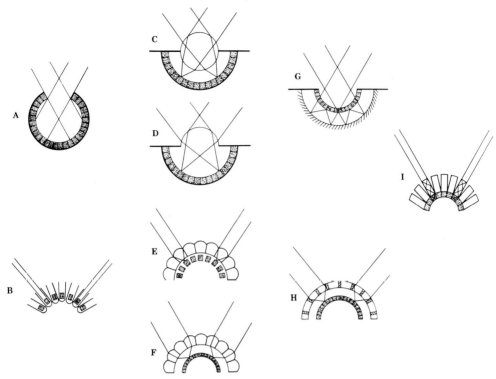

Fig. 15 A–I. The nine different mechanisms of image formation listed in Sect. C.I. **A** and **B** rely only on shadowing, **C–F** on refraction, **G** and **H** on reflection and **I** on total internal reflection. See also Table 4

across (Fig. 16). The receptor terminals are microvillous, the villi lining the inner wall of the pigment cup and oriented at right angles to its surface. Each such terminal is about 10 μm across and 6 μm deep; TALIAFERRO estimated that there are about 200 receptor terminals in each cup, although from the dimensions given this seems to be a slight overestimate. The receptor cell bodies are outside the eye and are joined to the terminals via dendrites passing through the aperture. This "inverted" retinal configuration is not found in all flatworms; in some the receptors point towards the light, and their cell bodies and axons penetrate the pigment cup in a manner much more typical of invertebrate simple eyes generally.

Not all pigment cup eyes have the spherical or ovoid shape seen in the planarian example. In limpets *(Patella)* and in certain leeches the pits are V-shaped or U-shaped, with no hint of a pigment ring or aperture around the opening. On the other hand, some of the ocelli of polychaete annelids have relatively much smaller openings than planarian eyes (HESSE, 1899), and there is even, in *Nereis*, a pupillary mechanism for altering the aperture (FISCHER and BRÖKELMANN, 1966). Most pigment cup eyes are very small, less than 100 μm in diameter, which is in keeping with the poor resolution they are capable of providing. There do, however, seem to be some interesting exceptions among the larger marine gastropods. HILGER (1885) described the eyes of several species (*Trochus, Turbo, Nerita,* and *Murex*) with eyes

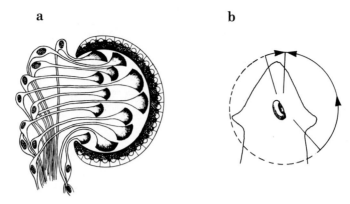

Fig. 16. a Pigment-cup eye of a planarian, *Euplanaria gonocephala*. The eye diameter is about 0.3 mm. (Redrawn from HESSE, 1899). **b** Demonstration that stimulation of different parts of the retina in *Planaria maculata* results in different behaviour. With one eye removed the animal turns to the left when a light is on the right, but to the right when the light is to left of the midline, illuminating the most posterior receptors only. (Redrawn from TALIAFERRO, 1920)

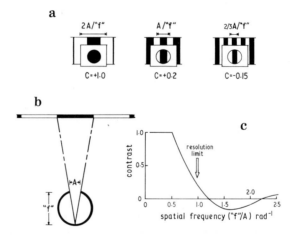

Fig. 17 a–c. The optics of eyes without lenses. **a** Stripe patterns of different periods as seen through an aperture. If one period of the pattern subtends an angle at the eye greater than $2 A/"f"$ (see **b**) the pattern will be fully resolved. Finer patterns rapidly lose image contrast, and this may even reverse, as in the third example where a retinal point "looking at" the dark stripe will actually be more strongly illuminated than its neighbours. **b** The geometry of **a**. **c** Graphical representation of **a**; image contrast for square gratings of different spatial frequencies as imaged by a circular aperture

1 mm or more across, but still with a wide pupil and an absent or ineffective lens. The resolution of these eyes can be no better than the smaller types, although they will, under the same conditions, secure a higher total retinal photon catch and so be usable at lower intensities.

The resolution of pigment cup eyes is obviously very poor. A distant point source will form an image which has the same diameter as the pupil, and two such images will not overlap on the retina if the angle between the sources is more than

$A/"f"$ radians, where $"f"$ is the axial length of the eye from the centre of the pupil to the receptors. In the planarian example this is about 69°. As explained in Fig. 17, similar considerations apply to striped patterns. If the period of such a pattern, expressed as an angle at the eye, is greater than $2\,A/"f"$ radians, the image contrast is the same as that of the object, and the grating is fully resolved. However, the image contrast falls to zero as the period of the pattern decreases to $A/"f"$, so for most purposes this is the limit of resolution; i.e. the highest spatial frequency is:

$$\mathscr{R} \simeq \frac{"f"}{A}. \tag{28}$$

In fact, at higher spatial frequencies than this, the contrast actually reverses; parts of the image that "ought" to be lighter, in fact, appear darker, but this effect is small – the maximum "reverse" contrast is only about 20% – and probably unimportant here. [This phenomenon and its implications are fully explored by GÖTZ (1965 a, b) in connexion with compound eye acuity]. One would expect from Eq. (28) that all the information this kind of eye can transmit would be extracted by receptors with an angular spacing of one-half $(A/"f")$ rad, and an actual spacing of one-half A. Thus, in a planarian eye with a 30-μm aperture, the minimum useful receptor spacing should be around 15 μm, and it is in fact 10 μm. However, some of the larger gastropod eye cups have receptor densities so high that they cannot possibly be explained by the need to exploit the available resolution.

Eyes of this simplicity are able to supply an animal with information about the general direction of light and about the presence of objects that subtend very large angles, and they can also mediate escape responses to shadow where only non-directional intensity changes are involved. For example, vision in *Planaria* is limited to (negative) phototaxis – the animal turning abruptly and accurately away from a light source. However, there is more to this behaviour than simply minimizing the stimulation on the two eyes. TALIAFERRO (1920) found that the posterior and anterior regions of the eye cup initiate slightly different responses, indicating a functional differentiation in the eye's connexions and also showing that some use is in fact made of the eye's limited resolution. He showed that whereas illuminating the eye cup from the side or behind, thereby stimulating the central and anterior receptors, results in a turn away from the stimulated side, when the receptors at the posterior end are stimulated by light from in front and slightly contralateral, the animal turns in the opposite direction, i.e. towards the side of the stimulated eye (Fig. 16b). This means that the posterior (contralaterally directed) region of one eye acts synergistically with the anterior region of the opposite eye, and the result is a turn of minimum size, wherever the light source appears.

2. Pinhole Eyes

The logical development of eyes which rely only on shadowing for image formation is towards a true "pinhole," if the resolution is to be improved. Making the eye larger and the aperture smaller will improve spatial resolution until the aperture becomes so small that the diffraction limit is reached. After that, smaller apertures will make the image worse, not better. The "ideal" pinhole eye, assuming that resolution rather than light capture is the most important consideration, would have a geometrical blur circle on the retina equal in diameter to that of the Airy disk. This would occur when the diameter of the aperture (A), which is also the size of the geometrical image for a distant point, is equal to 2.44 ($\lambda f/A$), the distance on the retina across the first dark ring of the Airy diffraction pattern. Reorganizing this expression gives:

$$A^2 = 2.44 \; \lambda \cdot f. \tag{29}$$

There appears to be only one real example of pinhole optics in the animal kingdom: in the eyes of the remarkable relict cephalopod mollusc *Nautilus* (Fig. 18). The gastropod mollusc *Haliotis* is sometimes regarded as having eyes of this kind (WEALE, 1974), but with a pupil 200 µm wide and an axial length of 1 mm (TONOSAKI, 1967), the resolution will be very poor – about 14° for gratings – and these eyes are probably best regarded as rather well-developed pigment cups. *Nautilus*, however, really is different. First, the eyes are large, about 1 cm in diameter and comparable in size to an octopus eye. This in turn implies that the eye is valuable to the animal and must represent a serious evolutionary attempt at image formation. Second, the aperture is small and almost certainly capable of changing size (see WELLS, 1966a). WELLS quotes ANNA BIDDER in 1964 as follows. "I have no evidence to give a lower limit to the diameter. My best photographs show a black spot about 1 mm in diameter, much of which I know to be pigment." More recently, HURLEY et al. (1978) have been able to show that the size of the aperture varies with ambient illumination from a lower limit of 0.4 mm to a maximum diameter of 2.8 mm. Equation (29) predicts that optimal resolution would be obtained with an aperture of about 0.1 mm, so even in bright light it seems that the resolution will be about four times worse than it could theoretically be for a pinhole eye of this size. The grating resolution (Eq. 28) should be about 25 cycles per radian with the pupil closed, and 3.6 when wide open. The corresponding angular subtenses for line pairs are 2.3 and 16 degrees. The former is comparable with the resolving power of a fairly typical insect eye. A third line of evidence indicating that the eyes are important to *Nautilus* is the presence of a compensatory reflex that stabilizes the eye against the pitching motion of the animal as it swims (HARTLINE et al., 1979). Such reflexes are found elsewhere only in animals (such as the other cephalopods) with a proven capacity to detect form or motion. Regretably, however, there is still no direct information about the function of vision in *Nautilus* itself.

The price to be paid for not having a lens, if relatively unimportant in terms of resolution, is enormous in its effect on retinal illuminance. For example, an octopus with a 1-cm diameter eye would have a maximum aperture of about 8 mm, compared with about 0.1 mm for an ideal pinhole eye of the same size. Since retinal illuminance, for a given focal length (f), is proportional to A^2 (Eq. 10), the ratio of retinal illuminances in a lens and pinhole eye can be as high as 6,400:1. Clearly a pinhole is a bad solution to the problem of achieving reasonable resolution in poor light – even in the shallow waters where *Nautilus* lives – and one can only marvel at the fact that such an eye has indeed survived for several hundred million years.

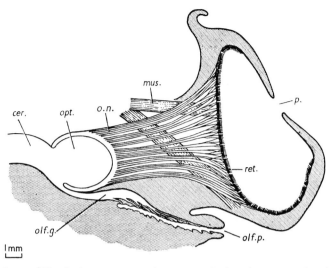

Fig. 18. Pinhole eye of *Nautilus* in transverse section. *cer.*: cerebral cord; *mus.*: muscles of eye stalk; *o.n.*: optic nerves; *olf.g.*: olfactory ganglion; *olf.p.*: olfactory pit; *opt.*: optic lobe; *p.*: pupil; *ret.*: retina. (YOUNG, 1964)

In neither *Haliotis* nor *Nautilus* can the dimensions of the receptors be said to match the resolution of the pinhole, where, as in the simpler pigment cups, one would not expect the receptor diameter to exceed half the diameter of the aperture. In both species the terminal microvillous regions of the receptors have diameters (and separations) in the range 5–10 μm (TONOSAKI, 1967; BARBER and WRIGHT, 1969a), where one might have expected diameters of 100 and 50 μm in the two species, respectively. Presumably in both species many receptors pool their responses at subsequent synapses, there being no resolution to be gained by not doing so, and sensitivity to intensity changes would otherwise be sacrificed.

3. Evolution of Lens Eyes in Aquatic Animals

a) Ideal Lens

For aquatic animals with simple (camera-like) eyes, the provision of a suitable lens is an obvious evolutionary advance over pigment cup or pinhole arrangements, since a lens permits all light from a given direction to reach a single small region of the retina, giving greatly improved resolution as well as an increase in retinal illuminance.

What would be the best construction for such a lens? Because it has to function in an external medium with a high refractive index, one would expect it to be spherical, as this shape gives the shortest focal length for a given difference in refractive index (Fig. 15C). Most such lenses are indeed spherical, the only important exceptions being in the eyes of certain copepod crustaceans (*Copilia, Corycaeus, Sapphirina*, Fig. 26) which have biconvex lenses with long focal lengths. However,

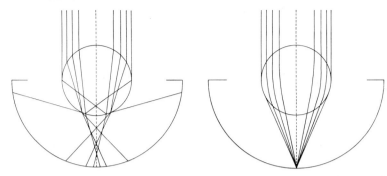

Fig. 19. Left: Spherical aberration of a homogeneous lens with a focal length-to-radius ratio of 2.5. The refractive index would need to be 1.67 (equivalent to hard flint glass). Right: Optically inhomogeneous lens of the fish type with a refractive index that decreases from the centre out. The spherical aberration can be reduced to zero, and the central refractive index can be as low as 1.52. (PUMPHREY, 1961)

a simple spherical lens with a homogeneous refractive index has two important drawbacks. Firstly, it will *still* have a relatively long focal length. This is given by:

$$f = \frac{r}{2}\left(\frac{n_2}{n_2 - n_1}\right) \tag{30}$$

for a sphere, where r is its radius, n_2 its refractive index and n_1 that of the medium around it. With $n_2 = 1.53$, the approximate refractive index of many *dry* biological materials, this gives $f = 3.8\,r$. In other words, the lens will be small in comparison with the eye itself, and the *F-number* relatively high (1.9). In fact the lenses of fish and most cephalopods have much shorter focal lengths than this, with $f \simeq 2.55\,r$ (Matthiessen's ratio) and an *F-number* of 1.3. The second and more serious drawback of a homogeneous spherical lens is its appalling spherical aberration, illustrated in Fig. 19. With a fully open pupil, such a lens would produce an image of very much poorer quality than is actually observed through fish or cephalopod lenses (PUMPHREY, 1961; SROCZYŃSKI, 1975, 1977).

The way in which both these problems – the long focal length and the aberration – have been overcome, in fish and cephalopods, is by the use of an inhomogeneous lens. If the refractive index of the lens decreases from centre to periphery, the focal length is shortened. This is because, instead of refraction occurring only at the two lens surfaces, it takes place continuously as a ray passes through the lens, and the total amount by which the ray is bent is much greater than two surface refractions alone would produce, given the same maximum refractive index. Also, because rays passing through the outer zones of the lens encounter lower refractive indices than those passing through the centre, the relative amount of bending is less for these peripheral rays. This counteracts the aberration problem of the homogeneous sphere, where the peripheral rays are brought to a focus much closer to the lens than are the central rays which form the ideal (gaussian) focus.

The discovery of this refractive index gradient, and the appreciation of its significance, goes back to MATTHIESSEN (1880, 1886). However, the solution of the problem of exactly what form the gradient should take for such a lens to be truly

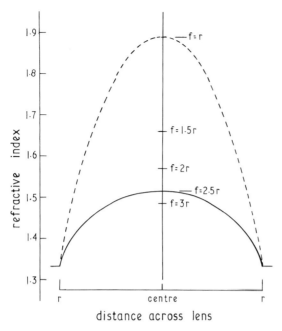

Fig. 20. The refractive index profile through a lens required to produce the aplanatic condition in Fig. 19. The solid line is for a Matthiessen's ratio lens ($f = 2.5\ r$), and the dashed curve for a lens which images on its rear surface. The central refractive indices for other f/r ratios are also indicated (Based on data from FLETCHER et al., 1954)

aberration-free (aplanatic) was not arrived at until a study by FLETCHER et al. in 1954. Their conclusions are reviewed by PUMPHREY (1961) and are shown in Fig. 20 which shows that an aplanatic lens with a focal length of 2.5 r can be obtained with a central refractive index of about 1.52. If the lens were homogeneous, however, Matthiessen's ratio would require a refractive index of 1.66, which is much higher than that of the sorts of material from which lenses are made.

b) Real Lenses

In the eyes of aquatic invertebrates, we are presented with a spectrum of lens types ranging from those that are little more than a jelly which fills the eye cup (*Füllmasse* was HESSE's term) to ones that are clearly of the "Matthiessen's ratio" type with low *F-numbers* and excellent imagery. Unfortunately, optical measurements on which to base optical quality judgements are rare in the literature, and we are forced to rely heavily upon inferences from anatomy.

One firm inference is that if the "lens" occupies the whole of the eye cup there is no way at all that it can form a good image. This is because, to form an image on its rear surface and hence the retina, the lens would need a refractive index of 2.66 (if homogeneous; Eq. 30) or 1.89 (if inhomogeneous; FLETCHER et al., 1954). Both figures are unrealistic. This means that for most of the lenses of polychaete annelid eyes (HESSE, 1899) where there is no space between lens and retina, and for

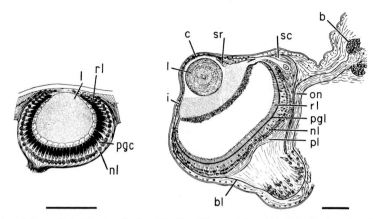

Fig. 21. Annelid eyes. Left: *Nereis cultrifera*. The "lens" is certainly optically ineffective. (Modified from HESSE, 1935). Right: *Vanadis formosa*. A large Alciopid polychaete with an exceptionally large pair of eyes. Although the lens has a high f/r ratio of about 4, it can be expected to form a good image (From HERMANS and EAKIN, 1974, after HESSE, 1899). The scale on both figures is 100 μm. *b*: brain; *bl*: basement lamina; *c*: cornea; *i*: iris; *l*: lens; *nl*: nuclear layer; *on*: optic nerve; *pgc*: pigment cell; *pgl*: pigmented layer; *pl*: plexiform layer; *rl*: layer of receptor endings; *sc*: secretory cell; *sr*: secondary retina

many gastropod mollusc eyes where the same condition exists, image formation will be little better than in the "pigment cup" eyes discussed in Sect. C.II.1.

However, the converse inference is also valuable. If there is a clearly demarcated lens, with a space between it and the retina of at least 1.5 lens radii, then it is reasonable to expect that a good image is formed. It is usually not possible, from gross anatomy, to tell quite how good the image formed by such eyes will be. If, for example the ratio f/r is 4 (measured as the lens centre to retina distance divided by the lens radius, and assuming the eye to be "in focus"), this might mean either that the lens is solid, with a refractive index around 1.52, or that it has a graded refractive index which reaches about 1.46 in the centre. The former lens will have serious spherical aberration, the latter is potentially perfect. Problems like this can only be settled by carefully examining image quality, or by measuring refractive index profiles (using frozen sections and interference microscopy), and no such invertebrate lenses have been subjected to either kind of examination. Nevertheless, both solid and graded lenses represent a great improvement over those of the *Füllmasse* kind. They occur in three invertebrate groups.

α) Annelids. Large eyes with distinct lenses have probably only evolved once in this phylum, in the Alciopidae, a family of carnivorous pelagic polychaetes. HESSE (1899) studied the eyes of *Alciopa cantrainii* and *Vanadis formosa*, and it is clear from his figures (Fig. 21) that although the eyes are small, about 0.5 mm in diameter, they are much more highly developed than in other polychaetes and that there is an adequate space behind the lens for image formation. If his figures are accurate, the ratio f/r is about 4. The receptors are long and narrow, about 80 μm by 6 μm (HERMANS and EAKIN, 1974), and are in many respects similar to those of cephalopod molluscs. The implication is that the resolution of the lens is good and that the fine-grain retina is exploiting its resolution. The species whose ultrastructure was studied by HERMANS and EAKIN, *Vanadis tangensis*, has slightly larger eyes than the other species, with a diameter of about 1 mm. Assuming a similar focal length, this gives an interreceptoral angle of approximately 21 min. PUMPHREY (1961) thought the large f/r ratio implied that the lens was homogeneous, but an observation by HERMANS and EAKIN suggests the contrary: "The density of vesicles near the surface of the lens varies, but toward the centre of the lens the granular material becomes uniformly and tightly packed, and the vesicular membranes lose their integrity." These worms are remarkable in a number of respects: they are large (up to 20 cm long), transparent and carnivorous. This suggests that they use their eyes in the capture of prey, rather than for the functions usually ascribed to the cephalic eyes in this phylum – orientation towards or away from light.

β) *Gastropod Molluscs*. The eyes of this class present a very confusing pattern. In pulmonate land snails like *Helix*, the "lens" is soft and fills the eye cavity (HESSE, 1908; RÖHLICH and TÖRÖK, 1963), but it may be that here the very small refractive power of the lens is supplemented by the curvature of the cornea, since this is in air. However, the same *Füllmasse* type of eye, often as large as 1 mm in diameter, seems to be present in a number of wholly marine prosobranchs (*Trochus*, *Turbo*, *Nerita*, and *Murex* species; HILGER, 1885). Conversely, some of the fresh-water pulmonates such as *Lymnaea stagnalis* have eyes with hard lenses with short focal lengths and a space behind them which is adequate for focussing. The ratio f/r is about 2.7 (personal observations, and also STOLL, 1973), implying that *Lymnaea* has a perfectly constructed lens. Similarly, the prosobranch sea snails *Littorina* and *Strombus* have convincing Mattiessen's ratio lenses. In *Littorina littorea*, NEWELL (1965) measured f/r as 2.8, the focal length 155 µm, and the receptor separation about 12 µm, giving an inter-receptor angle of 4.4° (in water). This is much greater than the diffraction limit for a lens of this size (22 min) indicating that the optical resolution is not fully exploited. GILLARY (1974) described the eye of the conch *Strombus* (Fig. 22). The eyes are large, up to 2 mm in diameter, with a well-defined fish-type lens. The lens shown in the figure is somewhat nearer the retina than it "ought" to be, i.e. less than 1.5 radii, but this appears to be due to distortion. The receptors are long and narrow (90 µm and 4 µm) giving a minimum inter-receptor angle of about 14 min for a 1-mm focal length lens. What the eye is used for, other than simple taxes for which it seems overadequate, remains a mystery. The small eyes of some opisthobranch gastropods like *Aplysia* seem to be intermediate between the Füllmasse and Matthiessen's ratio types, but there are no useful studies of their optics.

One group of gastropods, however, stands out as having remarkable eyes. These are the heteropod prosobranchs, large pelagic transparent carnivores whose life-style closely parallels that of the alciopid annelids. The paired eyes are relatively large (1–5 mm), with a spherical lens that is well separated from the retina. HESSE (1900) examined live specimens of several species, and from his data values of f/r can be obtained which range from 4.4 in *Pterotrachea mutica* down to 3.0 for *Oxygyrus keraudreinii*. My own measurement on living eyes of *Pterotrachea coronata* (Figs. 22 and 23) gave a focal length of 1,250 µm and a lens radius of 375 µm, with f/r about 3.3. The image formed by the lens was good, but not as good as that of a fish lens of similar size. Histologically, the lens appears to have a uni-

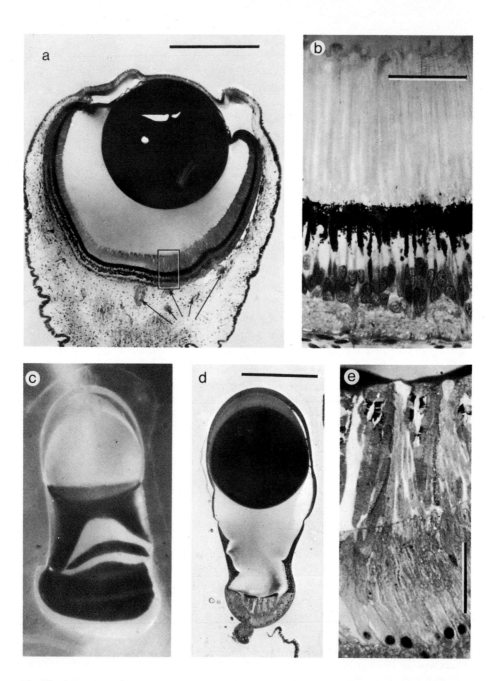

Fig. 22 a–e. Large eyes in gastropod molluscs. **a** Eye of the seasnail *Strombus luhuanus*. The arrows indicate components of the optic nerve. Scale 0.5 mm. (Courtesy of Dr. H. L. GILLARY, 1974). **b** Enlarged portion of the retina of *Strombus* (rectangle in **a**). The total number of receptors is more than 10^5. Scale 50 μm (From GILLARY, 1974). **c** Right eye of the heteropod *Pterotrachea coronata* seen from the dorsal side. The eye is tubular, with a characteristic pattern of reflecting bands around it that prevent non-image-forming light from reaching the retina. Scale as **d**. **d** Section at right angles to the plane of **c**. The six rows of receptor columns in the retina are visible at the bottom. Dorsal is on the left. Scale 0.5 mm. **e** Part of the retina at higher magnification showing how about five receptors contribute to each receptor column. Scale 50 μm

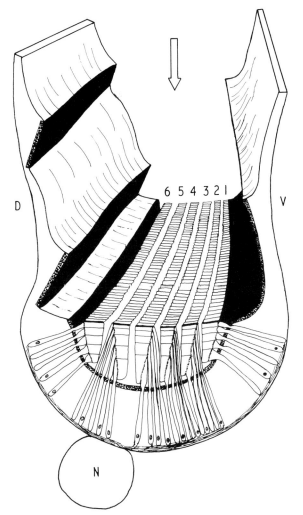

Fig. 23. Reconstruction of part of the retina of *Pterotrachea coronata*, showing the arrangement of receptors into columns and rows. (The numbering sequence is as given by HESSE, 1900). The significance of this peculiar multilayered organization is unknown. *D, V*: dorsal and ventral; *N*: nerve

formly dense centre, but a less dense cap. All of this suggests that these lenses are optically intermediate between the homogeneous and graded-index types.

The retina in these animals is even more remarkable. It is not the usual hemispherical cup of receptors, but a long flat ribbon (Fig. 23) which is straight in *P. coronata*, and bent into a horseshoe shape in *Carinaria* species. In *P. coronata* this ribbon contains six rows of "receptor columns," each about 22 μm wide, giving the ribbon a total width of 133 μm. Within each row the receptor columns are spaced much more closely, about 3.5 μm, and as the retina is about 1 mm long this means that there are roughly 286 columns in each row. The angular separation of each column is about 1.14° between rows (dorsoventrally with respect to the ani-

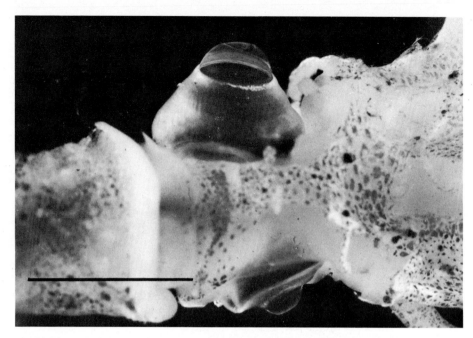

Fig. 24. The eyes of an unusual deep-sea squid, *Histioteuthis*. One eye is approximately twice the size of the other and the larger eye is somewhat tubular, as in some deep-sea fish. Partially dissected, from above. Scale 10 mm

mal) and 0.18° (11′) along the rows (lateromedially). "Column" is used rather than receptor to indicate another unique feature. The individual receptors are stacked up one above the other, so that light reaching one spot on the retina passes through a column containing the receptive segments of five cells whose *total* depth is about 100 μm. The arrangement of cell bodies is shown in Fig. 23; in the two dorsal rows the receptive segments are attached to the ventral side of each cell and to the dorsal side in the four ventral rows. All this was described with exemplary accuracy by Hesse in 1900.

The ultrastructure is peculiar as well. Dilly (1969) found that the receptive segments in *P. mutica* were made of stacks of membrane disks, like vertebrate receptors, and that these stacks were attached to the cell bodies by numerous ciliary basal bodies. I can confirm this, but would add that the receptive segments contain microvilli *as well*, and regions can be found where the one kind of array merges into the other. It would be particularly interesting to know whether these differences in membrane packing represent adaptation to different light levels.

All these features, together with considerable binocular overlap and some degree of eye mobility, imply that the eyes play an important role in the predatory life of these beautiful, enigmatic animals.

γ) Cephalopod Molluscs. The parallel evolution of the eyes of the advanced cephalopod molluscs (octopus, squid, cuttlefish) and those of fish is famous (see Packard, 1972). In both groups the eyes are large, spherical, possess Matthiessen's

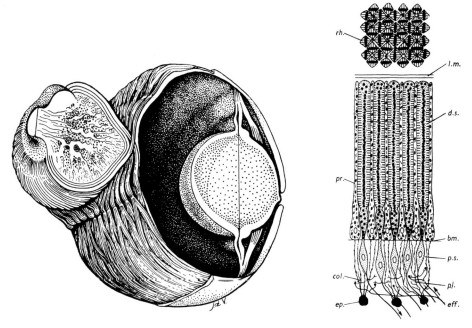

Fig. 25. Left: drawing of a dissection of the eye and optic lobe of *Octopus*. Right: diagrams of the structure of the retina of *Octopus*, in tangential section (above) and radial section. *bm*: basement membrane; *col*: collaterals of retinal axons; *ds*: distal segments of receptors; *aff*: efferent fibres to the retina; *ep*: epithelial (glial) cells; *l.m.*: limiting membrane; *p.s.*: proximal segments of receptors; *pl*: plexus of retinal fibres; *pr*: processes of supporting cells; *rh*: rhabdomeres of the receptors in which the microvilli of adjacent rhabdomeres are arranged at right angles to each other. (Both figures from YOUNG, 1964)

ratio lenses, have a mobile iris, a mechanism of accommodation for near vision, and a repertoire of essentially similar eye movements (COLLEWIJN, 1970) (Figs. 24 and 25). The world record for eye size is undoubtedly held by a cephalopod; BULLOCK and HORRIDGE (1965) quote BEER (1897) as recording an unidentified giant squid, taken off the Irish coast, with tentacles 10 m long and an eye 37 cm across. The principal differences between fish and cephalopod eyes are that in fish the retina is inverted whereas in cephalopods the receptors face the lens, and that in fish as in other vertebrates the receptors are made of stacks of tightly opposed membrane plates, whereas in cephalopods they are composed of arrays of microvilli, as in insects. A good general account of cephalopod eyes is given in WELLS (1966a), and only a few points will be considered here.

Because of the construction of the lens there is every reason to think that the eye produces a perfectly focussed image, *for monochromatic light*. Most available evidence points to the fact that these animals are colour-blind (MESSENGER et al., 1973) and this, coupled with the narrow wavelength range of light in the sea, implies that chromatic aberration may be unimportant (see Sect. B.III.6.b). How well is this good image exploited? The receptors are very narrow and densely packed. YOUNG (1962) estimates that *Octopus* has a receptor density of 70,000 per mm², or since the receptors are contiguous and packed in a square lattice, a receptor separation of 3.8 μm. HESS (1905) estimated 105,000 per mm² in *Sepia*, corresponding to a separation of 3.1 μm. For *Octopus*, with a focal length of approximately 1 cm, this gives an angular receptor separation of 1.3 min, which is very similar to that in man. The receptors are long – about 200 μm in *Octopus* – and their length and narrowness indicate that both photon capture and resolution are maximized.

There are, however, optical problems which prevent *simultaneous* optimization of resolution and sensitivity. If the receptive segments have a refractive index of about 1.37, the semi-angle of the cone of light that they will accept, and trap by total internal reflection, is about 13° (Sect. B.III.5). However, an unconstricted Matthiessen's ratio lens ($f/r = 2.55$) supplies them with a cone of semi-angle 21.4°, meaning that more than half the light from a point source reaching a receptor will escape from it, either into neighbouring receptors or into shielding pigment. When shielding pigment is withdrawn to achieve maximum sensitivity, the cone of light from a point image will intersect approximately 300 receptors and obviously spoil the quality of the received image. Conversely, with shielding pigment extended to isolate the receptors, most (63%) of the light would be absorbed by this and wasted. This emphasizes the role shielding pigment can have in improving resolution, as well as in reducing light flux in the receptors. It is worth noting that if the refractive index of the receptors were as great as 1.43 (which is unlikely), all light entering the lens would be trapped by the receptors and both the shielding pigment and the iris would, strictly speaking, not be necessary for improving resolution.

A final point of interest about the organization of the retina is the fact that adjacent receptors have their microvilli oriented at right angles (Fig. 25). This means that neighbouring receptors will respond best to light whose planes of polarization (*e*-vectors) are also at right angles (MOODY and PARRISS, 1961), and the whole retina can be said to consist of an analyser for polarized light. There may be many functional reasons for this, but one attractive possibility is that it is concerned with the detection of fish (like the herring) which camouflage themselves with a mirror surface. This makes them very nearly invisible in ordinary light, as the intensity reflected from their sides is almost the same as that of the background (DENTON, 1970). However, this reflected light is strongly polarized at most angles, so that a predator with an analyser – a squid, for example – would have no difficulty in detecting fish camouflaged in this way.

It hardly needs pointing out that cephalopods have a repertoire of visual behaviour comparable with that of higher vertebrates (WELLS, 1966b), and it is not surprising that they have large, high-resolution eyes, nor that the optic lobes of the brain contain more neurons than in the whole of the rest of the central nervous system (YOUNG, 1964). A review of cephalopod behaviour is given elsewhere in this handbook (MESSENGER, Vol. VII 6 C, Chap. 2).

c) Non-spherical Lenses: Copilia and Its Relatives

Some members of one group of copepod crustacea, the Cyclopoida, have eyes that are quite unique (Figs. 26 and 27, and see VAISSIERE, 1961). They break the general rule that aquatic lenses are spherical and instead have eyes containing two lenses, the anterior one large but thin, and the posterior small and pear-shaped. The arrangement of both eyes looks rather like a pair of binoculars (Fig. 26). The other

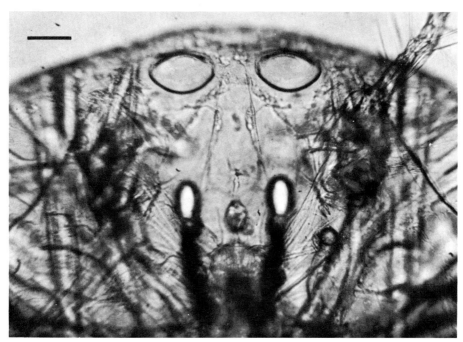

Fig. 26. Paired eyes of the copepod crustacean *Sapphirina*. The final image is formed behind the second (smaller) lens and falls onto a small number of rhabdoms contained in the long dark structures. In *Sapphirina* and its relatives the rear lenses and receptors can move laterally to scan the image formed by the front lenses. Photograph of living animal. Scale 100 μm

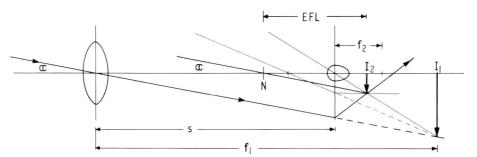

Fig. 27. Construction for finding the focal length of a combination of two lenses, such as that in the *Sapphirina* or *Copilia* eye. The first lens forms an image at I_1, which is intercepted by the second lens and imaged at I_2. The nodal point of the combination *(N)* can be found by drawing a line parallel to the original ray and passing through the final image; this line behaves like a ray passing through a single thin lens at N. The effective focal length of the system *(EFL)* is the distance from N to I_2

peculiar features are first that the number of receptors behind the second lens is very small [only five in *Copilia quadrata*, of which one is short and eccentric (WOLKEN and FLORIDA, 1969)], and second that in life the whole of the back part of the eye, including the receptors and second lens, "scans" from side to side. The rear sections of the two eyes move together, rapidly towards each other, then more slowly apart. The rate varies from 0.5–5 Hz (GREGORY et al., 1964).

At first sight, a thin lens in water seems a poor solution to the problem of light capture, as its relative aperture is bound to be low. The front lens of *Copilia*, on its own, has an *F-number* of about 5.4. However, the effect of the second lens is aptly referred to by WOLKEN and FLORIDA as "light amplification;" it condenses the partially focussed image from the first lens onto a much smaller area, thereby increasing the image brightness. The net effect is that the combination has the same aperture as the first lens (172 μm), but a much shorter effective focal length (EFL). It is not difficult to show that the combined focal length is given by

$$ \mathrm{EFL} = \frac{f_1 \cdot f_2}{f_1 + f_2 - s}, \tag{31} $$

where f_1 and f_2 are the focal lengths in water of the first and second lenses, and s is the separation of their centres. Using WOLKEN and FLORIDA's estimates ($f_1 = 0.93$ mm, $f_2 = 0.128$ mm, and $s = 0.65$ mm), the effective focal length is 0.27 mm. A construction showing this is given in Fig. 27. This brings the *F-number* down to 1.6, which is quite comparable with that of a fish lens (1.25–1.3).

The great drawback of this arrangement, compared with the spherical optical systems that it rivals in relative aperture, is the minute field of view of the receptor assembly. WOLKEN and FLORIDA give the surface dimensions of the *whole* receptor array in *Copilia* as 11×17 μm, and of individual receptors only 1.7×0.9 μm by 58 μm in length. With an EFL of 0.27 mm this means the entire field of vision is about 3° across, and the subtense of single receptors about 17 min. The construction of the eye, with a small mobile second lens, could not really be organized to give a wider field, and one is left with an interesting unresolved question. Do these eyes scan to increase the field of view of a very restricting optical system, or has the facility of scanning made possible this compact, high-aperture, high-resolution type of eye?

4. Simple Eyes in Terrestrial Animals

In air the interface between the eye and the outside can act as a refracting surface (as in Fig. 7), so that the spherical, short focal length lenses found in aquatic animals are no longer necessary (Fig. 15D). In man, for example, most of the power of the optical system is contributed by the cornea, not the lens. In only one group of invertebrates, the arachnids, have simple eyes with essentially the human eye form attained dominance. Insects, although often possessing simple eyes as larvae, invariably have compound eyes as the main organs of sight when adults. In some arthropods – centipedes, isopod crustacea and some of the smaller, more primitive insects – it is hard to tell whether the small collection of corneal facets is best thought of as a compound eye or a number of simple eyes (ocelli). Other simple eyes in which the cornea is important optically occur in land snails – although I do not think that the radius of the snail cornea *in life* has ever been measured, so its exact contribution is uncertain – and in the curious animal *Peripatus* which links the annelid and arthropod phyla.

a) Optics

The optics of an eye with a spherical air/tissue interface are shown in Fig. 7 and summarized in Eqs. (23) and (26). The focal length (or posterior nodal distance) of such a system is given by $f = r/(n-1)$, where r is the radius of curvature and n the internal refractive index. The image is situated at a distance f' from the refracting surface, where $f' = nf$, and the nodal point lies at the centre of curvature of the cornea. If we take 1.4 as a typical value for the refractive index of such an eye, this means that f' is 3.5 r and f is 2.5 r. The size of the image of an object of height h at a distance U is simply $h \cdot f/U$, provided U is large compared with f.

In nearly all the eyes discussed below there is actually more than one interface. The cornea is typically the front surface of a thickening of the cuticle whose rear surface is also spherical (Figs. 29 and 30). The power (reciprocal of focal length) of this second surface is usually less than that of the cornea, because the refractive index difference across it is smaller, but nevertheless it makes a contribution to shortening the focal length of the eye which increases light capture and, by spreading the refraction between two surfaces, it tends to reduce aberrations. Strictly, the properties of such lenses need to be evaluated one surface at a time, or by thick-lens optics. The general formula for the focal length (f) of a system with two surfaces (radii r_1 and r_2) separating three media (n_1, usually air; n_2, the lens; and n_3, the "vitreous" or cytoplasmic space behind the lens) is:

$$\frac{1}{f} = \frac{n_2 - n_1}{r_1} + \frac{n_3 - n_2}{r_2} - \frac{d(n_2 - n_1)(n_3 - n_2)}{n_2 r_1 r_2}, \tag{32}$$

where d is the distance separating the two surfaces. It is important to keep a Cartesian convention in which distances (such as radii of curvature) to the right of a surface are taken as positive and those to the left, negative. Equation (32) can also be written more simply in terms of the *powers* of the surfaces:

$$\frac{1}{f} = P = P_1 + P_2 - \frac{d}{n_2} P_1 P_2. \tag{32a}$$

In some eyes the optical system has two lenses (*Isia*, Fig. 29) somewhat like *Copilia* (Fig. 27), except that the first surface is in air. At this stage shortcuts probably have to be abandoned, and the system worked through by ray tracing, surface by surface.

b) Types of Eye

α) *Gastropods and Peripatus.* It has already been mentioned that land snails have soft lenses which nearly fill the eye cavity and that an effective cornea would be essential for them to focus properly. Assuming that the cornea is suitably curved, the eye of *Helix aspersa* would have a focal length of about 200 μm and, with receptors 15 μm wide (see SCHWALBACH et al., 1963; RÖHLICH and TÖRÖK, 1963), this would give an inter-receptor angle of 4.3°. In slugs this situation may well be different. According to NEWELL and NEWELL (1968), the lens of *Agriolimax reticulatus* has a focal length of 2.8 radii, which means that it must have a graded refractive index. There is a space behind the lens too, as in the shore-dwelling

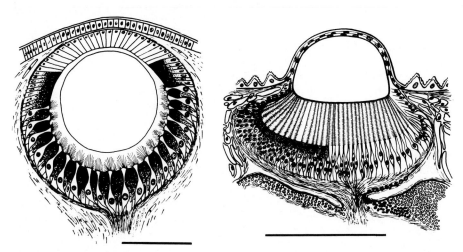

Fig. 28. Small terrestrial eyes. Left: the land snail *Helix pomatia*. A typical gastropod eye in which the lens, of unknown refractive index, is certainly unable to form an image on the retina by itself. The corneal surface may partially improve the imaging ability of the eye. (HESSE, 1908). Right: eye of the Onychophoran *Peripatoides occidentalis*. Here the cornea is prominent, but still not adequately curved to form an image on the retina which is situated only about one radius behind the corneal surface. (DAKIN, 1921). Scale bar 100 μm on both

prosobranch *Littorina*, so that an image would be formed on the receptor layer with only minimal assistance from the corneal surface. However, the eyes are very small ($f \simeq 100$ μm) and the receptors are large and widely spaced ($\simeq 20$ μm), so that in spite of an image that should be quite sharp, the resolution will be limited by the large inter-receptor angle of about 11°. The only known behaviour associated with the cephalic eyes in land gastropods is guidance towards dark objects or dark regions of the environment (HERMANN, 1968; BUDDENBROCK, 1919), but so far there is no clear information concerning their capacity for angular discrimination. Withdrawal responses evoked by shadowing the animal are apparently not mediated by the eyes, but by receptors located in more posterior regions of the mantle (FÖH, 1932).

The eyes of *Peripatus* are more like typical arthropod ocelli. DAKIN (1921) studied the eyes of *Peripatoides occidentalis*, and his description shows that they have a very pronounced, nearly hemispherical cornea bounding a non-cellular homogeneous structure whose flat rear surface is in contact with the layer of receptor outer segments. The whole eye is only about 200 μm wide by 150 μm deep, and the radius of curvature of the cornea is approximately 45 μm. This should produce a best image at a distance (f') from the cornea of about 160 μm. Unless DAKIN's sections were very badly distorted, which is unlikely, this means that the focal plane lies so far behind the retina ($\simeq 65$ μm) that sharp image reception is out of the question. Because of the wide aperture, the blur circle on the retina corresponding to a point object would cover roughly 300 receptors, out of a total of not more than 1,000. One would certainly not expect *Peripatus* to show visual behaviour that requires any degree of resolution. A recent account of the fine structure of these eyes is given by EAKIN and WESTFALL (1965a).

Isia   Euroleon   Perga

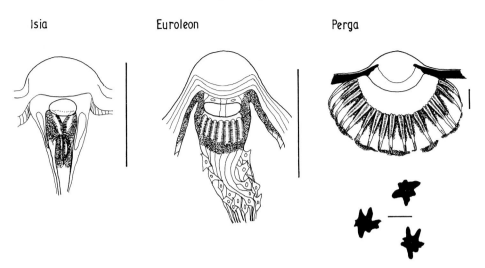

Fig. 29. Eyes of larval insects. Left: lateral ocellus (stemma) of a lepidopteran caterpillar, *Isia isabella*. There are six on each side, some having multiple lenses. The rhabdomeres all appear to share a common axis, implying little or no resolution within the field of view. (After DETHIER, 1943). Centre: ocellus of the ant-lion, *Euroleon nostras* (Neuroptera). There are 40–50 receptors per ocellus, lying in a single plane. Six ocelli share a single turret on each side of the head. (After JOCKUSCH, 1967). Right: sawfly larva, *Perga* sp. (Hymenoptera). There is only one ocellus on each side, and the image is fully exploited. Below: outline of rhabdoms in transverse section. (After MEYER-ROCHOW, 1974). Scales 100 μm on all ocelli, 10 μm on *Perga* rhabdoms

β) Ocelli of Insects. The larval ocelli of holometabolous insects present a spectrum from those that can be said to resemble a single ommatidium of a compound eye, and image only a small region of space with little or no resolution within this (*Isia*, Fig. 29), to others with extended retinae covering and resolving a wide field of view (*Perga*, Fig. 29).

Ocelli of the first type are typical of the larvae of Lepidoptera, Neuroptera, and Trichoptera. DETHIER (1942, 1943, 1963) made a particular study of the ocelli (or stemmata) of the caterpillar *Isia isabella*. There are six on each side of the head, some having a single lens, and the others having lenses divided radially into three segments, forming more or less separate images. Beneath the large ($\simeq 100$ μm diameter) corneal lens there is a second lens or crystalline body, and the combined action of the two lenses is to produce a focussed image close to the rear surface of the second lens. Most of the refraction occurs at the air-cornea surface. The receptors are arranged in two layers, three contributing to a distal rhabdom, and immediately beneath this another four producing the proximal rhabdom. The distal rhabdom forms a V-shaped cup around the base of the second lens, with the focal plane about halfway down the cup. The proximal rhabdom is completely fused and lies wholly behind the focal plane. It seems almost certain that there is no separate detection of different parts of the optical image and that the rhabdom is measuring the average light intensity over an angle which is quite wide, but which according to DETHIER does not overlap with the fields of view of adjacent stemmata. The whole group of 12 ocelli can probably be thought of as functioning as a compound eye with a very coarse 12-point mosaic. DETHIER suggests that the side-to-side swaying movements of caterpillars during locomotion compensate for the small number of sampling stations by allowing the ocelli to scan the intervening gaps. Behaviourally, however, little is known of their function other than that caterpillars are able to orient to light-dark boundaries, but they do not show any ability to detect small movements. The single advantage of stemmata appears to be their light-gathering power: DETHIER estimated an *F-number* of 0.5 for the largest ocellus in *Isia*, which is close to the minimum possible.

In complete contrast, the larvae of saw-flies (Hymenoptera) have a single pair of properly eye-like ocelli, each with a field of view approaching 180° and having a retina populated by clusters of receptors contributing to fused rhabdoms spaced at roughly 4°–6° intervals (MEYER-ROCHOW, 1974). Each such rhabdom is very like that of fused-rhabdom compound eyes; it is composed of eight rhabdomeres, has a total diameter of 12–15 µm, and the centre of one rhabdom is situated roughly 20 µm from the centre of its neighbour (Fig. 29, insert). Both the aperture and focal length in *Perga* are about 200 µm, and MEYER-ROCHOW found by ray tracing that the image produced by the corneal lens lies on or very close to the distal tips of the receptors. Presumably, each rhabdom traps much of the incident light by internal reflection preserving the "image" down its length; in any case each is isolated from its neighbours by screening pigment. MEYER-ROCHOW's study includes much interesting natural history of these animals' vision. They are vegetarian, and the eyes serve to guide them to new host trees (they will even mistake humans for trees and follow them). They also mediate a defense response in which the larva turns towards a close moving object, which can subtend an angle as small as 4°, and spits regurgitated sap. This value of 4° corresponds closely to the smallest acceptance angles measured electrophysiologically, as well as to the receptor subtense. It is quite clear that the resolution the eyes are capable of providing is fully utilized in the behaviour of the animal.

The larvae of certain beetles are rather similar to those of saw-flies. In the larvae of the tiger beetle, *Cicindela*, described by FRIEDERICHS (1931), the largest pair of the six functional ocelli contain more than 6,300 receptor cells each and are concerned in the detection of moving prey. These larvae live in burrows with their heads at the surface and shoot out their mandibles at any moving insect. Having caught it they then drop with it to the bottom of the burrow. "Ant lions," the larvae of certain Neuroptera, have a similar life-style, trapping insects that slip into a steep-sided pit, and they have ocelli intermediate between the lepidopteran and saw-fly type (JOCKUSCH, 1967 and Fig. 29). Again, there are six on each side, borne on a small turret behind the antennae, and each has a retina with 40–50 receptors. The resolution will be quite poor, since the inter-receptor angles are between 5° and 10°, but this would be adequate to detect a moving ant at a distance of about 1 cm.

The dorsal ocelli of adult insects are quite like the saw-fly ocelli in general construction, having a corneal lens up to 0.5 mm across and a cup-shaped retina made up of composite rhabdoms. They occur in most winged insects, almost always as a single group of three on the top of the head. The oddest aspect of their function is that there is almost universal agreement that they are out of focus, with the image falling some distance behind the receptor layer (see GOODMAN, 1970). In the blowfly *Calliphora*, for example, the image is 0.12 mm behind the lens, but the receptors

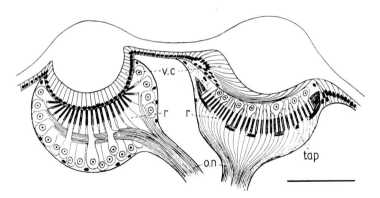

Fig. 30. The two types of eyes of spiders. Principal eye *(Hauptauge)*, left, and secondary eye *(Nebenauge)* of the house spider *Tegenaria domestica*. There is only one pair of principal eyes but two or three pairs of secondary eyes. In the principal eyes the receptor rhabdomeres (dark lines) lie distal to the cell body, but proximal to it in the secondary eyes. Tapeta are more common in the secondary eyes. Scale bar $\sim$ 100 μm. *o.n*: optic nerve; *r*: receptor cells; *tap*: tapetum (see Fig. 35); *v.c*: vitreous cells. (Redrawn by HESSE, 1935 from two figures of WIDMANN, 1908)

lie between 0.04 and 0.10 mm from the lens. A second argument against image transmission is the great convergence of the receptors onto second-order fibres; typically, 500–1,000 receptors make inhibitory synapses with only 25–30 neurons. Behavioural attempts to pin down the role of the ocelli in insect vision have been largely negative (GOODMAN, 1975), although recently WELLINGTON (1974) found that in bumblebees ocelli appear to mediate orientation to the pattern of sky polarization at low light intensities, and GOULD (1975) showed that in hive bees the ocelli extended the lower end of the range of intensities over which the bees could orient their dances to a light source by a factor of nearly 10 . These are perhaps the sorts of functions one would expect for upward-pointing wide-angle eyes with a high light-gathering capability (*F-numbers* in the range 1–2) but poor resolution (WILSON, 1978). However, more information is desirable, particularly because the anatomy of the ocellar nervous system is now becoming known in detail (GOODMAN, 1974).

γ) Eyes of Spiders. In spiders and their terrestrial relatives (phalangids and scorpions) the eyes are all of the simple corneal type. True spiders usually have eight eyes (sometimes six) and these are of two kinds: the principal eyes which point forwards and the secondary eyes which cover more peripheral fields of view (Figs. 30, 31 a, 32). The receptor arrangement in spiders differs from insect ocelli in that the receptors are not grouped into clusters that contribute to a single rhabdom, but are separate from each other and presumably functionally independent. In the principal eyes the outer segments lie distal to the cell body and the axon, as in cephalopods and most other invertebrates. However, in the secondary eyes it is usually the cell body that is distal, with the microvillous segment forming what is morphologically the first part of the axon, but the exact topology of the cells varies widely (Fig. 30; see also GRENACHER, 1879; WIDMANN, 1908, and HOMANN, 1971; an account of phalangid eyes is given by CURTIS, 1970).

The largest eyes are found in spiders which hunt their prey by sight rather than using webs as traps, in particular, wolf spiders (Lycosidae) and jumping spiders (Salticidae). In wolf spiders four of the secondary eyes are much larger than the rest, with corneal diameters of up to 400 μm in *Arctosa variana*. The focal length is similar to the eye diameter (*F-number* ≃ 1), and the rhabdomeric segments of the receptors are short (18–21 μm) but quite wide (4–6 μm) (BACCETTI and BEDINI, 1964). Each receptor is separated from the next by a narrow region of black pigment so that each is optically isolated from its neighbour, and the centre-to-centre separation is 8–10 μm, giving an inter-receptor angle of 1°–2°. Lycosids typically hunt at twilight, pouncing on their prey in a single, very rapid combined jump and turn. Only the four posterior eyes have fields of view large enough to initiate this pounce, which can be directed anywhere around the animal, and so these eyes are first and foremost movement detectors for detecting prey and probably predators as well. Besides having a wide aperture which would help vision at low intensities, the eyes also possess a reflecting tapetum which would have the function of doubling the effective length of the receptors (see Sect. C.II.5). It consists of many layers of very thin crystals (probably guanine) which form a long ribbon beneath the receptors (Fig. 35). Because the receptor axons continue down through the tapetal layer they have to be displaced laterally, so that the rhabdomeric portion "sits" on a tapetal strip as though it were a chair. HOMANN (1971) has produced photographs of the tapetum and receptors in lycosid and other spider species using an ophthalmoscopic technique. The principal eyes in lycosids are relatively small, with a much thinner tapetum, and although they are concerned with orientation to the pattern of polarized light in the sky (MAGNI et al., 1965), they are probably not involved in prey capture.

Salticids have basically similar eyes to lycosids, but they are mainly diurnal hunters and the eyes lack a tapetum. The way they catch prey is different too; instead of a single pounce they turn towards moving objects using the secondary eyes, and then stalk them using the principal eyes (HOMANN, 1928; DREES, 1952). DREES found that the principal eyes were also responsible for distinguishing between prey and potential mates and that this judgement was made on the basis of the geometry of the leg pattern of the target animal. Not surprisingly, in view of the need for fine discrimination, it is the principal eyes that are largest in salticids, with a corneal diameter of 580 μm and a focal length of 767 μm in one of the larger species, *Phidippus johnsoni* (LAND, 1969 a). By contrast, the posterolateral (secondary) eyes, which detect movement over a field of 135°, have a corneal diameter of 300 μm and a focal length of 254 μm. In addition, the receptors are narrower in the principal eyes, the smallest separation being 2.0 μm in the principal and 4.5 μm in the posterolateral eyes, corresponding to angular separations of 9′ and 1°, respectively. The principal eyes are specialized in two other ways. First, they each have a very narrow field of view (about 5° horizontally by 20° vertically), but this is offset by the fact that they "scan" targets, with a complex pattern of eye movements involving lateral, vertical, and rotational movements of the retinae (Fig. 32). Unlike vertebrate eyes, the lens itself remains still (LAND, 1969 b). Second, the retina is arranged in four layers, one behind the other (LAND, 1969 a; EAKIN and BRANDENBURGER, 1971). This is probably to compensate for the longitudinal chromatic aberration of the lens by arranging for receptors with different pigments to

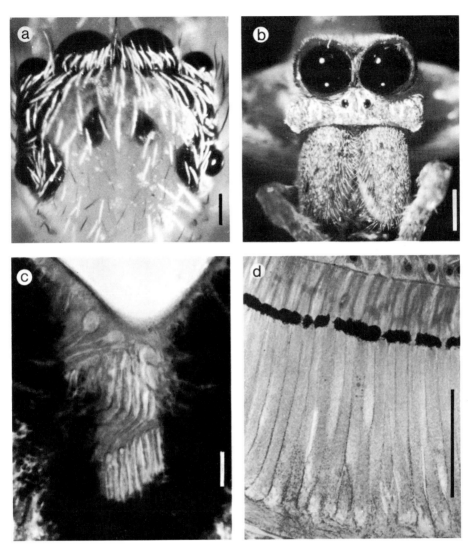

Fig. 31 a–d. Eyes of spiders, specialized for high resolution (**a, c**) and high sensitivity (**b, d**). **a** Prosoma of a juvenile jumping spider *(Metaphidippus harfordi)* from above, showing the three main pairs of eyes. The anteromedian (principal) eyes are largest and facing forwards. To the side of them are the anterolateral eyes, and behind these the posterolaterals. The posteromedian eyes are vestigial in this group. The rear surfaces of the principal eyes are visible near the midline in front of the posterolateral eyes. Note the differences in eye length. Scale bar 100 μm. **b** *Dinopis subrufus*, a nocturnal hunter, from in front. Here the largest eyes are the postero-medians (1.4 mm diameter); the principal eyes are the small dots below them. Scale bar 1 mm. **c** Longitudinal section through the retina of the right principal eye of a jumping spider *(M. aeneolus)* showing the multiple layering of the receptors. Scale bar 10 μm. **d** Massive receptor cells in *Dinopis*. The rhabdomeric region lies above the pigment layer. The cells are shown in the light-adapted state; in the dark the receptive parts double in length and fill with microvilli. Scale bar 100 μm. (**d** courtesy of Dr. A. D. BLEST)

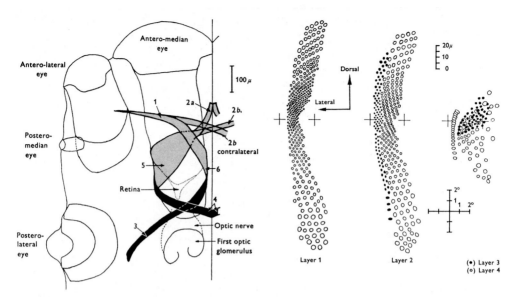

Fig. 32. Left: the six muscles that move the eyes in jumping spiders. Muscles below the eye are shown in lighter stipple. The retina can be moved laterally, or vertically, or can rotate around the long axis of the eye. (LAND, 1969 b; see also Fig. 31 a). Right: the arrangement of receptors in the four layers of the retina of a jumping spider *(Metaphidippus aeneolus)* as seen from the direction of incident light. *Layer 1* is the deepest (see Fig. 31 c). The closest receptor spacing is about 10 min of arc. (LAND, 1969 a)

be located in planes appropriate for their respective wavelengths of maximal sensitivity (Figs. 31 c, 32).

Of all the eyes considered in this section, the principal eyes of salticids are probably the only ones in which the full optical resolving power of the corneal lens is exploited. In all the others, including salticid secondary eyes, the fused rhabdoms have diameters that are considerably larger than the limit of about 2 μm below which optical cross-talk would begin to make them inefficient (Sect. B.III.2), and in no case is either diffraction or spherical aberration likely to be the limiting factor. However, in salticid principal eyes the retinal packing is probably denser than in any other eye (2-μm receptors with no space between them), and it is likely that a higher density would not improve the physiological resolution. Diffraction optics suggests that the image might contain more information than 2-μm receptors could fully utilize; Eqs. (19) and (20) imply that the receptor diameter could be as small as 0.5 μm, but so narrow a receptor would certainly be unusuably "leaky." In any case, spherical aberration cannot be ignored, and LAND (1969 a) has estimated that the blur caused by this defect seriously impairs the quality of images whose spatial periods are smaller than about two receptor diameters. It seems that, as in the human eye, image quality and receptor size are matched and optimal. Finally, it is worth noting that by confining high resolution to one pair of narrow, long focal length eyes, whilst using the secondary eyes for peripheral vision which requires less resolution and hence much smaller eyes, jumping spiders have saved a great deal of space. If the same eye performed both tasks (as in vertebrates), its volume would be at least ten times greater (LAND, 1972 a).

The largest eyes of any spider, and probably the largest simple eyes of any land invertebrate, are found in the genus *Dinopis* (Fig. 31 b). They are nocturnal hunters that ambush insects passing beneath them by pinning them to the substrate with a net of sticky silk; the trigger for this action is visually detected movement. The largest eyes are the posteromedians, not the principal eyes as in salticids (Fig. 31), and these have corneal diameters of up to 1.4 mm (BLEST and LAND, 1977). The focal length of such a lens is about 0.8 mm, and the *F-number* typically about 0.58, which is remarkable for an eye this big. The severe spherical aberration of an eye of this size and aperture is counteracted in part by the lens's having a double structure – a low index outer layer surrounding a more dense core – and, in addition, the core itself seems to have a graded refractive index, as in a fish-type lens (Sect. C.II.3). The receptors are very large, too, with receptive segments 20 μm wide and 55 μm long, lengthening in the dark to twice this (Fig. 31 d). The other remarkable feature of the receptors is that during the day the microvilli are almost completely resorbed into the proximal part of the cell and reconstituted to fill the rhabdomeres each night (BLEST, 1978). Similar large-scale diurnal changes in the amount of photoreceptor membrane have also been found in *Limulus* (BEHRENS and KREBS, 1976) and in crabs (NÄSSEL and WATERMAN, 1979). The net effect of these various heroic adaptations is that the sensitivity of these eyes is enormous. Compared with a salticid like *Phidippus*, the number of photons absorbed per receptor, for a given field luminance (Eq. 15), is roughly 2,000 times greater, although with an inter-receptor angle of about 1.5°, the resolution is about ten times coarser. It is interesting that this sensitivity difference is approximately the same as that between a diurnal insect with an apposition compound eye (e.g. a bee) and a nocturnal moth with an optical superposition eye (KIRSCHFELD, 1974).

5. Simple Eyes Containing Reflectors

One possible improvement in eyes of the simple pigment cup type would be the addition of a reflecting surface between the pigment and the receptors. The effect of this would be to increase the light flux through the receptors by a factor of up to 2. There would be no improvement in resolution.

Small eyes with reflectors are found in several groups. FAHRENBACH (1964) showed that each of the three median ocelli of the copepod *Macrocyclops albidus* (a crustacean) was backed by a reflector, and the median (nauplius) eyes of other copepods have a similar morphology (VAISSIÈRE, 1961). The cockle *Cardium edule*, a bivalve mollusc, has about 100 eyes borne on tentacles around the two siphons, and each of these consists of a cup of reflecting material surrounding a cluster of 12–20 receptors (BARBER and WRIGHT, 1969 b). The eye of a rotifer, *Asplanchna brightwelli*, is enclosed by a structure that *ought* to be a reflector from its morphology (EAKIN and WESTFALL, 1965 b; EAKIN, 1972), but its optical properties have not been examined. All the eyes mentioned so far are very small; the rotifer, for example, has only one receptor, and the whole eye is only 10 μm across.

Reflectors do occur, however, in much larger eyes with good image-forming powers, and there they can serve one of two functions. They can act as tapeta behind the retina, whose function is to return light back through the photoreceptor layer, providing a second opportunity for the retina to absorb photons not trapped on their first passage. This is the situation in cats' eyes and the secondary eyes of lycosid spiders. Alternatively, they serve in a very few instances as optical concave mirrors, actually forming the image on the retina (Fig. 37). The best known example of this unusual optical arrangement is in the eyes of scallops, bivalve molluscs of the genus *Pecten* and its close relatives (LAND, 1965). The way this optical system operates will be considered in detail in Sect. c. Before examining how mirrors of this kind are used, however, some consideration should be given to the problem of how biological materials can be used to produce a specular surface with a high reflectance.

a) Principle of Multilayer Reflexion

Surfaces made of metal do not occur in animals, and so mirrors must be produced in some other way. The commercial alternative to polished metal is a series of alternating high and low refractive index films, each of which has an optical thickness of a quarter-wavelength or a multiple of that. The principle is very much the same as that of reflexion from a thin oil film; light reflected at the upper surface interferes constructively with that reflected from the lower surface, if the optical thickness (actual thickness × refractive index) of the film produces a retardation of the light reflected from the lower surface of half the wavelength of the incident light. This is because light reflected at the top surface undergoes a half-wavelength phase change (this happens at low-to-high, but not high-to-low refractive index interfaces), and so constructive interference happens when the total optical path length in the film of light reflected from the lower interface is also half a wavelength (Fig. 33). Highly reflecting surfaces can be built up simply by stacking films of the appropriate thickness one above the other, so that light reflected at every interface emerges in phase, and the simplest way of achieving this is to alternate quarter-wavelength films of different refractive indices.

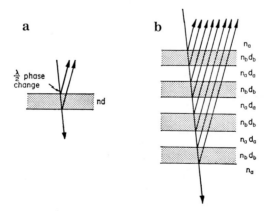

Fig. 33a, b. The principle of multilayer reflection. **a** Light reflected from both interfaces will interfere constructively if the optical thickness of the film (refractive index n × actual thickness d) is $^1/_4\,\lambda$, i.e. about 125 nm. **b** A high reflectance is produced when a stack is built up of alternating high and low refractive index layers $(n_a d_a = n_b d_b = {}^1/_4\,\lambda)$

Mirrors are made this way industrially by alternating vapour-deposited films of ZnS ($n = 2.4$) with MgF$_2$ ($n = 1.36$). Although the reflectance of a single interface is only a few percent, the reflectance of a stack increases very rapidly, approximately as the power of the number of interfaces. For a single interface the reflectance R (the ratio of reflected to incident light energy) is given by Fresnel's equation:

$$R = \left(\frac{n_b - n_a}{n_b + n_a}\right)^2 , \qquad (33)$$

where n_a and n_b are the refractive indices of the low and high index films. However, for a stack, R is given by:

$$R = \left(\frac{n_b^k - n_a^k}{n_b^k + n_a^k}\right)^2 , \qquad (34)$$

where k is the number of interfaces in the stack. This equation is only appropriate when all the films in the stack are a quarter-wavelength thick. When one inserts appropriate values for n_a and n_b, it becomes apparent that reflectances of greater than 90%, comparable with polished metal, can be achieved using biological materials (guanine, chitin) with only 10–20 interfaces, or 5–10 separate films (see LAND, 1972 b). In addition to being highly reflecting, multiple thin film surfaces of this kind are coloured because there is only a narrow range of wavelengths over which constructive interference occurs; such surfaces will appear black (due to destructive interference) if the incident wavelength is halved (Fig. 34). An account of the physical optics of these structures is given by HUXLEY (1968) and by LAND (1972 b).

Virtually all the reflectors found in animals are of this kind. They occur not only in eyes, but in other iridescent structures, such as the wings of some butterflies and moths (see FOX, 1953), and the reflecting external surfaces of fish and other marine animals (DENTON, 1970). In nearly all cases the structure consists of a series of alternating layers of different materials, each layer having a thickness of about 0.1 μm (if $n = 1.33$, for example, the wavelength best reflected will be 4 nt, or 532 nm, in the green part of the spectrum). The materials concerned vary considerably; in scallop eyes and fish scales they consist of guanine ($n \sim 1.83$) and cytoplasm ($n \sim 1.34$), and in insect structures they are commonly chitin ($n \sim 1.56$) and air, although in some cases like the coloured bands across the eyes of horseflies (Tabanidae) the layers are made of chitin of different densities (BERNARD and MILLER, 1968). In these flies and also in long-legged flies (Dolichopodidae), the function of the reflecting layers may not be reflexion as such, but to act as a selective transmission filter (wavelengths not reflected by multilayer structures are transmitted) modifying the spectral sensitivity of the underlying receptors (BERNARD, 1971).

b) Tapeta

The function of a tapetum is to increase the amount of light absorbed by retinal receptors, without increasing receptor length. Those of spiders have already been mentioned (Sect. C.II.4.b.γ). Ultrastructurally, they are very similar to the scallop

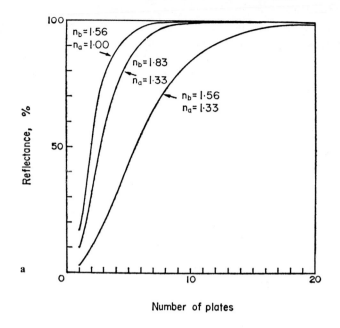

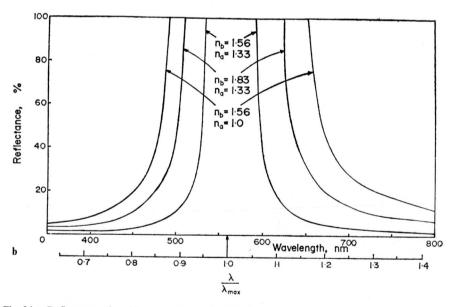

Fig. 34 a. Reflectance of multilayer stacks made of different materials. $n_a = 1.00$, $n_b = 1.56$: air and chitin; 1.83 and 1.33: guanine and water; 1.56 and 1.33: chitin (or protein) and water. The abscissa is the number of high refractive index layers in the stack. Reflectances given are for the wavelength of maximum reflectance. **b** Spectral distribution of reflectance in quarter-wavelength structures with a large number of layers (in practice, more than about 10). Refractive index combinations as in a. (Both figures from Land, 1972b)

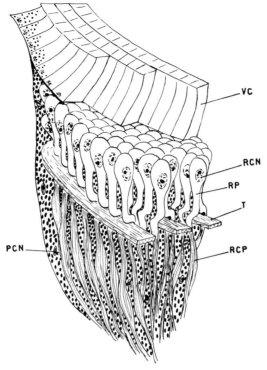

Fig. 35. Layout of the reflecting tapetum in a secondary eye of a wolf spider (Lycosidae). The tapetum is a long reflecting strip (guanine-cytoplasm multilayer) lying beneath the rhabdomeric part of the receptor cells. *VC*: vitreous cells; *RCN*: receptor cell nuclei; *RP*: rhabdomere-containing part of receptor cells; *PCN*: pigment cell nuclei; *RCP*: receptor cell prolongations (axons); *T*: tapetum. See also Fig. 30. (BACCETTI and BEDINI, 1964)

reflector or to iridescent fish scales, and contain a stack of thin flat crystals which are lost in preparation for electron microscopy, leaving clear "holes" separated by films of cytoplasm (BACCETTI and BEDINI, 1964). The dimensions of both crystals and spaces are compatible with quarter-wavelength reflexion. Because tapeta reflect light back more or less along its original path (Fig. 35), eyes containing them appear very bright when viewed from the direction of the illuminating source, but not other directions. This phenomenon is just as impressive in lycosid spiders as in cats, and the green reflexion from the tapeta makes them easily visible by light from a flashlight.

It is interesting that tapeta have not been reported in cephalopod molluscs, whose eyes resemble in so many other ways the eyes of fish, where tapeta are common (DENTON and NICOL, 1964). One would expect that the advantage of a tapetum to a deep-sea squid would be the same as for a fish, and the absence is the more striking because squid do have multilayer reflecting surface elsewhere, around the outside of the eye and around the ink sac (DENTON and LAND, 1971). It may be that in an eye with a non-inverted retina like a squid's, it is simply very difficult to lay out a flat tapetum – the problem has been solved in lycosid spiders, but it is clearly not easy (Fig. 35) – whereas the inverted retina of vertebrates does not present this problem.

Tapeta are also found in compound eyes. They lie behind each rhabdom in some butterflies and around it in moths. Miller and Bernard (1968) examined the tapeta of the butterfly *Anartia* and found that immediately beneath each rhabdom there was a highly modified tracheole, in which the taenidial ridges, whose usual function is to strengthen the walls of the tracheole, are extended to form a stack of about 40 plates, each 123 nm thick and separated from the next by an air gap of 88 nm. These dimensions are compatible with the observed bluish glow which is visible in a few of the eye's facets when viewed from the direction of illumination. In moths, which have superposition eyes, this eye shine is visible over a much larger region of the eye.

c) Image-Forming Reflectors

The eyes of scallops are the only eyes in which a well-resolved image is formed by reflexion (Fig. 15 G). In *Pecten maximus* there are about 60 eyes, each about 1 mm in diameter, distributed round the edges of the mantle (Fig. 36). Their most striking feature is the brilliant blue-green iridescence of the pupil which is caused by light reflected from the "argentea" lining the back of the eye. This mirror is composed of up to 30 layers of thin, square-faced crystals of guanine (1.1–1.3 μm square, by 80 nm thick) interspersed with cytoplasmic spaces 100 nm thick (Land, 1966a). The argentea is an accurately spherical surface, with a radius of curvature of about 410 μm. As early as 1886, Patten had noticed that it was possible to see an inverted image of the surroundings when the pupil of the eye was examined with a microscope, but he mistakenly believed that the image was actually formed by the lens and that the argentea reflected light back through the retina much as in the eye of a cat or wolf spider. However, in 1965, Land showed that the lens had a focal length which was at least twice as great as the entire depth of the eye, meaning that the image observed by Patten could only have been formed by reflexion at the spherical argentea. In fact, the lens/mirror combination has a focal length of about 270 μm, and the image lies 140 μm in front of the argentea. This places it on the more distal of the two retinal layers. Hartline (1938) had shown that receptors in this layer responded to the offset of light, whereas receptors in the proximal retina – which is adjacent to the argentea and does not receive a focussed image – responded to the onset. Land (1966b) confirmed that the distal cells would respond to movement of the image of a grating which produced no overall dimming, indicating that the function of the optical system was to permit responses to be made to moving objects which did not cast direct shadows. Buddenbrock and Moller-Racke (1953) had already shown that scallops would close their shells in response to very small movements in the environment. The smallest object capable of generating a response in the distal optic nerve must subtend an angle of about 2°, which corresponds closely to the angle subtended by one distal receptor ($\simeq 9$ μm diameter) at the nodal point.

The principal advantage of an eye of this type over one in which the lens forms the image is its compactness and large relative aperture. For the scallop A/f is about 1.7, compared with 0.8 for an eye with a Matthiessen's ratio lens, and the increase

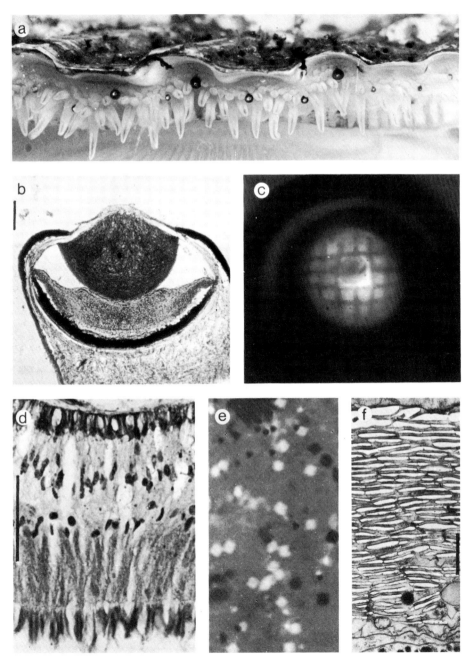

Fig. 36 a–f. Image-forming reflector in the scallop eye *(Pecten maximus)*. **a** View of the open shell, showing eyes and tentacles around the mantle. **b** Median frozen section through an eye. The eye cavity is almost completely filled by the lens and retina. The reflecting argentea lines the hemispherical inner surface of the pigmented back of the eye. Scale 100 µm. **c** Image of a grating, photographed in the pupil of an intact eye. The image lies close to the rear surface of the lens. **d** Silver-stained radial section through the retina. The distal receptors (top) have ciliary receptive regions, give "off" responses, and lie in the focal plane. The proximal cells have microvillous endings, give "on" responses, and are in contact with the reflector. Scale 50 µm. **e** Interference micrograph of isolated crystals from the reflector. Each crystal is about 1.2 µm square and 80 nm thick. **f** Electron micrograph of a section through the reflector. The spaces are the gaps left by crystals that have been dissolved or dislodged during preparation. Scale 1 µm. (**b** and **c** from LAND, 1965; **e** and **f** from LAND, 1966 b)

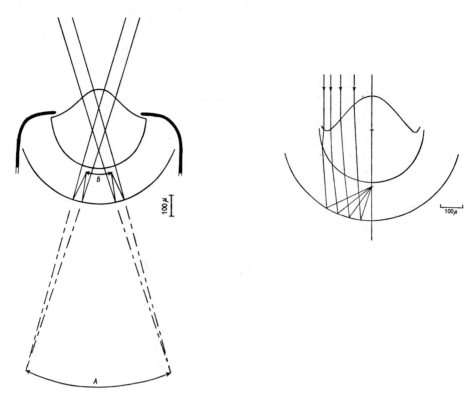

Fig. 37. Left: diagram of the optical system of the scallop eye. The lens on its own forms an image at *A*, but the final reflected image (Fig. 36c) lies at *B*. Right: construction of a lens profile that corrects for the axial spherical aberration of the reflector. The similarity between this and that of real lenses (Fig. 36b) suggests that this is the function of the lens. (Both from LAND, 1965)

in retinal illuminance is a factor of 4.5. Set against this there are two drawbacks. First a spherical reflector, like a homogeneous spherical lens, suffers from severe spherical aberration at large apertures. This is correctable, at least for axial points, by the use of a lens with a suitable profile (a "Cartesian oval," see Sect. B.III.6.a), and ray tracing indicates that the lens in *Pecten* eyes does have the right shape for reducing or even eliminating this defect (Fig. 37). The fact that this correction is only possible for points near the optic axis is possibly the reason why scallops have so many eyes; although each one has a field of view of about 90°, it is likely that resolution as good as the retinal mosaic is limited to the central 10° or so in each eye. The second drawback is perhaps the more serious, and that is that the image contrast is inevitably low. Before focussed light reaches the receptors it has already passed through the retina once as an unfocussed beam, so that unless the receptors are shielded in some way, the image contrast will be "diluted" by the unfocussed beam and will only be half that of an equivalent lens system.

The only other large eyes with optics at all similar to the scallop's are the median eyes of the giant deep-sea ostracods (Crustacea) of the genus *Gigantocypris* (Fig. 38). These animals live at depths where almost no daylight penetrates (700 m

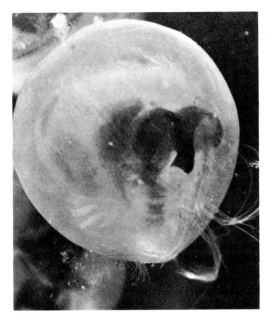 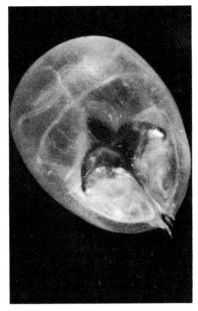

Fig. 38. Two views of the deep-sea Ostracod *Gigantocypris mülleri*. The animal has a diameter of about 1 cm. The paired reflectors are spherical when seen from the side, but parabolic from above (right). (Photographs by Dr. M. R. LONGBOTTOM)

and below), and the only function of their eyes would be to detect other luminous animals – prey, predators or possibly potential mates. The structure of the eyes has been described by LÜDERS (1909), and it is clear from his description that the only optical structures are the two large membranous reflectors, each about 3 mm across. HARDY (1956), who made a watercolour sketch of the animal, comments:

> The paired eyes have huge metallic-looking reflectors behind them, making them appear like the headlamps of a large car; they look out through glass-like windows in the otherwise orange carapace and no doubt these concave mirrors behind serve instead of a lens in front.

Here, however, the resemblance with scallop eyes ends. I had a recent opportunity to examine some live specimens of *G. mülleri*, and the following observations show that the formation of the image and its detection by the retina are quite unlike the simple situation in scallop eyes. In the first place, the reflector has a more complex shape: It is parabolic when viewed from above but from the side it has a spherical profile (Fig. 38). This means that there is no single focal point for a parallel beam of light, but rather an astigmatic line focus extending from the focal point of the parabolic profile (about 350 μm in front of the reflector) to the focus of the spherical profile (about 670 μm from the reflector) (LAND, 1978). Second, the retina is not so much a layer as a sausage-shaped structure, lying vertically down the centre of each eye, with its rear surface in contact with the reflector. The receptors are very large, about 25 μm in diameter by 700 μm long, with their long axes at right angles to the reflector. The geometry of the reflector dictates that most of the light reaching the receptors will enter them at right angles and, furthermore, light will pass through many receptors before reaching the one that corresponds to the geometrical image of the source. For this reason alone the quality of the *received* image is bound to be very poor indeed. The great virtue of these eyes must be their enormous light-gathering power; with an average focal length of about 0.5 mm and an aperture of at least 2 mm, the relative aperture (A/f) is about 4 (*F-number* 0.25!) and the retinal illuminance is 25 times that of an eye with a fish-type lens.

Both *Pecten* and *Gigantocypris* live in environments where the ambient light level is low, and it seems that the remarkable optical mechanisms they have evolved are solutions to the problem of securing an adequate light flux through the receptors. Mirrors are an intrinsically poor way of obtaining good resolution at higher light levels, because they provide low contrast images, and this is probably why reflecting eyes appear to be an evolutionary cul-de-sac.

There is another kind of optical system, this time in a compound eye, that is also based on multilayer reflexion (Fig. 15 H). This, however, will be considered in a later section (C.III.4.e).

III. Compound Eyes

In compound eyes, the image is formed not by a single lens system but by a large number of smaller optical systems. The characteristic form of these eyes, a nearly spherical array of minute facets overlying a layer of receptors, disguises the fact that the optical mechanisms involved are highly diverse; for example, the eyes of a butterfly and a crayfish look superficially similar, but whereas the first uses lenses to produce a large number of individual images, the latter uses mirrors to produce a single image.

Studies of the comparative optics of compound eyes had been in a state of near dormancy for about 70 years, from the time of the publication of SIGMUND EXNER'S famous treatise (1891) until the early 1960's when the subject revived, and since then many of the classical ideas have come to be challenged and revised. There have been many symposia and reviews devoted to the subject recently of which the following are only a selection: AUTRUM (1975); BERNHARD (1966); GOLDSMITH and BERNARD (1974); HORRIDGE (1975, 1978); MAZOKHIN-PORSHNYAKOV (1969); and KUNZE (1979) in this handbook (Vol. VII/6 A). The purpose of the present section is to outline and explore something of the diversity of compound eye types, to compare their optical performances (especially sensitivity and resolution) and to examine the similarities and differences between compound and simple eyes.

1. Basic Types

In the commonest (apposition) type of compound eye (Fig. 15 E), each lens or facet forms an image of a small region of the environment onto a single rhabdom, a structure composed of the receptive portions (rhabdomeres) of a small number of sense cells, typically about eight. There is general agreement that within the rhabdom of an apposition eye, light is free to pass from one rhabdomere to another, so that all the rhabdomeres contributing to the rhabdom share a common field

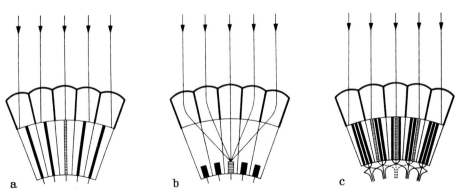

Fig. 39 a–c. Three basic types of compound eye. **a** Apposition eye in which single rhabdoms receive light from a small field through only one facet. **b** Superposition eye where light from many facets combines to form an erect image on a deep rhabdom layer. **c** Neural superposition eye, typical of dipteran flies, in which light from one direction stimulates different receptors in adjacent ommatidia. The axons of receptors that image the same point in space cross between ommatidia and synapse with the same second-order fibres in the lamina. (KIRSCHFELD, 1967)

of view, though not necessarily the same spectral or polarization sensitivities. The visual world of an animal with such an eye can thus be thought of as a mosaic of small solid angles, each monitored by one ommatidium (a rhabdom and its associated optics) with no further angular discrimination within ommatidia (Fig. 39). This is essentially the mosaic theory of insect vision proposed by MÜLLER (1826). The use of the term mosaic gives a slightly misleading impression, however, because the fields of view of adjacent ommatidia do overlap slightly, just as do those of adjacent receptors in the human eye – indeed, diffraction and optical imperfections make this inevitable. The literal implication of "mosaic," a world of small discrete patches, is neither more nor less true of a compound eye than a simple one.

A variation of the apposition eye occurs in dipteran flies (KIRSCHFELD, 1969 b; ZEIL, 1979) and some other insect groups, notably the Hemiptera (IOANNIDES and HORRIDGE, 1975). Here the rhabdomeres in each ommatidium are not fused together, but are physically and optically separate so that each samples a different part of the image produced by the corneal facet (Fig. 39 c). Thus, these eyes disobey the mosaic theory in that each facet does produce a resolved image, and the resolution provided in the image *is* exploited. This much was known at the turn of the century (VIGIER, 1907; DIETRICH, 1909). Only recently, however, was the full optical significance of this arrangement finally established (KIRSCHFELD, 1967). In brachyceran flies there are eight rhabdomeres in each ommatidium; two are narrow (typically ~ 1 μm diameter) and stacked one above the other, and the remaining six are wider (~ 1.5 μm) and arranged around the central pair in a characteristic pattern (Figs. 40 and 50 e). It turns out that each of the six larger rhabdomeres has a field of view that is the same as the central rhabdomere of an adjacent facet, so that optically each part of the visual field is sampled by seven detectors (counting the central pair as one). The reason for this apparent redundancy becomes clear when the connections of the receptors to the second-order neurons are mapped. All the receptors that image the same visual field send axons to the same laminar "cartridge," even though they originate in different ommatidia, so that at the level of

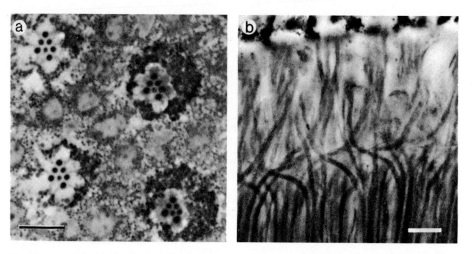

Fig. 40 a, b. The dipteran retina. **a** Characteristic arrangement of rhabdomeres in four ommatidia from the eye of the blowfly *Calliphora*. Light micrograph of a section taken very close to the distal tips of the receptors. Scale 10 μm. (See also Fig. 47 e) **b** Part of the crossover pattern of receptor axons between retina and lamina, responsible for channelling signals from all receptors imaging a single object point into a single lamina cartridge. Silver stain. Scale 10 μm

the lamina each cartridge "looks at" one region of space. The advantage of this system, which inevitably involves a complicated wiring pattern between the receptors and the lamina (Fig. 40), appears to be that signals from six receptors can be pooled in the lamina (the central pair pass straight through to the medulla), thereby improving the photon catch and hence the signal-to-noise ratio, without sacrificing optical resolution. Kirschfeld has coined the term "neural superposition" for eyes of this kind.

The third type of compound eye (optical superposition) is typical of nocturnal insects, especially moths and beetles. Here the rhabdom layer lies relatively deep, with a zone of clear material between it and the corneal facets (Figs. 39 and 55). Exner first showed that light from a distant point entering a large number of facets is bent in such a way that all rays arrive at or near a single point in the receptor layer. Thus, from an optical point of view the eye behaves rather like a simple eye, but with the facet array acting as the lens. The principal difference is that in these eyes the image is erect. The formation of a superposition image requires unconventional optics, either lenses with a graded refractive index in insects (Fig. 15 F) or a square array of radially arranged mirrors in decapod crustacea (Fig. 15 H). The properties of such systems will be considered in a later section. The important feature of these eyes, however constructed, is that they have a very large effective pupil, since many facets contribute light to the image of each region of space, and consequently the retinal illuminance is much greater than in apposition eyes. The receptors tend to be wide as well in these eyes (~ 8 μm in the moth *Ephestia*), and Kirschfeld (1974) has estimated that the number of photons reaching a rhabdom in a moth is greater by a factor of about 10^3 compared with an apposition eye like that of a bee, when both are looking at the same extended source.

It would be wrong to suppose that compound eyes divide neatly into these three classes. In particular the extent to which all eyes with "clear zones" between the lenses and receptors function as superposition eyes in EXNER's sense has been the subject of much controversy over the last 20 years (see HORRIDGE, 1975). There appears to be a spectrum of types from pure apposition to pure superposition, including some species with two populations of rhabdoms, one near the lenses and another much deeper, suggesting a dual mechanism in a single eye. In other types there may be movements of both rhabdoms and screening pigment, effectively converting an eye of one type into the other, depending on ambient light intensity (see KUNZE, this Handbook Vol. VII/6 A, Chap. 8).

2. Evolution

Compound eyes have evolved independently in three invertebrate phyla; the annelids, molluscs, and arthropods. In the annelids they are found in only one group, the sabellid tubeworms, and in molluscs too they are confined to two genera of bivalves, *Arca* and *Pectunculus*. Amongst the arthropods they are the dominant type of eye in the Crustacea and insects, but in the arachnids they are only found in *Limulus* – scorpions and spiders have only simple eyes. Well-developed compound eyes are found in trilobites, fossil arthropods which lived from the Lower Cambrian period (600 million years ago) to the Upper Permian (250 million), making them the most ancient type of eye known (LEVI-SETTI, 1975).

Annelid and molluscan compound eyes are shown in Fig. 41. The former are best known from *Branchiomma vesiculosum* (HESSE, 1899; KRASNE and LAWRENCE, 1966) although similar eyes occur throughout the Sabellidae (KERNEIS, 1975). These animals are tube-living filter feeders, with a fan-like crown of feeding tentacles some of which bears an eye at the tip. There are about 80 ommatidia per eye in *Branchiomma*, and each consists of a lens cell with a single receptor lying beneath it. The receptors have a ciliary lamellar structure reminiscent of the distal cells in *Pecten*, and the sensitivity of the animals to shadow and movement, but not to brightening, suggests that as in *Pecten* these cells are "off" receptors (NICOL, 1950). Optically, these are typical apposition eyes, with each element covering a field of between 5° and 10°. The compound eyes of the clams *Arca* and *Pectunculus* are similar to those of *Branchiomma*, although as yet no details of ultrastructure are available. They are borne in large numbers on the exposed part of the mantle; PATTEN (1886) counted 133 on one mantle edge and 102 on the other. The number of facets in each eye is very variable, from 10–80. There are, in addition, an even larger number of small pit-like eye spots of unknown structure and function. Descriptions of the compound eyes are given by PATTEN and by HESSE (1900). It is almost certain that the evolution of a modest optical system in these animals enables them to respond to movement of objects that do not cast direct shadows. BRAUN (1954) found that movement of a thin wire was sufficient to cause them to shut. The parallel here is again with the mirror eyes of *Pecten*: Movement detection becomes possible as the field of view of each receptor is restricted, but of course the optical arrangement producing this restriction is totally different in the two bivalve groups.

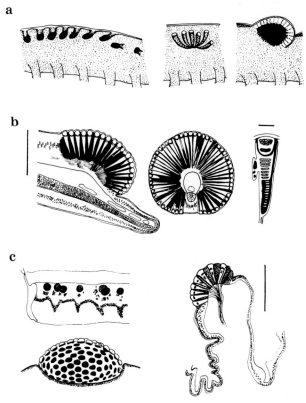

Fig. 41 a–c. Compound eyes outside the Arthropoda. **a** Epithelial pigment-tube eyes in some sabellid polychaete annelids. Left, *Hypsicomus*; middle, *Protula*; right, *Sabella*, which has a more clearly organized compound eye. (After HESSE, 1935) **b** Well-developed compound eye in the sabellid *Branchiomma vesiculosum*, in longitudinal and transverse section (left and middle; scale 100 μm) (Redrawn from HESSE, 1899). Right, single element in a *Branchiomma* eye. The receptive part is a stack of ciliary plates at the base of the cell. (Based on KRASNE and LAWRENCE, 1966) **c** Compound eyes round the mantle of the bivalve *Arca*. Left: eyes of *A. barbata* (above) and one eye of *A. noae* (below). (Both redrawn from PATTEN, 1886). Right: section through one eye of *A. noae*. Scale 100 μm. (Redrawn from HESSE, 1900)

Compound eyes in the tubeworms seem to have evolved from loose clusters of single receptors which became pigmented (Fig. 15 B), then acquired lenses and aggregated into distinct eyes (Fig. 41 a). HESSE (1935) illustrates such a series in existing forms. However, this may not have been the way compound eyes evolved in the different arthropod groups. They could equally well have arisen from the coalescence and reorganization of existing simple eyes. Amongst the Myriapoda the faster species like *Scutigera* with excellent vision have compound eyes with up to 250 ommatidia, each with a small number of receptors (12–16), whereas the less active and presumably more "ancestral" forms such as *Lithobius* have relatively small numbers of separated ocelli (up to 40), but these may have up to 110 receptors each (BÄHR, 1974). This suggests an evolution from simple to compound eyes. However, in insects and Crustacea no such inference is possible. Simpler, more "primitive" groups like apterygote insects have the same numbers of receptors in each ommatidium, (typically eight) as in other insects, even though the ommatidia are separated and few in number (PAULUS, 1975). Similarly the number of receptors in the ommatidia of "lower" Crustacea like the isopod *Porcellio*, with only 20 facets per eye, is the same (again eight) as in the Decapoda where each compound eye may have many thousands of ommatidia (NEMANIC, 1975). There is thus no obvious clue to the origins of the ommatidial unit in insects or Crustacea. Nor is there an obvious starting point for optical evolution in crustacea. In many ways the eye of the cladoceran *Daphnia* is very specialised (YOUNG and DOWNING, 1976), as are the eyes of many copepods (Sect. C.II.3.c.).

3. Optics of Apposition Eyes

a) Spherical Surfaces and Lens Cylinders

In most diurnal insects a small inverted image is formed at the distal tips of the receptors in each ommatidium. The usual method is spherical refraction, with the curved air/chitin interface of each corneal facet acting as the main refracting surface just as in a simple eye of the corneal type (Sect. C.II.4.a and Fig. 7). The optics of such eyes are perfectly straightforward, and there is no need to consider them again here.

There are, however, a few insects where the cornea is not facetted, for example the mantis *Cuilfina* (HORRIDGE and DUELLI, 1979), and this is also the situation in the crabs (Brachyura) and the king crab *Limulus* (Xiphosura). Spherical refraction alone cannot be responsible for image formation in such eyes, and an alternative mechanism must be sought. EXNER (1891) chose *Limulus* as the definitive example of such an eye, and from his studies came up with the idea of a lens-cylinder, a device conceptually not unlike the Matthiessen lens (Sect. C.II.3.a) in which ray bending is achieved by refractive index gradients within the bulk of the lens, or crystalline cone, and not by refraction at its surfaces. EXNER worked out that a flat-ended cylindrical lens would form an image on its posterior face if the structure contained a radially symmetrical refractive index gradient which was highest along the axis of the cylinder, and fell off roughly parabolically at increasing distances from the axis. If one imagines a ray striking the end of such a cylinder normally, at some distance from the axis, such a ray will encounter a zone in which the refractive index is higher towards the axis and lower away from it and, just as with refraction at a discrete interface the ray will be drawn into the higher index region, i.e. towards the axis. As the ray passes up the gradient, the degree of bending will increase, until finally the ray meets the axis. Given the appropriate index gradient, this will be the point where all parallel rays meet the axis, and so this is the position of the image (Fig. 42). This explanation of image formation in *Limulus* has been accepted as correct for almost a century (see KUNZE, 1979, this Handbook, Vol. VII/6 A), and it is interesting that in the last few years successful attempts have been made to manufacture similar lens cylinders commercially using glass and plastics (OHTSUKA, 1973; IGA and YAMAMOTO, 1977).

Recently, however, LEVI-SETTI et al. (1975) proposed that *Limulus* cones formed images not by refraction, but by reflection at their curved lateral surfaces. They

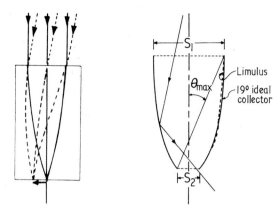

Fig. 42. Image formation in *Limulus* corneal cones according to EXNER (left) and LEVI-SETTI et al. (right). In EXNER's mechanism, rays are bent by refraction in the inhomogeneous core of the cone. In the LEVI-SETTI model image formation occurs by reflection at the parabolic walls of the cone. The dotted line shows the correspondence between the shape of a cone tip, and a light collector which accepts light up to an angle (θ_{max}) of 19°. All the light entering the pupil S_1 up to this angle passes through the lower aperture S_2. EXNER's mechanism is in fact the correct one in *Limulus* (LAND, 1979), but ideal collectors might exist elsewhere

pointed out the similarity in shape between *Limulus* cones and a device known as an "ideal light collector" (Fig. 42), a mirror with parabolic faces designed to concentrate faint radiation (WINSTON, 1970). They showed that such a device can form an image, and so it could be a real candidate mechanism not just for *Limulus* cones, but for any other biological focussing system that does not rely on spherical refracting optics.

It is now possible to say unequivocally that in *Limulus*, at least, EXNER's interpretation is the correct one (LAND, 1979). The proposal of LEVI-SETTI et al. (1975) requires first that the crystalline cones – which in *Limulus* are extensions of the cornea – should be optically homogeneous. Second, there should be an abrupt optical discontinuity between the cone and the matrix surrounding it; this is necessary if total internal reflection is to take place. Third, their mechanism predicts an erect image at the cone tip, whereas EXNER's predicts an inverted one. This is very simply tested. The images are indeed inverted (Fig. 43c). The first two points can be settled by interference microscopy. If a pattern of interference fringes is displayed in the object plane of an interference microscope, then parallel-sided sections placed in that plane will distort the fringe pattern laterally by an amount proportional to their local refractive index (see LAND, 1979). When a section of a *Limulus* cone is viewed in this way (Fig. 43b), the pattern of distortion is clearly parabolic, with the greatest distortion and hence the highest refractive index (1.51) on the cone axis. The refractive index decreases with no sudden discontinuities into the matrix between the cones, where the minimum index is 1.42 (Fig. 44a). Qualitatively these findings are entirely in accord with EXNER (1891).

They also fit quantitatively. An exact solution to the form of the refractive index gradient in a lens cylinder was produced by FLETCHER et al. in 1954, in the same paper in which they also gave the gradient required in a Matthiessen lens (see

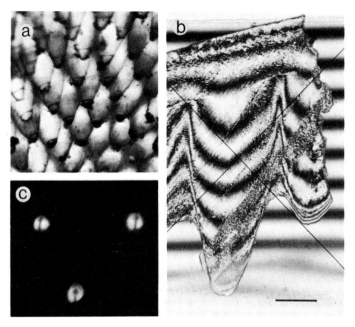

Fig. 43. a Inner surface of the cornea of *Limulus polyphemus* showing the tips of the crystalline cones. **b** Section (13 μm thick) through the cornea along the axis of a cone, as it appears in an interference microscope with a fringe field eyepiece. The straight interference fringes (at right) are distorted by the refractive index gradient in the specimen, and the higher the index the greater the fringe displacement. The uppermost fringe in the background reappears below the crosswires in the centre of the cone, and its displacement is four wavelengths. The parabolic form of the fringe distortion in the tissue indicates that the refractive index gradient is also parabolic (Fig. 44). Scale bar 100 μm. **c** Images of an arrowhead object visible at the tips of three corneal cones. The images are inverted, and the circular surround of the object subtended 8.9° at the eye surface. The average spacing of the cone tips is 255 μm. (From LAND, 1979)

Fig. 20). Their formula, for a lens cylinder that forms an image at a distance F from its front face is:

$$n_r = n_o \text{ sech } (\pi r / 2 \, F) \,, \tag{35}$$

where n_o is the refractive index on the axis, and n_r is the index at a radial distance r from the axis. The function is very similar to the parabolic approximation EXNER used. In Fig. 44 a, this function has been plotted out for lens cylinders of three different lengths (F), together with the measured refractive index gradient across a *Limulus* cone derived from the interference microscope measurements. The best fit is given by the $F = 600$ μm curve and, in fact, the length of the inhomogeneous part of the cone is 580 μm, so theory and measurement coincide very well indeed. FLETCHER et al. also predict the focal length (f) of a lens cylinder, where f corresponds to the posterior nodal distance of an ordinary lens, the length required to determine image magnification (see Fig. 7). They give:

$$f = 2 \, F / \pi n_o \,. \tag{36}$$

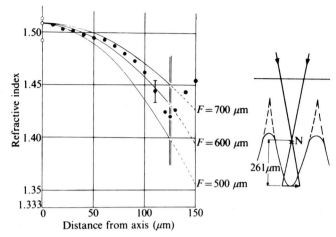

Fig. 44. Left: refractive index gradient in a corneal cone of *Limulus* determined by interference microscopy (points) and calculated for three different values of F using Eq. 35. The actual length of the inhomogeneous part of the cone is 580 μm, so there is good agreement between data and theory. Right: diagram of a cone showing the location of the nodal point (N) as determined from image magnification (Fig. 43c), and by calculation from Eq. (36) using measurements from interference microscopy. The calculated nodal point is the small cross just below the intersecting rays. The measured value of the focal length (f) is 261 μm, and the calculated value 253 μm. (Land, 1979)

From image magnification (Fig. 44b) the focal length was found to be 261 μm, compared with 253 μm by calculation (using $F=600$ μm and $n_0=1.51$). Again, there is good agreement, and this leaves no doubt at all about the correctness of Exner's original conjecture.

Lens cylinders of various kinds are probably a very common alternative to spherical surface optics in apposition eyes, especially in aquatic animals where there is very little optical power in the interface between the cornea and the world outside. They also occur in a modified form as the optical elements in most superposition eyes, but this is the subject of a later section (C.III.4.b).

b) Resolution

Each ommatidium in an apposition eye can be thought of optically as a simple eye of the corneal type, but containing effectively only one receptor and with a field of view limited to the subtense of the distal tip of this receptor (rhabdom) at the nodal point of the corneal lens. In practice, the acceptance angle will be slightly larger than this, partly because of blurring of the image by diffraction (and to a very minor extent by aberrations) and partly also because the waveguide properties of narrow receptors give them slightly wider acceptance functions than their geometrical width (see Sect. B.III.2 and Snyder, 1977).

Ultimately, it is the width of the acceptance function of each ommatidium ($\Delta\varrho$, Fig. 45) that determines the resolving power of the eye as a whole. However, a more obvious and accessible indication of resolving power is given by the inter-ommatidial angle ($\Delta\phi$), the angle between the line of sight of one ommatidium and

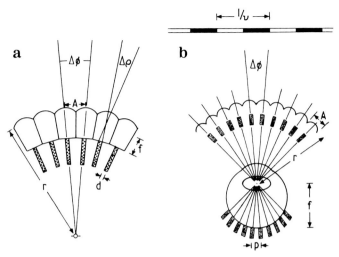

Fig. 45 a. Optical geometry of an apposition compound eye. The acceptance angle of a single rhabdom $(\Delta\varrho = d/f)$ is approximately the same as the inter-ommatidial angle $(\Delta\Phi = A/r)$, so that each ommatidium images a unique solid angle in external space. **b** Construction showing a compound eye and a simple eye with the same resolving power. $\mathscr{R} = v = 1/2\ \Delta\phi = r/2\ A = f/2\ p$. (Modified from KIRSCHFELD, 1976)

that adjacent to it. In a "well-designed" eye one would expect the fields of view of adjacent ommatidia to be contiguous, so that $\Delta\phi \simeq \Delta\varrho$ (ROSSEL, 1979). Thus, the structure of the eye as a whole and the optics of individual ommatidia should be closely related to each other. This is a point of critical importance in trying to understand why compound eyes have a particular size and shape.

Using an earlier argument (Sect. B.III.1) that it takes two receptors – or, in this case, ommatidia – to resolve each pair of stripes in a grating, one would expect that the finest grating an apposition eye can resolve would have a spatial period of 2 $\Delta\phi$ radians or a frequency ($\mathscr{R}$) given by:

$$\mathscr{R} = 1/2\ \Delta\Phi. \tag{37}$$

SNYDER (1977) has pointed out that the spacing of receptors between adjacent rows in a hexagonal lattice is slightly smaller than their spacing *along* rows (by a factor of $\sqrt{3}/2$), so that the highest spatial frequency might be expected to be closer to $1/\sqrt{3}\ \Delta\phi$. In fact, there is a very impressive correspondence between resolution measured behaviourally (usually by means of the optomotor turning response) and the value of $\Delta\phi$. In the bee the minimum inter-ommatidial angle is 0.9°, and the minimum width of a *single* stripe in an array (not the stripe *pair* which should correspond to 2 $\Delta\phi$) is 0.98°; in *Calliphora* the corresponding values are 2.4° and 2°; in *Drosophila*, 4.5° and 5°; and in *Chlorophanus*, 7° and 7° (all data from MAZOKHIN-PORSHNYAKOV, 1969). Some apposition eyes clearly operate close to their theoretical limit.

Compared with the human eye, which is able to resolve line pairs that subtend about 1′ of arc, the figures for insects just quoted all seem very high. Why are inter-ommatidial angles so large, and how might they be reduced? At first sight one might think that resolution could be improved by decreasing $\Delta\phi$, by making the facets smaller and packing the ommatidia more closely together. However, it quickly becomes clear that this cannot be done because usually the facets are so small that diffraction is a limiting factor. The spatial cut-off frequency, above which there is no contrast in the image, is given by Eq. (20):

$$v_c = A/\lambda \, , \tag{20}$$

where A is the facet diameter. The limiting condition occurs when the cut-off frequency for each ommatidium (Eq. 20) is equal to the frequency limit imposed by the inter-ommatidial angle (Eq. 37), so that:

$$A/\lambda = 1/2\,\Delta\Phi, \quad \text{or} \quad \Delta\Phi = \lambda/2\,A \, . \tag{38}$$

Equation 38 states that the inter-ommatidial angle can only be decreased if the aperture of each facet is *increased*. This result seems odd because large facets look as though they should be providing coarse resolution (see the photograph of a male fly, *Syritta*, in Fig. 48). Appearances, however, can be misleading, and the value of $\Delta\phi$ in the region of large (40 μm) facets in *Syritta* is 0.6°, although in the rest of the eye with small (18 μm) facets it is 1.5° (COLLETT and LAND, 1975).

c) Eye Parameter (P)

To what extent is diffraction the real limit to the resolving power of apposition eyes? This can be answered by determining the value of the product $A\Delta\phi$, which SNYDER (1977) has called the *eye parameter (P)*. If we reorganize Eq. (38) slightly we get, for a diffraction-limited eye, that:

$$P = A\Delta\phi = \lambda/2 \simeq 0.25 \text{ μm} \, . \tag{39}$$

Both A and $\Delta\phi$ are usually easy to determine from external measurements. If the product $A\Delta\phi$ approaches 0.25 μm, then diffraction is limiting; if on the other hand it is substantially larger than this (more than, e.g. 0.5 μm), then other factors are likely to be involved. In particular, where an eye has evolved to operate at low light intensities it is an advantage for $A\Delta\phi$ to be large since big facets coupled with large acceptance angles will mean that each rhabdom receives a greater number of photons than would be the case if $A\Delta\phi$ were at the diffraction limit. The theoretical implications of differences in $A\Delta\phi$ have been explored in detail by SNYDER (1977) and SNYDER et al. (1977 b), and HORRIDGE (1978) has examined the way the eye parameter differs between arthropod eyes and also varies from place to place within individual eyes. At one extreme one finds that day-flying insects, especially those that hover, have eye parameters close to the diffraction limit; in the sand wasp *Bembix*, $A\Delta\phi$ has a minimum value of 0.32 μm; in the hover-fly *Syritta* the value is 0.42 μm in the large facet region and 0.47 μm elsewhere. Other insects, however, have larger eye parameters inconsistent with the diffraction limit. The nearly nocturnal dragon-fly *Zyxomma* has eye parameter values between 1 and 2 μm (HOR-

RIDGE, 1978), and I have found that in the twilight hunting larva of the dragon-fly *Cordulegaster annulatus*, $A\Delta\phi$ is around 2.4 µm. No insects are known that "do better" than the diffraction limit, which encourages our belief that this is *the* fundamental constraint on compound eye design, but some have appreciably larger facets and/or inter-ommatidial angles than diffraction alone can account for. The relation between the eye parameter and sensitivity will be examined further in Sect. *f*.

d) Eye Size

The small diameter of individual facets in a compound eye, compared to the large aperture of most simple eyes, makes the compound eye design unsuitable for high resolution. The reason again is the diffraction limit. To resolve 1 min of arc (1/3,440 radians) an optical system would require, according to Eq. (20), an aperture of 1.7 mm. This resolution and this aperture are similar to those of the human eye in bright conditions. If, however, we try to make a compound eye with this resolution, it is clear that *every* facet must have a diameter of 1.7 mm, and this makes the eye impossibly large. If the eye is spherical and symmetrical, simple geometry shows that the inter-ommatidial angle is equal to A/r radians, where r is the radius of the eye. Combining this with Eq. (38) then gives:

$$A/r = \Delta\phi = \lambda/2\, A, \text{ or } r = \frac{2\,A^2}{\lambda}. \tag{40}$$

If A is a minimum of 1.7 mm, this means that the radius r of the eye will be about 12 *metres*! By contrast the human eye has a focal length – not much different from its radius – of about 16.7 mm. The absurdity of a high resolution compound eye is beautifully illustrated by the figure from KIRSCHFELD (1976) reproduced in Fig. 46. KIRSCHFELD has in fact been kind to the compound eye and has taken into account the way that resolution falls off at increasing distances from the fovea in the human eye. This reduces the diameter to about 1 m, but nevertheless the inappropriateness of the design is clear enough.

Besides showing why compound eyes are not capable of supplying high resolution, Eq. (40) also predicts a relation between facet diameter and eye size (r) which ought to hold true between one insect and another. The facet diameter ought to be proportional to the square root of the linear size of the eye. BARLOW (1952) showed that this was true for 27 species of diurnal Hymenoptera ranging in body length from 1–60 mm. Intuitively it is easy to see why this should be so. If a compound eye is diffraction limited, a doubling of its resolution requires a doubling of the size of each facet, but the doubled resolution also means that the *number* of facets can be doubled, so that the radius of the eye, or any other linear dimension, must be quadrupled. The same point is made in Fig. 47 which shows the heads of a large and a small fly (*Volucella* and *Drosophila*) enlarged so that the head diameters appear the same. It is clear that the larger fly is not just a "scaled-up" version of the smaller fly; it has many more facets and, although not immediately apparent from the photograph, these are larger. The radius of curvature of the *Volucella* eye is about 1,650 µm and only 270 µm in *Drosophila*, a ratio of 6.1:1. The corresponding facet diameters, however, are 40 µm (average) and 16 µm, the ratio being 2.5:1. As Eq. (40) predicts, the ratio of radii is almost exactly equal to the

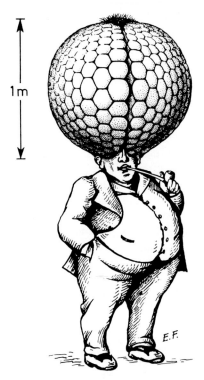

Fig. 46. A man with a compound eye whose resolving power is the same as that of the human eye. Each "facet" represents 10⁴ actual facets. Further details in the text. (KIRSCHFELD, 1976)

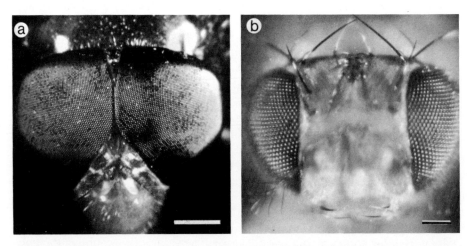

Fig. 47 a, b. Eyes of a large fly (**a**: *Volucella pellucens*) and a small fly (**b**: *Drosophila melanogaster*) scaled up to the same size to show that one is not a simple enlargement of the other. Although the *Volucella* eye contains more facets, they are larger than those of *Drosophila* by a factor of 2.5. The eyes themselves differ in radius by a factor of 6:1. Scales 1 mm on **a**, 0.1 mm on **b**

square of the ratio of facet diameters. It is interesting that this rule holds even for eyes that are *not* strictly diffraction limited; in *Drosophila* for example, $\Delta A\phi$ is about 1.25, which is similar to the housefly *Musca* (1.3; STAVENGA, 1975) and about five times greater than the diffraction limit. It seems that the square-root scaling rule applies across species whenever the value of the eye parameter is constant between them, and it does not matter whether it is diffraction or some other feature of eye design that sets the eye parameter's value (see Sect. *f* below).

e) "Foveas" in Compound Eyes

Differences in resolution in different parts of compound eyes are not uncommon, just as in simple eyes, and frequently this variation takes the form of a quite sharply defined forward or upward region of the eye surface in which the facet size is greater than elsewhere. It seems reasonable to refer to this as a fovea, by analogy with vertebrate eyes, in spite of the fact already mentioned that the increased resolution is often not achieved by packing receptors closer together, but by moving them further apart! Some of the most striking examples are in the Diptera, and are usually connected with the need for males to detect and track small females. Consequently, it is only the male eye that has a foveal modification. Two examples are given in Fig. 48. The upper photographs show a male and female bibionid fly, where the transition from the large (27 µm) facet region to the rather inconspicuous small (15 µm) facet part is quite abrupt, and where the large facet region is simply absent in the female (ZEIL, 1979). Similar "double eyes" are also found in male simuliid flies where the males have to detect and track females (1×3 mm) at a distance of 50 cm against the dawn sky, when they subtend an angle of only $0.2°$ – considerably less than the acceptance angle of even the largest (40 µm) facets (KIRSCHFELD and WENK, 1976). Divided eyes are also found in other dipteran groups, notably the Tabanidae (see DIETRICH, 1909), and also in the Ephemeroptera (WOLBURG-BUCHHOLZ, 1976; HORRIDGE, 1976) where the specialized male eye seems to be a hybrid between apposition and superposition types. A less pronounced fovea is found in many syrphids (Fig. 48c and d) where the large facets of the male merge gradually into the surrounding region, but the contrast between the sexes is still quite marked. In *Syritta pipiens* some of the optical modifications of the fovea can be seen in Fig. 48e; as the facets enlarge their focal lengths increase proportionately, but interestingly the diameters and separations of the receptors stay the same. This means that the subtense of each receptor ($\Delta\varrho = d/f$) decreases in the foveal region, but the light received by each receptor proportional to $(A/f)^2 \cdot d^2$ stays the same. The other point worth noting is that the presence of a fovea necessitates a pronounced distortion of the ommatidia surrounding it, so that the 20th ommatidium from the midline has its visual axis displaced by about $30°$ from the optical axis of the facet, or from a normal to the eye surface.

In all the preceding examples the presence of a fovea was related to a behavioural sexual dimorphism. However, this is not always so; in insects that prey on other insects (e.g. Asilid flies, mantids, sand wasps, dragon-flies, and damsel-flies), a frontal region of high acuity is present, usually in both sexes (see HORRIDGE, 1977, 1978). In dragon-flies there may actually be several higher resolution regions in each eye: frontal, lateral, and dorsal (SHERK, 1978a, b).

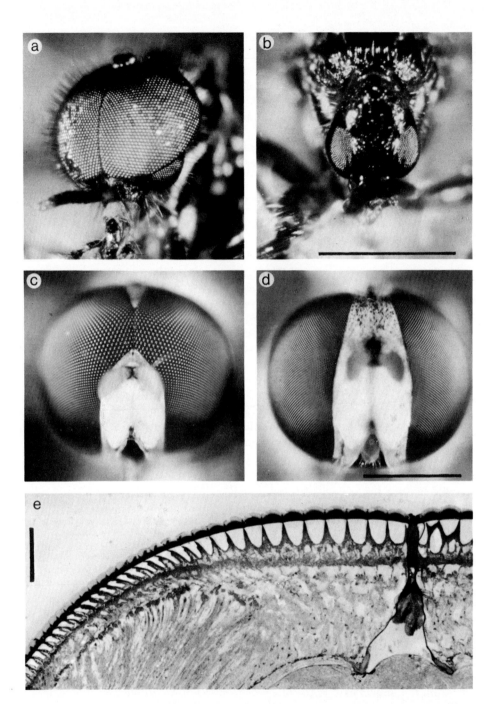

Fig. 48 a–e. Foveae in the eyes of dipteran flies. **a** and **b** Heads of male and female Bibionid flies *(Dilophus febrilis)*, showing the large separate region of enlarged facets present only in the male. Scale for **a** and **b** 1 mm. **c** and **d** More gradual transition from large to small facets in the eye of a male syrphid *(Syritta pipiens)*. The female **(d)** has no fovea. Scale 100 μm. **e** Section along a horizontal facet row in the fovea of a male *Syritta*. The individual optical systems double in both aperture and focal length in the central region. In the transitional region between large and small facets the visual axes make large angles with normals to the eye surface. Scale 100 μm

Although in most of these examples the fovea has larger facets – presumably because it is necessary to overcome the limit to resolving power imposed principally by diffraction – there are some exceptions. One of the oddest is the locust *Schistocerca gregaria* which, being a herbivore, has no need to see other small insects, and in which the facet diameters are nearly identical throughout the eye (36–40 μm). Nevertheless, it has a region of high resolution *in the vertical plane only* situated frontally on the horizontal midline of the eye. One of the manifestations of this is the enlargement and vertical elongation of the pseudopupil (see Sect. g) visible in Fig. 50 a. My own measurements, based on the shift of the pseudopupil position with eye rotation, give the vertical inter-ommatidial angle in this region as 0.59° and the corresponding horizontal angle as 1.82°. In the parts of the eye furthest from the frontal region the vertical/horizontal asymmetry gradually decreases and the inter-ommatidial angle lies between 2.5° and 3°. It is interesting that where the inter-ommatidial angle is smallest, the eye parameter is very close to the diffraction limit ($A\Delta\phi=0.37$), but around the periphery it is much larger (~ 1.7). It is as though the facet diameter, and ultimately the size of the locust eye, is set by the highest resolution region, in marked contrast to, e.g. *Syritta*, where a small high resolution part has been "squeezed" into an eye of small size and relatively low resolution. Alternatively, it may be that the high value of the eye parameter in peripheral parts of the locust eye really means that these regions are designed to work at lower light intensities than the front; or it may be, as SNYDER (1977) suggests, that they are designed for faster image movement.

f) Sensitivity

The amount of light caught by single rhabdoms in an apposition eye follows the same rule as for a simple eye (Eq. 14 and 15), as each ommatidium is optically equivalent to a simple eye. If the receptors are of adequate length to absorb most of the light imaged on them, then the proportion of photons received from an extended source will be proportional to $(A/f)^2 \cdot d^2$. However, $d/f = \Delta\varrho \simeq \Delta\phi$, so that the sensitivity is given by:

$$\mathscr{S} \propto A^2 \Delta\Phi^2 = P^2 . \tag{41}$$

SNYDER's eye parameter is thus a useful indicator not only of how close a compound eye is to the diffraction limit, but also of its absolute sensitivity. A high value means that the eye is specialized for relatively dim light conditions. SNYDER (1977) has calculated *optimal* values for P for different illumination conditions. These calculations are based on similar arguments to those developed in Sect. B.II, and the "optimal" eye design is the one that provides the highest spatial resolution for a given signal-to-noise ratio in the receptors, which is itself a function of the value of P, of the mean luminance of the surroundings, and of the contrast (taken as 50%) in the environmental patterns. The results are given in Fig. 49, and show that a value of P close to the diffraction limit (0.25 μm) is only to be expected in animals that operate within the range of intensities that would be thought of as daylight. Below this P rises steeply or, put another way, one would expect facet sizes to increase and inter-ommatidial angles to increase too. This is, qualitatively at least, exactly what one finds.

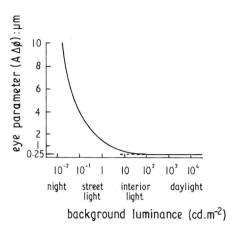

Fig. 49. Optimal values of the eye parameter ($P = A\Delta\phi$) for apposition compound eyes under different illumination conditions. Only when the eyes have evolved for use in full daylight will the eye parameter come close to the diffraction-limited condition ($P \sim 0.25$ μm). (Modified from SNYDER, 1977)

A further point made by SNYDER (1977) is that if an animal moves rapidly, particularly if it rotates, this is equivalent to living in a dim environment. This is in fact clear from Eq. (4), where the photon sample size from any region of space is a function not only of the retinal illuminance, but also of the sampling time t. If the image is not to be blurred by motion, t must be short, and so to obtain the same photon count – and hence the same contrast sensitivity and signal reliability – the amount of light reaching the rhabdoms, i.e. P^2 (Eq. 41), must be correspondingly increased. This probably explains why some diurnal flies like *Musca* or *Fannia* which are both fast and highly manoeuverable, have values of P of around 1.3, compared with 0.25 at the diffraction limit. It is also important to remember that dipteran flies have effectively seven receptors looking at the same part of the visual world through seven different facets, so that the total photon gain compared with a fused rhabdom eye like that of *Bembix*, operating near the diffraction limit, is something like $(1.3/0.3)^2 \times 7$, or 190 times.

The same line of reasoning may also help to explain the vertical/horizontal asymmetries in the inter-ommatidial angles in other insects, especially in the locusts mentioned in the preceding section. An animal in level flight, or when walking, experiences much greater velocities around its eye's horizontal than its vertical circumference, and it is a reasonable assumption that this is why the eye parameter is so much greater horizontally than vertically.

g) Pseudopupil

Many insect eyes of the apposition type show a black spot which moves around the surface of the eye in a slightly alarming way and always appears to be facing the observer (Figs. 50 and 52). This dark spot, the pseudopupil, so-called because of its superficial resemblance to the pupil of a human eye, is the virtual image of the rhabdoms and their surrounding pigment in those ommatidia that share a common line of sight with the observer. The situation is the same as occurs when a

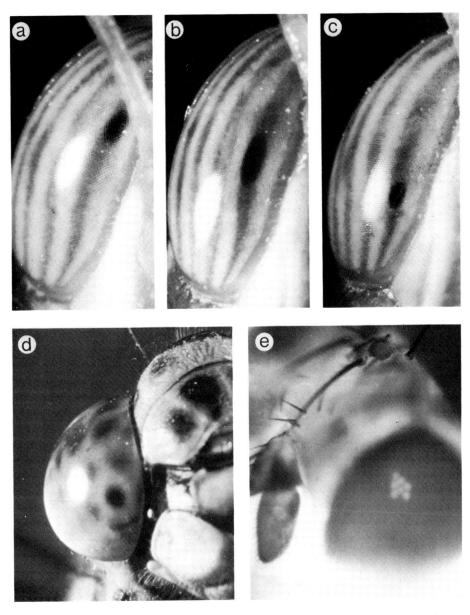

Fig. 50 a–e. The pseudopupil in apposition eyes. **a–c** The frontal region of the eye of the locust *Schistocerca gregaria*; in **a** the head is tilted down by 20°, in **b** it is horizontal, and in **c** it is tilted up by 20°. The vertical enlargement of the pseudopupil on the horizontal equator is accompanied by a large difference in inter-ommatidial angle (0.6° vertically, 1.8° horizontally). **d** Multiple pseudopupils in the ventral region of the eye of the dragon-fly *Aeschna cyanea* (Odonata). The secondary pseudopupils are best explained by assuming that they are the virtual images of the receptors and screening pigment as seen through the optics of *neighbouring* ommatidia. **e** Antidromic deep pseudopupil in the upper part of the left eye of *Drosophila melanogaster*. This is produced by illuminating the receptors from inside the head. The image has the same geometry as that of the open rhabdomere pattern in single ommatidia (Fig. 40 a), but is about ten times larger

small black object is placed at the focal point of a lens and that lens is viewed from a distance; when the object, the nodal point of the lens and the observer's eye are on the same line, the whole of the lens appears black. Another way of putting this is to say that an ommatidium acts as a light sink (and so appears dark) over that angular range over which it is actually absorbing photons (see STAVENGA, this Handbook, Vol. VII/6 A, Chap. 7).

The pseudopupil is not a pupil in the sense of a variable diaphragm and has no significance for the animal. However, it can be a useful tool for someone examining an eye, because its position indicates accurately the direction of the visual axes in each eye region. Inter-ommatidial angles can be simply measured using it; for example if when an insect is rotated 15° the pseudopupil moves across five facets, the inter-ommatidial angle is 3°. This method is more accurate than histological measurements or estimates from radii of curvature, because it measures the true line of sight of ommatidia rather than normals to the surface, etc. Figure 48 e shows how the latter might be misleading. Details of these methods can be found in HORRIDGE (1978) and STAVENGA (this Handbook, Vol. VII/6 A, Chap. 7). The form of the pseudopupil can also be significant. If, for example, it is elongated vertically (Fig. 50 a), this usually means that a larger number of ommatidia is devoted to a given angle in the vertical rather than the horizontal dimension and hence that the inter-ommatidial angles differ in the two planes.

In the eyes of dipteran flies, and other eyes with open rhabdoms, the pseudopupil takes the form of the pattern of receptor endings in the focal plane of each facet – the typical 6+1 arrangement (Fig. 50 e). Because of the precise alignment of the visual axes of different receptors in adjacent ommatidia (see Fig. 40), the virtual images of many receptors merge in the depths of the eye to give a single deep pseudopupil, the formation of which has been examined in detail by FRANCESCHINI and KIRSCHFELD (1971). These authors also invented a technique whereby the eye is illuminated from behind ("antidromic illumination") so that the receptor endings appear as illuminated points, rather than dark spots. Both "ortho-" and "antidromic" methods have been useful in studying light flux control by pigment migration as well as the spectral and polarization sensitivities of the separate receptor sub-systems (1–6 and 7–8) in single ommatidia (see FRANCESCHINI, 1975).

Although in many eyes the presence of peripheral shielding pigment makes it difficult or impossible to see the pseudopupil, where one can be seen this is a fairly safe indication that the eye is of the apposition type. In superposition eyes a pseudopupil is rarely if ever visible, but the corresponding "diagnostic feature," at least when the eye is dark adapted, is a patch of "glow" when the eye is illuminated from the direction of viewing (Fig. 62 c and d).

h) Pupil Mechanisms

Receptors can respond over an intensity range as great as 5 log units (LAUGHLIN, 1976), but if this range is to be extended upwards mechanisms must exist for restricting the light reaching them. In simple eyes there seem to be only two: decreasing the aperture of the optical system by means of an iris, and shielding the receptors from off-axis light by the use of opaque pigment brought up into the spaces between them. These may be supplemented by changes in the amount of re-

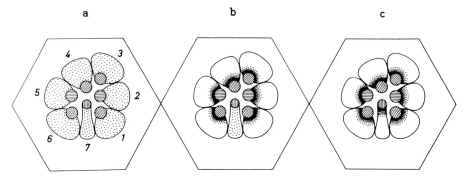

Fig. 51 a–c. Pupil mechanism in the dipteran retina in three stages of light adaptation. In **a** the eye is dark adapted and the small pigment granules are dispersed in the cytoplasm of the retinula cells. In **b** they have moved into contact with the rhabdomeres of the outer (1–6) system, and "bleed" light from them by reducing the internal/external refractive index difference. In **c** the inner receptors (7) are light adapted in the same way. (FRANCESCHINI and KIRSCHFELD, 1976)

ceptor membrane (Sect. C.II.4.b.γ). In compound eyes all these mechanisms exist, and they may also be accompanied by changes in the positions of the rhabdoms relative to the optical structures of the ommatidium that are not easy to interpret (WALCOTT, 1975). However, one additional mechanism stands out as being particularly interesting, and so far at least seems to be restricted to apposition eyes. This is an arrangement whereby high refractive index material is moved "radially" towards each rhabdom or rhabdomere, thus lowering the refractive index difference between receptive segment and surrounding cytoplasm, increasing the critical angle for total internal reflexion (Sect. B.III.5) and "bleeding" the receptors of light that has already entered them (Fig. 51). In locusts, HORRIDGE and BARNARD (1965) showed that during the light a palisade of mitochondria with a refractive index similar to that of the rhabdom (1.39–1.40) moves into contact with the rhabdom, and vice versa in the dark.

In flies a similar phenomenon was demonstrated by KIRSCHFELD and FRANCESCHINI (1969), but here the high index material consists of minute (∼0.15 μm) pigment granules. The mobilization of these granules is very fast, complete within 10 s after illumination of the 1–6 receptor system (FRANCESCHINI and KIRSCHFELD, 1976), and this seems to be a quick and very effective light-attenuating device linked directly to the response of the receptors themselves which contain both the photopigment and the absorbing pigment.

i) Light Guide Optics in Amphipods

In the deep-sea amphipod crustacean *Phronima*, and several related genera such as *Phrosina* and *Streetsia*, apposition eyes are found in which each ommatidium has a long light guide joining the deeply situated rhabdom to a light-collecting cone just beneath the surface of the carapace (Fig. 15 I). *Phronima* itself is a remarkable animal (BALL, 1977); it makes a barrel from a chewed-off part of a salp (colonial tunicate) and in such a barrel the females raise their young (Fig. 52 a). The eyes are double; a small ventral eye has a nearly hemispherical field of view,

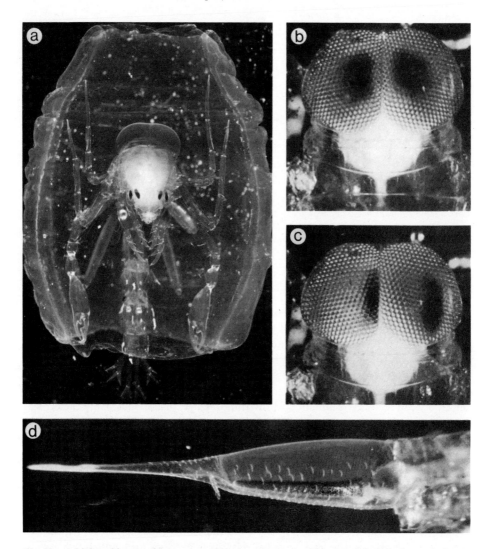

Fig. 52a–d. Light guide eyes of deep-sea amphipod crustaceans. **a** *Phronima sedentaria*, in a typical posture in its barrel. The four black spots near the base of the head are the retinae. The outer pair are the retinae of the two small "tear-like" eyes surrounding them. The inner pair receive light guides from the whole of the upper surface of the head, 5 mm distant. The animal is about 3 cm long. **b** and **c** Two views of the pseudopupils in the dorsal eyes of *Phronima*. The whole head surface is about 5.5 mm across, and single cone ends are 135 μm in diameter. **d** *Streetsia challengeri*. The eye occupies the whole of the posterior half of the spike-like head and is about 5 mm long. As in *Phronima*, it is made up of radially arranged light guides linking the surface to the retina, which is the long dark structure in the ventral region of the eye. The dorsal visual field of the eye in the anteroposterior direction is only about 30°, the angle over which a pseudopupil is visible. All photographs are of live animals

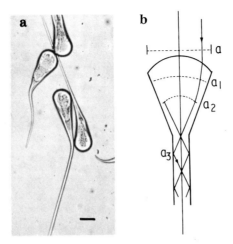

Fig. 53 a. Fresh cones from the dorsal eye of *Phronima sedentaria*, dispersed from the eye and photographed in sea-water. Their average diameter is 135 µm, and the 13-µm light guide that emerges from them has a total length of 5 mm. Scale bar 100 µm. **b** EXNER's (1891) suggestion for the way the cones funnel light. A plane wave (*a*) is partially focussed by spherical refraction (a_1) and focussed further by inhomogeneities in the cone (a_2) so that rays reaching the light guide make angles that are small enough for total internal reflexion to occur. The refractive index of the light guide part is about 1.375 so that rays will only be trapped by the guide if they make initial angles of less than 14° with its walls

and a much larger dorsal eye has a very small field of about 10°. The surface of the dorsal eyes occupies the whole of the top of the head, and each is made up of roughly 400 gelatinous cone-like structures which send narrow threads to the retina. In *P. sedentaria* this lies fully 5 mm away, next to the retina of the ventral eyes (Fig. 52 a). The dorsal and ventral eyes share a common lamina (BALL, 1977).

Optically the cones are the most interesting features of the eyes, since they operate as devices that concentrate light from their surface (diameter, 135 µm) into light guides of roughly one-tenth this diameter (13 µm), giving an increase in the "catchment area" of each light guide of about 100 times. [The unpublished measurements were made by the author on fresh animals and are rather larger than those given by BALL (1977); it seems that fixation and particularly dehydration has a dramatic shrinking effect on these very soft tissues.] That the cones do act as light concentrators is shown by the uniform blackness of the pseudopupil (Fig. 52 b), each cone acting as an efficient light "sink" when the otherwise quite transparent animal is lit with diffuse light. There are three possible mechanisms involved. Total internal reflexion certainly plays a part, but as EXNER himself pointed out in connexion with *Phronima*, a conical structure is not a good light concentrator since at each successive reflexion from the wall, the angle of incidence a ray makes increases, and in this case most of the light not already close to the axis would escape. The hemispherical distal tip (Fig. 53) looks as though it could focus light into the thread, but again for a surface of 70-µm radius to form an image 400 µm away would require a refractive index of 1.62, which is very much greater than the value of 1.37 I obtained by measuring the focal lengths of transversely illuminated cone tips. The only remaining mechanism which, it seems, must be invoked, is for the cone to have an inhomogeneous refractive index, greatest in the centre as in *Limulus* lens cylinders, and this is precisely what EXNER proposed (1891). Pseudopupil measurements show that each cone has an acceptance angle of about 3°, although the inter-cone separation is much less than this (about 0.5°), and it would appear from this that each point in space is viewed simultaneously by at least 30 rhabdoms, or 60 if the point lies within the 7° region of binocular overlap between the eyes. Unfortunately nothing is known of the behaviour of these animals that might explain the extraordinary structure of the eyes.

The eye of *Streetsia*, another midwater amphipod, is even more bizarre (Fig. 52d), with the array of light guides forming an almost cylindrical tube along the animal's rostrum. The eyes are not double, as in *Phronima*, but nevertheless there is a gradation between upper and lower regions, the dorsal elements being larger, longer, and subtending *smaller* visual angles than the lateral and ventral ones. Pseudopupil measurements indicated that in spite of its almost flat appearance, the dorsal surface views an anteroposterior arc of about 29°. The only major optical difference between *Streetsia* and *Phronima* is that in the former the cones are flat topped, so that light concentration can *only* be due to internal reflexion and inhomogeneities in the medium of the cones.

4. Optics of Superposition Eyes

a) Ray Paths

Behind the cleaned cornea of the eye of the firefly *Lampyris* it is possible to see and photograph a *single erect* image (the most famous photograph is the frontispiece to EXNER's monograph of 1891; another by H. E. ELTRINGHAM is given in

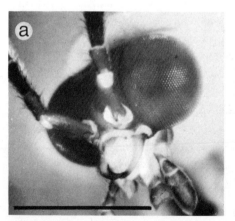
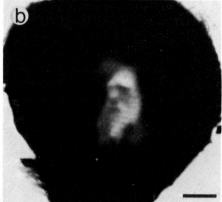

Fig. 54 a. Head of a firefly, showing the large superposition eyes. Scale bar 1 mm. **b** Photograph of a famous nineteenth century naturalist taken through the eye of the firefly shown in **a**. The cornea was cleaned to expose the tips of all the corneal cones, but leaving the pigment between them. The subject was, in fact, a transparency of the famous portrait by Julia Cameron (1869). The eye was placed in a hanging drop of saline with the outside of the cornea in air, 10 cm in front of the illuminated photograph. The photograph of the image was made using an ordinary microscope with a × 10 objective. Scale bar 100 μm

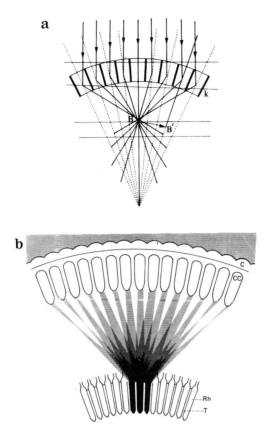

Fig. 55. a Diagram from EXNER (1891) showing the paths of rays contributing to the image in a super-position eye. Parallel light entering the eye from above is imaged at *B*. A spatially extended object forms an erect image along *BB'*. **b** Reconstruction, based on ray tracing through individual cones whose optical properties are known, of the distribution of image-forming light in the eye of the moth *Ephestia kühniella. C*: cornea; *CC*: crystalline cone; *Rh*: rhabdom; *T*: tapetum. (CLEARY et al., 1977)

IMMS, 1956). It is not difficult to replicate this observation, and my own attempt to do so is given in Fig. 54. It is not possible to do this with most insects that have this type of eye because the crystalline cones that form the image are separate from the cornea and come away when the eye is prepared. In the fire-flies (Lampyridae) and some other beetles, however, the optical elements are physically part of the cornea (just as in *Limulus*, Fig. 43 a), and they survive maltreatment. The presence of a single image formed by the superposition of light entering many facets distinguishes eyes of this type from apposition eyes, where typically only small inverted images are visible behind each facet. The other important feature of superposition eyes is the presence of a *clear zone* of transparent material between the superficial optical array and the rhabdom layer. The rhabdoms usually lie about halfway out from the centre of curvature of the eye, with the clear zone filling most of the region beyond this. It is across this clear zone that image-forming rays travel to a focus on the rhabdom layer (Fig. 55).

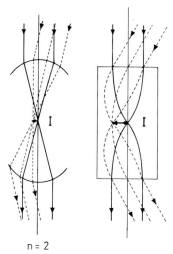

n = 2

Fig. 56. Two devices with the properties required for contributing to a superposition image, as in Fig. 55. Left: two-interface telescope with a focal plane between the faces and an overall magnification of −1. For a device with the proportions shown the refractive index would need to be 2.0, with air outside both faces. Right: lens cylinder with a refractive index gradient decreasing from the axis to the periphery. The result is the continuous bending of light rays, which allows the same result as with the telescope, but with much lower refractive indices. (EXNER, 1891)

The problem of the erect image is shown in Fig. 55a. In each optical element, axial rays pass straight through undeviated, but those making an angle with the axis must be bent in such a way that they emerge in a direction opposite to that of the incident ray. This, however, is not a property that can be achieved with a simple optical component – a single interface or a thin lens. Such structures always have a nodal point through which rays pass undeviated, which means that one ray from each direction emerges in the *same* direction as the incident ray, and an image is formed on the opposite side of the axis from the object. The optical elements contributing to superposition images do not have an internal nodal point, nor in general do they individually produce external images. They are said to be *afocal*, and as CLEARY et al. (1977) point out they are analogous in their properties to a Kepler telescope; that is to say, they are equivalent to a two-lens system where the first lens produces an image inside the instrument, at the front focal plane of the second (Fig. 56a). If the lenses have equal power the final image will be at infinity and the magnification −1, which is the same as saying that the emerging rays make an angle with the axis that is equal and opposite to the original angle of incidence. This is the property required for the production of a superposition image. HORRIDGE (1975) and KUNZE (1979, this Handbook Vol. VII/6 A) review this subject thoroughly.

b) Lens Cylinders

Although in theory a very thick lens – a two interface system with a focus in the middle (Fig. 56a) – would provide the appropriate ray paths for superposition imagery, EXNER was forced to reject this idea because, among other things, it required implausibly high refractive indices (see HORRIDGE, 1975). EXNER proposed instead that the same final ray paths could be attained if refraction occurred not at the interfaces but within the media between them (Fig. 56 b), just as in the lens cylinders discussed in Sect. C.III.3.a. The crucial difference between the lens cylinders required in superposition eyes and those of apposition eyes like *Limulus* (Fig. 42 a) is that the superposition kind should be twice as long [2 *F* rather than *F* in Eq. (35)]. This will give them a focus in the middle, just as in the telescope equivalent, and rays from that focus will emerge parallel to each other. Furthermore, provided the structure is symmetrical about its central focus, rays making an initial angle (α) with the distal surface of the structure will be bent through a total angle (2 α), and will emerge from the proximal end still making an angle (α) with the cylinder axis, but this time on the opposite side. In other words, such a lens cylinder will behave as a telescope with a magnification of -1. The axial refractive index gradient in a lens cylinder of this kind will be exactly the same as in an image-forming lens cylinder half as long, and the formula of FLETCHER et al. (1954) still applies Eq. (35).

In the past decade, interference microscopy has made it possible to measure refractive indices in small structures accurately and directly, and where this has been done and lens cylinder-like structures found, Eq. (35) gives a close fit to the observed gradient (MEYER-ROCHOW, 1975; LAND and BURTON, 1979).

c) Objections to Exner's Theory

After enjoying half a century as the standard textbook account of image formation in nocturnal insects and certain crustacea, EXNER's ideas met with serious criticism in the 1960 s. This criticism was directed both at the superposition principle in general and the lens cylinder mechanism in particular. Both have survived, but it is interesting to see how close they came to being abandoned.

The term "superposition" implies that the images formed by the cones are superimposed on each other. There is no reason to suppose that this is true for any compound eye, and there are several reasons, given above, why the superposition image of the firefly is no more than an artefact of the cleaned retina (HORRIDGE, 1969).

It seems very doubtful if "lens cylinder" properties will ever be found in a compound eye and therefore it would probably be better to discard the idea (KUIPER, 1962).

The objections that led to these statements were the following:

1) The clear zones of many intact eyes are not homogeneous, but are crossed by crystalline threads or tracts joining each optical element to a corresponding rhabdom. These could function as light guides, thereby making an apposition eye of what appeared to be a superposition eye. This is undoubtedly a serious argument, but the question is: How much light is actually trapped by these structures compared with the amount that is not so trapped? This will depend on the refractive index of the guide, and to trap *all* the light that would go to form a superposition image, emerging at angles of up to 30° from the axis of each cone, the refractive index required would be 1.33/sin 60°, or about 1.54 (see Sect. B.III.5). This would mean that the tracts should be solid rods, and this they are certainly not. However, in fire-flies and some moths the cones and tracts become lined with absorbing pigment in the light-adapted state (HORRIDGE, 1975; HÖGLUND, 1966), implying that in bright conditions it is only that fraction of

the light which manages to enter a tract that finally reaches a rhabdom. Further, as KUIPER (1962) first suggested, even that light is liable to attenuation by loss into the pigment surrounding the tract, which acts as a "longitudinal pupil." This is the same mechanism as is found to operate on the *receptors* of some apposition eyes (Sect. C.III.3.h). In the dark-adapted state, however, with the pigment retracted, there is good reason to suppose that only a small fraction of the light reaching the rhabdoms does so via the tracts.

2) The refractive index gradients required for lens cylinder optics are not present in the optical structures. Both the authors quoted above asserted this, but as interference microscopy improved it turned out that they were wrong, at least in *insects* with clear-zone eyes. SEITZ (1969) first showed that the corneal cones of fire-flies had a gradient similar to that proposed by EXNER, with a maximum index of 1.520 in the centre falling to 1.356 at the periphery. Similar findings were reported for a moth by KUNZE and HAUSEN (1971) and for a skipper butterfly by HORRIDGE et al. (1972). Lens cylinder optics certainly do exist, sometimes in the cornea (fire-flies and some other beetles) and sometimes in the underlying crystalline cone (moths and skipper butterflies). However, except in water beetles where the cornea is flat – and in any case optically irrelevant in water – the lens cylinder mechanism is supplemented by ordinary refraction at the curved corneal surface, and to some extent at the proximal tip of the cone. It seems that the optical systems of most insect superposition eyes are hybrid. In fairness it should be said that the rehabilitation of EXNER's ideas is very largely due to HORRIDGE, both for his unequivocal demonstration with GIDDINGS and STANGE (HORRIDGE et al., 1972) of the existence of a well-focussed superposition image in skipper butterflies *and* the presence of lens cylinder optics, as well as for a thorough study of possible mechanisms of superposition imagery (HORRIDGE, 1975). Furthermore, KUIPER (1962) was quite correct about decapod crustacean superposition eyes; they do not have lens cylinders, but employ an optical system based on mirrors that was not discovered until 1975 (see Sect. e below).

d) Eyes of Euphausiids

Refracting superposition eyes in insects have been so thoroughly reviewed recently (see KUNZE, 1979 this Handbook Vol. VII/6 Part A) that it would be of no service to go over that ground again. Instead I shall illustrate some of the attributes of this kind of eye by examining the eyes of a group of Crustacea, the euphausiids, which make use of the same optical system. The Euphausiacea is a family of shrimp-like animals that abound in the rather dim light conditions of the deep sea. They are better known as "krill" – a major part of the diet of the great whales. They are distantly related to the true decapod shrimps, but in spite of their close resemblance to them they have a completely different eye structure (see Sect. e below). The eyes were first studied in detail by CHUN (1896) whose descriptions were so good that very little has been added to them since (KAMPA, 1965; MEYER-ROCHOW and WALSH, 1978). Figure 57 shows sections through the eye of a large euphausiid, *Meganyctiphanes norvegica*, and illustrates the main features. Around the surface of the eye is a corneal layer which is presumably of negligible optical importance since it has water on its outer face. Beneath this lie the crystalline cones. These are

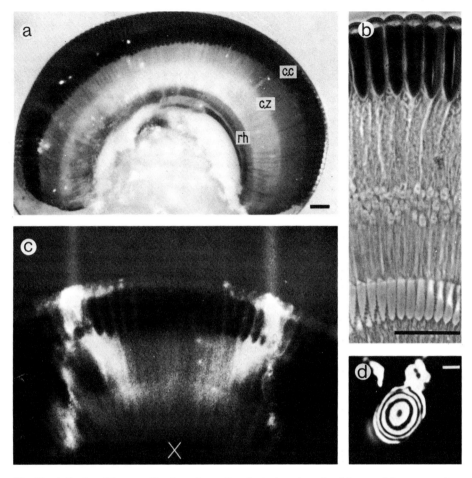

Fig. 57 a–d. Euphausiid eyes. **a** Hemisected eye of a spherical-eyed species, *Meganyctiphanes norvegica*, showing the layer of crystalline cones *(c.c)*, the wide clear zone *(c.z)* and the rhabdom layer *(rh)*. Scale bar 100 μm. **b** Part of a 1-μm section of the same eye in phase contrast. The receptor cell nuclei lie in the middle of the clear zone. The rhabdoms are banded. Bar 100 μm. **c** Demonstration of ray-bending by the cones. Two light beams, made visible with fluorescein in the bathing fluid, intersect the cut surface of a hemisected eye. Their initial paths in the fixed clear zone show up clearly. The light paths are bent by the cones through twice the angle of incidence at the eye surface, as in Fig. 55. The white cross marks the point in the rhabdom layer where the refracted beams would meet when extrapolated (LAND et al., 1979). **d** Interference micrograph of an 11 μm-thick section through the central region of a crystalline cone. The centre shows a path difference (in water) of four wavelengths, decreasing to one wavelength at the periphery. The spacing of the rings shows an approximately parabolic refractive index gradient. Scale bar 10 μm. (LAND and BURTON, 1979)

large structures, 115 μm long by 39 μm wide, and they form a close-packed hexagonal lattice. The spaces between are occupied by screening pigment, but only for the distal two-thirds of their length; it never reaches the proximal tips. Below the cones is a wide clear zone occupied mainly by the cell bodies of the receptors, and there is no evidence that it is crossed by light guide structures of any kind (MEYER-

Rochow and Walsh, 1978; Land et al., 1979). The rhabdoms, each of which is made up of microvilli from seven receptors, occupy a near perfect hemisphere situated about half an eye radius out from the centre of the eye (this is where one would expect it to be located if the crystalline cones have a magnification factor of -1; see Fig. 55). Each rhabdom is about 63 μm long and 17 μm wide. The overall similarity of this arrangement to the geometrical layout of moth eyes led Chun (1896) to the conclusion that they employed Exner's superposition mechanism, and in this he was certainly correct (Land et al., 1979). The resemblance in shape between the crystalline cones of moths and euphausiids is very striking (Fig. 57 b), and given that the two groups are totally unrelated, this must mean that there is only one good way of designing such structures.

A demonstration that the crystalline cones do bend light across their axes in the way required for superposition image formation is given in Fig. 57 c. It shows two beams of light, made visible with fluorescein, intersecting the cut surface of a hemisected eye. The beams are bent through almost exactly twice the angle at which they were incident at the corneal surface (Land et al., 1979). Interference microscopy also confirmed that the refractive index gradient in euphausiid cones is what one would predict for double length lens cylinders (Fig. 57 d). The central refractive index is 1.52, falling parabolically to 1.36 in 15 μm, the radius of a cone near its centre (Land and Burton, 1979). These values, substituted into Eq. (35) predict that the structure should behave as a lens cylinder whose length to its first focus (F) is 49 μm, and it should have a total length $(2F)$ of 98 μm if it is to behave as an afocal telescope. In fact, these particular cones were about 100 μm long, so there is no doubt at all that their optical properties arise from the lens cylinder refractive index profile.

The diversity of the shapes of euphausiid eyes is probably the most intriguing feature of the group. Although they are all clearly built on the basic superposition plan, not all are spherically symmetrical. Double eyes are common (Fig. 58), and whilst the lower eye of the pair is usually spherical the upper eye has a different geometry, with the eye surface typically centred in the receptor layer but the cones pointing towards a much deeper part of the eye. It is interesting that this geometrical configuration is one that would remove spherical aberration from the centre of the image (Land et al., 1979). What seems most likely is that the upper eyes – which usually have a small field of view, a long focal length and small values for $\Delta\phi$, as well as partially "corrected" optical systems – are acting as superposition "foveae," providing a limited, upward-pointing region of high resolution. The spherical part of the eye is presumably responsible for all-round vision, but with lower resolution.

The upper eyes of some species have a remarkably small number of crystalline cones; only four in *Stylocheiron microphthalma* and seven in *S. suhmii* (Fig. 58 b). Some larval eyes are reduced in the same sort of way, as in the furcilia larva of *Thysanopoda tricuspidata* (Fig. 58 d), a species whose adult has a spherical eye. There are only seven large cones, but they image light onto a retina with approximately 90 receptors, giving a field of view of about 70° by 20°, with a value for $\Delta\phi$ of 4° (see Fig. 64). In theory, an image could be obtained from a single crystalline cone, since a ray from a particular direction in object space will have a unique direction in image space as well. The problem with such an eye would presumably

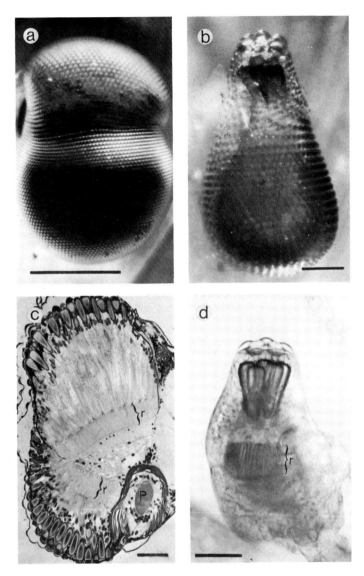

Fig. 58 a–d. Double eyes and larval eyes of euphausiids. **a** Large double eye of *Nematoscelis megalops*. Front of the eye is to the right. Live animal. **b** Eye of *Stylocheiron suhmii*, with a very reduced upper eye containing only seven crystalline cones. The lower eye is almost spherical. Around the cone region of the upper eye are numerous corneal facets that are functionless. **c** 1-μm transverse section through the eye of *Nematoscelis atlantica*. Note that the upper eye is not spherically symmetrical, with the cones pointing to a region much deeper than the centre of curvature of the eye surface, and the almost flat retina *(r)*. There is also a downward-pointing light organ or photophore *(p)*. **d** Eye of the furcilia larval stage of *Thysanopoda tricuspidata*, whose adult has a spherical eye. There are only seven crystalline cones, but a retina with about 90 rhabdoms. **b** and **d** are fixed unstained specimens kindly supplied by Dr. Arthur Baker of the Institute of Oceanographic Sciences, Wormley. Scale bars **a** 1 mm; **b–d** 100 μm

not be low resolution or small field of view, but rather that its aperture would be very small and the image correspondingly dim. As far as I know, this "limiting case" of a one-cone superposition eye is never reached but, with cone numbers as low as four and seven, some euphausiids approach it quite closely. With the possible exception of the mayflies (Ephemeroptera; see WOLBURG-BUCHHOLZ, 1976), there seem to be no parallels amongst insects with the asymmetrical and reduced superposition eyes of euphausiids. Similar eyes are, however, found in one other related crustacean group, the Mysidacea (CHUN, 1896).

e) Superposition Imagery by a Reflecting Mechanism

The Macrura, the group of decapod Crustacea that include shrimps, prawns, crayfish and lobsters, have eyes that are not unlike those of moths, with a pronounced clear zone crossed by crystalline tracts. In many species there is an inward migration of pigment along these tracts during light adaptation. On the face of it these should be superposition eyes, as EXNER supposed, but attempts to find appropriate inhomogeneities in the square-sided crystalline cones (better, pyramids) persistently failed to reveal them (KUIPER, 1962; CARRICABURU, 1975). In fact, CARRICABURU, using interference microscopy, found that *Astacus* pyramids have a uniform refractive index of 1.425, which in water is too low for any useful refraction to occur, and he concluded: "Therefore the eye cannot give superposition images." The question, however, remained: If this is not a superposition eye, what is the function of the clear zone?

The solution was first given in a brief note on *Astacus* eyes by VOGT (1975) who stated: "Rays from an object point entering through different facets are superimposed not by refracting systems as in other superposition eyes but by a radial arrangement of orthogonal reflecting planes which are formed by the sides of the crystalline cones and purine layers surrounding them." Aware of the problem, but not VOGT's paper, I came to exactly the same conclusion after noticing the iridescent appearance of the inner surfaces of the cones of a deep-sea shrimp, *Oplophorus spinosus* (LAND, 1976). The principle is so simple (Figs. 59 and 60c) that it requires little explanation. The sides of the pyramids act as plane mirrors, and as it is in the nature of mirrors to reflect light through twice the angle between the incident ray and the plane of the mirror, the condition for obtaining a superposition image (that rays should emerge at an equal but opposite angle to the incident ray) is precisely met. Some detailed points are interesting. It is important that the reflecting surfaces

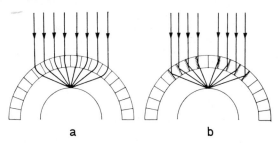

                        a   b

Fig. 59 a, b. Diagram showing that essentially the same ray paths as those in Fig. 55 can be attained by replacing the refracting optical components with plane mirrors oriented radially

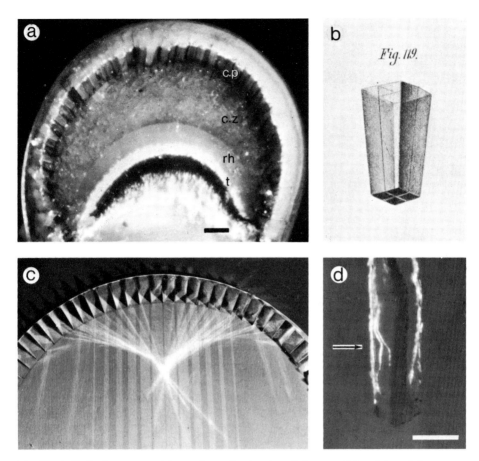

Fig. 60 a–d. Reflecting superposition optics. **a** Hemisection of the eye of the shrimp *Palaemonetes varians* in the fully dark-adapted state, showing the layer of crystalline pyramids *(c.p)*, clear zone *(c.z)* containing cell bodies, rhabdom layer *(rh)*, and the tapetal layer *(t)* of reflecting pigment behind it. The geometry is essentially the same as in the refracting superposition eye (Fig. 57 a). Scale bar 100 μm. **b** The square box-like optical devices of macruran Crustacea are not a new discovery. This careful drawing of a crystalline pyramid from *Palaemon squilla* is from GRENACHER (1879). **c** Demonstration of image formation by a series of radially arranged mirrors. The mirrors in this model are small strips of card lined with metallized adhesive tape. The model is illuminated by a parallel beam from a projector located above the top of the page. Compare with Fig. 59. **d** The multilayer coating of the walls of the crystalline pyramids of the deep-sea shrimp *Oplophorus spinosus*. In this imperfect section the three layers have separated from each other (arrow). The principle of multilayer reflection is outlined in Sect. C.II.5.a. Scale bar 10 μm

have the right dimensions; if they are too short radially, most of the light will pass straight through without reflexion and, if they are too long, multiple reflexions will occur, and these too will degrade the image. The ideal height-to-width ratio for each reflecting "box," which maximizes image-forming and minimizes non-image-forming light, lies somewhere near 2:1. VOGT's second paper (1977) explains why the facets of macruran eyes are square (Figs. 60 b and 62) rather than hexagonal, as in all other compound eyes (e.g. Fig. 62 d). The diagram in Fig. 59 only shows

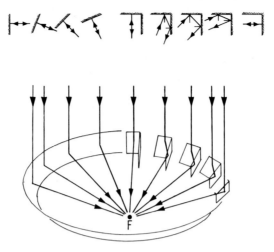

Fig. 61. Ray paths for off-axis light in a crustacean superposition eye. The diagram illustrates the principle that a series of reflecting planes, at right angles to each other and to the eye surface (right), behave optically as a single reflecting surface that is always at right angles to the plane of the incident and reflected ray (left). The upper part of the figure shows typical ray paths as seen from along the axis of individual pyramids. *F*: focus; *C*: centre of curvature of the eye. (Based on Vogt, 1977)

light reflected in a plane at right angles to the reflecting surfaces in the pyramids; if the figure were rotated into the page, about its central axis, by any angle other than 90°, the rays would encounter more than one reflecting surface on their passage through each box. Fortunately, a pair of reflecting surfaces set at right angles to each other reflects light along a direction that is very nearly in the original plane of incidence (i.e. they behave as a single reflecting surface perpendicular to the plane of incidence), and for this reason all rays incident on the cornea of a square-facetted eye reach the same focus (Fig. 61). A hexagonal reflecting box would not have this convenient property, and this leads to a useful diagnostic conclusion: *Where compound eyes are composed almost entirely of square facets, it is highly probable that they behave optically as reflecting superposition eyes.* The converse is also true. So far, only one completely square-facetted eye has been found outside the Decapoda. This is in the mayfly *Atalophlebia* (Horridge and McLean, 1978), but its optics are not yet well understood. A full account of the optics of crayfish eyes is now available (Vogt, 1980).

Vogt (1977) gives both polarization and electron micrographs of the reflecting structures in *Astacus*, and the latter show that the mirrors are composed of three to four layers of 0.2 μm thick crystals with similar spacings between them. Given the high angles of incidence ($> 60°$), this structure is just the kind of multilayer interference reflector one would expect to find (Sect. C.II.5.a). Part of the reflecting layer around a pyramid from *Oplophorus spinosus* is shown in Fig. 60 d, and again it can be seen to have three layers. The nature of the reflecting material is not known with certainty. The only relevant study is that of Zyznar and Nicol (1971) who found that the principal reflecting pigment in the appropriate parts of the eye of the white shrimp *Penaeus setiferus* was isoxanthopterin, a pteridine.

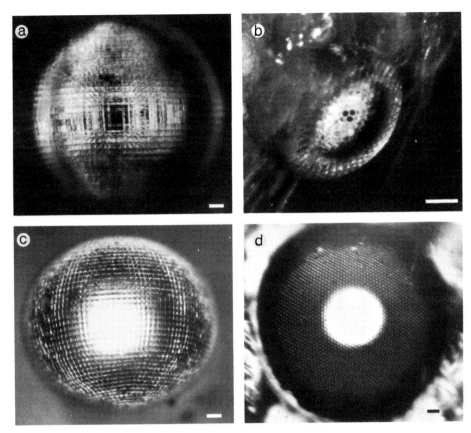

Fig. 62. a Light-adapted eye of the shrimp *Palaemonetes varians*, showing a square, black pseudopupil. **b** First instar larva of a related shrimp *Palaemon serratus*. A similar three-facet pseudopupil is visible, but here the facet geometry is hexagonal, and the eye cannot possibly be acting by reflecting superposition. **c** Fully dark-adapted eye of *P. varians*, illuminated from in front in the same way as **a**. The appearance is totally changed; there is no pseudopupil, but a large patch of glow (eye-shine) instead which originates from light reflected from the tapetal layer behind the receptors (Fig. 60 a). **d** The same eye-shine phenomenon in the refracting superposition eye of the skipper butterfly *Ochlodes venatus*. In **c** and **d** the size of the patch of glow corresponds roughly with the diameter of the superposition pupil. The eyes shown in **a** and **b** are both behaving optically as apposition eyes. Scale bars on all figures 100 μm. All living animals except **c** which was freshly killed with hot water

Because this mechanism is a new discovery, it will be some time before all the possible variations on the "reflecting superposition" theme have been worked out, but there are several lines of enquiry that suggest themselves as potentially interesting. First, it is not yet clear whether all such eyes have multilayer mirrors. The pyramids have a quite high refractive index (1.41–1.43), and total internal reflexion alone would be adequate to produce reflexion from the pyramid sides for angles of incidence on the eye surface of up to about 20°. Coating the pyramids with a multilayer could increase this to about 30°, thereby roughly doubling the pupil area and hence the image brightness. It looks at present as though some of the shallow-water shrimps, like *Palaemonetes varians* (Fig. 62), do not employ a reflecting coating on the pyramid walls but rely on total internal reflexion instead. They do possess reflecting pigment, but this seems to be involved more with the exclusion of light when the eye is light adapted, rather than with image formation in the dark. Second, the whole question of light and dark adaptation in these eyes needs further study. There is, in fact, a large literature on the subject, reviewed by KLEINHOLZ (1961); it is clear that there are movements of both reflecting and absorbing pigment, and that these vary in detail depending on the species (Fig. 63). There is evidence for both direct control by light and indirect control via circulating hormones linked to circadian rhythms (e.g. BARRERA-MERA and BERDEJA-GARCÍA, 1979). All these phenomena need re-evaluating now that the mechanism of image formation is better understood. Finally, there are interesting developmental problems. The first instar larvae of palaemonid shrimps do *not* have square facets, but hexagonal ones (Fig. 62 b). They cannot, therefore, be using reflecting superposition optics. The very clear three-facet pseudopupil indicates that the eye is behaving as an apposition eye, and histological examination shows that there is nothing, at this stage, corresponding to the square-sided reflecting pyramids of the adult. The reflecting pigment forms a sheet around the eye, punctuated by tubes down which lie the rhabdoms. This is, in fact, the same configuration as in the adult, light-adapted eye (Fig. 62 a). It seems that in this shrimp the eyes change from apposition to superposition during development, and also daily in the adult between day and night! It is likely that amongst the macruran groups there may be a very wide variety of adaptation mechanisms.

f) "Glow" and the Pupil in Superposition Eyes

In both the refracting and reflecting types of superposition eyes there is usually a tapetum just proximal to the rhabdoms which, like the tapetum in the eye of a cat or a spider, serves to double the effective path of light through the receptor layer. The externally visible sign of this is that light directed at the eye emerges, after tapetal reflection, along very much the same path that it entered, resulting in a large patch of the eye surface that appears to glow brightly when viewed from the direction of the incident light (Fig. 62 c and d). Provided the superposition image is reasonably well focussed in the first place, so that the light emerging from the eye can be thought of as coming from a point source in the image plane, the area of eye over which glow is visible will be the same as the entrance pupil of the eye. The fact that light entering a single facet can produce glow over the whole pupil area (KUNZE, 1972, 1979) indicates that the tapetum acts as a diffuser rather than a specular reflector, and also shows that the *emerging* light follows the classic superposition ray paths rather than being intercepted by light guides.

In skipper butterflies (a diurnal exception to the general rule that superposition eyes are only found in nocturnal animals), the patch admitting light subtends about 35° at the centre of the eye (HORRIDGE, 1975 and Fig. 62 d), and as the focal length (the distance from the centre of the eye to the focus) is roughly half the radius of the eye, the aperture of the system, expressed as the *F-number*, comes to 4/tan 17.5°, i.e. 1.27 (see Fig. 64). This is probably a smaller aperture than in nocturnal moths, and certainly smaller than in deep-water Crustacea, where the entrance pupil is

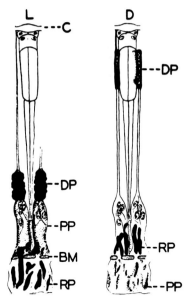

Fig. 63. Light and dark adaptation in the shrimp *Palaemonetes*, modified from KLEINHOLZ (1961). In the light *(L)* the distal pigment *(DP)* is withdrawn, and the space around the rhabdoms is occupied by the proximal pigment *(PP)*. In the dark *(D)* the distal pigment, which consists of both reflecting and absorbing material, moves out into the spaces between the crystalline pyramids. The proximal pigment is withdrawn beneath the basement membrane *(BM)*, and the reflecting pigment *(RP)* that forms the tapetum moves into position around the rhabdoms. Compare Figs. 60a and 62a and c

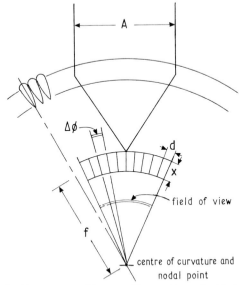

Fig. 64. Definitions applicable to superposition eyes. The most important feature is that the nodal point (through which rays pass undeviated; cf. Fig. 7) lies at the centre of curvature of the eye, defined as the intersection point of the axes of the crystalline cones. The focal length *(f)* as in other eyes is the distance from the nodal point to the image, and the inter-receptor angle *(Δφ)* is the angle subtended by the centres of adjacent rhabdoms (equal to *d* if they are contiguous) at the nodal point. (LAND et al., 1979)

larger than the radius of the eye, giving *F-numbers* less than 0.5 (LAND, 1976). It is clear that the raison d'être for superposition optics is the high retinal illuminance such systems provide. However, it is equally true that high aperture systems of whatever kind bring the attendant disadvantages of poor geometrical image quality (aberrations) and scattered, non-image-forming light. What little we know of superposition eyes suggests that the same sorts of evolutionary "trade-off" exist as with simple eyes: Where photon capture is all important, resolution is sacrificed for the sake of a wide aperture and vice versa.

Superposition eyes can have variable apertures. In moths a decrease in the diameter of the glow patch is very clearly visible as soon as the animal is brought into the light. The mechanism responsible is a movement of the distal pigment (around the crystalline cones in the dark) inwards, radial to the eye surface. The effect seems to be double; first the pigment collects around the rear of each cone, restricting its exit pupil, and then it migrates further inwards, occluding rays tending to pass across the clear zone and so restricting the aperture of the eye *as a whole* (HÖGLUND, 1966; HORRIDGE, 1975). Similar mechanisms exist in Crustacea. In *Astacus*, light adaptation causes an inward radial movement of pigment into the clear zone (BERNHARDS, 1916; WATERMAN, 1961), and in the prawn *Palaemonetes*, this pigment may be drawn right down into a region just above the rhabdoms (KLEINHOLZ, 1961) not completely occluding the clear zone but, presumably, restricting the entry of peripheral rays into the rhabdom itself (Fig. 63).

g) Terminology

It was quite proper, during the 1960 s and early 1970 s when the very existence of superposition imagery was in some doubt, that a new and more neutral anatomical term should have been introduced to describe those eyes for which superposition optics had formerly been assumed. The term "clear zone" eye was introduced by HORRIDGE (1971). It is now widely agreed that where there is a clear zone there is nearly always a superposition image. There are exceptions (such as *Phronima*; Sect. C.III.3.i), considerable anatomical diversity, two different principles of image formation, and differences in image quality in different animals, but nevertheless the superposition principle of EXNER has survived, for all those eyes to which it was originally applied. Superposition is an optically precise term and should be retained in preference to clear zone to describe those crustacean and insect eyes with an adequate transparent space for this kind of image formation, except where some other mechanism has been clearly demonstrated to exist.

IV. Comparisons

1. Resolving Power and Sensitivity

The many different types of eyes described in the preceding sections are all different evolutionary solutions to the same pair of problems: how to divide the world up into an appropriate number of separately resolved sectors, and how to ensure that enough light is received from each sector for differences between sectors to be detectable. All eyes can be compared with each other in relation to how well they have solved these problems, by using as criteria their resolving power ($\mathscr{R}$; Eq. 16) and absolute sensitivity ($\mathscr{S}$; Eq. 15). Almost all the information needed to make these comparisons is available from simple anatomical measurements of the eyes and their receptors and a knowledge of the optical principle on which each eye is based. There is, however, one important unknown, which is the extent of neural pooling. Where this is extensive, and the signals from many receptors are combined, the resolving power will be lower than that given by the calculations, and the sensitivity higher, and furthermore this trade-off is likely to be variable depending on the light intensity. How many of the eyes characterized in Tables 5 and 6 are capable (like man's) of making this kind of reciprocal adjustment is not known – possibly only *Octopus* which has resolution to spare but a need for high sensitivity, but even here there is no firm information. The estimates of $\mathscr{S}$ given in Table 6 also take no account of light loss in the ocular media, and it has also been necessary to assume that the extinction coefficient of visual pigment in situ is the same for all invertebrate receptors. This should be more or less true for rhabdomeric receptors, and the value for lobster rhabdoms of 0.0069 μm^{-1} (from BRUNO et al., 1977) has been used throughout. Table 6 should thus be taken as a guide to the relative capabilities of different eyes, but the values for $\mathscr{R}$ and $\mathscr{S}$ should not be taken as exact.

Probably the most striking feature of the two scales shown in Table 6 is their range. The difference in resolving power that separates the simple pigment-cup eye of a planarian from the large-lens eye of *Octopus* is about 3.5 log units, and the span in sensitivity is 5 log units. In terms of the availability of light in the environment, this sensitivity range nearly covers the difference between sunlight and moonlight (5–6 log units) or alternatively represents a depth difference in clear ocean water of about 350 m. It is significant that all the high-resolution eyes shown (*Octopus*, a jumping spider and the carnivorous worm *Vanadis*) are camera-type simple eyes; the bee *Apis*, whose resolving power is typical of animals with apposition compound eyes, is halfway down the list, nearly 2 log units "worse" than *Octopus* or man. The reasons why apposition eyes are fundamentally incapable of providing high resolution are discussed elsewhere (Sect. C.III.3.b). Below *Apis* comes a very mixed series of eyes, most of which are specialized for dim-light vision, and the simplest (and phylogenetically most common) type of eye, represented by *Planaria*, has by far the lowest resolving power as would be expected in an eye with essentially no optics. The sensitivity scale reflects fairly accurately the ways of life of the different animals. *Oplophorus* is a deep-sea crustacean, and both *Dinopis* and *Ephestia* are nocturnal. The high sensitivity of these animals is due to a combination of a very wide aperture (*F-numbers* around 0.5) and very large receptors. High sensitivity can be attained by both simple eyes *(Dinopis)* as well as by both types of superposition compound eye. At the other end of the scale, *Apis* and *Phidippus* are strictly diurnal, and one would have to infer too that the shore snail *Littorina* only uses its eyes in daylight. Similarly, whatever assumptions one makes about the size of the pinhole aperture of *Nautilus*, there is no way this eye could function effectively in lighting conditions much dimmer than shallow water in daylight.

Table 5. Resolving power ($\mathcal{R}$: Eq. 16) and absolute sensitivity ($\mathcal{S}$: Eq. 15) of different types of eye

Animal	Type of eye	Focal length f μm	Aperture A μm	Receptor separation (diameter) $p(d)$ μm	Receptor length x μm	Absorption coefficient k μm⁻¹	Resolving power $\mathcal{R}$ $f/2p$ rad⁻¹	Effective angular receptor separation $\Delta\phi$ p/f deg	Absolute sensitivity $\mathcal{S}$ $\left(\frac{\pi}{4}\right)^2\left(\frac{A}{f}\right)^2 d^2(1-e^{-kx})$ μm²	Principal source of data
Planaria (platyhelminth)	Simple pit	25	30	10	6	0.0067	0.83[a]	35[a]	3.2	TALIAFERRO, 1920
Nautilus (cephalopod mollusc)	Pinhole	10^4	$2.8 \times 10^{3\,b}$ (0.4×10^3)	7.5	450	0.0067	3.6[a] (25)	8.0[a] (1.15)	2.6 (0.053)	BARBER and WRIGHT, 1969a
Littorina (gastropod mollusc)	Small lens in water	155	55	12(3.5)	10	0.0067	6.5	4.5	0.062	NEWELL, 1965
Vanadis (polychaete annelid)	Lens in water	10^3	250	6	80	0.0067	83	0.35	0.58	HERMANS and EAKIN, 1974
Octopus (cephalopod mollusc)	Large lens in water	10^4	8×10^3	3.8	200	0.0067	2,632	0.011	4.23	YOUNG, 1962
Perga (insect larva)	Small corneal lens eye in air	200	200	20(10)	120	0.0067	5	5.7	34.3	MEYER-ROCHOW, 1974
Phidippus (diurnal spider: AM eye)	Corneal lens eye in air	767	380	2.0	23	0.0067	192	0.15	0.087	LAND, 1969a

									Source
Dinopis (nocturnal spider: PM eye)	Corneal lens eye in air	771	1,325	20	55	0.0067	19.3	1.5	225.3	BLEST and LAND, 1977
Man (fovea in daylight)	Cornea and lens in air	16.7×10^3	2×10^3	2	30	0.035	4,175	0.007	0.023 ⎫	Various sources
Man (peripheral rod pool at night)	Cornea and lens in air	16.7×10^3	8×10^3	20[c]	30	0.035	417.5	0.07	37.1 ⎭	
Pecten (bivalve mollusc)	Simple reflector eye	270	450	7.5	15	0.0067	18	1.6	9.3	LAND, 1965
Apis (worker) (diurnal insect)	Apposition compound eye	60	25	2(1)[d]	200	0.0067	30	0.95	0.318	KIRSCHFELD, 1974
Ephestia (nocturnal insect)	Superposition compound eye	170	340	8	110[e]	0.0067	10.6	2.7	82.8	CLEARY et al., 1977
Oplophorus (deep-sea crustacean)	Reflecting superposition eye	226	600[f]	32	200[e]	0.0067	3.5	8.1	3,303	LAND, 1976

[a] Since there is no lens, $\mathscr{R}$ is taken as "f"$/A$, and $\Delta\phi$ as $A/2 \cdot f$" (C.II.1)

[b] These figures represent plausible upper and lower figures for aperture diameter (HURLEY et al., 1978)

[c] Based on the anatomical observation that about 100 rods converge on one ganglion cell; psychophysical measurements suggest a higher value

[d] Based on inter-ommatidial angle, not actual anatomy

[e] Twice measured value because tapetum doubles light path

[f] Excludes the small contribution from outer partly reflecting facets

Table 6

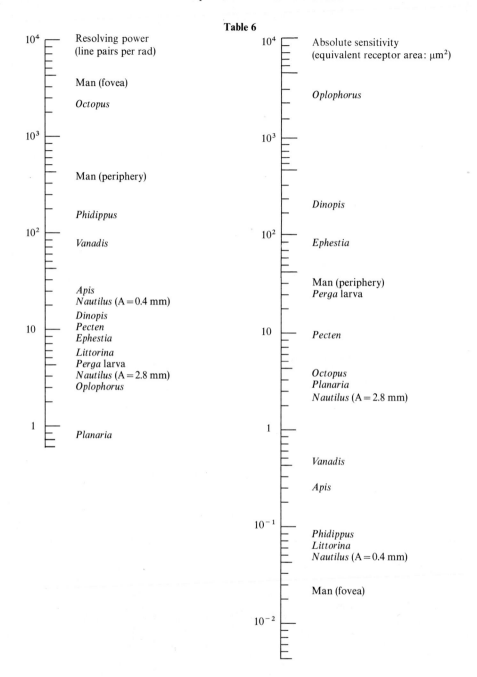

2. Eye Size and Body Size

It could be argued that all animals inhabit more or less the same world, with similar objects at similar distances subtending similar visual angles, and that therefore the need for clear vision would be much the same across the spectrum of animal types. If this were true, however, one would expect most animals to possess similar large eyes, since by whatever criterion one chooses larger eyes are better. For simple eyes both resolution and sensitivity are functions of the focal length (f) (see Sect. B.IV.3):

$$f \alpha \mathscr{R} \sqrt{\mathscr{S}} . \tag{42}$$

This relationship also holds for superposition compound eyes. For apposition eyes, however, the considerations in Sect. C.III.3 indicate a slightly different relationship between size (expressed as the radius r), resolution and sensitivity:

$$r \alpha \mathscr{R}^2 \sqrt{\mathscr{S}} . \tag{43}$$

Both expressions indicate that an improvement in resolution is relatively more "expensive" in terms of eye size than an increase in sensitivity, and this is expecially true for apposition eyes (although the fact that such eyes are generally a shell with a usable interior does tend to compensate for their necessarily large dimensions). However, whatever compromise a particular animal strikes between resolution and sensitivity in the design of its eye, the quality of vision is always limited by the eye's *absolute* size.

This being the case, one might expect smaller animals to have disproportionately large eyes, but this does not seem to be generally true. Both within taxonomic groups and to a lesser extent between them, eye size appears to increase approximately in proportion to body size. There are obvious exceptions to this rule such as the salticid and dinopid spiders (Fig. 31) which for opposite reasons have atypically large eyes, but these *are* exceptions and it is usually easy to discover the reasons behind them. The conclusion must therefore be that smaller animals have worse vision than larger ones.

There may be obvious reasons for this; for example, large eyes may be physically too unwieldy or metabolically expensive for a small animal to maintain. However, KIRSCHFELD (1976) has suggested a more interesting reason, which is basically a negation of the first sentence of this section. Smaller animals need to act at shorter distances than larger animals, so that it is unreasonable to suppose that they need the same absolute resolving power. We, for example, may need to begin to take some action about the presence of an obstacle in our path when it is several metres away, but for a fly the appropriate distance might be centimetres. KIRSCHFELD suggests that it is more instructive to think of visual angles less in terms of absolute quantities (object height divided by distance) but rather in relative ones (object height divided by *distance in units of body height*). It turns out that if one compares resolution in this way, not in terms of inter-receptor angle ($\Delta\phi$) but ($\Delta\phi \times$ body height), this latter quantity, which KIRSCHFELD calls *subjective resolution*[1], is remarkably constant across a wide range of animals from *Drosophila* to

---

[1] Resolution, in the sense used here, is a function of $\Delta\phi$ and so *decreases* as it improves. A low value of ($\Delta\phi \times$ body height) indicates a high subjective resolution.

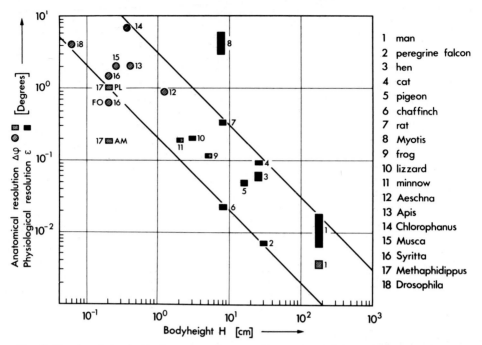

Fig. 65. Visual resolution ($\Delta\phi$ in degrees) as a function of body height *(H)* for a wide range of different animals, some with compound and some with simple eyes. For most animals the "subjective resolution" ($\Delta\phi \cdot$ H) lies in the range 0.2–3 deg × cm. (KIRSCHFELD, 1976)

man, and has a value that is usually in the range 0.2–3 deg · cm (Fig. 65). There are, of course, exceptions to this norm: The jumping spider *Metaphidippus* has an unusually high subjective resolution (because it is a visual predator) and in the bat *Myotis* it is low (echolocation is used for navigation and prey capture), but again these exceptions are of a kind one would predict. There are obvious problems with this idea if too generally applied – a slow snail and a fast bee would not be expected to have similar subjective resolution even if their body heights were the same – but it does nevertheless go part of the way towards explaining why eyes are related to the size of their owners, rather than to physical ideals.

3. Relations of Optical Structure to Behaviour

Why do some animals need better eyes than others, and what have been the evolutionary stimuli that have caused, in particular, improvements in optical design that have led to increased resolving power? These are not simple questions to answer because brains and eyes have co-evolved, and it is usually impossible to tell whether an optical "discovery" by a particular animal group has led in turn to an improvement in the ability to digest and use the new information provided, or whether the reverse has occurred and the exploitation of a new habitat – insects taking to the air, for example – has led simply to improvements in the form and function of whatever eye type was present before. Despite this, it is worth a brief attempt to piece together some of the possible steps in eye evolution, as they relate to behaviour.

Simple pigment cups (A; Fig. 15) are found in almost all the main phyla except where they have been supplanted by something better, and presumably they represent the starting point in the evolution of all other eye types. The resolving power they provide is necessarily poor ($\Delta\phi > 10°$), but they are adequate for mediating behaviour in which only the general direction of light and dark areas is important (klinotaxis, tropotaxis, simple menotaxis; see FRAENKEL and GUNN, 1961). Strictly speaking, kineses and shadow responses do not require eyes at all, just photoreceptors with no particular directional preference. Pigment-cup eyes cannot be improved to the point that they become usable in visually more demanding types of behaviour, because (as in *Nautilus*) retaining or improving resolution by keeping the aperture small involves an appalling decrease in sensitivity as the eye enlarges. New types of visual behaviour require better optical mechanisms.

In older textbooks the division that is drawn is usually between image-forming and non-image-forming eyes, often with the suggestion that the former are capable of "pattern vision" or "form perception," but the latter are not. This is almost certainly a grossly over-simplified view of why improvements in eye design occurred. In the first place, there is no clear break in the spectrum of resolving power that different eyes show, and second, the capacity to distinguish form (the geometrical disposition of parts of an object) is probably a quite late development, and is known with certainty only in cephalopod molluscs, some insects, and by implication from the complexity of their mating displays, fiddler crabs (*Uca*) and jumping spiders (Salticidae). There are plenty of reasons why an animal might require good resolution that have nothing to do with the appreciation of geometrical form.

To begin with, improvements in resolution probably accompanied not form but movement perception. If one examines some of the types of eye produced outside the mainstreams of arthropod and cephalopod evolution, for example the compound eyes of sabellid tube worms, the compound eyes of the clam *Arca*, or the mirror eyes of scallops, one finds that what all these animals have in common is an ability to respond to the presence of a small moving object. This ability does require reasonable resolution, because small movements in large angular fields simply will not be registered, but it requires no great neural sophistication. The behaviour can evolve quite naturally from a shadow response, like that of the clam *Spisula* (KENNEDY, 1960) which has no eyes at all but simply an "off" responding receptor in the mantle nerve. A retina of such receptors, together with an optical system of some kind, gives an animal the chance to react if a change occurs in any small sector of the surroundings, which means that predators can be seen well before they get the chance to cast a shadow. The better the resolution of the eye the further the detection distance. In scallops, at least, movement and local dimming are not distinguished (LAND, 1966 b), which is what one would expect; the animal is not really responding to movement itself, but to local change.

The animals just mentioned are usually sedentary, and their eyes are concerned with the detection of movements of creatures other than themselves. This need was probably also the stimulus for the unusual enlargement of the eyes of some of the predatory worms (Alciopidae) and heteropod snails *(Pterotrachea, Carinaria)*, although here of course it is prey that is being detected and the eyes must provide more than just an indication of the presence of an object; presumably they must guide as well.

Prey capture and predator avoidance may also have played a part in the evolutionary development of arthropod compound eyes. There is, however, another reason, also involving movement perception, for improving resolving power in an active animal. This concerns the role of the eyes in monitoring self-initiated movement. Almost all arthropods (as well as cephalopod molluscs and vertebrates) show some kind of "optomotor response." When placed in a rotating striped drum they move their bodies, heads, eyes or all three around in the direction of drum movement. As many have realized, the meaning of this behaviour must be that the moving animal is attempting to maintain a constant relationship with a visual world that its nervous system has every reason to suppose is still. Formally, the animal is part of feedback loop in which self-initiated activity causes movement of the image across the retina; this is detected and evokes a compensatory movement (Mittelstaedt, 1964; Horridge, 1966). This reflex can help to keep an animal on course (Wilson and Hoy, 1968) or keep its eyes stable during motion, and hence its vision clear (Collett and Land, 1975). Unlike the predator avoidance responses of worms and molluscs, this kind of behaviour involves the extraction of true movement – *systematic* changes in the pattern of light and dark across the retina, not just local intensity changes – and so requires not only improved eyes, but a real innovation in the visual nervous system as well. The evolution of a nervous system with a capacity to detect direction and speed of movement must have paralleled the development of improved eyes, since the better the resolution the greater the accuracy with which the optomotor loop can be employed. The formal nature of movement perception in arthropods is discussed by Reichardt (1961) and Thorson (1966). Judging from the ubiquity of optomotor behaviour, it must be a particularly important element in the visual guidance system of animals, and it probably developed early in the evolution of the visual systems in at least three phyla.

A related development is the ability of animals to localize much smaller targets than can be done with pigment-cup eyes. As Schöne (1975) has pointed out, in a valuable recent review of orientation mechanisms, the older concept of tropotaxis, in which orientation is achieved by balancing the outputs of two symmetrical but only weakly directional receptors, is not in principle different from orientation using e.g. a compound eye with an array of many narrowly directional receptors (telotaxis). Both are basically ways of fixating a target, large or small as the case may be, using a feedback loop that translates seen position with respect to the midline into a turn. The difference is in the size of object that can be fixated and the precision of the initial position measurement. Both differ from classic optomotor responses where image velocity, not image position, constitutes the stimulus for turning.

These mechanisms, the developing abilities of early nervous systems to extract movement and position information from retinal images, were probably the initial reasons why eyes themselves improved and new optical designs evolved. More than this it is not possible to say. A bee still has poor resolution compared with man or *Octopus* (a degree compared to a minute of arc), but that does not seem to have prevented it from evolving high powers of pattern recognition, pattern learning, place learning, celestial navigation, and so on. There seems to be no particular class of behaviour that is precluded by having a resolving power 60 times worse than our own. Better resolution makes possible finer judgements at longer distances, but that seems to be all.

Acknowledgements. I am indebted to many friends in Sussex University and elsewhere for helping me, both with my biology and my physics. Special thanks are due to John Lythgoe and Jochen Zeil for giving the manuscript a critical reading, and to Gay Gibson who was new to the field and helped me to avoid too much incomprehensibility in Sect. B. Original work in this chapter was largely supported by the Science Research Council, and the Institute of Oceanographic Sciences made it possible for me to go to sea to study the eyes of deep-water invertebrates. Frances Burton has helped throughout with histological and photographic expertise.

References

Autrum, H.: Die Belichtungspotentiale und das Sehen der Insekten (Untersuchungen an *Calliphora* und *Dixippus*). Z. Vergl. Physiol. **32**, 176–227 (1950)

Autrum, H.: Les yeux et la vision des insectes. In: Traité de Zoologie. VIII, fasc. III. Paris: Masson 1975

Baccetti, B., Bedini, C.: Research on the structure and physiology of the eyes of a lycosid spider. I. Microscopic and ultramicroscopic structure. Arch. Ital. Biol. **102**, 97–122 (1964)

Bähr, R. R.: Contribution to the morphology of chilopod eyes. Symp. Zool. Soc. Lond. **32**, 383–404 (1974)

Ball, E. E.: Fine structure of the compound eyes of the midwater amphipod *Phronima* in relation to behavior and habitat. Tissue Cell **9**, 521–536 (1977)

Barber, V. C., Wright, D. E.: The fine structure of the sense organs of the cephalopod mollusc *Nautilus*. Z. Zellforsch. **102**, 293–312 (1969 a)

Barber, V. C., Wright, D. E.: The fine structure of the eye and optic tentacle of the mollusc *Cardium edule*. J. Ultrastruct. Res. **26**, 515–528 (1969 b)

Barlow, H. B.: The size of ommatidia in apposition eyes. J. Exp. Biol. **29**, 667–674 (1952)

Barlow, H. B.: The physical limits of visual discrimination. In: Photophysiology **2** (ed. A. C. Giese), pp. 163–202. New York: Academic Press 1964

Barrera-Mera, B., Berdeja-García, G. Y.: Bilateral effects on retinal shielding pigments during monocular photic stimulation in the crayfish, *Procambarus*. J. Exp. Biol. **79**, 163–168 (1979)

Beer, T.: Die Accommodation des Kephalopodenauges. Pflügers. Arch. **67**, 541–586 (1897)

Behrens, M., Krebs, W.: The effect of light-dark adaptation on the ultrastructure of *Limulus* lateral eye retinular cells. J. Comp. Physiol. **107**, 77–96 (1976)

Bernard, G. D.: Evidence for visual function of corneal interference filters. J. Insect Physiol. **17**, 287–300 (1971)

Bernard, G. D., Miller, W. H.: Interference filters in the corneas of Diptera. Invest. Ophthalmol. **7**, 416–434 (1968)

Bernhard, C. G. (ed.): The functional organization of the compound eye. Oxford: Pergamon Press 1966

Bernhards, H.: Der Bau des Komplexauges von *Astacus fluviatilis* (*Potamobius astacus* L.). Z. Wiss. Zool. **116**, 649–707 (1916)

Blest, A. D.: The rapid synthesis and destruction of photoreceptor membrane by a dinopid spider. I. The daily cycle. Proc. R. Soc. Lond. B. **200**, 463–483 (1978)

Blest, A. D., Land, M. F.: The physiological optics of *Dinopis subrufus* L. Koch: a fish-lens in a spider. Proc. R. Soc. Lond. B. **196**, 197–222 (1977)

Born, M., Wolf, E.: Principles of optics. Oxford: Pergamon Press 1965

Braun, R.: Zum Lichtsinn facettenaugentragender Muscheln. Zool. Jahrb. Abt. Allg. Zool. Physiol. **65**, 91–125 (1954)

Brown, J. L.: Flicker and intermittent stimulation. In: Vision and visual perception (ed. C. H. Graham), pp. 251–320. New York: Wiley 1965

Bruno, M. S., Barnes, S. N., Goldsmith, T. H.: The visual pigment and visual cycle of the lobster *Homarus*. J. Comp. Physiol. **120**, 123–142 (1977)

Buddenbrock, W. von: Versuch einer Analyse der Lichtreaktionen der Heliciden. Zool. Jahrb. Abt. Allg. Zool. Physiol. **37**, 313–360 (1919)

Buddenbrock, W. von: Vergleichende Physiologie. Bd. 1. Sinnesphysiologie. Basel: Birkhäuser 1952

Buddenbrock, W. von, Moller-Racke, I.: Über den Lichtsinn von *Pecten*. Pubbl. Zool. Staz. Napoli **24**, 217–245 (1953)

Bullock, T. H., Horridge, G. A.: Structure and function in the nervous systems of invertebrates. 2 Vols. San Francisco: Freeman 1965

Carricaburu, P.: Examination of the classical optics of ideal apposition and superposition eyes. In: The compound eye and vision of insects (ed. G. A. Horridge), pp. 236–254. Oxford: Clarendon 1975

Chun, C.: Atlantis. Biologische Studien über pelagische Organismen. Zoologica (Stuttg.) **7**, 1–260 (1896)

Clarkson, E. N. K., Levi-Setti, R.: Trilobite eyes and the optics of DesCartes and Huygens. Nature (Lond.) **254**, 663–667 (1975)

Cleary, P., Deichsel, G., Kunze, P.: The superposition image in the eye of *Ephestia kühniella*. J. Comp. Physiol. **119**, 73–84 (1977)

Collett, T. S., Land, M. F.: Visual control of flight behaviour in the hoverfly, *Syritta pipiens* L. J. Comp. Physiol. **99**, 1–66 (1975)

Collewijn, H.: Oculomotor reactions in the cuttlefish, *Sepia officinalis*. J. Exp. Biol. **52**, 369–384 (1970)

Curtis, D. J.: Comparative aspects of the fine structure of the eyes of Phalangida (Arachnida) and certain correlations with habitat. J. Zool. (Lond.) **160**, 231–265 (1970)

Dakin, W. J.: The eye of *Peripatus*. Q. J. Microsc. Sci. **65**, 163–172 (1921)

Denton, E. J.: On the organization of the reflecting surfaces in some marine animals. Philos. Trans. R. Soc. Lond. (Biol.) **258**, 285–313 (1970)

Denton, E. J., Land, M. F.: Mechanism of reflexion in silvery layers of fish and cephalopods. Proc. R. Soc. Lond. (Biol.) **178**, 43–61 (1971)

Denton, E. J., Nicol, J. A. C.: The chorioidal tapeta of some cartilaginous fishes (Chondrichthyes). J. Mar. Biol. Assoc. U.K. **44**, 219–258 (1964)

Denton, E. J., Wyllie, J. H.: Study of the photosensitive pigments in the pink and green rods of the frog. J. Physiol. (Lond.) **127**, 81–89 (1955)

Dethier, V. G.: The dioptric apparatus of lateral ocelli. I. The corneal lens. J. Cell. Comp. Physiol. **19**, 301–313 (1942)

Dethier, V. G.: The dioptric apparatus of lateral ocelli. II. Visual capacities of the ocellus. J. Cell. Comp. Physiol. **22**, 115–126 (1943)

Dethier, V. G.: The physiology of insect senses. London: Methuen 1963

DeVoe, R. D.: Ultraviolet and green receptors in principal eyes of jumping spiders. J. Gen. Physiol. **66**, 193–207 (1975)

Dietrich, W.: Die Facettenaugen der Dipteren. Z. Wiss. Zool. **92**, 465–539 (1909)

Dilly, P. N.: The structure of a photoreceptor organelle in the eye of *Pterotrachea mutica*. Z. Zellforsch. **99**, 420–429 (1969)

Drees, O.: Untersuchungen über die angeborenen Verhaltensweisen bei Springspinnen (Salticidae). Z. Tierpsychol. **9**, 169–207 (1952)

Duke-Elder, S.: System of ophthalmology. Vol. 1. The eye in evolution. London: Henry Kimpton 1958

Eakin, R. M.: Structure of invertebrate photoreceptors. In: Handbook of sensory physiology, Vol. VII/1 (ed. H. J. A. Dartnall), pp. 625–684. Berlin-Heidelberg-New York: Springer 1972

Eakin, R. M., Brandenburger, J. L.: Fine structure of the eyes of jumping spiders. J. Ultrastruct. Res. **37**, 618–663 (1971)

Eakin, R. M., Westfall, J. A.: Fine structure of the eye of *Peripatus* (Onychophora). Z. Zellforsch. **68**, 278–300 (1965a)

Eakin, R. M., Westfall, J. A.: Ultrastructure of the eye of the rotifer *Asplanchna brightwelli*. J. Ultrastruct. Res. **12**, 46–62 (1965 b)

Eberle, H.: Cone length and chromatic aberration in the eye of *Lebistes reticulatus*. Z. Vergl. Physiol. **57**, 172–173 (1967)

Exner, S.: Die Physiologie der facettirten Augen von Krebsen und Insecten. Leipzig-Wien: Deuticke 1891

Fahrenbach, W. H.: Fine structure of a nauplius eye. Z. Zellfosch. **62**, 182–197 (1964)

Fischer, A., Brökelmann, J.: Das Auge von *Platynereis dumerilii* (Polychaeta): Sein Feinbau im ontogenetischen und adaptiven Wandel. Z. Zellforsch. **71**, 217–244 (1966)

Fletcher, A., Murphy, T., Young, A.: Solutions of two optical problems. Proc. R. Soc. Lond. A. **223**, 216–225 (1954)

Föh, H.: Der Schattenreflex bei *Helix pomatia*. Zool. Jahrb. Abt. Allg. Zool. Physiol. **52**, 1–78 (1932)

Fox, D. L.: Animal biochromes and structural colours. Cambridge: Cambridge Univ. Press 1953

Fraenkel, G. S., Gunn, D. L.: The orientation of animals. New York: Dover 1961

Franceschini, N.: Sampling of the visual environment by the compound eye of the fly: fundamentals and applications. In: Photoreceptor optics (eds. A. W. Snyder, R. Menzel), pp. 98–125. Berlin-Heidelberg-New York: Springer 1975

Franceschini, N., Kirschfeld, K.: Les phénomènes de pseudopupille dans l'oeil composé de *Drosophila*. Kybernetik **9**, 159–182 (1971)

Franceschini, N., Kirschfeld, K.: Le contrôle automatique du flux lumineux dans l'oeil composé des Diptères. Biol. Cybern. **21**, 181–203 (1976)

Friederichs, H. F.: Beiträge zur Morphologie und Physiologie der Sehorgane der Cicindeliden (Col.). Z. Morphol. Ökol. Tiere **21**, 1–172 (1931)

Fuortes, M. G. F.: Transduction of single-quantum effects. Electrophysiological data. In: Processing of optical data by organisms and by machines (ed. W. Reichardt), pp. 167–175. New York: Academic Press 1969

Gillary, H. L.: Light-evoked potentials from the eye and optic nerve of *Strombus*: response waveform and spectral sensitivity. J. Exp. Biol. **60**, 383–396 (1974)

Goldsmith, T. H., Bernard, G. D.: The visual system of insects. In: The physiology of insecta. 2nd edn., Vol. II (ed. M. Rockstein), pp. 165–272. New York: Academic Press 1974

Goodman, C.: Anatomy of locust ocellar interneurons: constancy and variability. J. Comp. Physiol. **95**, 185–201 (1974)

Goodman, L. J.: The structure and function of the insect dorsal ocellus. Adv. Insect Physiol. **7**, 97–195 (1970)

Goodman, L. J.: The neural organization and physiology of the insect dorsal ocellus. In: The compound eye and vision of insects (ed. G. A. Horridge), pp. 515–548. Oxford: Clarendon 1975

Götz, K. G.: Die optischen Übertragungseigenschaften der Komplexaugen von *Drosophila*. Kybernetik **2**, 215–221 (1965 a)

Götz, K. G.: Behavioral analysis of the visual system of the fruitfly *Drosophila*. In: Information processing in sight sensory systems (ed. P. W. Nye), pp. 85–100. Pasadena: California Institute of Technology 1965 b

Gould, J. L.: Communication of distance information by honeybees. J. Comp. Physiol. **104**, 161–173 (1975)

Gregory, R. L., Ross, H. E., Moray, N.: The curious eye of *Copilia*. Nature (Lond.) **201**, 1166 (1964)

Grenacher, H.: Untersuchungen über das Sehorgan der Arthropoden, insbesondere der Spinnen, Insecten und Crustaceen. Göttingen: Vandenhoeck und Ruprecht 1879

Hagins, W. A.: Electrical signs of information flow in photoreceptors. Cold Spring Harbor Symp. Quant. Biol. **30**, 403–418 (1965)

Hardy, A. C.: The open sea. Part 1. London: Collins 1956

Hartline, H. K.: The discharge of impulses in the optic nerve of *Pecten* in response to illumination of the eye. J. Cell. Comp. Physiol. **11**, 465–477 (1938)

Hartline, P. H., Hurley, A. C., Lange, G. D.: Eye stabilization by statocyst mediated oculomotor reflex in *Nautilus*. J. Comp. Physiol. **132**, 117–126 (1979)

Hartridge, H.: Recent advances in the physiology of vision. London: Churchill 1950

Hecht, S., Shlaer, S., Pirenne, M. H.: Energy, quanta, and vision. J. Gen. Physiol. **25**, 819–840 (1942)

Helmholtz, H. von: The recent progress of the theory of vision (1868). Republished in: Popular scientific lectures by Hermann von Helmholtz. New York: Dover 1962

Hermann, H. T.: Optic guidance of locomotor behavior in the land snail, *Otala lactea*. Vision Res. **8**, 601–612 (1968)

Hermans, C. O., Eakin, R. M.: Fine structure of the eyes of an alciopid polychaete, *Vanadis tagensis* (Annelida). Z. Morphol. Tiere **79**, 245–267 (1974)

Hess, C.: Beiträge zur Physiologie und Anatomie des Cephalopodenauges. Pflügers Arch. **109**, 393–439 (1905)

Hesse, R.: Untersuchungen über die Organe der Lichtempfindung bei niederen Thieren. II. Die Augen der Plathelminthen, insonderheit der tricladen Turbellarien. Z. Wiss. Zool. **62**, 527–582 (1897)

Hesse, R.: Untersuchungen über die Organe der Lichtempfindung bei niederen Thieren. V. Die Augen der polychäten Anneliden. Z. Wiss. Zool. **65**, 446–516 (1899)

Hesse, R.: Untersuchungen über die Organe der Lichtempfindung bei niederen Thieren. VI. Die Augen einiger Mollusken. Z. Wiss. Zool. **68**, 379–477 (1900)

Hesse, R.: Das Sehen der niederen Tiere. Jena: Fischer 1908

Hesse, R.: Tierbau und Tierleben, 2nd ed. Band 1. Die Tierkörper als selbständiger Organismus (eds. R. Hesse, F. Doflein). Jena: Fischer 1935

Hilger, C.: Beiträge zur Kenntnis des Gastropodenauges. Morphol. Jahrb. **10**, 351–371 (1885)

Höglund, G.: Pigment migration and retinular sensitivity. In: The functional organization of the compound eye (ed. C. G. Bernhard), pp. 77–101. Oxford: Pergamon Press 1966

Homann, H.: Beiträge zur Physiologie der Spinnenaugen. Z. Vergl. Physiol. **7**, 201–268 (1928)

Homann, H.: Die Augen der Araneae. Z. Morphol. Tiere **69**, 201–272 (1971)

Horridge, G. A.: Study of a system, as illustrated by the optokinetic response. Symp. Soc. Exp. Biol. **20**, 179–198 (1966)

Horridge, G. A.: The eye of the firefly *Photuris*. Proc. R. Soc. Lond. B. **171**, 445–463 (1969)

Horridge, G. A.: Alternatives to superposition images in clear zone compound eyes. Proc. R. Soc. Lond. B. **179**, 97–124 (1971)

Horridge, G. A.: Optical mechanisms of clear zone eyes. In: The compound eye and vision of insects (ed. G. A. Horridge), pp. 255–298. Oxford: Clarendon 1975

Horridge, G. A.: The ommatidium of the dorsal eye of *Cloeon* as a specialization for photoreisomerization. Proc. R. Soc. Lond. B **193**, 17–29 (1976)

Horridge, G. A.: The compound eye of insects. Sci. Am. **237**(1), 108–120 (1977)

Horridge, G. A.: The separation of visual axes in apposition compound eyes. Phil. Trans. R. Soc. Lond. B **285**, 1–59 (1978)

Horridge, G. A., Barnard, P. B. T.: Movement of palisade in locust retinula cells when illuminated. Q. J. Microsc. Sci. **106**, 131–135 (1965)

Horridge, G. A., Duelli, P.: Anatomy of the regional differences in the eye of the mantis *Cuilfina*. J. Exp. Biol. **80**, 165–190 (1979)

Horridge, G. A., Giddings, C., Stange, G.: The superposition eye of skipper butterflies. Proc. R. Soc. Lond. B **182**, 457–495 (1972)

Horridge, G. A., McLean, M.: The dorsal eye of the mayfly *Atalophlebia* (Ephemeroptera). Proc. R. Soc. Lond. B **200**, 137–150 (1978)

Hurley, A. C., Lange, G. D., Hartline, P. H.: The adjustable "pin-hole camera" eye of *Nautilus*. J. Exp. Zool. **205**, 37–44 (1978)

Huxley, A. F.: A theoretical treatment of the reflexion of light by multilayer structures. J. Exp. Biol. **48**, 227–245 (1968)

Iga, K., Yamamoto, N.: Plastic focusing fibre for imaging applications. Appl. Optics **16**, 1305–1310 (1977)

Imms, A. D.: Insect natural history, 2nd. ed. London: Collins 1956

Ioannides, A. C., Horridge, G. A.: The organization of visual fields in the hemipteran acone eye. Proc. R. Soc. Lond. B **190**, 373–391 (1975)

Jockusch, B.: Bau und Funktion eines larvalen Insektenauges. Untersuchungen am Ameisenlöwen (*Euroleon nostras* Fourcroy, Planip., Myrmel.). Z. Vergl. Physiol. **56**, 171–198 (1967)

Kampa, E. M.: The euphausiid eye – a re-evaluation. Vision Res. **5**, 475–481 (1965)

Kennedy, D.: Neural photoreception in a lamellibranch mollusc. J. Gen. Physiol. **44**, 277–299 (1960)

Kerneis, A.: Etude comparée d'organes photorécepteurs de Sabellidae (Annélides Polychètes). J. Ultrastruct. Res. **53**, 164–179 (1975)

Kirschfeld, K.: Die Projektion der optischen Umwelt auf das Raster der Rhabdomere im Komplexauge von *Musca*. Exp. Brain Res. **3**, 248–270 (1967)

Kirschfeld, K.: Absorption properties of photopigments in single rods, cones, and rhabdomeres. In: Processing of optical data by organisms and by machines (ed. W. Reichardt), pp. 116–136. New York: Academic Press 1969a

Kirschfeld, K.: Optics of the compound eye. In: Processing of optical data by organisms and by machines (ed. W. Reichardt), pp. 144–166. New York: Academic Press 1969b

Kirschfeld, K.: The absolute sensitivity of lens and compound eyes. Z. Naturforsch. **29**c, 592–596 (1974)

Kirschfeld, K.: The resolution of lens and compound eyes. In: Neural principles in vision (eds. F. Zettler, R. Weiler), pp. 354–370. Berlin-Heidelberg-New York: Springer 1976

Kirschfeld, K., Franceschini, N.: Ein Mechanismus zur Steuerung des Lichtflusses in den Rhabdomeren des Komplexauges von *Musca*. Kybernetik **6**, 13–22 (1969)

Kirschfeld, K., Snyder, A. W.: Waveguide mode effects, birefringence and dichroism in fly photoreceptors. In: Photoreceptor optics (eds. A. W. Snyder, R. Menzel), pp. 56–77. Berlin-Heidelberg-New York: Springer 1975

Kirschfeld, K., Wenk, P.: The dorsal compound eye of simuliid flies: an eye specialized for the detection of small, rapidly moving objects. Z. Naturforsch. **31**c, 764–765 (1976)

Kleinholz, L. H.: Pigmentary effectors. In: The physiology of Crustacea, Vol. II (ed. T. H. Waterman), pp. 133–169. New York: Academic Press 1961

Krasne, F. B., Lawrence, P. A.: Structure of the photoreceptors in the compound eyespots of *Branchiomma vesiculosum*. J. Cell Sci. **1**, 239–248 (1966)

Kuiper, J. W.: The optics of the compound eye. Symp. Soc. Exp. Biol. **16**, 58–71 (1962)

Kunze, P.: Comparative studies of arthropod superposition eyes. Z. Vergl. Physiol. **76**, 347–357 (1972)

Kunze, P., Hausen, K.: Inhomogeneous refractive index in the crystalline cone of a moth eye. Nature **231**, 392–393 (1971)

Kunze, P.: Apposition and Superposition Eyes. In: Handbook of Sensory Physiology Vol. VII/6A (ed. H. Autrum) 441–502. Berlin-Heidelberg-New York: Springer 1979

Land, M. F.: Image formation by a concave reflector in the eye of the scallop *Pecten maximus*. J. Physiol. (Lond.) **179**, 138–153 (1965)

Land, M. F.: A multilayer interference reflector in the eye of the scallop, *Pecten maximus*. J. Exp. Biol. **45**, 433–447 (1966a)

Land, M. F.: Activity in the optic nerve of *Pecten maximus* in response to changes in light intensity, and to pattern and movement in the optical environment. J. Exp. Biol. **45**, 83–99 (1966b)

Land, M. F.: Structure of the principal eyes of jumping spiders (Salticidae: Dendryphantinae) in relation to visual optics. J. Exp. Biol. **51**, 443–470 (1969a)

Land, M. F.: Movements of the retinae of jumping spiders (Salticidae: Dendryphantinae) in response to visual stimuli. J. Exp. Biol. **51**, 471–493 (1969b)

Land, M. F.: Mechanisms of orientation and pattern recognition by jumping spiders (Salticidae). In: Information processing in the visual systems of arthropods (ed. R. Wehner), pp. 231–247. Berlin-Heidelberg-New York: Springer 1972a

Land, M. F.: The physics and biology of animal reflectors. Prog. Biophys. Mol. Biol. **24**, 75–106 (1972b)

Land, M. F.: Superposition images are formed by reflection in the eyes of some oceanic decapod crustacea. Nature (Lond.) **263**, 764–765 (1976)

Land, M. F.: Animal eyes with mirror optics. Sci. Am. **239**(6), 126–134 (1978)

Land, M. F.: The optical mechanism of the eye of *Limulus*. Nature (London) **280**, 396–397 (1979)

Land, M. F., Burton, F. A.: The refractive index gradient in the crystalline cones of the eyes of an euphausiid crustacean. J. Exp. Biol. **82**, 395–398 (1979)

Land, M. F., Burton, F. A., Meyer-Rochow, V. B.: The optical geometry of euphausiid eyes. J. Comp. Physiol. **130**, 49–62 (1979)

Land, M. F., Collett, T. S.: Chasing behaviour of houseflies *(Fannia canicularis)*. A description and analysis. J. Comp. Physiol. **89**, 331–357 (1974)

Laughlin, S. B.: Adaptation of the dragonfly retina for contrast detection and the elucidation of neural principles in the peripheral visual system. In: Neural principles in vision (eds. F. Zettler, R. Weiler), pp. 175–193. Berlin-Heidelberg-New York: Springer 1976

Levi-Setti, R.: Trilobites. A photographic atlas. Chicago-London: University of Chicago Press 1975

Levi-Setti, R., Park, D. A., Winston, R.: The corneal cones of *Limulus* as optimised light concentrators. Nature (Lond.) **253**, 115–116 (1975)

Lillywhite, P. G.: Single photon signals and transduction in an insect eye. J. Comp. Physiol. **122**, 189–200 (1977)

Lüders, L.: *Gigantocypris agassizii*. Z. Wiss. Zool. **92**, 103–158 (1909)

Magni, F., Papi, F., Savely, H. E., Tongiorgi, P.: Research on the structure and physiology of the eyes of a lycosid spider. III. Electroretinographic responses to polarised light. Arch. Ital. Biol. **103**, 146–158 (1965)

Matthiessen, L.: Untersuchungen über den Aplanatismus und die Periscopie der Kristallinsen in den Augen der Fische. Pflügers Arch. **21**, 287–307 (1880)

Matthiessen, L.: Ueber den physikalisch-optischen Bau des Auges der Cetaceen und der Fische. Pflügers Arch. **38**, 521–528 (1886)

Mazokhin-Porshnyakov, G. A.: Insect vision. New York: Plenum Press 1969

Menzel, R.: Spectral Sensitivity and Colour Vision in Invertebrates. In: Handbook of Sensory Physiology Vol. VII/6A (ed. H. Aurum) 503–580. Berlin-Heidelberg-New York: Springer 1979

Messenger, J. B., Wilson, A. P., Hedge, A.: Some evidence for colour-blindness in *Octopus*. J. Exp. Biol. **59**, 77–94 (1973)

Meyer-Rochow, V. B.: Structure and function of the larval eye of the sawfly, *Perga* (Hymenoptera). J. Insect Physiol. **20**, 1565–1591 (1974)

Meyer-Rochow, V. B.: The dioptric system in beetle compound eyes. In: The compound eye and vision of insects (ed. G. A. Horridge), pp. 299–313. Oxford: Clarendon 1975

Meyer-Rochow, V. B., Walsh, S.: The eyes of mesopelagic crustaceans: III. *Thysanopoda tricuspidata* (Euphausiacea). Cell Tissue Res. **195**, 59–79 (1978)

Miller, W. H., Bernard, G. D.: Butterfly glow. J. Ultrastruct. Res. **24**, 286–294 (1968)

Milne, L. J., Milne, M.: Photosensitivity in invertebrates. In: Handbook of physiology. Section 1 (Neurophysiology), Vol. 1 (ed. J. Field), pp. 621–645. Washington, D.C.: Am. Physiol. Soc. 1959

Mittelstaedt, H.: Basic control patterns of orientational homeostasis. Symp. Soc. Exp. Biol. **18**, 365–385 (1964)

Moody, M. F., Parriss, J. R.: The discrimination of polarised light by *Octopus:* a behavioural and morphological study. Z. Vergl. Physiol. **44**, 268–291 (1961)

Müller, J.: Zur vergleichenden Physiologie des Gesichtsinnes. Leipzig: Cnobloch 1826

Nässel, D. R., Waterman, T. H.: Massive diurnally modulated photoreceptor membrane turnover in crab light and dark adaptation. J. Comp. Physiol. **131**, 205–216 (1979)

Nemanic, P.: Fine structure of the compound eye of *Porcellio scaber* in light and dark adaptation. Tissue Cell **7**, 453–468 (1975)

Newell, G. E.: The eye of *Littorina littorea*. Proc. Zool. Soc. Lond. **144**, 75–86 (1965)

Newell, P. F., Newell, G. E.: The eye of the slug, *Agriolimax reticulatus* (Müll.). Symp. Zool. Soc. Lond. **23**, 97–111 (1968)

Nicol, J. A. C.: Responses of *Branchiomma vesiculosum* (Montagu) to photic stimulation. J. Mar. Biol. Assoc. U.K. **29**, 303–320 (1950)

Ohtsuka, Y.: Light-focusing plastic rod prepared from diallyl isophalate-methylmethacrylate copolymerisation. Appl. Phys. Letters **23**, 247–248 (1973)

Packard, A.: Cephalopods and fish: the limits of convergence. Biol. Rev. **47**, 241–307 (1972)

Patten, W.: Eyes of molluscs and arthropods. Mitt. Zool. Staz. Neapel **6**, 542–756 (1886)

Paulus, H. F.: The compound eyes of apterygote insects. In: The compound eye and vision of insects (ed. G. A. Horridge), pp. 3–19. Oxford: Clarendon 1975

Pirenne, M. H.: Vision and the eye. London: Chapman and Hall 1967

Plate, L.: Allgemeine Zoologie und Abstammungslehre. Teil 2: Die Sinnesorgane der Tiere. Jena: Fischer 1924

Pumphrey, R. J.: Concerning vision. In: The cell and the organism (eds. J. A. Ramsay, V. B. Wigglesworth), pp. 193–208. Cambridge: Cambridge Univ. Press 1961

Reichardt, W.: Autocorrelation, a principle for the evaluation of sensory information by the central nervous system. In: Sensory communication (ed. W. A. Rosenblith), pp. 303–317. New York: M.I.T. and Wiley 1961

Reichardt, W.: Quantum sensitivity of light receptors in the compound eye of the fly *Musca*. Cold Spring Harb. Symp. Quant. Biol. **30**, 505–515 (1965)

Reichardt, W.: Transduction of single-quantum effects. (Evidence from behavioral experiments on the fly *Musca*). In: Processing of optical data by organisms and by machines (ed. W. Reichardt), pp. 176–186. New York: Academic Press 1969

Robinson, D. A.: Eye movement control in primates. Science **161**, 1219–1224 (1968)

Röhlich, P., Török, L. J.: Elektronenmikroskopische Untersuchungen des Auges von Planarien. Z. Zellforsch. **54**, 362–381 (1961)

Röhlich, P., Török, L. J.: Die Feinstruktur des Auges der Weinbergschnecke. Z. Zellforsch. **60**, 348–368 (1963)

Rossel, S.: Regional differences in photoreceptor performance in the eye of the praying mantis. J. Comp. Physiol. **131**, 95–112 (1979)

Schöne, H.: Orientation in space: animals. In: Marine ecology II (ed. O. Kinne), pp. 499–553. London: Wiley 1975

Schwalbach, G., Lickfeld, K. G., Hahn, M.: Der mikromorphologische Aufbau des Linsenauges der Weinbergschnecke (*Helix pomatia* L.). Protoplasma **56**, 242–273 (1963)

Seitz, G.: Untersuchungen am dioptrischen Apparat des Leuchtkäferauges. Z. Vergl. Physiol. **62**, 61–74 (1969)

Sherk, T. E.: Development of the compound eyes of dragonflies (Odonata). III. Adult compound eyes. J. Exp. Zool. **203**, 61–80 (1978a)

Sherk, T. S.: Development of the compound eyes of dragonflies (Odonata). IV. Development of the adult compound eyes. J. Exp. Zool. **203**, 183–199 (1978b)

Sidman, R. L.: The structure and concentration of solids in photoreceptive cells studied by refractometry and interference microscopy. J. Biophys. Biochem. Cytol. **3**, 15–30 (1957)

Snyder, A. W.: Optical properties of invertebrate photoreceptors. In: The compound eye and vision of insects (ed. G. A. Horridge), pp. 179–235. Oxford: Clarendon 1975a

Snyder, A. W.: Photoreceptor optics – theoretical principles. In: Photoreceptor optics (eds. A. W. Snyder, R. Menzel), pp. 38–55. Berlin-Heidelberg-New York: Springer 1975b

Snyder, A. W.: Acuity of compound eyes: physical limitations and design. J. Comp. Physiol. **116**, 161–182 (1977)

Snyder, A. W., Laughlin, S. B., Stavenga, D. G.: Information capacity of eyes. Vision Res. **17**, 1163–1175 (1977a)

Snyder, A. W., Stavenga, D. G., Laughlin, S. B.: Spatial information capacity of compound eyes. J. Comp. Physiol. **116**, 183–207 (1977b)

Sroczyński, S.: Die sphärische Aberration der Augenlinse der Regenbogenforelle (*Salmo gairdneri* Rich.). Zool. Jahrb. Physiol. **79**, 204–212 (1975)

Sroczyński, S.: Spherical aberration of crystalline lens in the roach, *Rutilus rutilus* L. J. Comp. Physiol. **121**, 135–144 (1977)

Stavenga, D. G.: Optical qualities of the fly eye. An approach from the side of geometrical, physical, and waveguide optics. In: Photoreceptor optics (eds. A. W. Snyder, R. Menzel), pp. 126–144. Berlin-Heidelberg-New York: Springer 1975

Stavenga, D. G.: Pseudopupils of Compound Eyes. In: Handbook of Sensory Physiology Vol. VII/6A (ed. H. Autrum) 357–439. Berlin-Heidelberg-New York: Springer 1979

Stoll, C. J.: Observations on the ultrastructure of the eye of the basommatophoran snail *Lymnaea stagnalis* (L.). Proc. Kon. Ned. Akad. Wet. C, **76**, 1–11 (1973)

Taliaferro, W. H.: Reactions to light in *Planaria maculata*, with special reference to the function and structure of the eyes. J. Exp. Zool. **31**, 59–116 (1920)

Thorson, J.: Small signal analysis of a visual reflex in the locust. I and II. Kybernetik **3**, 41–66 (1966)

Tonosaki, A.: Fine structure of the retina in *Haliotis discus*. Z. Zellforsch. **79**, 469–480 (1967)

Vaissière, R.: Morphologie et histologie comparées des yeux des crustacés copépodes. Arch. Zool. Exp. Gén. **100**, 1–125 (1961)

Vigier, P.: Sur la réception de l'excitant lumineux dans les yeux composés des insectes, en particulier les Muscides. Comptes Rendues **145**, 633–636 (1907)

Vogt, K.: Zur Optik des Flußkrebsauges. Z. Naturforsch. **30**c, 691 (1975)

Vogt, K.: Ray path and reflection mechanisms in crayfish eyes. Z. Naturforsch. **32**c, 466–468 (1977)

Vogt, K.: Die Spiegeloptik des Flußkrebsauges. The optical system of the crayfish eye. J. Comp. Physiol. **135**, 1–19 (1980)

Walcott, B.: Anatomical changes during light-adaptation in insect compound eyes. In: The compound eye and vision of insects (ed. G. A. Horridge), pp. 20–33. Oxford: Clarendon 1975

Wald, G., Brown, P. K., Gibbons, I. R.: Visual excitation: a chemo-anatomical study. Symp. Soc. Exp. Biol. **16**, 32–57 (1962)

Waterman, T. H.: Light sensitivity and vision. In: The physiology of crustacea, Vol. II (ed. T. H. Waterman), pp. 1–64. New York: Academic Press 1961

Weale, R. A.: Natural history of optics. In: The eye, Vol. 6 (eds. H. Davson, L. T. Graham), pp. 1–110. New York: Academic Press 1974

Wellington, W. G.: Bumblebee ocelli and navigation at dusk. Science **183**, 550–551 (1974)

Wells, M. J.: Cephalopod sense organs. In: Physiology of mollusca, Vol. 2 (eds. K. M. Wilbur, C. M. Yonge), pp. 523–545. New York: Academic Press 1966a

Wells, M. J.: The brain and behavior of cephalopods. In: Physiology of mollusca, Vol. 2 (eds. K. M. Wilbur, C. M. Yonge), pp. 547–590. New York: Academic Press 1966b

Westheimer, G.: Pupil size and visual resolution. Vision Res. **4**, 39–45 (1964)

Westheimer, G.: Optical properties of vertebrate eyes. In: Physiology of photoreceptor organs. Handbook of sensory physiology VII/2 (ed. M. G. M. Fuortes), Chapter 11. Berlin-Heidelberg-New York: Springer 1972

Widmann, E.: Über den feineren Bau der Augen einiger Spinnen. Z. Wiss. Zool. **90**, 258–312 (1908)

Wilson, D. M., Hoy, R. R.: Optomotor reaction, locomotory bias and reactive inhibition in the milkweed bug *Oncopeltus* and the beetle *Zophobas*. Z. Vergl. Physiol. **58**, 136–152 (1968)

Wilson, M.: The functional organisation of locust ocelli. J. Comp. Physiol. **124**, 297–316 (1978)

Winston, R.: Light collection within the framework of geometrical optics. J. Opt. Soc. Amer. **60**, 245–247

Wolburg-Buchholz, K.: The dorsal eye of *Cloëon dipterum* (Ephemeroptera). A light- and electronmicroscopical study. Z. Naturforsch. **31**c, 335–336 (1976)

Wolken, J. J.: Invertebrate photoreceptors: a comparative analysis. New York: Academic Press 1971

Wolken, J. J.: Comparative structure of invertebrate photoreceptors. In: The eye, Vol. 6 (eds. H. Davson, L. T. Graham), pp. 111–154. New York: Academic Press 1974

Wolken, J. J., Florida, R. G.: The eye structure and optical system of the crustacean copepod, *Copilia*. J. Cell Biol. **40**, 279–285 (1969)

Yamashita, S., Tateda, H.: Spectral sensitivities of jumping spider eyes. J. Comp. Physiol. **105**, 29–41 (1976)

Young, S., Downing, A. C.: The receptive fields of *Daphnia* ommatidia. J. Exp. Biol. **64**, 185–202 (1976)

Young, J. Z.: The retina of cephalopods and its degeneration after optic nerve section. Philos. Trans. R. Soc. Lond. B. **245**, 1–18 (1962)

Young, J. Z.: A model of the brain. Oxford: Clarendon 1964

Zeil, J.: A new kind of neural superposition eye: the compound eye of male Bibionidae. Nature (Lond.) **278**, 249–250 (1979)

Zyznar, E. J., Nicol, J. A. C.: Ocular reflecting pigments of some malacostraca. J. Exp. Mar. Biol. Ecol. **6**, 235–248 (1971)

Addendum to Chapter 1

Note Added in Proof

This review has not included data about connexions between neurons and glia cells, and amongst glia, in the optic lobes. Two recent papers by CHI and CARLSON (1980a,b) which are based on conventional electron microscopy and electron microscopy of freeze-fracture replicas, describe glial structures in the fly *(Musca)* lamina. CHI and CARLSON have demonstrated special junctions other than chemical synapses between neurons, between neurons and glia, and between glia. They discuss the relevance of these with respect to lamina electrophysiology in the locust and fly (SHAW, 1975, 1978, 1979) and the insect blood-brain barrier (see LANE et al., 1977). CHI and CARLSON emphasize that interneuronal membrane specializations, particularly gap junctions, should be considered in schemes of functional connexions. Other junctions, such as desmosomes, septate junctions and tight junctions, are probably important for maintaining structural coherence and for maintaining barriers to ion diffusion.

References

Chi, C., Carlson, S.D.: Membrane specializations in the first optic neuropil of the housefly, *Musca domestica* L. I. Junctions between neurons. J. Neurocytol. **9**, 429–449 (1980a)

Chi, C., Carlson, S.D.: Membrane specializations in the first optic neuropil of the housefly, *Musca domestica* L. II. Junctions between glial cells. J. Neurocytol. **9**, 451–469 (1980b)

Lane, N.J., Skaer, H.le B., Swales, L.S.: Intercellular junctions in the central nervous system of insects. J. Cell Sci. **26**, 175–199 (1977)

Shaw, S.R.: Retinal resistance barriers and electrical lateral inhibition. Nature **255**, 480–483 (1975)

Shaw, S.R.: The extracellular space and blood-eye barrier in the insect retina: an ultrastructural study. Cell Tiss. Res. **188**, 35–61 (1978)

Shaw, S.R.: Photoreceptor interaction of the lamina synapse of the fly's compound eye. In: Association for Research in Vision and Ophthalmology. Florida (abstracts p.6) (1979)

Author Index

Page numbers *in italics* refer to bibliography

Subject Index

Contents Parts 6A and 6C

Reviews of Physiology, Biochemistry and Pharmacology

formerly
Ergebnisse der Physiologie,
biochemischen Chemie und
experimentellen Pharmakologie

Editors:
R. H. Adrian, E. Helmreich,
H. Holzer, R. Jung, O. Krayer,
R. J. Linden, F. Lynen,
P. A. Miescher, J. Piiper,
H. Rasmussen, A. E. Renold,
U. Trendelenburg, K. Ullrich,
W. Vogt, A. Weber

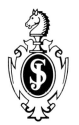

Springer-Verlag
Berlin
Heidelberg
New York

Volume 85

1979. 64 figures, 7 tables. III, 231 pages (58 pages in German)
ISBN 3-540-09225-0

Contents:
M. Lindauer: Orientierung der Tiere in Raum und Zeit. –
U. E. Nydegger: Biological Properties and Dedection of Immune
Complexes in Animal and Human Pathology. – S. Matern, W. Gerok:
Pathophysiology of the Enterohepatic Circulation of Bile Acids. –
Author Index. – Subject Index.

Volume 86

1979. 44 figures, 3 tables. III, 206 pages

ISBN 3-540-09488-1

1979. 44 figures. III, 206 pages
ISBN 3-540-09488-1

Contents:
P. Thóren: **Role of Cardial Vagal C-Fibers in Cardiovascular Control:**
Morphological Considerations. – Characteristics of Atrial and Ventri-
cular C-Fibers Endings. – Reflex Effects of Cardiac Vagal C-Fibers. –
Role of Cardiac Vagal C-Fibers in the Control of Heart Rate and
Peripheral Circulation. – Role of Cardiac Vagal C-Fibers in the
Control of Blood Volume. – The Role of Cardiopulmonary
Afferents in the Control of Circulation in Man. – Pathophysiologi-
cal Implications of Cardiac Vagal C-Fibers.
R. J. Hogg, J. P. Kokko: **Renal Countercurrent Multiplication System:**
Overview of the Countercurrent Multiplication System. – Morpho-
logy. – Physiology of the Various Nephron Segments.
P. Scheid: **Mechanism of Gas Exchange in Bird Lungs:** Anatomy
of the respiratory System. – Ventilation of Respiratory Tract. – Gas
Transport Properties of Blood. – Basic Concepts for Parabronchial
Gas Excahnge. – Cross-Current Model for Gas Exchange in the
Ideal Parabronchus. – Applicability of Cross-Current Model to the
Parabronchial Lung. – Measurement of Gas Exchange Under Various
Conditions.

Volume 87

1980. 26 figures, 6 tables. V, 232 pages (8 pages in German)
ISBN 3-540-09944-1

Contents:
G. Moruzzi: In Memoriam Lord Adrian. – D. E. W. Trincker:
Wilhelm Steinhausen. – U. Trendelenburg: A Kinetic Analysis of
the Extraneuronal Uptake and Metabolism of Catecholamines. –
J. T. Fitzsimons: Angitensin Stimulation of the Central Nervous
System. – L. D. Strawser, O. Touster: The Cellular Processing of
Lysosomal Enzymes and Related Proteins. – Author Index. –
Subject Index.

Pflügers Archiv
European Journal of Physiology

ISSN 0031-6768 Title No. 424

Coordinating Editor: F. Kreuzer, Nijmegen

Subject Editors: E. Gerlach, München; P. Deetjen, Innsbruck; O. Pompeiano, Pisa

Field Editors: P.-O. Åstrand, T. Brismar, E. E. Carmeliet, R. Casteels, J. Crabbé, C. de Rouffignac, J. Durand, J. Hasselbach, H. Hensel, K. Hierholzer, W. D. Keidel, N. A. Lassen, H. H. Loeschke, S. Mellander, H. Meves, R. B. Moreton, H. Murer, A. Nizet, M. I. M. Noble, O. H. Perten, W. Precht, H. Seller, E. Simon, L. Tauc, G. Thews, K. Thurau, W. Trautwein, K. J. Ullrich, E. Wetterer, M. Wiesendanger, J. Zachar, W. G. Zijlstra

Pflügers Archiv is the oldest still existing physiological journal in the world (founded in 1868). The name was changed into Pflügers Archiv – European Journal of Physiology in 1968.
The recent development of physiology is characterized by increasing spezialization and, within the physiological specialties, by extensive interdisciplinary collaboration with other fields, for example, biochemistry, biophysics, and bioengineering.

While still remaining a comprehensive journal of Physiology, Pflügers Archiv has taken the modern developments into account and has introduced a subdivision into three subject groups:
A) Heart, circulation, respiration and blood; environmental and exercise physiology;
B) Transport processes, metabolism and endocrinology; kidney gastrointestinal tract, and exocrine glands;
C) Excitable tissues and central nervous physiology.
In addition to the original research reports each subject group includes sections on "Instruments and Techniques" as well as "Letters and Notes".

Subscription Information and/or sample copies upon request.

Send your order to your bookseller or directly to:
Springer-Verlag, Promotion Department,
P. O. Box 105 280, D-6900 Heidelberg, FRG
North America: Springer-Verlag New York Inc.,
Journal Sales Dept., 44 Hartz Way, Secaucus, NJ 07094, USA

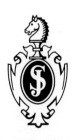

Springer
International